Care of the Critically Ill Patient in the Tropics

Second edition

David A.K. Watters   ChM, FRCS, FRACS
Iain H. Wilson   MB, ChB, FRCA
Richard J. Leaver   MB, ChB, DA, MRCP
Antonia Bagshawe   FRCP

Second edition revised by
David A.K. Watters
and
Iain H. Wilson

Paediatric revisions advised by
John D. Vince

Illustrated by Bernard M. Chipanta

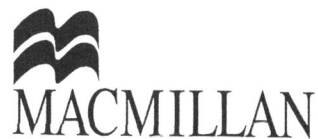

Macmillan Education
Between Towns Road, Oxford OX4 3PP
A division of Macmillan Publishers Limited
Companies and representatives throughout the world

www.macmillan-africa.com
www.macmillan-caribbean.com

ISBN 978 0 333 91501 1

Text © David A.K. Watters, Iain H. Wilson, Richard J. Leaver
and Antonia Bagshawe 2004
Illustrations © the authors and Bernard M. Chipanta 2004
Design © Macmillan Publishers Limited 2004

First published 1991
Second edition 2004

All rights reserved; no part of this publication may be
reproduced, stored in a retrieval system, transmitted in any
form or by any means, electronic, mechanical, photocopying,
recording, or otherwise, without prior written permission
of the publishers.

Designed by Wendy Bann
Typeset by EXPO Holdings Ltd, Malaysia
Illustrated by Bernard M. Chipanta
Cover design by Gary Fielder, AC Design
Cover illustrations by the authors

The content of and information contained in this publication is
intended as an aid only. Macmillan Publishers Limited and its agents
accept no liability for any loss, cost, claim or expense arising from
reliance upon any data, opinion or statement contained in this
publication. Any information or content should be independently
verified before reliance upon it.

Printed and bound in Malaysia

2016 2015 2014 2013 2012 2011 2010 2009
10 9 8 7 6 5 4 3 2

Contents

Authors and contributors	vi
Foreword *Professor J.O.M. Pobee*	viii
Foreword *Professor J.S.M. Zorab*	ix
Acknowledgements	x
Introduction to first edition	xi
Introduction to second edition	xii

1 Respiratory failure — 1
J.R. Sinclair, D.A.K. Watters and I.H. Wilson

What is respiratory failure?	1
Clinical recognition	1
How to determine the cause	3
Management	6
Specific respiratory problems	11

2 Shock — 20
D.A.K Watters, A. Bagshawe and B.M. Kawimbe

Hypovolaemic shock	20
Anaphylactic shock	30
Blood transfusion	31
Coagulation failure	34
Haemolytic crisis *A. Bagshawe*	35
Gastrointestinal haemorrhage *B.M. Kawimbe*	40
Acute pancreatitis	44

3 Cardiovascular disease — 46
H. De Baetselier, R.J. Leaver and A. Bagshawe

Cardiac failure	46
Specific problems	56
Non-cardiac problems	71

4 Fluid and electrolytes — 76
D.A.K. Watters, J.D. Vince

Definitions	76
Clinical recognition	77
Management	78
Intravenous fluid therapy in children *J.D. Vince*	80
Specific problems	82

5 Renal failure — 87
R.J. Leaver and A. Bagshawe

Definitions	87
Clinical recognition	88
How to determine the cause	90
Management	91

6 Metabolic and endocrine problems — 97
T. Bennike, R.J. Leaver and D.A.K. Watters

Acute liver failure	97
Diabetes	101
Management of diabetics undergoing surgery *D.A.K. Watters*	107
Heat disorders	110
Other metabolic crises	115
Delirium tremens	116

7 Poisoning — 118
A. Bagshawe and D.A.K. Watters

Definition	118
Recognition	118
Management	118
Specific poisons	121
Snake bite *D.A.K. Watters*	127
Spider bites and scorpion stings	130
Venomous stings in the sea	131

8 Infections 133
A. Bagshawe, D.A.K. Watters, T. Bennike, R.J. Leaver and E. Athan

Definition and introduction	133
Septicaemia *D.A.K. Watters*	133
Pneumonia *A. Bagshawe and E. Athan*	135
Infections causing paralysis *A. Bagshawe*	137
Viral haemorrhagic fevers *A. Bagshawe*	139
Life-threatening malaria *A. Bagshawe*	140
Tetanus *T. Bennike*	148
Complicated typhoid *T. Bennike*	152
Meningitis and encephalitis *R.J. Leaver*	154
Peritonitis *D.A.K. Watters*	158
Necrotising fasciitis *D.A.K. Watters*	163
HIV infection and AIDS *E. Athan*	164

9 Coma 166
D.A.K. Watters

Definitions	166
Clinical recognition	166
How to determine the cause	170
Management	175
Specific problems	177

10 Head injuries 185
D.A.K. Watters

Introduction	185
Clinical recognition	185
Management	187
Specific problems	190
Assessment of prognosis	192

11 Trauma 196
D.A.K. Watters

Introduction	196
Multiple injuries: Immediate management	196
Further management of specific problems in trauma	201
Mass accidents and disasters	222

12 Burns 226
A.J. Heywood and D.A.K. Watters

Introduction	226
Clinical assessment	229
Planning and starting treatment	232
Monitoring and further treatment	241
Conclusions	245

13 Perioperative care 248
I.H. Wilson and D.A.K. Watters

Preoperative care	248
Postoperative recovery from anaesthesia	253
Postoperative recovery from surgery	256

14 Critical illness in obstetrics and gynaecology 264
D.R. Clegg, D.M. Chikamata, I.H. Wilson

Pre-eclampsia and eclampsia *D.M. Chikamata and I.H. Wilson*	264
Obstetrical haemorrhage *D.R. Clegg*	270
Obstetrical and gynaecological sepsis *D.R. Clegg*	276
Management of the newborn baby *J.D. Vince*	279

15 Nutritional support in the critically ill 284
D.A.K. Watters and A. Bagshawe

Definitions	284
Recognition of malnutrition	284
Nutritional support	286
The child with critical malnutrition *I.D. Campbell*	290

16	**Nursing critically ill patients** *A. Bagshawe*	291	

Problems of nursing critical
   illness ... 291
Standard nursing care ... 291
Special nursing procedures ... 295
Monitoring progress ... 299
Administration of drugs ... 301
Investigations ... 302
Prevention of infection ... 303
Cardiorespiratory arrest ... 308
The patient's family ... 308
Reporting to the next shift ... 310
Housekeeping ... 310

17 **Organisation and
   management** ... 312
   D.A.K. Watters

Definitions ... 312
Benefits of and ICU ... 312
Planning and costs ... 313
Design and location ... 314
Organisation of care ... 316
Patient selection ... 323
Measuring effectiveness ... 323
Teaching and training ... 324
Specific requirements ... 325

Practical procedures ... 329
Endotracheal intubation
   J.R. Sinclair and I.H. Wilson ... 329
Ventilation *J.R. Sinclair and
   I.H. Wilson* ... 336
Oxygen therapy *I.H. Wilson* ... 345
Chest physiotherapy *B. Nkowe
   and A. Bagshawe* ... 349
Airway suction *I.H. Wilson* ... 352
Blood gas analysis *I.H. Wilson* ... 355
Tracheostomy *D.A.K. Watters
   and I.H. Wilson* ... 359
Insertion of a intercostal drain
   D.A.K. Watters ... 365
Giving oxygen by nasopharyngeal
   catheter *F. Shann* ... 369
Peritoneal dialysis and lavage
   R.J. Leaver ... 371

Insertion of a nasogastric tube
   D.A.K. Watters ... 374
Puncture suprapubic cystotomy
   B. Elem ... 376
Venous access and central venous
   pressure measurement (CVP)
   *A.J. Heywood, I.H. Wilson,
   D.A.K. Watters* ... 379
Pericardial aspiration
   R.J. Leaver ... 394
Management of cardiac arrest
   I.H. Wilson and A. Bagshawe ... 396
Autotransfusion *R. Page* ... 401
Carotid angiography at the
   bedside *L. Levy* ... 403
Burr holes *L. Levy* ... 407
Managing the serious head injury
   with a GCS <9 and intracranial
   pressure monitoring *D.A.K. Watters
   and J.V. Rosenfeld* ... 415
Advanced investigative and
   monitoring techniques in shock
   D.A.K. Watters ... 418
Arterial cannulation and direct
   pressure measurement
   I.H. Wilson ... 420

A to Z of ventilation ... 422
I.H. Wilson

Drugs for critical care ... 435
I.H. Wilson

Drugs in critical care ... 435
Doses ... 435
Key points in drug administration ... 436
Principles of antibiotic therapy
   D.A.K. Watters ... 436
Local anaesthetics in critical care ... 437

A to Z of drugs ... 439
I.H. Wilson and R.J. Leaver

Table of normal values ... 457

Further reading ... 458

Index ... 459

Authors and contributors

Principal authors

David A.K. Watters ChM FRCSEd FRACS
Professor of Surgery,
University of Melbourne and Barwon Health,
Geelong Hospital, Geelong, Victoria 3220,
Australia
Formerly Professor of Surgery,
University of Papua New Guinea 1992–2000
Formerly Senior Lecturer in Surgery,
University Teaching Hospital, Lusaka,
Zambia 1985–1991

Iain Wilson MB ChB FRCA
Consultant Anaesthetist and
Joint Medical Director, Royal Devon and
Exeter Hospital, Exeter, UK.
Formerly Lecturer in Anaesthesia,
University Teaching Hospital, Lusaka,
Zambia

Dr Richard Leaver MB ChB DA MRCP
General Practitioner,
The Borders, Scotland
Langlea Mains Farmhouse,
Galasheils, TD1 2NZ, UK
Fomerly Lecturer in Medicine,
University of Zambia

Antonia Bagshawe
Consulting Physician,
Aramadale Kelmscott Memorial Hospital,
Armadale, WA 6112, Australia.
Formerly Professor of Medicine,
University Teaching Hospital, Lusaka,
Zambia 1987–1994

Also previously Lecturer and Senior Lecturer
in Medicine, and Private Physician,
University of Nairobi, Nairobi and Aga Khan
Hospitals 1967–1982
Senior Lecturer
Menzies School of Health Research,
Australia 1994–1997
Director of Postgraduate Medical Education
and Consultant Physician,
Charles Gardiner Hospital, Perth WA,
Australia 1997–2004

The second edition (2004) was revised by
David Watters and Iain Wilson

Paediatric revisions for the second edition
were advised by
John D. Vince
Professor of Paediatrics,
University of Papua New Guinea and
Port Moresby General Hospital,
PO Box 5623 Boroko, Papua New Guinea

Invited contributors

E. Athan
Director, Department of Infectious Diseases,
Barwon Health,
Geelong, Australia

H. De Baetselier MD
Formerly Lecturer in Medicine,
University Teaching Hospital,
Lusaka, Zambia

T. Bennike
Formerly Professor of Medicine,
University of Teaching Hospital,
Lusaka, Zambia

I.D. Campbell MRCP
Formerly Senior Medical Officer,
Chikankata Salvation Army Hospital,
Zambia

D.M. Chikamata MRCOG
Formerly Senior Lecturer in Obstetrics,
University Teaching Hospital,
Lusaka, Zambia

D.R. Clegg FRCOG
Formerly Senior Lecturer in Obstetrics,
University Teaching Hospital,
Lusaka, Zambia

B. Elem FRCS
Formerly Senior Lecturer in Surgery,
University Teaching Hospital,
Lusaka, Zambia

A.J. Heywood FRCS(Ed)
Specialist Plastic Surgeon
Formerly Lecturer in Surgery,
University Teaching Hospital,
Lusaka, Zambia

B.M. Kawimbe FRCS(Ed)
Formerly Senior Lecturer in Surgery,
University Teaching Hospital,
Lusaka, Zambia

L.F. Levy FRCS
Professor of Neurosurgery,
University of Zimbabwe,
Harare, Zimbabwe

R. Page FRCA
Consultant Anaesthetist,
Royal Cornwall Hospital,
Truro, UK
Formerly Lecturer in Anaesthesia,
Kumasi, Ghana

Frank Shann FRACP
Professor and Director of Intensive Care
Royal Children's Hospital, Melbourne,
Australia

J.R. Sinclair FRCA
Consultant Anaesthetist, Royal Cornwall
Hospital, Truro, UK
Formerly Lecturer in Anaesthesia,
University Teaching Hospital,
Lusaka, Zambia

J.D. Vince
Professor of Child Health,
University of Papua New Guinea,
PO Box 5623 Boroko,
Port Moresby, Papua New Guinea

Illustrator

Bernard M. Chipanta

Foreword to first edition

Professor J.O.M. Pobee

Written by doctors working in Africa for other professionals working in the tropics, this book is no high-flown text for super-specialists in sophisticated practice. Such a book would be quite out of touch with reality, given the medical developing world in which, and for which, this book is written. Indeed, that world stands at a crossroads: on the one hand, infections, parasitic disorders and malnutrition have yet to be conquered, while on the other, non-communicable, chronic and degenerative disorders are emerging fast, and we see large numbers of patients suffering from both categories of disease. These patients are critically ill, but because they are rescuable, they ought not to die.

Such patients will *not* be rescuable if relatively meagre resources in equipment and personnel are dispersed; however, when such resources are concentrated in one place and available to all the critically ill, then the chances of survival are bound to increase; this is proved by experience. The cerebral malaria patients, the cardiac in cardiogenic shock, the badly burnt patient and the fitting eclamptic lady are rescuable and must have the benefit of the expertise available.

Throughout this book, the emphasis that is placed on recognising the problem without fluffing about acknowledges a basic fact of critical care: there is always little time to waste. Each section contains a discussion of the pathological basis of the condition in question which, however brief, by going back to basics makes for an intelligent understanding of what one is doing, as well as rebuttressing the foundations of one's own practice. The sections on therapy are straightforward and to the point.

It may seem at first glance that the book contains too much, but in fact every condition mentioned is common somewhere, and if it is not seen in one hospital or one area it will occur in another. The references have been kept to a minimum simply to suit the busy and harrassed practitioner.

It is not intended that this book should replace traditional textbooks of medicine, but, rather, add to them, so strengthening the capacity of the health professional to serve his or her patients the better. I expect it to have a wide readership, from consultants at main referral hospitals, through postgraduate and undergraduate students, to nurses: in fact curing and caring health professionals of all grades. Everything in the book points to the fact that it deserves their support and ownership.

J.O.M. Pobee
Professor of Medicine
University of Ghana
Accra, Ghana

Foreword to first edition

Professor J.S.M. Zorab

Critical care medicine is widely thought of as being confined to highly developed countries. Those who have suggested that such a discipline might have a role in developing countries have often been accused of failing to understand the medical priorities outside the main centres.

That this is not so has been clearly demonstrated by experience and research in a number of developing countries including the unit where the authors of this book work. With their ability in medical care, teaching, organisation and administration, they have been able to adapt the principles of critical care medicine to the available facilities, and yet still be highly effective. Their experience is incorporated in this book.

The text gives sound, commonsense advice on the management of a wide range of conditions. The theoretical background of each problem is adequately covered and accompanied by detailed, practical advice.

Because the authors write from personal experience, it is hoped that doctors and nurses confronted by critically ill patients, in whatever environment, will find the necessary guidance in *Care of the Critically Ill Patient in the Tropics*. Indeed, there may be times in 'developed' nations when easy access to this book will enable less-experienced doctors to handle critical situations with confidence.

I would like to take this opportunity of congratulating all those how have contributed to this remarkable book. The World Federation of Societies of Anesthesiologists was delighted to be able to assist in the distribution of the first edition.

John S.M. Zorab, FCAnaes
President, WFSA

Acknowledgements

First edition

The authors and publishers gratefully acknowledge the receipt of a generous grant from The Beit Trust to support a lower price for the sale of this book in developing countries.

The authors would also like to thank the following for their advice: Professor I.D.A. Johnston, Dr J. Bion, Dr I. Cross, Mr P. Bewes, Mr M. King, Dr J. Searle, Dr A. Ansary, Dr A. Sinclair, Dr A. Tomkin, Professor C. Chintu, Dr P. Nunn, Dr Shilalukey-Ngoma, Mrs H.I. Chirwa, Ms B. Nkowe and Ms L. Dunstall.

Thanks are also due to Mr Michael King FRCS for drawing and supplying the illustrations in the Introduction and on p. 313.

Second edition

Chapter 8 was revised by Eugene Athan, Director, Department of Infectious Diseases, Barwon Health, Geelong, Victoria 3220, Australia. The obstetric sections of Chapter 14 were reviewed by Dr A.B. Amoa, Port Moresby General Hospital, Papua New Guinea. Chapter 16 was reviewed by Ms Lesley Dunstall.

The authors and publishers are very grateful to Papuan Oil Search and St Vincent's Health, Melbourne for their purchase of 400 copies of the second edition.

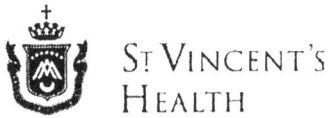

Introduction to first edition

The medical officer felt frustrated and isolated. He was 45 km from the nearest tar road and 230 km from his teaching hospital. The ambulance had a faulty gearbox, and anyway, the road was flooded. There were three patients who were worrying him. The first was a male aged 32 who was becoming progressively more confused and more breathless, and today had developed uraemic frost. The second was a 24-year-old nurse who was 38 weeks pregnant, hypertensive and who had just had a fit. The third patient was a 45-year-old man with abdominal distension from whom pus had been aspirated from peritoneal cavity. There was no working laboratory, so he could order no further tests to help his decision making. How then should he deploy his team of one doctor, two clinical officers and a handful of senior nurses? He thought of the intensive care unit in the teaching hospital. It might as well be in outer space.

He picked up a copy of *Care of the Critically Ill Patient in the Tropics and Sub-tropics*. Would it be of any help?

Meanwhile the teaching hospital was having a busy night. It was the end of the month, pay-day, with petrol and alcohol freely available. Three severe head injuries had been admitted, one of whom was fitting, another had a ruptured spleen and the conscious level of the third was deteriorating. The on-call medical team were resuscitating a diabetic in ketoacidotic coma, performing a lumbar puncture in another comatose patient with fever and at the same time trying to cope with 43 other admissions since midnight. The obstetricians were on their fifth Caesarean section having just performed a laparotomy and hysterectomy for a 19-year-old with ruptured uterus. The casualty officer looked up the indications for burr holes in *Care of the Critically Ill Patient in the Tropics and Sub-tropics*.

The tired medical intern searched for the management protocol for diabetic ketoacidosis. The nurse in charge of the intensive care unit discovered that the postoperative hysterectomy patient was not passing urine. She looked up the guidelines for the management of oliguria.

Intensive care of the critically ill means doing your best for the patient with the available resources. All hospitals have critically ill patients. It is inexcusable that a hospital fails to do its 'best', although what is 'best' will vary from hospital to hospital and from country to country. The debate in the tropics should not be 'Is intensive care appropriate?' but rather 'What is appropriate?'. The term *intensive care* has been wrongly associated with technology and machines, and indeed, machines such as ventilators can be lifesaving. However, it is the integration of technology and the concentration of available skills and resources that will enable you to save the rescuable patient. Such management is often simple in design although intensive in effort. Delay, ignorance and wastage are the stumbling blocks to effective and appropriate care.

This book has been written for those who must treat critically ill patients in the tropics. Explanations of pathophysiology have been kept to a minimum. The emphasis is on recognising and solving the problem. We hope that what you find will guide your treatment of patients whether you work in a district or a central hospital. Although technical details have been simplified to make them easily understood, their inclusion should enable the reader to progress to a more advanced text when facilities allow.

Many of the problems in the treatment of individual patients can be solved only by organisation and planning of care for the critically ill in advance. Good airway management cannot be carried out if the suction machine is broken. Disasters with infusions of potent but life-saving drugs such as insulin can be avoided only if enough nurses are allocated for the critically ill patients. In intensive care, as in so many other disciplines in medicine, prevention is just as important as cure. We hope that you will find principles, protocols, facts and figures that will allow you to decide what is appropriate in your hospital for the care of the critically ill.

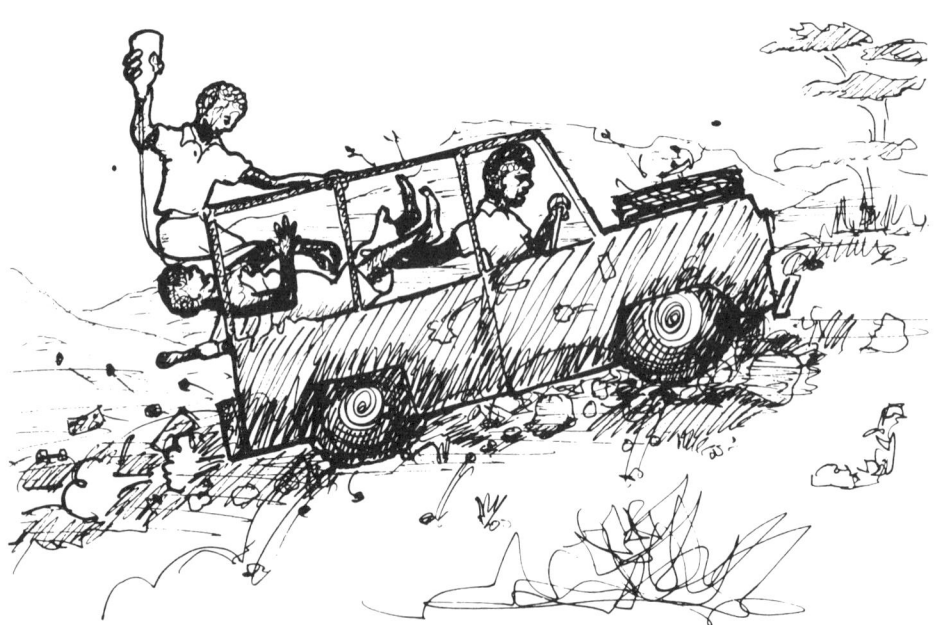

Figure I.1 Transferring the patient is not always in his best interests.

Introduction to second edition

It is over a decade since this book was first conceived, written and published by a group of clinicians working in Zambia. Since then there have been some significant changes in the practice of medicine in both the Western world and the tropics. However, the lack of resources to manage disease in the developing world has persisted and there are many limitations to 'best practice'. Our original definition of intensive care, 'doing the best for critically ill patients with the resources that are available', remains appropriate. Perhaps the greatest advance in the past decade has been the Internet, which makes information available to anyone with a phone and computer. Guidelines can be accessed from anywhere. Sadly many of the steps in the guidelines will not be feasible in a Third World hospital and guidelines always need to be adapted to the local situation. We offer this second edition for those who must still manage the sick patients described above with conditions like eclampsia (now termed pregnancy-induced hypertension), peritonitis (still peritonitis), coma, uraemia and diabetic ketoacidosis. The incidence and prevalence of co-existent HIV infection has increased in tropical countries in the last decade. We assume that most tropical clinicians need to be much more broadly trained than their Western counterparts. The options available to manage critically ill patients in many developing countries today are similar to what we have described in the text. There have been few inexpensive improvements to medical care in the last decade although there is a greater ability to diagnose and manage disease through portable medical imaging such as ultrasound. However, the majority of preventable deaths still occur because simple things are not done. Examples of simple interventions that save lives include making an early decision to do a laparotomy for intra-abdominal sepsis, securing the airway, giving oxygen and ventilatory support early to patients developing respiratory failure, effective resuscitation of patients in hypovolaemic shock, caring for major burns with a dedicated team in an environment which limits cross-infection, organising the care of critically ill so that the limited expertise and resources in a tropical hospital are available for the patients who most need them. Both editions of this book have been written with the view that good organisation, communication and prompt decision-making combined with simple, widely available treatments will save the majority of critically ill, salvageable patients.

1
Respiratory failure

What is respiratory failure?

The respiratory system is responsible for the body's intake of oxygen and excretion of carbon dioxide. The respiratory system fails whenever the exchange of oxygen and/or carbon dioxide across the alevolar membrane is insufficient for the body's needs.

Impaired oxygenation results in hypoxia and cyanosis and the impaired carbon dioxide excretion results in a raised carbon dioxide level in the blood (hypercarbia) and acidosis.

Hypercarbia does not always occur in respiratory failure because carbon dioxide diffuses across the alveolar membrane more easily than oxygen.

Causes of respiratory failure

These are as follows:

Inadequate breathing

This results from:
1. depression of the respiratory centre due to drugs, alcohol or intracranial disease including head injury;
2. neuromuscular dysfunction due to fractured ribs, muscle paralysis (e.g. polio) or tetanus;
3. pleural or chest wall disease, e.g. pneumothorax, empyema, scoliosis.

Obstructed airway

Causes are:
1. upper airway – foreign bodies, epiglottitis, or compression of the airway by an extrinsic lesion;
2. lower airway – bronchospasm.

Inadequate gas exchange

This occurs if there is a problem affecting the exchange of gases between alveolar gas and the blood. It may be due to inadequate diffusion of oxygen and carbon dioxide as in pulmonary oedema or pneumonia or to inadequate perfusion of the lung as in a large pulmonary embolus.

Respiratory failure may be acute or chronic. Most critically ill patients have acute respiratory failure or else an acute problem such as pneumonia or fractured ribs which has complicated chronic respiratory disease.

Clinical recognition

The underlying problem in most cases of respiratory failure is hypoxia, and this is recognised by tachypnoea, tachycardia, sweating, peripheral vasoconstriction, hypotension, central and peripheral cyanosis, restlessness and some mental confusion. Tracheal tug is a sign of severe distress. Just before death the patient in respiratory failure develops a bradycardia accompanied

Table 1.1 Signs of respiratory failure
The signs of hypoxia and hypercarbia are often combined.

Hypoxia	Hypercarbia
Cyanosis	Pink tongue
Tachycardia	Bounding pulse
Dyspnoea	Warm peripheries
Peripheral vasoconstriction	Peripheral vasodilatation
Sweating	Pupil dilatation
Hypotension	Drowsiness, coma
Agitation, confusion	Hypertension (sometimes)
Bradycardia (end stage)	Muscle twitching

by gasping respirations which warn of the impending cardiac arrest.

Some patients with respiratory failure show signs of carbon dioxide retention. These are peripheral vasodilatation, a full bounding pulse (possibly with hypertension), sweating, dilatation of the pupils, drowsiness, muscle twitching and coma (Table 1.1).

Rapid, shallow breathing, gross abdominal movement with breathing and the use of accessory muscles including intercostal indrawing (and sternal indrawing in children) are signs of respiratory distress. However, patients unable to breathe because of muscle paralysis, end-stage exhaustion or central depression may be in respiratory failure without dyspnoea.

> **KEYPOINT**
>
> Respiratory failure may be present without obvious dyspnoea.

When respiratory failure is due to inadequate gas exchange hypoxia dominates the clinical picture (Table 1.1). The respiratory rate rises and if this fails to allow adequate oxygenation the patient becomes cyanosed. Figure 1.1 shows the respiratory rate in an imaginary patient with pneumonia. Early in the disease the respiratory rate

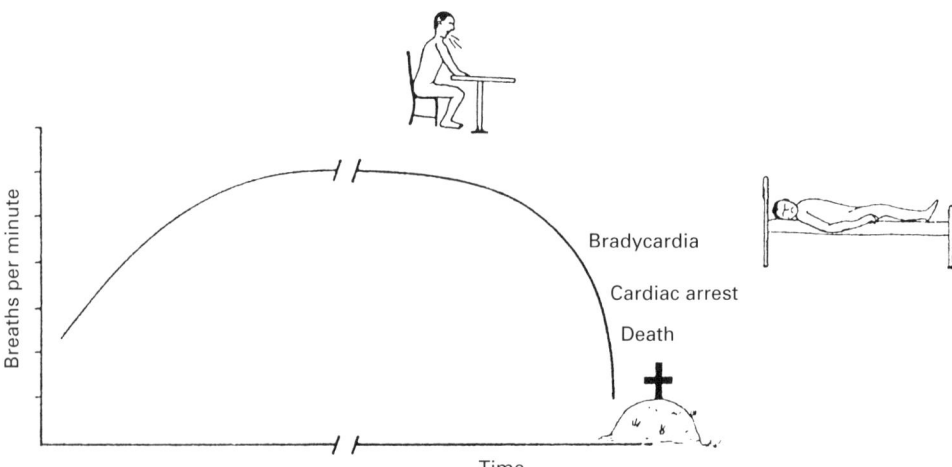

Figure 1.1 Progression of respiratory failure according to respiratory rate. The duration of the plateau varies but may be short in the elderly, and those with chronic cardiac disease, sepsis, shock or chest trauma.

starts to rise and in an adult will plateau between 40 and 60 breaths per minute (adults cannot breathe much faster than once a second). The duration of this plateau will vary depending upon the severity of the underlying disease, progress of the disease, general fitness of the patient and the response to treatment. Successful treatment will result in the respiratory rate falling and signs of hypoxia lessening. If treatment fails the patient will eventually become exhausted and the respiratory rate start to fall. This fall in respiratory rate is accompanied by worsening hypoxia but now signs of hypercarbia also develop as breathing becomes insufficient even to allow carbon dioxide excretion.

> **KEYPOINT**
>
> It is important to recognise whether a fall in respiratory rate is due to improvement or to deterioration and exhaustion.

How to determine the cause

Respiratory failure may be due to inadequate breathing, an obstructed airway or inadequate gas exchange. Some common causes of acute respiratory failure are shown in Figure 1.2. Some of the signs and symptoms of respiratory failure are common to circulatory and cardiac failure which are described in Chapters 2 and 3.

The cause is usually determined from a good history, careful examination and a chest X-ray. Several problems may coexist: for example, pulmonary infection, chest trauma or major surgery may cause acute respiratory failure in patients with underlying chronic respiratory disease such as chronic bronchitis, emphysema or chest wall deformities.

Inadequate breathing

The problem here is inadequate movement of air in and out of the lungs. The clinical picture will depend upon the cause.

Slow or shallow respirations may be due to central depression caused by brain stem ischaemia, trauma, or drugs such as opiates, diazepam, barbiturates, tranquillisers or alcohol. Check an in-patient's drug chart and enquire from the patient or attendants whether the patient has taken drugs or poisons. The patient will usually be unconscious with a respiratory rate of less than 12 per minute. There may be signs of hypercarbia (Table 1.1) and in the late stages a gasping pattern of respiration with tracheal tug will occur.

If inadequate breathing is due to a neuromuscular cause, the patient will be conscious (unless severely hypoxic), with a more rapid but ineffective respiratory pattern and chest wall movement.

Examine for inadequate or unequal movement of the chest wall, paradoxical movement with a flail segment, deviation of the trachea from the midline. Percuss and auscultate the chest: poor air entry with a stony dull percussion sound may indicate a pleural effusion, empyema or haemothorax; poor air entry associated with hyperresonance suggests pneumothorax. Pneumothorax and tracheal deviation together suggest a tension pneumothorax.

Obstructed airway

Upper airway

The commonest cause of upper airway obstruction is coma. Loss of tone in the muscles of the tongue causes it to fall back into the pharynx.

There is noisy breathing similar to snoring. In other causes of airway obstruction the clinical picture depends upon the severity of the obstruction and on whether respiratory failure is in its early or late

Inadequate breathing*
A. Central nervous system depression
1. Brain stem compression or ischaemia.
2. Drugs such as opiates, diazepam, tranquillisers, barbiturates and alcohol.

B. Neuromuscular dysfunction
1. Muscle paralysis – Guillain–Barré syndrome, poliomyelitis, diphtheria.
2. Drugs: muscle relaxants, organophosphate poison.
3. Muscle spasm – tetanus.
4. Neurological – fracture cervical spine.

C. Pleural and chest wall problems
1. Pneumothorax, haemothorax, effusion, empyema.
2. Fractured ribs including flail chest.
3. Diaphragmatic injury.

Obstructed breathing ●
A. Upper airway
1. Fractured jaw, tongue falling back, false teeth, foreign body, epiglottitis.
2. Laryngeal oedema (trauma, inflammation or anaphylaxis).
3. Laryngeal tumours.
4. External compression from neck tumours, e.g. thyroid, Burkitt's, lymphoma or from cellulitis.
5. Blocked endotracheal tube or tracheostomy.

B. Lower airway
1. Bronchospasm – asthma, allergy.
2. Foreign body.

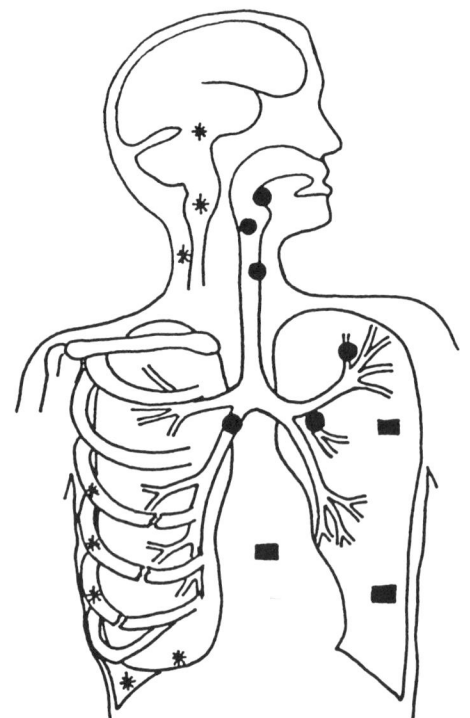

Inadequate gas exchange ■
A. Pulmonary
1. Pneumonia.
2. Pulmonary oedema e.g. due to fluid overload or cardiac failure.
3. Acute respiratory distress syndrome (shock lung), fat embolism.
4. Inflammatory lung disease e.g. pulmonary fibrosis, alveolitis.

B. Circulatory (not discussed in this chapter)
1. Pulmonary embolus.
2. Shock.
3. Heart failure.
4. Haemoglobin abnormalities including carbon monoxide poisoning.

Figure 1.2 Some causes of acute respiratory failure.

stage. The clinical picture often includes stridor (noisy breathing, particularly on inspiration).

Early

In conscious patients with inspiratory stridor the patient will prefer to sit up and lean forward and is likely to be distressed. The respiratory rate will be above 25 per minute and there may be signs of hypoxia and/or hypercarbia.

Late

The patient will be exhausted and drowsy and will eventually lose consciousness. There will be signs of hypoxia and hypercarbia.

Lower airway

The commonest cause is asthma, which presents a similar picture to upper-airway obstruction except that there is expiratory wheeze rather than inspiratory stridor. Coarse crepitations suggest copious airway secretions or aspiration of vomit, saliva or blood, which not only obstruct the airway but also interfere with gas exchange. Always consider the possibility of an inhaled foreign body in a child with unexplained dyspnoea, stridor, wheeze or pneumonia.

Inadequate gas exchange

This presents as respiratory failure associated with dyspnoea (Figure 1.1) despite good air flow in and out of the lungs. Signs of hypoxia (Table 1.1) dominate the clinical picture. Failure of oxygen and carbon dioxide to diffuse across the alveolar membrane may be due to infection, oedema, aspiration pneumonia or pulmonary embolism. Circulatory causes of inadequate gas exchange are not discussed in this chapter.

Pyrexia may indicate pulmonary or pleural infection. A chest X-ray may be diagnostic. When respiratory failure develops 1–2 days after severe shock suspect acute respiratory distress syndrome (ARDS), which is characterised by stiff (non-compliant) lungs, dyspnoea and a characteristic chest X-ray appearance (Figure 1.3). When dyspnoea develops within a few days of a fractured femur consider fat embolism.

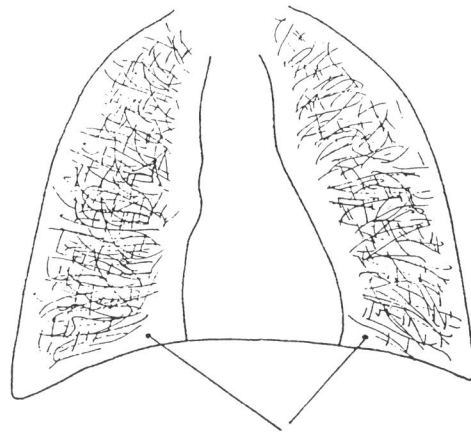

Bilateral diffuse patchy opacities

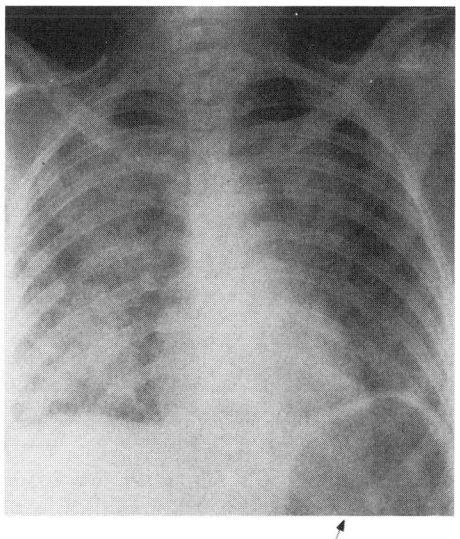

Distension of stomach with air

Figure 1.3 Acute respiratory distress syndrome (ARDS).

Relevant investigations

Chest X-ray

Always examine the patient carefully and treat life-threatening problems *before* ordering a chest radiograph. The chest X-ray may confirm clinical findings but in some patients clinical examination is misleading, so that a chest X-ray should be taken once the patient's condition is stabilised. Do not leave a patient in respiratory failure unattended nor allow the taking of a radiograph to interrupt the treatment of the respiratory failure.

Blood gases

Although most cases of respiratory failure can be recognised by careful clinical examination, arterial blood gas analysis gives an accurate measure of the severity of respiratory failure and of the response to treatment. Respiratory failure is defined according to blood gases as a $PaO_2 < 8$ kPa (60 mmHg) and/or $PaCO_2 > 7.3$ kPa (55 mmHg). There may also be acidosis (pH < 7.35), the degree of which will depend on the $PaCO_2$ and the degree of compensation. A full description on how to interpret blood gas analysis is given on p. 355. The level of oxygen saturation in the blood may be measured using a pulse oximeter. Oxygen saturation is normally above 95%; below 90% represents severe hypoxia. (See Table 1.2.)

Table 1.2 Blood gases in respiratory failure

Hypoxia	Hypercarbia
PaO_2 low < 8 kPa	PaO_2 usually low unless on oxygen
$PaCO_2$ may be normal, low or high	$PaCO_2$ high, > 7.3 kPa
Oxygen saturation low < 90%	Oxygen saturation low unless on oxygen
	Respiratory acidosis

Lung function tests

These are used normally in the assessment of chronic chest diseases and their use in acute respiratory failure is limited. However, measurements of vital capacity using a Wright's respirometer (p. 434) is an excellent method of assessing the progress of a patient with neuromuscular problems, such as a patient with polio. Adult patients with a vital capacity (volume measured from maximal inspiration to expiration) of less than 1 litre are likely to need support from a ventilator. Peak flow rate is a useful measurement in asthma and serial measurements will help monitor progress of treatment. (Normal peak flow is 300–700 l/min.) More sophisticated lung tests are rarely available.

Management

In the preceding section the major problems causing respiratory failure were described. More than one problem may be present and the development of a second problem may cause respiratory function to deteriorate from subnormal but adequate to dangerously inadequate. One example of this would be pneumonia developing in a patient with tetanus, the respiratory function of which is already compromised by muscle fixation.

Management may be divided into supportive (general measures) and specific to the underlying disease process (see Table 1.3 and specific problems).

Supportive management

Do not leave a patient in respiratory failure unattended. Supportive therapy should begin in the admission room and continue until the patient has been stabilised. Transfer the patient to a ward or critical care area where a suitably qualified nurse, clinical officer, anaesthetist or doctor can monitor progress and commence specific therapy.

Supportive management is needed in all patients and must include the following:
1. airway management;
2. oxygen therapy;
3. posture;
4. hydration;
5. physiotherapy;
6. the decision to ventilate or not.

Airway management

In an unconscious patient, airway obstruction can occur owing to loss of tone in the muscles of the pharynx, jaw and tongue. These patients have depressed laryngeal reflexes and do not cough or swallow. The airway might also be obstructed by dislodged false teeth or food particles. Airway obstruction will be worsened by the presence of secretions in the airway. Unconscious patients are also at risk of aspiration.

First clear the upper airway using suction and your fingers if necessary (a laryngoscope will help you see what you are doing if the patient is deeply unconscious). The airway must then be supported by extending the neck and pulling the jaw forward. If the patient is breathing, start oxygen therapy using a face mask and position him in the coma position (Figure 9.5). If spontaneous respirations are inadequate, ventilate using an Ambu bag and face mask and intubate as soon as possible (p. 329). Patients in whom it is difficult to maintain a clear airway, or who are at risk of aspiration, should be intubated.

The management of conscious patients with severe airway obstruction can be very difficult as intubation may be difficult or impossible.

Conscious patients with upper airway obstruction should not be sedated and must be given oxygen as soon as they are admitted. Once the obstruction has been relieved ventilation is not necessary and the patient can breathe spontaneously through an endotracheal tube or tracheostomy.

Patients who are not deteriorating rapidly should be transferred to theatre and anaesthetised by an experienced anaesthetist using a gaseous induction with halothane and the airway inspected and intubation performed under controlled conditions with a doctor scrubbed and ready to perform an immediate tracheostomy if the airway is lost or intubation is impossible. This should not be attempted by inexperienced staff. If there is no suitable anaesthetist available it is safer to perform an emergency tracheostomy under local anaesthesia.

If you fail to intubate you must perform an emergency cricothyroidotomy using a 14 or 12 gauge cannula (p. 197) or minitracheostomy (p. 362). Withdraw the needle from the cannula and ventilate via the cannula using a high pressure oxygen source. The patient will not be able to breathe spontaneously through the cannula. A formal tracheostomy will be immediately required.

Once the patient's airway is secure clear the lower airway by suction, coughing, postural drainage or chest physiotherapy as appropriate. The method will depend on whether or not the patient is conscious and whether or not he is intubated.

In children, airway obstruction due to an inhaled foreign body is common, and it is important to be aware that this is not always evident from the history. First aid and immediate management is to hold the child upside down and slap him on the back in the hope of dislodging the obstructing object. If this fails or the child presents late, the foreign body should be removed by bronchoscopy under general anaesthesia.

KEYPOINT
Always consider an airway foreign body if there are unexplained respiratory problems in a child.

Oxygen therapy

Whatever the cause of respiratory failure there will be hypoxia. Oxygen should therefore be given to all patients. Oxygen therapy is described as a practical procedure on p. 345.

Posture

Any patient with a respiratory problem needs correct positioning (i.e. sit up if conscious or postural drainage for secretions or coma position to protect the airway – Figure 9.5) and chest physiotherapy.

Hydration

Patients with acute respiratory failure are unable to eat or drink adequate fluids. They require intravenous fluids and careful monitoring of fluid balance (Chapter 4). Avoid overhydration, which can cause pulmonary oedema and reduce oxygen transfer across the alveolar membrane. Once dehydration has been corrected, restrict fluid intake to about 75% of normal requirements, providing adequate urine output is maintained (>0.5 ml/kg/h).

Chest physiotherapy

This is discussed as a practical procedure on p. 349. The aim of chest physiotherapy is to clear the airways of secretions and improve airflow to the alveoli. It may avoid the need for intubation and ventilation but in postoperative or traumatised patients requires adequate analgesia. Chest physiotherapy may tire the patient and cause hypoxaemia, so that repeated assessment of the strength of the patient, his ability to cooperate and the response to physiotherapy must be made.

Ventilation

The decision to ventilate will depend upon the cause of the respiratory failure, the response to simple management and oxygen therapy. These will often be enough to allow the specific therapy for the cause to work. If the above are unsuccessful and the patient's prognosis is reasonable, ventilate.

Patients with severe tetanus, neuromuscular paralysis, flail chest, postoperative respiratory failure, poisoning, drug-related central depression, septicaemia, fat

Table 1.3 Specific treatment for different causes of respiratory failure

Cause	Treatment
Inadequate breathing	
Central depression	Reverse opiates with naloxone.
	Other causes – ventilate.
Muscle paralysis	Ventilate.
Pleural space collections	Intercostal drain.
Flail chest	Analgesia; physiotherapy; ventilate if large or respiratory distress.
Obstructed airway	
Upper airway	Clear airway; correct position; intubate; tracheostomy.
Foreign body	Clear by suction, physiotherapy, drainage, bronchoscopy.
Bronchospasm	Nebulise with salbutamol; aminophylline and hydrocortisone.
Inadequate gas exchange	
Pneumonia	Antibiotics, oxygen.
Pulmonary oedema	Diuretics if renal function normal; dialysis if renal failure.
ARDS	Ventilation and positive end expiratory pressure (PEEP).
Pulmonary embolus	Anticoagulation, oxygen, morphine.

embolism and ARDS of any cause should be given ventilatory support if available.

Patients with severe head injuries, cerebrovascular accident (CVA), hypertensive encephalopathy, and terminal disease are unlikely to benefit from ventilation unless respiratory failure is due to some other, but correctable, cause (e.g. flail chest in a patient with a head injury).

The mortality of mechanical ventilation remains around 30–50% in intensive care units (ICUs) in the developed world since in many patients the disease leading to respiratory failure is incurable. In the rural or district hospital in the tropics, the decision whether or not to ventilate a patient must take into account the best use of available resources. Avoid ventilating patients with a poor prognosis when equipment and skills are limited.

The practical aspects of endotracheal intubation and ventilation are discussed in detail on pp. 329–344.

Specific therapy

Inadequate breathing

Naloxone may be used to reverse the action of opiate drugs such as pethidine or morphine. Other causes of central depression will probably require treatment by assisted ventilation.

Intercostal or diaphragmatic muscle paralysis must be treated by mechanical ventilation once respiratory failure develops. There may be a stage where the breathing is subnormal but adequate. The patient must be closely monitored because further loss of muscle power or the development of pneumonia may result in severe hypoxia without dyspnoea.

Drain pleural space collections of air (Figure 1.4), fluid, blood (Figure 1.5), or pus (Figure 1.6). A tension pneumothorax (Figure 1.7) will be made worse by ventilation. Insertion of an intercostal drain is described on p. 365.

Good pain relief using an intercostal nerve block, pethidine infusion or epidural or intrapleural analgesia may enable the patient with multiple fractured ribs and/or a flail segment of the chest wall to breathe adequately. Physiotherapy and oxygen should be given. If these measures fail the patient will need to be ventilated or the flail segment fixed.

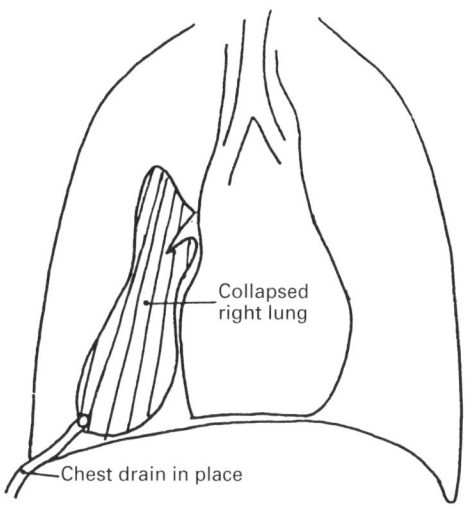

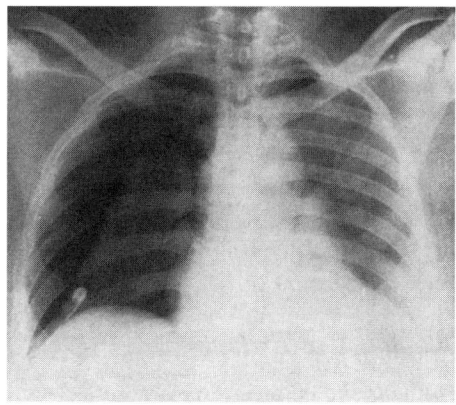

Figure 1.4 Pneumothorax in the right chest. Despite the underwater seal drain the lung remained collapsed and the drain continued to bubble. The cause of the pneumothorax was a bronchopleural fistula following trauma.

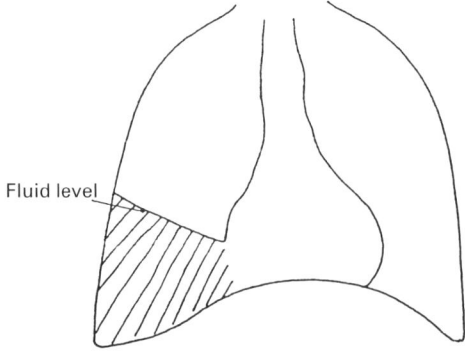

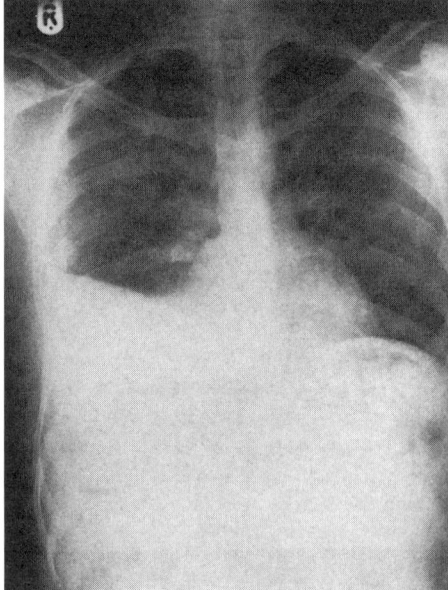

Figure 1.5 Haemothorax of the right chest. The fluid level would be consistent with any type of fluid: effusion, blood or pus.

Patients with pulmonary oedema and normal renal function will benefit from diuretic therapy when the underlying problem is fluid overload or cardiac failure. When pulmonary oedema is due to renal failure then peritoneal or haemodialysis is urgently required.

If these measures fail to prevent respiratory failure then mechanical ventilation will need to be commenced. In acute respiratory distress syndrome (ARDS), fat embolism, and diffuse lung disease, positive end expiratory pressure (PEEP) will help to maintain the patency of small airways and so keep more alveoli open for gas exchange.

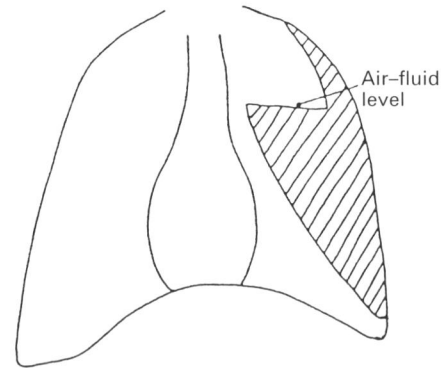

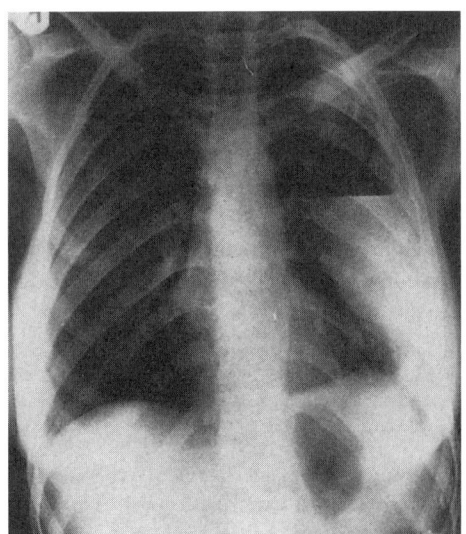

Figure 1.6 Loculated empyema left chest.

Obstructed airway

This has already been discussed under airway management (p. 7).

Inadequate gas exchange

All patients should be given oxygen therapy as described above.

Aspiration should be treated by chest physiotherapy and suction as described on p. 14. Pneumonia will require appropriate antibiotics (pp. 135–137).

Respiratory failure

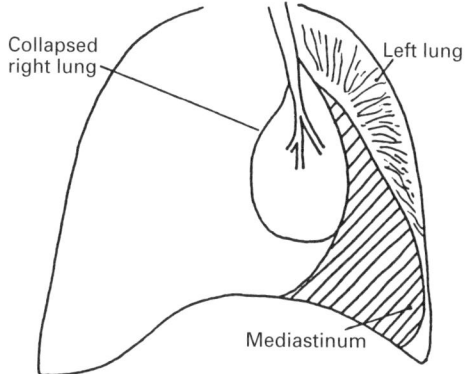

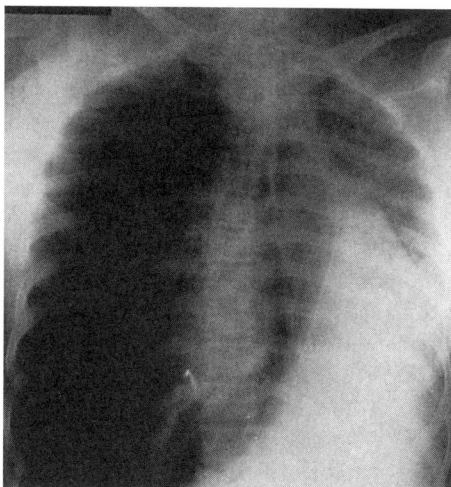

Figure 1.7 Tension pneumothorax: the tension pneumothorax on the right is pushing the mediastinum into the left chest and compressing the left lung.

Further reading

SINCLAIR JR, WATTERS DAK DAVISON M. Outcome of mechanical ventilation in Central Africa. *Ann R Coll Surg Engl* 1988;70:76–9.

Specific respiratory problems

This section details the specific management of the commoner causes of respiratory failure, which should be used in association with the supportive management mentioned earlier.

Asthma

Asthma is caused by reversible airflow obstruction due to constriction of smooth muscle in the airways. Bronchial wall inflammation is a fundamental component and results in mucus hypersecretion and epithelial damage as well as an increased tendency for airways to constrict. Bronchoconstriction may be triggered by a number of different mechanisms.

Symptoms of acute asthma are most frequently a combination of shortness of breath, wheeze, cough and sputum production. Many episodes of asthma will be controlled by inhaled bronchodilators and some patients will need steroids.

A patient presenting with acute severe asthma is usually distressed, frightened and dyspnoeic. The patient may be cyanosed and have audible wheeze. They will be unable to talk in complete sentences, respiration rate >25/min, pulse >110 beats/min and their peak expiratory flow rate will be <50% of predicted. Life-threatening features include silent chest, bradycardia, hypotension, exhaustion or coma, low oxygen saturation or a rising $PaCO_2$ on blood gases. Severe asthma in children is discussed on p. 18.

Management

- oxygen 60% by face mask;
- salbutamol 5 mg or terbutaline 10 mg by nebuliser – repeat as required;
- prednisolone 30–60 mg orally daily or hydrocortisone 200 mg intravenously then 100 mg 6 hourly for 24 h, then oral prednisolone;
- chest X-ray to exclude pneumothorax;
- monitor closely including oxygen saturation if possible;
- regular medical review;

- no sedatives;
- antibiotics are not required unless evidence of infection is present.

If life-threatening features are present:
- Add ipratropium 500 micrograms to the nebulised beta agonists and repeat 6 hourly.
- Give aminophylline 250 mg intravenously over 20 min followed by an infusion. Do not give a bolus of aminophylline if the patient is taking it orally. Alternatively an infusion of salbutamol or terbutaline may be tried.
- Magnesium 2 g intravenously is sometimes effective.
- Adrenaline 0.5 mg intramuscularly may be tried, or in the absence of salbutamol for nebulisation, adrenaline may be nebulised (2.5–5 mg).
- Transfer to ICU or high dependancy unit (HDU) as ventilation may become necessary.

On ICU most patients do not require ventilation for severe asthma and settle with medical therapy. Ventilation in severe asthma is often difficult due to the high inspiratory pressures required to overcome the airways resistance, and the tendency for the patient to develop air trapping within their lungs as full expiration is not possible. Hypotension and a reduced cardiac output may result.

Ventilation is indicated when the patient continues to deteriorate despite maximal medical therapy. It is a usually a clinical decision, although a falling oxygen saturation or deteriorating blood gases are informative. Ketamine and suxamethonium are useful for induction and intubation, and then the patient should be sedated (and often paralysed) until the bronchospasm resolves. Sedation should avoid drugs that may release histamine (morphine, curare). Ketamine, midazolam, pethidine, fentanyl, propofol, vecuronium and pancuronium have all been used.

A slow ventilation rate should be set, with a prolonged expiratory phase aiming to improve oxygenation but accepting a rise in $PaCO_2$. Initially ventilation may have to be by hand using 100% oxygen to produce adequate inspiration. A prolonged expiratory phase should then be allowed to prevent air trapping. If ventilation proves very difficult, even by hand, an infusion of adrenaline or salbutamol may be effective. Hypotension in severe asthma is most likely to be due to excess gas trapping. Volatile anaesthetic agents have been used in severe asthma with varying effectiveness.

Tension pneumothorax is a recognised complication of ventilation in acute severe asthma and should be watched for.

Further reading

Guidelines on the Management of Asthma. *Thorax* 1993;48:1S–24S.

CORBRIDGE TC, HALL JB. The assessment and management of adults with status asthmaticus. *Am J Respir Crit Care Med* 1995; 151:1296–316.

Pneumonia (Figure 1.8a, b)

The patient has respiratory failure due to inadequate gas exchange. Oxygen therapy is essential; physiotherapy is useful but should not be allowed to exhaust the patient. If there is no response to broad-spectrum antibiotic therapy and oxygen, ventilation is indicated if the long-term prognosis is good.

It is rare for a bacterial pneumonia such as a pneumococcal lobar pneumonia to present as respiratory failure unless adequate treatment has been delayed or there is a severe cavitating pneumonia due to staphylocci or klebsiella infection. In such circumstances ventilation can be successful. Pneumonia presenting with respiratory failure may be due to atypical infections,

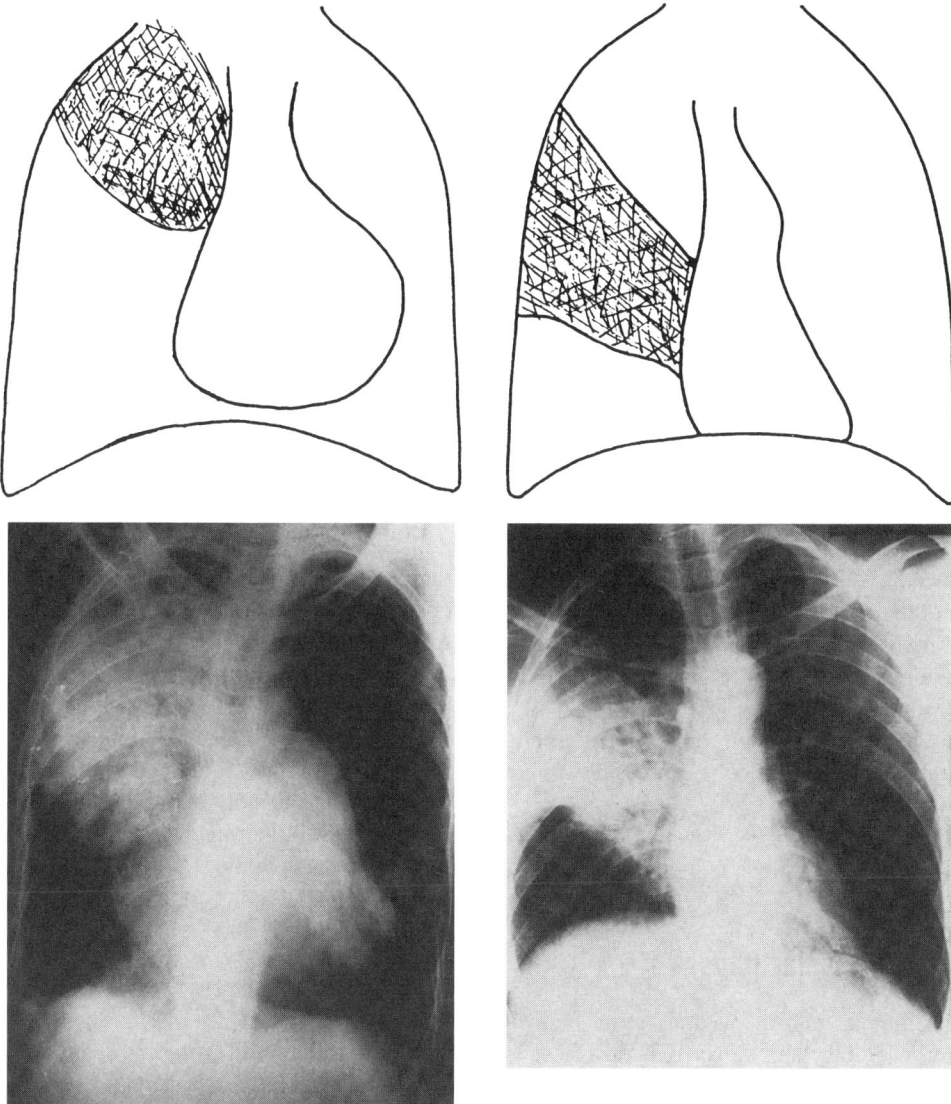

Figure 1.8 (a) Right upper lobe pneumonia.

Figure 1.8 (b) Right middle lobe pneumonia.

especially those with immunosuppression including AIDS. These patients have a poor prognosis so that ventilation is often ineffective.

Aspiration

Aspiration pneumonia may be caused by inhalation of stomach contents, blood or saliva. It may also follow spontaneous rupture of a lung or pharyngeal abscess. It is recognised by coarse crepitations heard throughout the lung fields. The chest X-ray may be similar to ARDS or bronchopneumonia (Figure 1.3). Sometimes only one area of the lung is affected, fluid flowing into the dependent lobe according to the position of the patient. There may be a history of maxillo-facial trauma, coma, hypersalivation (as in organophosphate poisoning), or vomiting under anaesthesia.

Aspiration often results in chemical damage causing an acute inflammatory response and pulmonary oedema. Although the aspirate is usually sterile, secondary infection may develop later.

Antibiotics are indicated for aspiration of infected material. Emergency management includes suction, postural drainage, physiotherapy and sometimes intubation or bronchoscopy. Prevent further aspiration by correct positioning of the patient (Figure 9.5 on p. 175) or intubation.

Ventilation may be required if severe pulmonary oedema or secondary infection develops.

Neuromuscular causes

Respiratory failure secondary to neuromuscular blocking drugs is almost always due to residual block following anaesthesia and is best dealt with by an anaesthetist. Reversal of the block with neostigmine and atropine may be all that is required, although a short period of ventilation is often necessary. Organophosphate poisoning is another cause and is dealt with on p. 122. Both of these groups of patients should recover if ventilated.

Patients with fractures of the cervical spine breathe using the diaphragm since the intercostal muscles may be paralysed. Abdominal distension or chest infection may cause respiratory failure. Polio, diphtheria and Guillain–Barré syndrome are discussed on pp. 137–139.

Such patients tend to present in respiratory failure with inadequate breathing rather than dyspnoea. Involvement of the respiratory muscles may develop quickly during the progression of paralysis, so they should be closely observed for signs of respiratory failure. The patient is unable to cough and retains secretions. Sweating, tachycardia, restlessness, diminished chest movement, and diaphragmatic (abdominal) breathing are the earliest signs. Respiratory failure should be detected before cyanosis and hypoxaemia occur. With oxygen therapy these patients may develop signs of CO_2 retention (bounding pulse, vasodilatation, warm peripheries, tracheal tug) rather than of hypoxia. If respiratory failure is precipitated by pneumonia then dyspnoea will be present.

Pneumonia may cause a patient whose breathing is just adequate to develop respiratory failure. Once respiratory failure is expected or has developed mechanical ventilation is the only possible treatment. Ventilation will then need to be continued until the patient can breathe adequately on his own.

Tetanus

This is described fully on p. 148. Respiratory failure occurs because of intercostal muscle fixation, which results in both underventilation and failure to cough. Spasms on disturbance make chest physiotherapy difficult. If there is laryngospasm the patient should be intubated. If bronchopneumonia develops, ventilatory support may be necessary, but it is often better to intubate and ventilate before bronchopneumonia has occurred. Diazepam and chlorpromazine have muscle relaxant as well as sedative effects and these can help to reduce muscle rigidity in patients still breathing spontaneously.

Acute respiratory distress syndrome (ARDS)

ARDS (shock lung) was first described in 1967 and became more widely recognised as a cause of respiratory failure in the battle casualties of the Vietnam war when it was called Danang Lung. It described a picture of pulmonary oedema without heart failure in traumatised casualties who had received large blood transfusions for hypovolaemic shock. The mortality rate was high. The underlying pathology is damage to the pulmonary alveolar-capillary membrane, which leads to leakage of plasma from the pulmonary circulation into the alveoli and results in severe hypoxia with a clinical picture similar to severe pneumonia.

ARDS may develop in any patient who has suffered hypovolaemic or septic shock. Other causes are listed in Table 1.4. The patient is tachypnoeic. There may be marked abdominal movement with respiration, minimal chest expansion and use of other accessory muscles. The oedematous lungs are stiff and difficult to expand. Signs of hypoxia are evident (Table 1.1).

Changes are often not seen on a chest X-ray until 24–36 h after the episode of shock. The appearance is similar to severe pulmonary oedema, with fluffy shadowing throughout both lung fields (Figure 1.3).

The principles of treatment are the same in all cases: oxygen therapy and, as in pneumonia, it may be necessary to use high concentrations of oxygen. As the underlying cause is pulmonary oedema, fluid restriction to 70% of the normal requirement is advisable, providing the patient is adequately resuscitated. Furosemide (frusemide) may also help if the kidneys are normal. Always monitor the urine output hourly, as these patients are at risk of renal impairment. If the urine output drops below 30 ml/h the fluid intake must be increased. This may cause a deterioration in respiratory function so that ventilation becomes necessary. Central venous pressure (CVP) monitoring may guide fluid therapy. In ICUs in the developed world where the full range of high-technology medicine is available, the mortality of ARDS requiring ventilation is at least 50% no matter what the cause. The decision to ventilate should be made with this in mind. Ventilation requires high inflation pressures due to the stiff lungs and positive end expiratory pressure (PEEP; p. 431) to maintain adequate oxygenation. Ventilation is usually required for at least a week and should be continued until PEEP is no longer required to maintain oxygenation on 40% oxygen or less (see management of ventilated patient and weaning). The commonest causes of death on the ventilator are pneumonia and renal failure. Steroids may be of benefit in some patients. Patients who survive ventilation recover normal lung function after a year.

Table 1.4 Causes of ARDS

Hypovolaemic shock
Anaphylactic shock
Septic shock
Acid aspiration (Mendelson's syndrome)
Fat embolism
Amniotic fluid embolus
Near-drowning

Further reading

WYNCOLL DL, EVANS TW. Acute respiratory distress syndrome. *Lancet* 1999;354:497–501.

Pulmonary oedema

Cardiac failure and pulmonary oedema are discussed in Chapter 3. Ventilation may be lifesaving in pulmonary oedema secondary to treatable cardiac failure. Ventilation may be complicated by hypotension due to reduced venous return in patients with heart failure.

Near-drowning

If possible discover the time of the accident, the type of fluid (fresh water, salt water, sewage, cattle dip, etc.) and what attempts have already been made at cardiopulmonary resuscitation.

Nurse the unconscious but breathing patient in the coma position. Clear the airway and give oxygen. The victim will have swallowed as well as aspirated the fluid in which he was immersed.

When the patient is not breathing ventilate using mouth-to-mouth resuscitation, an Ambu bag or mechanical ventilation according to what is available. Give chest compressions if there is no pulse (p. 396). Most of those who will survive make their first respiratory gasp within 5 min of resuscitation. High pressures will be needed to inflate the lung.

When the body temperature is less than 28°C attempts to regain sinus rhythm from asystole or ventricular fibrillation will fail.

Aggressive warming is recommended: warm water baths, warming inspiratory gases and warm saline peritoneal dialysis may be tried, but are often ineffective.

Secondary problems may develop owing to loss of surfactant in the lungs or damage to the alveoli due to the toxicity of the fluid aspirated. Always take a chest X-ray. Check serum electrolytes in patients who are not fully conscious after an episode of near-drowning.

Consider primary medical problems that may have led to the incident and treat as appropriate: e.g. epilepsy, alcohol, drug overdose, spinal injury.

Further reading

GOLDEN FS, TIPTON MJ, SCOTT RC. Immersion, near-drowning and drowning. *Br J Anaesth* 1997;79:214–25.

PEARN J. The management of near drowning. *BMJ* 1985;291:1447–50.

Chest trauma

Respiratory failure may be due to one or more of the following:
1. the chest wall injury;
2. a pleural space collection of air or blood; or
3. lung contusion.

Good analgesia is required if the patient is to breathe adequately. This can be provided by an intercostal nerve block, a pethidine infusion, or epidural analgesia. Physiotherapy will be required to remove secretions and prevent atelectasis. Oxygen therapy should be given.

If the above measures fail to prevent respiratory distress (which frequently develops on the second or third day after chest trauma), mechanical ventilation will be needed for 10 days or so until the rib fractures begin to unite. If there is a large flail segment, or severe lung contusion or associated injuries and a ventilator is available it is advisable to ventilate the patient from admission.

An alternative to ventilation for a large flail segment is to fix the rib fractures using stainless steel wire.

Respiratory problems in children

Inhaled foreign body, epiglottitis and acute laryngotracheobronchitis lead to severe respiratory problems in children which require careful management. Senior staff should be involved in their care from the outset and because these children can deteriorate rapidly they should never be left unattended. They all present with stridor (noisy breathing) and respiratory distress.

KEYPOINT
Never sedate a child with stridor.

Inhaled foreign body

A child of any age can present with a foreign body in the airway and a careful history will usually establish the diagnosis and the nature and size of the foreign body. A sudden attack of coughing and choking is usual, although the absence of such a history does not exclude the possibility. Buttons, coins and stones tend to be inhaled by infants, who may put anything in their mouths. Older children tend to inhale peanuts and other types of food. Vegetative matter such as peanuts irritate the mucosa of the airway causing oedema and a chemical pneumonia. The size of the object will determine whether it gets stuck in the proximal airway (pharynx, larynx or trachea), or the distal airway (right or left main bronchus or lower).

The narrowest part of the proximal airway in young children is at the cricoid cartilage. Proximal airway obstruction can be rapidly fatal and presents as severe respiratory distress with cyanosis. If you are present as the child inhales the foreign body, immediately turn the child upside down and hit him across the back or compress the abdomen in an attempt to expel the foreign body. If this fails, try to remove the foreign body using a laryngoscope and Margill's forceps.

If this fails and the child is deteriorating, perform a tracheostomy (p. 359). Under these circumstances you must not waste time on getting a chest X-ray.

If the obstruction is less severe the foreign body is likely to be in the distal airway and bronchoscopy under general anaesthesia is required. Clinical examination will determine which main bronchus the object is in. An X-ray may also define the site but do not leave the child alone as the object can dislodge and obstruct the trachea and the child may die. Bronchoscopy requires an experienced operator, an anaesthetist, and the correct instruments. The trachea is approximately the diameter of the patient's thumb and the size of bronchoscope required is the size of the child's little finger. A good light source, forceps and suction which will pass down the paediatric bronchoscope are needed for a successful removal. General anaesthesia should be used with good pre-oxygenation and continued oxygenation during the procedure. Some foreign bodies may need to be removed at thoracotomy.

Once the foreign body is removed recovery is rapid. In cases of distal airway blockage by organic material, pneumonia is expected to occur and the child should be treated with antibiotics. If the foreign body has been in the airway for some days, the child will present with pneumonia and collapse of the distal lung, or even empyema.

Epiglottitis

Epiglottitis is due to *Haemophilus* influenza B and causes upper airway obstruction in children aged 2–5 years when the epiglottis becomes grossly oedematous and inflamed. The onset is rapid over a few hours and the child has a sore throat, high fever, may be drooling at the mouth, and is severely toxic. The child will have stridor and difficulty in swallowing. Oral feeding should be stopped for fear of provoking laryngospasm. Inspection of the larynx may precipitate laryngospasm, so should be avoided unless you are prepared for emergency intubation or tracheostomy. A drip should be inserted for hydration and administration of i.v. antibiotics.

Specific investigations

Exclude other conditions by chest radiograph. A throat swab may induce laryngospasm, so should not be taken until the condition is settling.

Treatment

1. Humidified oxygen.
2. Ampicillin is active against *Haemophilus influenzae* (62.5 mg q.i.d. under 1 year, 1–5 years 125 mg q.i.d.).
3. If the airway obstruction is not improving the child will need to be intubated. Intubation may be difficult, so use

inhalational anaesthesia and get skilled anaesthetic help if possible. Sometimes intubation is impossible, in which case tracheostomy should be performed.
4. Do not sedate a restless child. Restlessness is a sign of hypoxia and the child may need to be intubated.

Recovery is as rapid as the onset once antibiotics have been started and the child can usually be extubated after 24–48 h. Again this is best done under anaesthesia in theatre to allow inspection of the epiglotis. The major hazard in the management of intubated patients with epiglottitis is hypoxia from a blocked endotracheal tube. Adequate humidification is essential and if a blocked tube is suspected then a rapid extubation and change of tube are required.

Laryngotracheobronchitis (Croup)

This is characterised by cough, fever and inspiratory stridor in a child aged 6 months to 2 years. The onset of symptoms is not as rapid as in epiglottitis. It may complicate measles and other upper respiratory tract viral infections. Nurse in a warm, moist atmosphere and observe for deterioration. Be prepared to intubate (a small endotracheal tube may be necessary) to maintain the airway. Antibiotics and steroids are given (either dexamethasone or inhaled budesonide).

Nebulised adrenaline (up to 5 mg) can be used and reduces the need for intubation in severe cases. This is due to its vasoconstrictive effect, which reduces the oedema. Stop the nebuliser if the pulse rate exceeds 180.

When intubation has been performed the child should be restrained to prevent extubation, sedated, and ventilated, with well-humidified air and oxygen. The humidification is essential owing to the copious secretions and if these are allowed to dry they can block the endotracheal tube, which is rapidly fatal. The swelling of the airway subsides after 2–5 days but extubation should be performed only when a leak is present round the endotracheal tube, and the child weaned from the ventilator. Croup is often complicated by lung atelectasis after intubation. Regular suctioning via the endotracheal tube is essential.

Severe asthma in children

Asthma is severe if the child is:
- too breathless to talk;
- too breathless to feed;
- breathing at >50 breaths/min;
- tachycardic (pulse >140/min).

Asthma is life threatening if the child is:
- cyanosed;
- making poor respiratory effort;
- very tired or exhausted;
- agitated or with reduced consciousness.

Management

Oxygen should be given, if available, at 10 l/min through a face mask, or at 2 l/min through a nasal cannula. (It is possible that the attempt to put in a nasal cannula may make the child more agitated and cause deterioration. If this is so, give nebulised salbutamol first.) Nebulised salbutamol should be given as soon as possible (5 mg to older children, 2.5 mg to those less than 1 year or less than 10 kg). A metered dose inhaler with a spacing device is equally effective. Give one puff every few seconds until improvement occurs – up to a maximum of 20 puffs. Commence steroids immediately with either intravenous hydrocortisone 4 mg/kg 6 hourly or oral prednisolone at 1 mg/kg twice daily.

These measures will usually be sufficient to control the attack. Nebulised salbutamol or salbutamol via multidose inhaler (MDI) and spacer should be continued 1–4 hourly as indicated by the child's condition, and steroids are continued for 4–5 days.

If, however, there is no improvement, give nebulised salbutamol (0.5% solution) continuously and give a loading dose of aminophylline of 5 mg/kg over 20 min followed by an infusion of 1 mg/kg/h or 6 mg/kg 6 hourly infused over 1 h. (Omit the loading dose if the child is already taking oral aminophylline or other theophylline preparation.)

If available nebulised ipratroprium 125–250 micrograms given 6 hourly may be of benefit.

Notes

Insertion of a venous line, while desirable in severely ill children, may be difficult and may cause deterioration. Administration of inhaled beta agonists is the most important part of treatment and steroids can be given orally. Intravenous access can be established, if necessary, once the inhaled beta agonists have been given, and, hopefully, the child's condition has improved. Use 4.3% dextrose and 0.18% N saline at two-thirds maintenance rates.

In the absence of inhaled beta agonists, subcutaneous 1/1000 adrenaline in a dose of 0.01 ml/kg should be given.

In older children the diagnosis of asthma is usually straightforward. However, in infancy, bronchiolitis presents in almost identical fashion to asthma, and inhaled salbutamol may be harmful rather than beneficial. Children with bronchiolitis should not be given salbutamol or aminophylline. Children less than 2 years old with recurrent 'bronchiolitis' may of, course, have asthma. In these children, a trial of salbutamol should be given but if there is no response it should not be continued.

2
Shock

Hypovolaemic shock

Definitions

The term *shock* is used to describe a variety of disorders in which there is a failure of oxygen supply to the tissues.

Oxygen supply to the tissues may be impaired because of:
1. respiratory failure (Chapter 1);
2. cardiac failure (Chapter 3); or
3. inadequate circulating blood volume (hypovolaemia).
4. hypothermia (p. 114)

The underlying problem in shock, whatever the cause, is tissue hypoxia. Hypoxia causes the metabolism of the cell to fail, which results in acidosis and the release of toxic metabolites.

Hypoxia stimulates the secretion of hormones (adrenaline, noradrenaline, glucagon and glucocorticoids) which increase the heart rate and force of contraction in an attempt to improve cardiac output and thus oxygen supply. Adrenaline and noradrenaline also cause constriction of the blood vessels in the skin, skeletal muscle, gastrointestinal tract and kidney. This diverts blood away from less essential tissues to the heart and brain whose vessels dilate in response to hypoxia in an effort to preserve life.

Prolonged hypoxia damages the endothelial cells lining the arterioles and capillaries of the microcirculation, leading to leakage of fluid out of the intravascular compartment into the interstitial spaces. Endothelial damage occurs early in septic shock (which has a higher mortality than other types) because the destruction of white cells and activation of other blood constituents such as complement and clotting factors releases products that damage the endothelial cells. Once fluid begins to leak through the capillaries the blood becomes thicker and the flow more sluggish, which increases the resistance to blood flow and worsens the hypovolaemia.

Clinical recognition

Table 2.1 Signs of shock

Tachycardia
Cold and clammy peripheries
Droplets of sweat on the face and hands
Restlessness, anxiety and confusion
Hypotension
Tachypnoea
Oliguria

The earliest clinical sign of hypovolaemia is a *tachycardia*. The heart rate is increased before the blood pressure falls. The pulse is usually rapid and of low volume, although in septic shock it may be rapid and bounding.

As tissue hypoxia persists the patient becomes *cold, clammy* and *confused*. The 'cold' is due to vasoconstriction in the skin microcirculation. 'Clammy' means a damp feel to the skin, which also appears pale.

Droplets of sweat appear on the face and hands. 'Confusion' may be evident from anxiety, restlessness or unco-operative behaviour and is due to toxic metabolites and hypoxia affecting the brain. Peripheral vasoconstriction may be sufficient to maintain the blood pressure to near-normal levels for some hours, despite considerable blood loss, particularly in young people. The respiratory rate is increased in an attempt to provide more oxygen and reduce the carbon dioxide in the blood to compensate for the acidosis. The patient may complain of thirst and feel faint on trying to sit up.

Urine output falls owing to reduced renal perfusion and also because there is stimulation of antidiuretic hormone and aldosterone secretion, which promote resorption of sodium and water in the kidney. These are compensatory mechanisms aimed at conserving the intravascular volume. The amount of urine produced is an important measure of the response to treatment in shock.

Early in septic shock there may be an increased flow of blood throughout the peripheral circulation owing to opening of the precapillary sphincters. This is the so-called 'warm' phase of septic shock. The peripheries feel warm and the pulse may be 'bounding', but the effect is usually short-lived and vasoconstriction soon develops, so that the patient becomes cold and clammy.

Unfortunately many patients are first seen after they have been in shock for some time. The blood pressure may be unrecordable and there may already be little or no urine output. Late in shock the patient may appear sedated.

The term *irreversible* shock has been used to describe an advanced stage when cellular hypoxia is so severe that death is inevitable. Although some patients will die despite aggressive resuscitation it is not normally possible to predict which patients are in irreversible shock. Therefore treat all shocked patients as if they are rescuable. Irreversible shock may only be diagnosed at death.

Investigations

Shock is essentially a clinical diagnosis. Blood gases and invasive monitoring procedures (for example central venous pressure) only measure the severity and may help to monitor the response to treatment. Most of the hormones secreted antagonise the action of insulin so that the blood glucose may be raised, particularly in septic patients.

How to determine the cause

The signs of shock may be present in respiratory failure, which is discussed in Chapter 1, or in circulatory failure, when the problem is either inadequate cardiac output (Chapter 3) or lack of circulating blood volume (Table 2.2).

Table 2.2 Different types of shock and their causes

Cardiogenic shock	*Hypovolaemic shock*
Cardiac muscle failure	Blood loss
Arrhythmias	Fluid loss
Valvular heart disease	Severe diarrhoea
Cardiac tamponade	Intestinal obstruction
Obstruction to blood flow	Peritonitis
Pulmonary embolus	Burns
Valve stenosis	Fluid maldistribution
Shunting of blood	Septicaemic shock
Congenital heart disease	Anaphylactic shock

Hypovolaemia may be due to loss of blood or fluid from the circulation. Fluid may be lost from the body in patients with diarrhoea, vomiting or burns, or else it may lie in body cavities such as the peritoneum and lumen of the bowel. Fluid may also leak out of the vascular space into the interstitial spaces (fluid maldistribution), and this is the main reason for the development of hypovolaemia in septic and anaphylactic shock.

The underlying cause is usually obvious from taking a history and examining the patient. Table 2.3 gives guidelines for differentiating cardiogenic from hypovolaemic shock. When shock is prolonged or affects patients with underlying cardiovascular disease there may be a combination of both forms. Similarly, in septic or anaphylactic shock cardiac failure may complicate hypovolaemia.

If the cause is not obvious search carefully for a focus of infection on the assumption that the most likely diagnosis is septicaemia (p. 133). Alternatively, consider the possibility of a severe reaction to a snake bite or herbal medicine. A low blood pressure and weak pulse are also found in patients suffering from hypothermia.

Management

The immediate aim is to supply the tissues with oxygenated blood by restoring the circulation as fast as possible. Thereafter, further treatment depends upon the response to the initial resuscitation and the underlying cause of hypovolaemic shock.

Table 2.3 Features which help to distinguish hypovolaemia from cardiac failure as a cause of shock

	Hypovolaemic shock	*Cardiogenic shock*
Pulse rate	High	Usually high
Pulse volume	Low	Usually low
Blood pressure	Low	Low
Neck veins	Not raised	Distended
Central venous pressure	Low	High
Cardiac output	Low	Low
Clinical heart disease	Not apparent	Often apparent

KEYPOINT
Never leave the shocked patient unattended at any time during the initial period of resuscitation.

Immediate management

The initial management of hypovolaemic shock is shown in Figure 2.1.

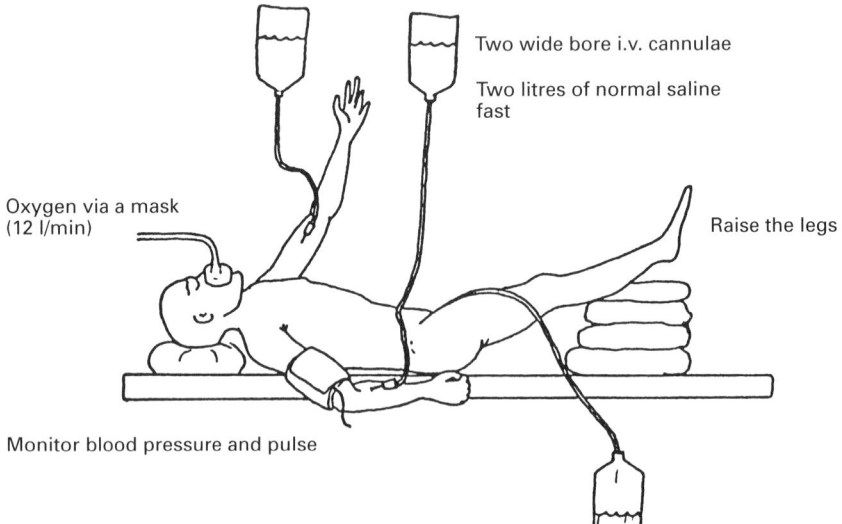

Figure 2.1 The immediate management of hypovolaemic shock. In children give 20 ml/kg as a rapid crystalloid infusion rather than the 2 litres shown here.

1. **Give oxygen** at 12 l/min as the cells are hypoxic.
2. **Restore intravascular volume.** To do this:

First raise the legs by 30° which will increase the venous return.

Second, insert two large-bore venous cannulae into a vein for rapid infusion of large volumes of fluids. Use 14 gauge cannulae in adults and as large ones as possible in children. A cutdown should be done quickly if good venous access cannot be obtained (p. 379). The i.v. giving set tubing can be inserted directly into the upper end of the saphenous vein in the thigh if necessary to allow very rapid volume replacement. The quicker the intravascular volume is replaced the quicker the restoration of oxygen to the cells and thus the less acidosis and risk of cell death. Take blood for cross-matching at the time of inserting the intravenous lines.

KEYPOINT
In hypovolaemic shock too little fluid is too often given too late.

Third, infuse 2 litres of crystalloid (Table 2.4) as quickly as possible, preferably within 10 min. Open the drip fully and do not leave the patient during this period. The crystalloid restores circulatory volume rapidly and improves blood flow. Thereafter choose the correct fluid for replacement. Unfortunately this is often determined by what is available. The choice lies between crystalloids, colloids and blood (Table 2.4).

At first monitor the pulse rate, peripheral circulation and blood pressure every 5–10 min. Insert a urinary catheter and aim to obtain 50 ml urine per hour in an adult (0.5–1 ml/kg/h in a child). The urine output will subsequently act as an indication of the state of renal perfusion and the intravascular volume.

Resuscitation for children in hypovolaemic shock

A single, free-flowing drip should be established. If a large peripheral vein cannot be cannulated percutaneously then a cutdown (pp. 379–381) or intraosseus cannula (p. 392) should be established. An alternative is a large cannula inserted into the femoral vein (p. 388). Calculate the normal circulating blood volume, which is 80 ml/kg (Figure 2.2). Give 20 ml/kg as crystalloid quickly. Thereafter resuscitation can continue with 10 ml/kg aliquots. With the most appropriate fluid (Table 2.4). Once resuscitation is complete continue with intravenous fluids according to the maintenance requirements (pp. 79–80).

Table 2.4 Choice of fluids for resuscitation in shock

	Type of solution		
	Crystalloids	Colloids	Blood products[1]
Duration in vascular space	30 min–2 h	2–24 h	Days
Amount equivalent to 1 litre blood loss	3.0 litre	1.0 litre	1.0 litre
	0.9% Saline	Dextran 70[2]	Whole blood
	Ringer's lactate	Haemaccel	Packed cells
	Plasmalyte B	Gelafundin	Fresh frozen plasma

1 If shock is due to coagulation failure the patient will need to be given clotting factors. These are present in fresh whole blood, in fresh frozen plasma and in cryoprecipitate. If bleeding is due to platelet deficiency give platelets or fresh whole blood if platelets are not available.
2 Note that dextran 70 may interfere with blood cross-matching, so samples for cross-match should be taken before giving dextran 70.

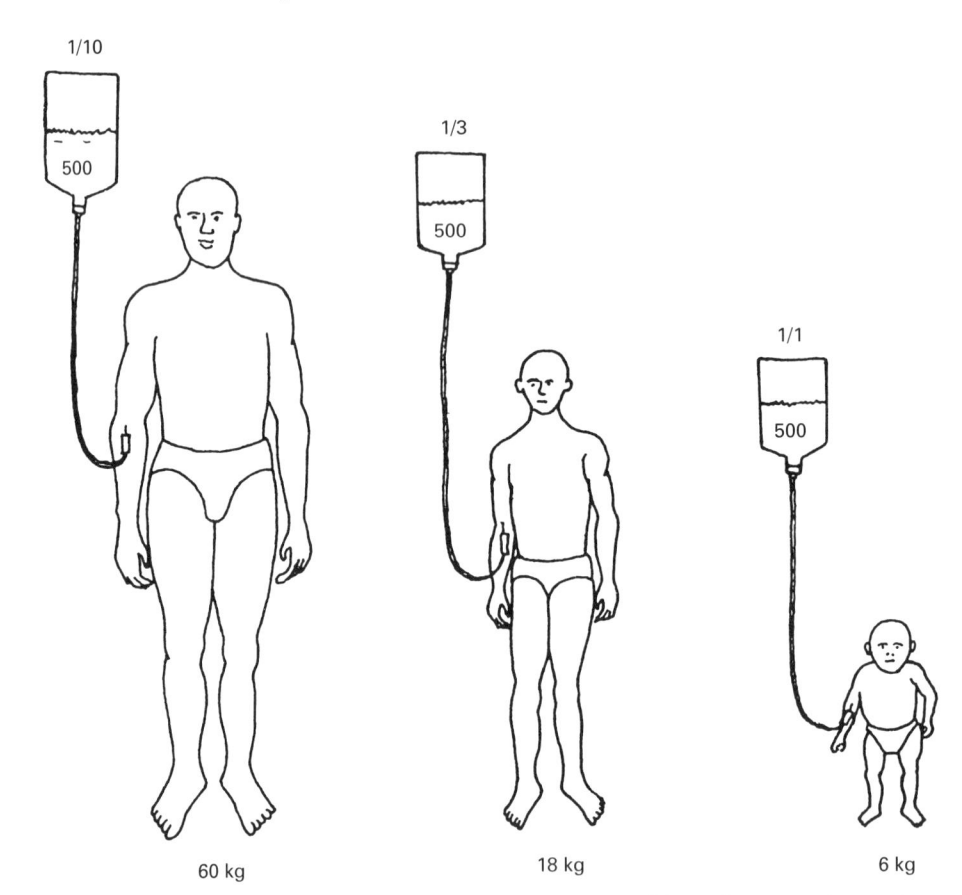

Figure 2.2 The importance of blood volume calculation in children. Always estimate the normal circulating blood volume (80 ml/kg) before resuscitating a shocked child. In a 60 kg adult 500 ml of fluid is about one-tenth of the blood volume but in a 6 kg child 500 ml represents the entire blood volume.

EXAMPLE

A 5-year-old child running across a road is knocked down by a car. He is admitted shocked with a suspected ruptured spleen and a fractured femur. His airway and breathing are satisfactory. The child is estimated to weigh 20 kg. How should the child be resuscitated on admission?

ANSWER The child is given oxygen by face mask, his legs are raised on pillows and a reliable intravenous line is inserted while blood is taken for emergency cross-match. The child's blood volume is calculated to be 1600 ml. Twenty ml/kg is 400 ml, so this is given as quickly as possible as normal saline. A doctor or nurse stays with the patient while the infusion is running to ensure the drip remains patent. Further treatment depends on the response to this initial therapy.

After the initial 2 litres of crystalloid the choice of fluid largely depends upon what the patient has lost; thus replace blood if there is a ruptured spleen, fluid and electrolytes in intestinal obstruction, and plasma in burns. Figure 2.3 shows the fluid compartments of the body. Blood and blood products stay within the 5 litre vas-

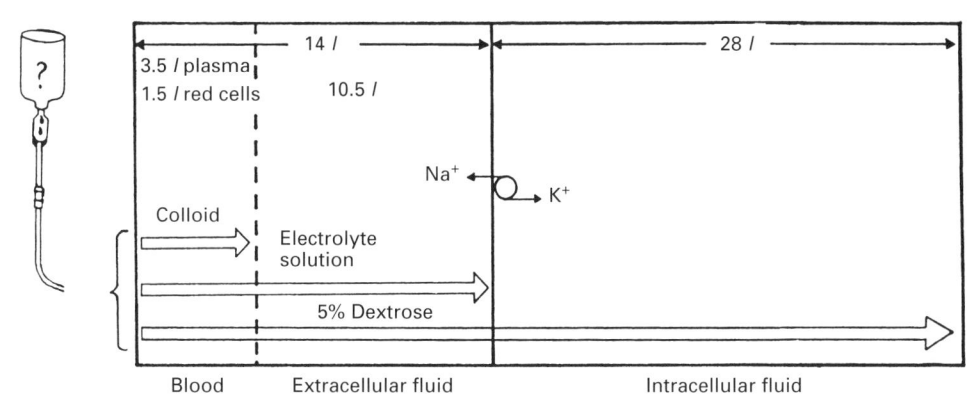

Figure 2.3 The distribution of resuscitation fluids in the body's fluid compartments. Note that colloid remains in the intravascular compartment, normal saline and Ringer's lactate are distributed throughout the extracellular space whilst 5% dextrose water passes even into the intracellular space.

cular compartment for days (Table 2.4). Colloid solutions remain for 6–48 h unless there is gross capillary leak (as in septic shock). Crystalloid solutions pass fairly freely between the intravascular compartment and the extracellular fluid and so only remain within the circulation for 30 min to 2 h. Since the total extracellular space is about three times the blood volume, about three times as much crystalloid as colloid is needed to resuscitate a patient. Figure 2.3 also shows that 5% dextrose is useless in resuscitation because it passes freely into the intracellular fluid and so eight times more 5% dextrose is needed than colloid. Do not use 5% dextrose for resuscitation unless nothing else is available.

O-negative or group-specific blood can be given if there is insufficient time for even an emergency cross-match. If there is time, shocked patients should be cross-matched on an emergency time scale, which takes 20–30 min rather than the normal cross-match, which takes 2 h. However, patients should not be allowed to die from blood loss while waiting for a cross-match to be done.

The technique of autotransfusion is described on p. 401. It is feasible where the blood lost has not been contaminated, such as in a ruptured ectopic, ruptured spleen or haemothorax, and when the blood is less than 6 h old.

Further management

Further management depends on the patient's response to the initial resuscitation (Figure 2.4). Most patients will show some improvement with 2 litres of crystalloid infusion. If there is no improvement continue resuscitation using colloids, plasma or blood, giving these as rapidly as possible providing there is no cardiac failure. Use O-negative or group-specific blood if cross-matched blood is not available but blood transfusion is needed urgently.

If there is an improvement then the choice of resuscitation fluid depends on the underlying cause of shock. Thus when shock is due to blood loss give blood or colloid. If the cause of hypovolaemia is fluid and electrolyte loss due to intestinal obstruction or peritonitis continue crystalloid resuscitation. In a shocked adult there will be little danger of fluid overload until at least 4 litres of crystalloid have been given. Observe the neck veins during resuscitation. Once the jugular venous pressure (JVP) becomes visible you know

26 Care of the Critically Ill Patient in the Tropics

SHOCK

Recognition:
- Tachycardia
- Low BP
- Cold + clammy
- Sweating
- Confused
- Restless

Initial management:
- Raise legs
- O₂ by mask
- 2 Iv lines
- 2 l crystalloid fast
- X-match
- Catheterise

Response → ? Blood loss
- Yes → Give blood
- No → Give Crystalloid

No response → ? Blood loss
- Yes → Give blood
- No → Give colloid

Response:
- pulse volume improving
- rate slowing down
- BP rising
- warm peripheries
- urine output 1/2 ml/kg/h

No response or remains hypotensive:
- Are neck veins distended?
- ? Cardiac failure

CVP:
- 0–5 cm → Continue resuscitation
- 5–8 cm → Fluid challenge
- >8 cm → Cardiac failure likely

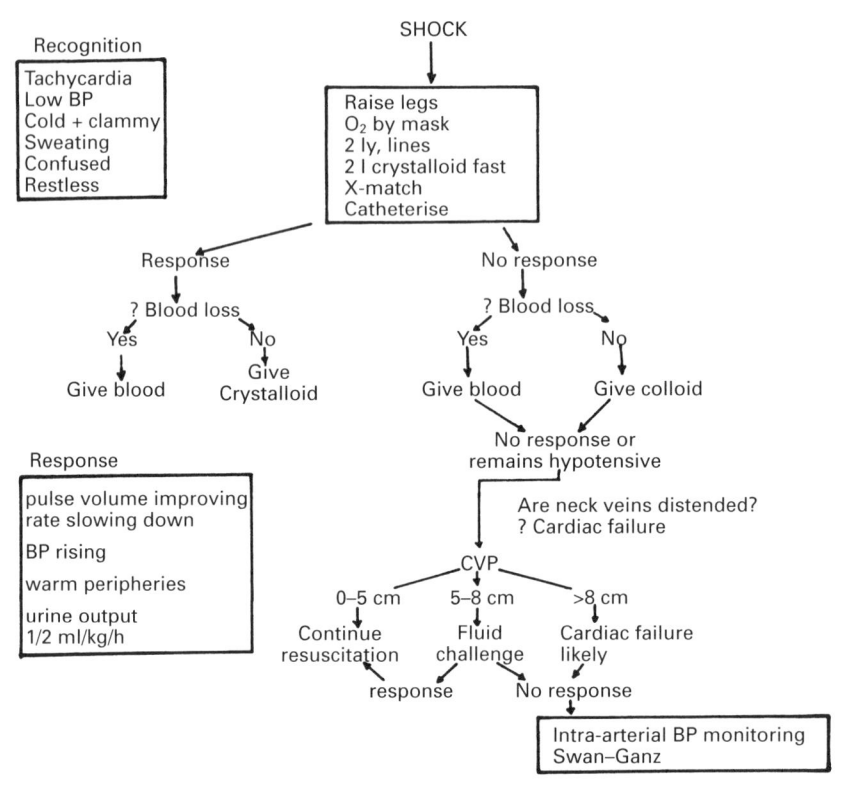

Fluid challenge → response / No response
No response → Intra-arterial BP monitoring, Swan–Ganz

Figure 2.4 Management of hypovolaemic shock.

that the venous side of the circulation is filling up. There will still be marked venoconstriction so that resuscitation should still continue but at a slower rate.

Whenever there is doubt about how much fluid to give, a central venous pressure (CVP) line can help to monitor progress in resuscitation. Since 70% of the blood volume is normally on the venous side of the circulation, the CVP reflects venous return (preload) to the heart. It is reliable providing the heart is pumping normally and the tip of the catheter is correctly placed in a central vein. Aim to restore the CVP to between 5 and 10 cm saline above the right atrium (see pp. 381–392), although in septic shock 15 cm may be required.

When oliguria (urine output less than 0.5 ml/kg/h) persists despite resuscitation insert a CVP line and follow the flowchart (Figure 5.2). Oliguria suggests either that there is still a low circulating volume or that renal failure is developing.

A patient with a normal CVP may still require further fluid resuscitation because venous constriction may maintain a normal venous pressure despite hypovolaemia. Thus in patients who have been shocked and who remain oliguric a fluid challenge with 5–10% of blood volume is normally indicated (Figure 5.2). Hypothermia developing during resuscitation needs to be corrected but is best avoided as hypothermia impairs perfusion, oxygenation and resistance to infection.

Do not give steroids in shock unless there is anaphylaxis. Steroids have not been shown to be beneficial. Too many doctors give steroids in shock while failing to attend to the important matters of volume replacement and proper monitoring.

Treatment of the underlying cause

Once resuscitation has restored the peripheral circulation and blood pressure, treatment should be directed to the underlying cause. Surgery should normally be delayed until the patient is fully resuscitated unless there is uncontrollable bleeding as may be the case with postpartum haemorrhage or a ruptured spleen. Septic foci in the peritoneal cavity or elsewhere should be drained once the blood volume has been restored.

Shock due to anaphylaxis or diabetic ketoacidosis requires specific therapy, which should commence at the same time as resuscitation.

Anaphylactic shock (p. 30)

This is treated by stopping the administration of the causal agent. Bronchospasm may require treatment with a bronchodilator so that adequate breathing can be maintained and the circulation must be supported.

Diabetic ketoacidosis

Hypovolaemia and poor cellular utilisation of oxygen both contribute to the condition of the patient, which is fully discussed on p. 101. In addition to fluid replacement, which in an adult often needs to be in excess of 5 litres, intravenous insulin infusion should be given. Subcutaneous insulin will not be absorbed in shock because of poor tissue perfusion. Underlying vascular disease or nephropathy may complicate the management.

Septic shock

The first aim of treatment as with other forms of hypovolaemic shock is to restore the circulating volume. A blood culture should be taken to identify the causative organism, although the 'best guess' antibiotics must be prescribed until the results of culture are known. Surgical intervention to remove or drain the source of sepsis should follow resuscitation. If resuscitation is unsuccessful despite adequate volumes of crystalloid and colloid, then inotropic support with vasoactive amines such as dopamine, dobutamine, adrenaline and isoprenaline should be considered. In septic shock there is tissue shunting, causing low peripheral vascular resistance, and inotropic support may be indicated, in sufficient dosage to raise the cardiac output and the systemic vascular resistance. This may also be beneficial in improving oxygen extraction by the tissues. Destruction of blood constituents and activation of complement and the coagulation cascade may cause disseminated intravascular coagulation (p. 34). The widespread endothelial damage with consequent capillary leak and sludging of blood flow in septic shock impairs organ function. Acute respiratory distress syndrome (ARDS; p. 14) and renal failure may complicate the picture and consequently the mortality of septic shock is high, usually above 50%.

Cholera

When gastrointestinal fluid loss is responsible for shock in cholera, continue to replace intravenous fluids and wait for the disease to run its course, as there is no effective specific therapy. Antibiotics such as chloramphenicol or tetracycline are effective in reducing the duration of diarrhoea (and probably of infectivity) but make no impact on survival if fluids are not managed properly.

Gastroenteritis in children

See p. 82.

Gastrointestinal haemorrhage

See p. 40.

Management of those who fail to respond to treatment

Despite achieving a good circulating volume some patients remain hypotensive and oliguric. The reasons for this include the following:

1. Not enough blood replacement despite adequate fluid resuscitation. If the patient has lost blood or had pre-existing anaemia treat with blood transfusion.
2. Tissue shunting causing low peripheral resistance in septic shock. If available dobutamine combined with noradrenaline may be indicated.
3. Coexistent cardiac failure. Late in shock acidosis, ionic disturbance, toxic metabolites and increased cardiac work may result in cardiac failure. Pre-existing cardiac disease will limit the capacity of the heart to respond to shock. Cardiac failure in shock should be treated with drugs which improve the contractility of the heart such as dopamine, dobutamine, isoprenaline or adrenaline, and afterload should be reduced with vasodilators when peripheral resistance is responsible for reducing the cardiac output (see below under complications of hypovolaemic shock).
4. The underlying cause of shock has not been successfully treated: for example, continuing bleeding or persistent sepsis. The patient may need to go to theatre.
5. Persistent peripheral vasoconstriction. This will be recognised by a central (femoral or carotid) pulse of good volume but a low-volume radial pulse and cold peripheries. Dobutamine or dopamine may be tried at low dose. Vasodilators can be used to dilate the blood vessels and reduce the resistance to cardiac output.
6. Irreversible shock – this should not be diagnosed until all available measures have been tried and failed.

Further assessment

Although intra-arterial blood pressure monitoring is not normally necessary it does give a more accurate assessment of low blood pressures than a sphygmomanometer when blood pressures are changing rapidly such as during major surgery or when using vasoactive drugs. The main indication is when hypotension persists despite a normal CVP. It can be measured without complex monitors or transducers using an i.v. cannula inserted directly into an artery such as the radial, femoral or brachial (p. 420), a three-way tap for flushing, and an aneroid sphygmomanometer or mercury column. Electronic methods of recording intra-arterial pressure using transducers are widely used in developed countries but the monitors are expensive. Intra-arterial blood pressure recording may soon be replaced by ultrasonic, non-invasive methods.

Pulse oximetry provides important information on oxygen saturation. Blood gases will allow monitoring of arterial oxygenation and acid–base status. In the tropics shocked patients can usually be adequately treated without blood gases. Unnecessary deaths occur not because of lack of monitoring equipment but rather because of failure to resuscitate swiftly or if there is insufficient blood available for transfusion.

Core–peripheral temperature, Swan–Ganz catheters, measurement of cardiac output and lung water are monitoring techniques which are expensive and require special equipment. Their role is discussed on pp. 418–422.

Complications

All organs of the body suffer from the effects of shock. This damage is caused by poor tissue perfusion resulting in hypoxia and the effects of inflammatory mediators, complement and coagulation cascade activation, cytokine release, intravascular cell lysis, endotoxaemia and deposition of antigen–antibody complexes in the microcirculation. As fluid leaks through the damaged endothelial cells the flow of blood becomes increasingly sluggish, worsening the vicious circle of hypoxia. Prompt resuscitation of the shocked patient aims, if possible, to prevent the complications of organ failure by restoring the supply of oxygenated blood.

Kidney

The reduction in blood flow to the kidney leads to poor oxygen delivery. The failing kidney cannot improve its own perfusion by autoregulation, so that if hypovolaemia persists the renal tubules will necrose.

In hypovolaemic shock oliguria may be due to a low circulating blood volume (pre-renal renal failure), or tubular necrosis (a cause of renal failure) may have occurred. Thus renal support is directed first towards restoring the intravascular volume in the hope of improving renal perfusion before tubular necrosis occurs. A better blood flow will also help to minimise the renal damage, which occurs due to antigen–antibody complexes, complement activation and microvascular coagulation.

Sometimes it is difficult to be certain whether oliguria is due to pre-renal failure (i.e. low circulating blood volume) or to renal failure (i.e. acute tubular necrosis from renal cell hypoxia). Measurement of urine specific gravity and urea and electrolytes may then help (Table 5.3). In pre-renal failure the specific gravity is high (> 1020) and sodium is conserved by the still-healthy tubules (urine sodium < 20 mmol/l). In renal failure there is sodium leak through the tubules (urine sodium > 20 mmol/l) and the concentrating ability is lost (specific gravity < 1010).

> **KEYPOINT**
>
> Always monitor the urine output and try to treat oliguria before acute tubular necrosis occurs.

Oliguria

This can be managed according to the flow chart (Figure 5.2). Once *tubular necrosis* is established it is important to avoid overloading the patient with fluid. Acute renal failure must be treated conservatively, by peritoneal or haemodialysis or haemofiltration according to the facilities available. The management of acute renal failure is discussed on p. 91.

Lung

Capillary endothelial damage leads to a leak of fluid into the interstitial spaces making the lungs stiff and difficult to expand. Oxygen diffusion across the alveolar–capillary membrane is impaired. The breathing becomes rapid and shallow, with increasing use of accessory muscles of respiration and ultimately dependence on diaphragmatic movement for breathing. Alveolar collapse and inequalities between ventilation and perfusion mean the blood returning to heart from the pulmonary circulation is inadequately oxygenated. The typical chest X-ray signs of 'shock lung' or acute respiratory distress syndrome (ARDS) are not usually apparent until after 24 h (Figure 1.3).

Treatment consists of oxygen therapy, intermittent positive pressure ventilation and positive end expiratory pressure (PEEP). ARDS is described in greater detail in Chapter 1 (p. 15).

Intestine

The two most serious consequences of a poorly perfused gastrointestinal tract are stress ulceration and bacteraemia. Stress ulceration occurs because gastric mucus production decreases while at the same time acid production is increased in response to stress. It should be suspected if a critically ill patient develops gastrointestinal bleeding. Antacids, histamine H_2 receptor antagonists such as cimetidine or ranitidine, or mucosal protective agents such as sucralfate may be given for treatment or prophylaxis. Antacids by nasogastric tube seem as effective as H_2 receptor antagonists or protein pump inhibitors given intravenously. Magnesium trisilicate (15 ml) alternated with aluminium hydroxide 2-hourly via nasogastric tube is normally sufficient. Whenever possible the diagnosis should be confirmed by upper gastrointestinal endoscopy. Emergency surgery to under-run a bleeding ulcer is sometimes required. In Lusaka we did not find stress ulceration to be common and therefore did not give antacids routinely to prevent it.

Late in shock the hypoxic intestinal mucosa fails to act as a barrier to bacterial invasion. Once bacteria enter the blood endotoxaemia occurs, accelerating the demise of the patient.

Heart

Cardiac failure as the primary cause of circulatory failure is discussed in Chapter 3. This section deals with cardiac failure complicating hypovolaemic shock.

The method of supporting a failing heart depends upon whether failure is due to preload, contractility or afterload. Preload (circulating volume) is assessed by examining for signs of hypovolaemia or fluid overload but is best measured by using CVP. Poor contractility (the force of cardiac contraction) must often be deduced from signs of left heart failure, the heart rate, rhythm and blood pressure. A more objective assessment of the function of the left side of the heart can be made from measurements of pulmonary capillary wedge pressure and cardiac output using a Swan–Ganz catheter (Figure P49, p. 418). Afterload (the resistance to cardiac output) is a function of peripheral vascular resistance and blood pressure.

Preload

Low circulating volume is treated by volume replacement. High preload is treated by diuretics or vasodilators, and occasionally blood may be removed.

Contractility

This may be improved by infusions of vasoactive amines, the most commonly used being dopamine (5–10 µg/kg/min) and dobutamine (5–10 µg/kg/min), although adrenaline may also be used and is more widely available (0.05–0.5 µg/kg/min).

Afterload

Vasodilators are used to improve tissue perfusion and/or cardiac output once circulating blood volume is normal. Both glyceryl trinitrate and sodium nitroprusside are capable of producing significant improvement in cardiac performance in patients with myocardial infarction and cardiogenic shock by inducing a fall in pulmonary capillary wedge pressure without reducing cardiac output. Noradrenaline may be used to increase peripheral resistance in patients where persistent shock is due to a low peripheral resistance.

Anaphylactic shock

Definition

Anaphylactic shock occurs following a type I (immediate) hypersensitivity reaction mediated by immunoglobulin E (IgE). The IgE–antigen complex provokes the mast cell to release vasoactive amines into the microcirculations in the various tissues of the body.

Recognition

Anaphylactoid reactions vary from mild to severe but may progress so that patients who initially have a mild reaction can deteriorate. Any unexpected reaction to the administration of a drug or diagnostic agent should be suspected as being anaphylactic. Deterioration is often rapid.

Early symptoms are sensations of warmth, itching and a feeling of anxiety. These may progress to an urticarial rash and oedema of the face, neck and soft tissues.

Evidence of a severe reaction is as follows:
1. bronchospasm which is recognised by wheezing and ronchi on auscultation of the chest;
2. laryngeal oedema, which is recognised by dyspnoea, stridor and drooling at the mouth;
3. hypovolaemic shock; and
4. arrhythmias and cardiac arrest.

Management

1. Stop the administration of the causal agent.
2. Secure the airway if severe laryngeal oedema is leading to obstruction.
3. Treat as for hypovolaemic shock by raising the legs, expanding the circulating volume and giving oxygen therapy (p. 345).
4. In severe reactions give 0.5 mg adrenaline (5 ml 1/10 000 or 0.5 ml 1/1000 diluted in 10 ml saline) intravenously over 10 min or by bolus if cardiac arrest is imminent.
   In children give 0.1 ml/kg of 1/10 000 adrenaline. Start cardiac massage if indicated.
5. Intravenous steroids do not act as rapidly as adrenaline but should also be given: 2–6 mg/kg hydrocortisone i.v.
6. Treat bronchospasm with bronchodilators (salbutamol or terbutaline) and/or aminophylline i.v., 5 mg/kg over 10 min followed by an infusion of 0.5 mg/kg/h (p. 440).

> **KEYPOINT**
>
> Adrenaline is the most important drug in the treatment of anaphylactic reactions. Give it early: it is effective and safe.

Severe blood transfusion reactions are treated as above and are discussed further on p. 33.

Prevention

Always ask about a history of allergy before prescribing treatment. Patients with a history of allergy or blood transfusion reactions or who have asthma or eczema are more likely to react to a drug or diagnostic agent. A dilute subcutaneous or intradermal test dose is indicated whenever an anaphylactoid reaction is likely, particularly when snake anti-venom is being given.

Blood transfusion

Blood is normally transfused to provide haemoglobin for transportation of oxygen to the tissues and vital organs. Sometimes blood or blood products are given to provide clotting factors or platelets in patients with coagulation failure.

Indications

1. Acute blood loss.
2. Chronic blood loss and severe anaemia.
3. Preoperatively in a patient with a low haemoglobin and in whom blood loss during surgery is anticipated.
4. To provide plasma, platelets or clotting factors.

Blood and blood products may be given in the following forms:

Autologous blood transfusion
(p. 401)

1. Blood can be removed from a patient 2–7 days before elective surgery and retransfused if necessary. If the patient's haemoglobin is above 13 g/dl (39% haematocrit) the operation can be performed 2–5 days after donation. Patients in whom the haemoglobin is above 9.3 g (28% haematrocrit) are also suitable for autologous transfusion, but wait 5–7 days between donation and surgery and give the patient ferrous sulphate.
2. The patient's own blood can be retransfused during surgery. This is called *autotransfusion* and is safe where blood in the peritoneal cavity is less than 6 h old and not contaminated by bile or intestinal contents. Patients with a ruptured spleen, ruptured ectopic pregnancy or thoraco-abdominal vascular injury are the most suitable. Do not autotransfuse blood from a ruptured liver as it is contaminated with bile.

Heterologous blood transfusion

This is the most frequently practised method of transfusion, and involves giving the patient someone else's blood. To avoid incompatibility and transfusion reaction, cross-matched (or in an emergency, group-specific or O-negative) blood is given. Never leave a unit of blood out of the fridge for longer than 30 min if you plan to send it back to the blood bank.

Before transfusion:
1. Check that the blood is the correct group and the name and number on both the label and the form match the patient.
2. Check that the i.v. line is patent and of sufficient calibre (19 gauge or wider). Use 22 gauge in babies.

During transfusion:
1. Check that the blood is running in at the correct speed.
2. Observe for signs of transfusion reaction (see below) by recording the temperature and pulse every 15 min during transfusion.

Red cells may be given as:
1. Whole blood – all the constituents of the blood are present.
2. Packed cells where most of the plasma has been removed. Packed cells can usually be transfused directly using a wide bore cannula.
3. Red cell concentrate – these must be reconstituted in saline before transfusion.

When the aim of transfusion is to increase haemoglobin content there is no need to transfuse whole blood. In some hospitals in the tropics whole blood may be the only form of red cells available. It is, however, much cheaper and more efficient for a blood bank to supply packed cells after having separated and stored the plasma for other uses.

Blood products

Plasma

This provides colloid, protein or clotting factors and is available as fresh frozen plasma (FFP) from a blood bank. It may still transmit hepatitis B or HIV infection. Freeze-dried plasma (FDP) is available commercially but does not contain clotting factors.

Platelets

In some situations in which the platelet count falls below 30 000 *and* there is active bleeding these may be indicated. Patients with a bleeding crisis due to platelet consumption from hypersplenism should be transfused if possible once the spleen is removed, otherwise the transfused platelets will also be consumed by the spleen.

Platelet infusions carry a risk of HIV and hepatitis B infection.

Cryoprecipitate

This contains concentrated clotting factors including factor VIII. It is indicated in coagulation failure. Cryoprecipitate may also transmit HIV, and in the 1980s resulted in a number of haemophiliacs becoming infected. Haemophiliacs can also be given factor VIII concentrate.

Albumin solutions

These are used to give colloid. They are pasteurised at 60°C for 1 h and have no risk of transmitting hepatitis B or HIV. 4, 10 and 20% solutions are the most common.

Blood substitutes

Synthetic compounds called *perfluorocarbons* are being developed that will transport oxygen to the tissues. It will be some years before they are widely available. Stroma-free haemoglobin is another alternative.

Side effects

Transmission of infection

HIV
Hepatitis B and C (non-A-non-B)
Malaria
Cytomegalovirus
Staphylococci and other bacteria

Careful selection of donors, screening of blood before infusion and proper storage aim to minimise these risks, but there is always some risk of transmitted infection with a blood transfusion. In areas where HIV infection is widespread, blood transfusions should only be given when absolutely essential.

Transfusion reaction

Cross-matching reduces the risk of transfusion reactions. The risk of a transfusion reaction is greater when an emergency cross-match as opposed to a full cross-match is carried out. Emergency cross-match is safer than giving group-specific blood without any form of cross-matching. No patient, however, should be allowed to die from blood loss because of fear of a transfusion reaction. Patients with a history of allergy, hypersensitivity or rhesus incompatibility during pregnancy are more likely to suffer from transfusion reaction.

A transfusion reaction is characterised by the following signs in increasing order of severity:
1. Pyrexia (>38°C) and rigors.
2. Tachycardia.
3. Itchiness and petechial rash.
4. Loin pain.
5. Tachypnoea.
6. Haemoglobinuria (due to intravascular haemolysis).
7. Confusion, hypotension and anaphylactic shock (see p. 30).

Whenever there are signs of a transfusion reaction the following actions should be taken:
1. Stop the blood transfusion.
2. Give 200 mg hydrocortisone i.v.
3. Check the number on the blood tag and the form to make sure the correct unit is being transfused.
4. Send the blood back to the blood bank together with a further sample of the patient's blood.
5. Test the patient's urine for haemoglobin.
6. Send patient and donor blood for blood culture.

Any further blood should be transfused with caution.

Cardiac failure due to circulatory overload

This is most likely in severely anaemic patients, and those with underlying cardiac or renal disease. Packed cells rather than whole blood should be given in those at risk and 20 mg furosemide can be given with each unit.

Changes to blood due to storage

1. Oxygen-carrying capacity is reduced due to deteriorating red cell function during storage. Fresh blood has the best oxygen-carrying capacity.
2. Platelet function declines rapidly so that after 48–72 h of storage the platelets will not assist in coagulation.
3. Hyperkalaemia: during storage potassium is released from damaged red blood cells. Red cell membranes become less efficient with increasing length of storage.
4. Deterioration of coagulation factors.
5. Acidosis from stored blood. During transfusion this is rapidly dealt with by the body and needs no treatment.
6. Citrate toxicity. During rapid transfusion (> 1 unit per 5 min) hypocalcaemia may occur causing myocardial depression which is best treated with calcium.
7. Hypothermia. Since blood is stored at 4°C, large transfusions may produce hypothermia. There is no need for the first unit of blood to be warmed. Warming can be done by placing a sealed bag or bottle of blood in water at 35–40°C for 7 min for subsequent units. If the water temperature is above 45°C haemolysis will occur. No shocked patient should have blood transfusion delayed simply because the blood is being warmed.

Coagulation failure

Normally blood should clot within 5–7 min of being placed in a sterile glass tube.

If the normal coagulation pathways are deranged then patients may present with bleeding. The common sites for bleeding are the gastrointestinal tract, mouth, nose and skin. The patient may also develop haemoptysis and/or haematuria. Skin bleeding is manifest as petechiae. Retinal haemorrhages may occur. Patients undergoing surgery may ooze persistently at operation or bleed postoperatively.

Common causes of bleeding disorders

1. Congenital deficiencies of clotting factors, e.g. haemophilia (factor VIII) or Christmas disease (factor IX).
2. Low platelet count (thrombocytopaenia) due to:
    (a) hypersplenism;
    (b) cytotoxic drugs;
    (c) leukaemia;
    (d) bone marrow suppression due to other drugs, e.g. chloramphenicol.
3. Massive blood transfusion with blood more than 4 days old which is platelet, calcium and clotting factor deficient.
4. Disseminated intravascular coagulation (DIC), which is most commonly due to septicaemia but may occur in any patient with shock. The commonest obstetric causes of DIC are pre-eclampsia, abruptio placentae and amniotic fluid embolism.
5. Anticoagulant overdose due to the patient taking the wrong dose or due to potentiation of the effect of warfarin by another drug (e.g. aspirin or tetracycline) or liver disease.
6. Chronic liver disease resulting in a failure of the liver to synthesise clotting factors II, VII, IX and X.
7. Patient with malabsorption or obstructive jaundice which results in a failure to absorb the fat-soluble vitamin K necessary for liver synthesis of factors II, VII, IX and X.

Bleeding disorders in the critically ill present in two main ways:
1. persistent bleeding in a postoperative patient;
2. spontaneous bleeding from the mouth, gastrointestinal tract, lungs or urinary tract.

Management of bleeding disorders

1. Determine the likely cause.
2. Give fresh whole blood, plasma, platelets or clotting factors as appropriate. If the patient has already had many units of blood which have been rapidly infused, give 10 mmol calcium gluconate for every 4 units of blood because the citrate in the blood may bind ionised calcium.
3. Avoid surgery whenever possible. Exceptions to this rule include splenectomy where massive hypersplenism is contributing to platelet consumption or when an abrupted placenta must be evacuated. Surgery is indicated where the primary condition will be improved by surgery, for example drainage of septic foci.
4. Treat septicaemia, optimise oxygenation and circulating blood volume.

The response to treatment can be monitored by measuring the clotting of blood in a sterile glass tube when there are no other coagulation tests available.

More specialised laboratories will be able to measure fibrinogen levels, fibrin degradation products (FDPs), prothrombin and thrombin times.

The above tests will allow both diagnosis and monitoring of the response to therapy. Therapeutic options are however limited and we recommend that low doses of heparin should not be used in the tropics for suspected DIC. Recombinant factor VII, an expensive but effective agent can be used when other measures have failed but is unlikely to be available.

EXAMPLE

A 25-year-old female presented with massive ante-partum haemorrhage necessitating emergency Caesarean section. Following delivery of the fetus there was difficulty in stopping uterine bleeding. Bleeding continued despite 6 units of blood being transfused. The units that had been given were donated 6–10 days previously and were thus deficient in clotting factors. A coagulopathy was suspected although no laboratory facilities were available to confirm this. Two units of fresh frozen plasma (which contains clotting factors) were given and the bleeding stopped. Two more units of fresh blood were transfused and the woman made a slow but steady recovery.

Haemolytic crisis

Definition

Haemolysis is the breakdown of red cells and is a normal process, but if excessive it may cause anaemia, jaundice and renal failure. Haemolytic disease may be acute or chronic. This section is limited to the problems of acute severe haemolysis and standard medical texts should be consulted for additional information on chronic haemolytic disease. Common causes of haemolysis are listed in Table 2.5 and while severe haemolysis can occur in virtually all these conditions, infections, particularly malaria and septicaemia, are the commonest causes in developing countries.

Severe haemolysis during or soon after blood transfusion is usually due to administration of blood of the wrong group but can also occur as a result of poor storage, overheating or administration of old or infected blood. Haemolytic disease of the newborn is due to blood group (ABO or rhesus) incompatibility between the blood of the mother and the fetus. Rhesus incompatibility occurs only in infants of rhesus-negative women if the infant is rhesus positive and only after the mother has been sensitised by a previous pregnancy or by a rhesus-positive blood transfusion.

Deficiency of the enzyme glucose-6-phosphate dehydrogenase (G6PD) in red cells is inherited and occurs frequently in peoples from Africa, Mediterranean coun-

Table 2.5 The main causes of excess haemolysis

Infections
    Malaria
    Septicaemia
    Gas gangrene
    Endocarditis
Drugs and chemicals (see also Table 2.6)
    Dose-dependent toxicity
    Hypersensitivity/autoimmunity
    Red cell deficiency of glucose-6-phosphate dehydrogenase
Incompatible blood
    Rhesus and ABO incompatibility in the newborn
    Incompatible blood transfusion
Immune
    Primary autoimmune haemolytic anaemia
    Secondary autoimmune haemolytic anaemia – e.g. systemic lupus erythematosis, polyarteritis nodosa, lymphomas
    Hyper-reactive malarial splenomegaly
Haemoglobinopathies
    e.g. sickle cell disease
Microangiopathic haemolytic anaemia
    Haemolytic-uraemic syndrome, e.g. from septicaemia
    Pre-eclampsia, malignant hypertension, renal disease
    Collagen diseases
    Carcinomatosis
Trauma
    Burns
    Fresh water near-drowning
    Snake bite

tries and Asia. Affected people are usually without symptoms unless haemolysis is precipitated by ingestion of drugs (Table 2.6), fava beans (broad beans; *Vicia faba*) or chemicals. Drugs and chemicals commonly incriminated in haemolysis are listed in Table 2.6.

Haemolysis that occurs in autoimmune disease is seldom severe enough to cause a crisis but in pregnant women with the hyper-reactive malarial splenomegaly (tropical splenomegaly syndrome) very rapid haemolysis may occur. The condition is due to an abnormal immune response to malaria and it is probable that malaria triggers this acute haemolysis, but it is unclear why it seldom occurs except in pregnancy.

Microangiopathic haemolytic anaemia describes mechanical destruction of red cells due to damage in small blood vessels. In acute disease fibrin deposition in small vessels may be contributory. It is sometimes associated with disseminated intravascular coagulation and may complicate a number of conditions (Table 2.5).

Sickle cell disease is inherited and is widely distributed in Africa and parts of Asia. The abnormal red cell predisposes to thrombosis as well as haemolysis and severe illness may result from anaemia or infarction in vital organs. Some of the more severe manifestations of this condition are described below and similar problems are encountered with some other abnormal haemoglobins such as haemoglobin C.

Table 2.6 Some drugs and chemicals that can cause haemolysis

Analgesics
   Phenacetin[1]
   Aspirin[2]
   Mefenamic acid
   Amidopyrine
Antibacterials
   Penicillins
   Cephalosporins
   Chloramphenicol[2]
   Sulphonamides[1] and sulphones[1]
   Nitrofurantoin[2]
   Isoniazid
Para-amino salicylic acid[1]
   Rifampicin
Antimalarials
   Chloroquine[2]
   Primaquine[2]
   Quinine[2] and quinidine[1]
Miscellaneous
   Vitamin K (water-soluble analogues)[2]
   Probenacid[2]
   Dimercaprol
   Sulphonylureas
   Stibophen
   Insulin
   Methyldopa
Chemicals
   Insecticides
   Some weedkillers
   Naphthalene
   Nitrobenzene derivatives
Traditional herbs

1 May cause haemolysis in normal and in G6PD-deficient red cells.
2 Only cause haemolysis in G6PD-deficient red cells.

Recognition

Severe haemolysis rapidly leads to anaemia and jaundice. The rate at which anaemia develops depends on the rate of red cell destruction and haemoglobin may fall by as much as 4.0 g/dl per day. Similarly the rate of bilirubin rise depends on the rate of bilirubin production from destroyed red cells in relation to the ability of the liver to conjugate and excrete it. The accumulated bilirubin is unconjugated and is not excreted in the urine but urinary urobilinogen is increased. The spleen is usually enlarged (except in adults with sickle cell disease) and in hyper-reactive malarial splenomegaly it is usually below the level of the umbilicus. If haemolysis takes place within the blood vessels (intravascular) haemoglobin is released into the blood (haemoglobinaemia) and passes through the glomeruli to the urine (haemoglobinuria). Serum may become pink or murky brown in haemoglobinaemia. Haemoglobinuria is characterised by dark-brown or black urine which gives a positive chemical test for blood but does not contain red cells. Acute renal failure may complicate haemolysis associated with haemoglobinuria.

Additional laboratory evidence is seldom required to establish the presence of severe acute haemolysis but may be useful to monitor progress. Increased reticulocytes and the appearance of nucleated red cells in the peripheral blood is evidence of compensatory increase in bone marrow activity. In addition serum haptoglobin will be diminished and, in intravascular haemolysis, the presence of methaemalbumin or free haemoglobin in the serum or urine can be measured spectrophotometrically.

The cause of the haemolytic crisis may be apparent from the history and clinical examination but its elucidation may require additional investigations. Malaria and septicaemia should always be considered. The history should be explored for any evidence of sickle cell disease and a sickling test or haemoglobin electrophoresis done if necessary. Recent ingestion of traditional or conventional drugs and previous episodes of anaemia should also be sought from the history. Tests for red cell G6PD deficiency may be negative immediately after an episode of haemolysis and should be repeated after 2 months. A blood transfusion reaction is suggested by the signs discussed on p. 33. The transfusion should be stopped and the remaining blood sent back to the laboratory to be retested. The indirect Coombs' test may be positive in haemolysis due to autoimmune disease. Microangiopathic haemolytic anaemia is suggested by the appearance of fragmented red cells in the peripheral blood and if it is associated with disseminated intravascular coagulation there may be spontaneous bleeding with reduced clotting factors and platelets and increased products of fibrin degradation in serum.

Management

Management is directed at removing the cause, controlling the anaemia, dealing with renal failure if it occurs and occasionally administering specific treatment to control the haemolysis. In neonates hyperbilirubinaemia above 340 mmol/l must be prevented because of the danger of kernicterus.

All suspect drugs should be discontinued and underlying causes such as malaria and septicaemia treated. The haemoglobin should be monitored daily. Transfusion is the only way to correct anaemia and blood may need to be given as packed red cells or with a small dose of a diuretic to avoid precipitating cardiac failure. Difficulties may be encountered in cross-matching blood in some autoimmune haemolytic states. Folic acid supplements (5.0 mg daily) may be given to prevent acute folate deficiency. Iron supplements are not usually indicated unless there is coincidental iron deficiency. Renal failure is treated in the usual way (p. 91).

In neonates serum bilirubin should be monitored daily and if unconjugated bilirubin threatens to exceed 340 mmol/l exchange transfusion is necessary. Exchange transfusion may also be used in severe sickling crisis, preoperatively in sickle cell anaemia and occasionally in haemolytic crises of other causes. The principle of exchange transfusion is to gradually replace a proportion of the patient's blood with fresh normal blood. It requires a relatively large intravenous cannula and blood is removed from the patient and replaced in equal amounts: 10–20 ml aliquots in neonates and larger volumes in adults. Hypovolaemia must be avoided. More detail of the technique is available in paediatric or haematology books.

Specific treatment to reduce the rate of haemolysis is seldom available. Corticosteroids are effective in autoimmune haemolytic anaemia, in blackwater fever (p. 144) and in the haemolytic crisis of hyper-reactive malaria splenomegaly. The initial dose of prednisolone for an adult is 80 mg daily (1.0 mg/kg/day in children) and it is reduced rapidly once haemolysis diminishes. Heparin has been given in microangiopathic haemolysis associated with disseminated intravascular coagulation but its effect is unpredictable and removal of the underlying cause is of greater importance. Heparin should not be used unless coagulation tests are available to control the dose.

Special problem: Crises in sickle cell disease

Low-grade continuous haemolysis is a constant feature of sickle cell disease. If there is a significant increase in sickling haemolysis will increase, as will clumping of sickled cells leading to small-vessel occlusion. This will increase tissue hypoxia and may lead to a sickling crisis. Sickling is increased by infections, dehydration, hypoxaemia and hypotension – all conditions which may decrease tissue oxygenation. Minor illness such as flu or transient diarrhoea may precipitate a crisis or it may start spontaneously. Patients with sickle cell disease may have reduced ability to concentrate their urine and are therefore particularly susceptible to dehydration. They are also more susceptible to infections, particularly pneumonia, meningitis, septicaemia and osteomyelitis, and while the carrier of sickle cell disease is relatively less likely to die from severe malaria than those with normal haemoglobin, malaria is a severe illness in patients with sickle cell disease and may precipitate a crisis.

Recognition

Most adults are aware of their disease but young children may present with a sickling crisis. The crisis may be predominantly due to anaemia or to infarction but in many situations both problems are present.

Haemoglobin levels in the order of 6.0–8.0 g/dl are usual in patients with sickle cell disease, but a small increase in haemolysis or decrease in haemoglobin production can rapidly lead to dangerous anaemia. Usually worsening anaemia is due to haemolysis from increased sickling and it is then accompanied by an increase in jaundice, peripheral blood reticulocytes and urinary urobilinogen. Less commonly, severe anaemia is the result of bone marrow failure (aplastic crisis), which is thought to follow asymptomatic parvovirus infection, but bone marrow function is also reduced by infection and by renal failure. When this happens reticulocytes and nucleated red cells are reduced or absent from the peripheral blood. Acute sequestration of red cells in the spleen occurs in children and causes a profound fall in haemoglobin, rapid enlargement of the spleen and sometimes peripheral circulatory failure.

Pain and disturbed function are the major manifestations of tissue ischaemia, which may be transient or followed by infarction and tissue necrosis. The clinical features vary with the major site or sites affected. Acute pulmonary episodes present with chest pain, cough, fever and dyspnoea and it is often not possible to differentiate pulmonary infarction (due to thrombosis *in situ* or embolism) from pneumonia, but in both hypoxia may occur and will increase sickling. Painful abdominal crises are particularly common in children and they may simulate an acute abdomen. However they often settle with conservative management and bowel infarction is uncommon. Cerebral involvement may present with acute confusion, fits, coma or focal signs including hemiplegia, vertigo, impaired vision and impaired hearing. Lesions in the spinal cord may cause a paraplegia. Focal neurological signs are often transient. Severe limb pain is the commonest form of vaso-occlusive crisis.

The diagnosis requires a high index of suspicion, confirmation of sickle cell disease by a sickling test and haemoglobin electrophoresis if this is available, and exclusion of other possible causes of the clinical problem. Infection needs to be excluded by appropriate examination and investigations, as it is the usual precipitant of a crisis and may be difficult to recognise in the presence of a crisis.

Management

There is no treatment that reduces or reverses the sickling process and management relies on supportive care, including control of pain, correction of anaemia, prevention of dehydration and avoidance of any factor known to aggravate the sickling tendency. Specific treatment is required for infections.

Pain is severe in vaso-occlusive crisis and will often need narcotic analgesics which can be given by intravenous infusion; the risk of addiction is low and is not a justification for failing to control pain.

Transfusion may be needed for severe anaemia but it is probably unwise to try and raise the haemoglobin above 7.0 to 8.0 g/dl as patients are well adapted to this level and higher levels may, by increasing blood viscosity, further impede blood flow through small vessels.

In vaso-occlusive crisis, intravenous infusion of dextrose 5%, even in well-hydrated patients, may reduce the duration (possibly by reducing blood viscosity), but care should be taken not to precipitate cardiac failure. Fluid intake and signs of dehydration should be monitored as well as the urinary output as the inability of these patients to concentrate urine reduces the value of urine output as a guide to hydration.

If general anaesthesia is necessary hypoxia must be avoided by pre-induction oxygenation, high concentrations of oxygen (30–50%) throughout the anaesthetic and continuing oxygen postoperatively. Oxygen should also be given whenever there is a possibility of impaired oxygenation and in acute pulmonary crisis respiratory support may be needed and should not be delayed. During surgery, hypotension, dehydration and limb tourniquets must be avoided. Anticoagulants are not beneficial except in pulmonary infarction, owing to embolism from peripheral veins (p. 69). If infection is suspected antibiotics and/or antimalarials should be given after appropriate samples have been collected for the laboratory.

If sufficient blood is available exchange transfusion can be considered in severe crisis. It has been shown to be useful particularly in crises affecting the central nervous system, the abdomen and the lungs and before general anaesthesia. In adults 100 ml aliquots can be alternatingly withdrawn and transfused or it can be carried out by concurrent withdrawal and transfusion of equal volumes through two different venous access points. In children smaller aliqots are exchanged.

Gastrointestinal haemorrhage

Approximately 80% of patients with severe gastrointestinal haemorrhage stop bleeding spontaneously. The remaining 20% will require some form of surgical intervention. Unfortunately, in any particular patient it is impossible to know at the outset whether the bleeding will stop or not. The principles of management are as follows:

Restore circulating blood volume

Treat the patient as for hypovolaemic shock due to blood loss (p. 22). Crossmatch and transfuse blood as soon as possible. If the patient is shocked he will certainly require a blood transfusion. All patients with major gastrointestinal haemorrhage will need a urinary catheter to monitor urine output.

If the patient cannot be resuscitated or is haemodynamically unstable, operate if you suspect a surgically correctable lesion.

Reduce the risk of continuing bleeding

The presence of blood in the stomach promotes further bleeding from a duodenal or gastric ulcer. Insert a widebore nasogastric tube and lavage the stomach with icecold water or saline until all the blood is removed. Give antacids (15 ml hourly) or sucralfate down the nasogastric tube or an H_2 antagonist by i.v. infusion. Sedate the patient with pethidine unless he is hypotensive.

KEYPOINT
Resuscitation and emergency surgery are the priorities in gastrointestinal haemorrhage and these should not be delayed or interrupted by efforts to make a diagnosis.

Determine the source of the bleeding

Upper gastrointestinal bleeding

Mallory–Weiss tears and gastritis are common causes of bleeding but this is rarely

severe. Severe bleeding is more likely to be due to:
1. oesophaegeal varices;
2. duodenal, gastric or stress ulcer;
3. gastric erosions; or
4. coagulation failure.

The diagnosis is first suspected by history and clinical examination. The medical history may suggest a peptic ulcer or examination may yield hepatomegaly, jaundice and signs of liver disease, which would point to oesophageal varices being the source of the bleeding. Endoscopy will reveal the actual cause of the bleeding in most cases and is the investigation of choice. The introduction of endoscopy has not, however, reduced the mortality of upper gastrointestinal bleeding in developed countries, which suggests that resuscitation and well-timed surgical intervention are more important factors in determining mortality. Endoscopy also offers the opportunity to inject a bleeding ulcer with adrenaline (1 in 1000) while medical therapy with proton pump inhibitors (e.g. omeprazole) and antihelicobacter antibiotics are given.

Lower gastrointestinal bleeding

Bleeding from haemorrhoids is very rarely severe unless there is coagulation failure. Severe bleeding may be due to:
1. intussusception in children;
2. amoebic colitis in endemic areas;
3. typhoid fever;
4. vascular malformations and angiodysplasia in the elderly;
5. ischaemic bowel in those with atherosclerosis;
6. inflammatory bowel disease;
7. diverticular disease and carcinoma of the colon or rectum in Caucasians;
8. Meckel's diverticulum in children;
9. a rectal or colonic polyp
10. coagulation failure.

The diagnosis is made first by history and examination. Examination should include proctoscopy and sigmoidoscopy.

When to operate

Where the cause of bleeding is unknown then colonoscopy, arteriography and radiosotope scans (technetium or tagged red blood cells) may be indicated. Bleeding has to occur at a rate of 1 ml/min for arteriography or scans to have a reasonable chance of localising the correct site. If this technology is not available or the patient is deteriorating despite resuscitation and coagulation failure is not the problem then emergency laparotomy is indicated.

In cases of upper gastrointestinal bleeding the stomach and pylorus ought to be opened to look for a duodenal ulcer, which should be undersewn with silk if present. Vagotomy and pyloroplasty should also be performed if the patient can tolerate a slightly longer procedure and the surgeon is capable. Bleeding gastric ulcers should be excised either by local resection or by partial gastrectomy. Bleeding oesophageal varices can be treated by emergency transection if injection sclerotherapy is not available and tamponade of the varices with a Sengstaken–Blakemore tube is unsuccessful.

When lower gastrointestinal bleeding is the cause but no source can be located at laparotomy, a right hemicolectomy should be performed in the hope of removing a vascular malformation or angiodysplastic lesion. Total colectomy may have to be performed for bleeding amoebic colitis, although with other complications of amoebic colitis, colectomy should be avoided if possible.

Rebleeding is dangerous where blood is in short supply, and the following categories of patients tolerate rebleeding badly:
1. the elderly;
2. those with chronic medical diseases,

particularly hypertension, cardiac failure, anaemia, renal failure, cirrhosis of the liver and chronic bronchitis;
3. those who were severely shocked when they initially presented; and
4. those who required more than 4 units of blood for resuscitation.

In the above patients the timing of surgery is crucial to outcome. If there is a surgically correctable cause of the bleeding (e.g. an ulcer) surgery is safer for the patient than rebleeding so that, whenever possible, a surgeon should be involved in management of the patient at the start. Surgery should be timed once the patient has been successfully resuscitated. A visible vessel or clot in the bed of an ulcer on endoscopy indicates that bleeding is more likely to recur.

Oesophageal varices

These are commonly due to underlying hepatic cirrhosis. Patients with oesophageal varices and ascites, jaundice or encephalopathy have a worse prognosis.

The aims of treatment in bleeding oesophageal varices are to:
1. resuscitate the patient;
2. stop the bleeding; and
3. protect the failing liver.

Resuscitation

See p. 22.

Stopping the bleeding

Bleeding may stop spontaneously. If it does not then the choice of treatment includes drugs to reduce portal venous pressure, balloon tamponade of the varices, sclerotherapy or operative transection of the oesophagus.

VASOPRESSIN
Give 20 units in 100 ml 5% dextrose over 15 min followed by 0.4 units/min until the bleeding stops. In patients with coronary artery disease nitroglycerine should also be given.

Octreotide – a somatostatin analogue (250 mg bolus followed by an infusion of 250 mg/h) will also produce splanchnic vasoconstriction without any significant systemic vascular effect or complications. It is safer than and as effective as vasopressin.

BALLOON TAMPONADE USING A SENGSTAKEN–BLAKEMORE TUBE
This tube has a gastric and oesophageal balloon which enables the oesophageal varices to be compressed by the oesophageal balloon (Figure 2.5). Bleeding commonly recurs and complications such as pulmonary aspiration, cardiac arrest and misplacement of the tube into the trachea are fairly common, particularly when used by the inexperienced. This method of stopping the bleeding is not recommended unless you are familiar with the technique and the patient can be closely observed while balloon tamponade is being applied.

EMERGENCY ENDOSCOPIC TREATMENT
This requires a trained endoscopist with appropriate equipment. The varices are injected with sclerosant or, preferably, banded and these procedures repeated at weekly intervals until the varices are ablated.

OESOPHAGEAL TRANSECTION
This should be reserved for patients with a reasonable prognosis and in whom other treatments have failed.

Once the acute bleed has settled the subsequent treatment of oesophageal varices to prevent further bleeding can be planned. The best choice of treatment requires specialist advice. Intragastric ligation of the varices via a gastrotomy is an alternative that is easier for the non-oesophageal surgeon.

Protecting the failing liver (p. 99)

Blood in the gastrointestinal tract results in a raised urea and blood ammonia with deterioration of mental function. Therefore, blood should be cleared out of the gastrointestinal tract by giving lactulose and magnesium sulphate to promote diarrhoea.

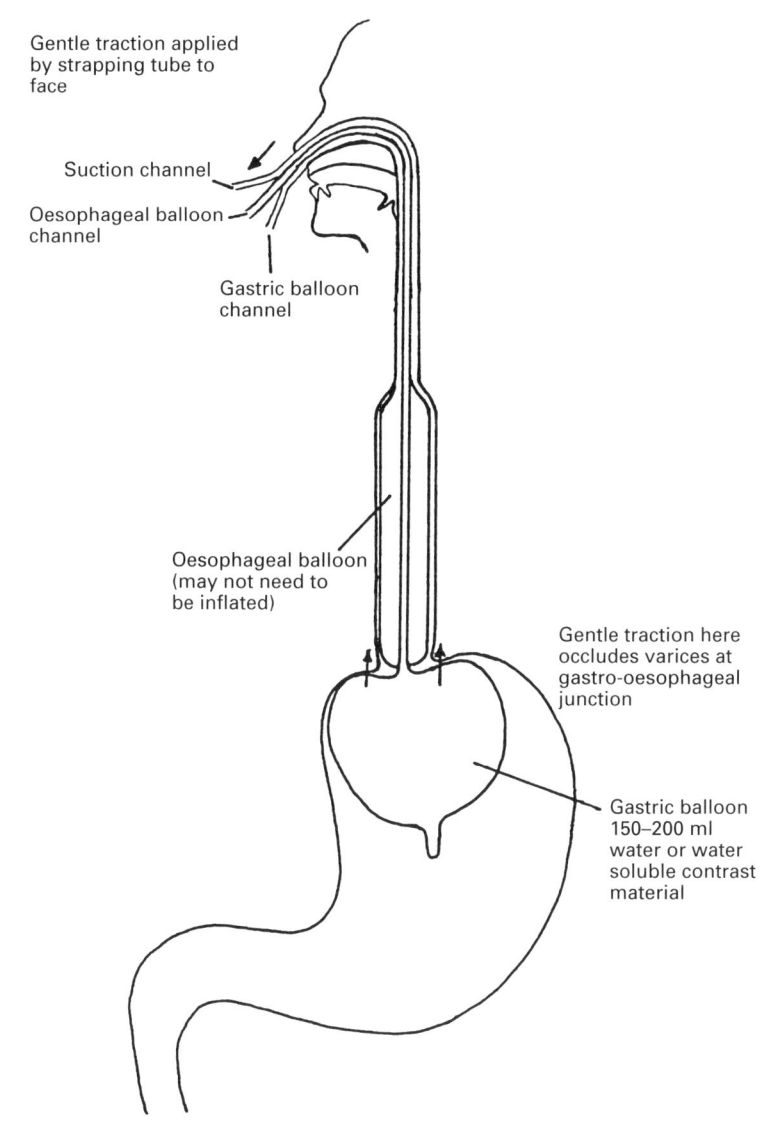

Figure 2.5 Use of the Sengstaken–Blakemore tube to stop bleeding from oesophageal varices.

Antibiotics should be given to reduce bacterial content in the bowel (neomycin 1 g 8-hourly and metronidazole 400 mg 8-hourly, both via the nasogastric tube).

Prevention of stress ulceration (p. 29)

We have not found routine prophylactic methods to be necessary in Zambia. In Western countries stress ulceration is more common in critically ill patients, particularly those with severe head injuries, burns and multisystem failure. We recommend that prophylaxis against stress ulceration be given only if it is a common problem in your hospital.

Acute pancreatitis

Acute pancreatitis is defined as an acute and potentially reversible inflammation of the pancreas. Patients with severe acute pancreatitis often present critically ill with hypovolaemic shock or respiratory failure.

The most common causes are alcohol and gallstones. Trauma, mumps, hyperlipidaemia and hyperparathyroidism also account for a small proportion of cases.

Clinical recognition

Upper abdominal pain is usually severe and may radiate through to the back. Nausea, vomiting and hiccoughs often accompany the pain. There may be a recent history of heavy alcohol ingestion or chronic alcoholism. The abdomen is rigid, tense, distended and tender. Acute pancreatitis may mimic any other cause of an acute abdomen. The diagnosis is confirmed by detecting a raised serum amylase and lipase. Serum lipase remains elevated for longer than serum amylase, which may only be raised for about 24 h as it rapidly cleared from the blood, but the urine amylase is increased for longer than this. If the diagnosis of pancreatitis is uncertain it may be safer to perform a laparotomy in patients with marked abdominal signs.

Attacks of acute pancreatitis range from mild to severe. Hypovolaemic shock may dominate the clinical picture and respiratory impairment is usually more severe than at first suspected.

Management

The treatment is essentially supportive rather than surgical.

The aims of management are to:
1. resuscitate the patient and treat respiratory failure;
2. establish the diagnosis;
3. rest the pancreas and relieve pain;
4. grade the severity of the attack;
5. monitor for complications.

1. Treat hypovolaemic shock with fluid replacement as described in Chapter 2. Assume there is respiratory impairment if you do not have blood gas analysis available and give the patient oxygen. If respiration deteriorates despite oxygen therapy the patient may be developing acute respiratory distress syndrome and may require ventilation (p. 336). Monitor urine output in case there is renal failure.

2. Establish the diagnosis by urine or serum amylase and/or lipase measurement or by laparotomy where the diagnosis is uncertain. Peritoneal aspiration may yield dark haemorrhagic fluid, which has a high amylase content (many thousand i.u./l). Exclude other causes of acute abdomen which require early surgical intervention such as perforated duodenal ulcer, ischaemic bowel or intestinal obstruction. Ultrasound will show whether or not pancreatitis is due to gallstones.

3. Rest the pancreas by inserting a nasogastric tube and giving intravenous fluids. Give generous analgesia, e.g. pethidine 100 mg 3–4-hourly. Antibiotics are indicated if the patient is febrile but probably have little effect on the outcome.

4. Grade the severity of the attack to assess the prognosis: if one or more of the following risk factors are present the attack is severe:

    BP <100 mmHg systolic;
    hypocalcaemia <2.0 mmol/l;
    PaO_2 <8 kPa;
    dark peritoneal aspirate.

    Other findings such as raised white blood count (>20 × 10^9/l), raised liver enzymes, high blood urea (>14 mmol/l) blood glucose (>10 mmol/l) and a low serum albumin (<30 g/l) imply a severe attack and a worse prognosis. The prognosis is also worst in those above 60 years of age.

5. Monitor for complications: respiratory and renal failure, deep venous thrombosis and hyperglycaemia may occur. Thus respiration, urine output and blood glucose should be monitored. The treatment of these complications is discussed in the appropriate chapters. If pyrexia persists for a few days or the abdominal signs do not improve with the above treatment then a pseudocyst or pancreatic abscess may be developing. Ultrasound is an accurate means of diagnosing pseudocyst and abscess. CT scanning is a more accurate means of assessing the pancreas than ultrasound particularly identifying pancreatic necrosis.

Surgical treatment

The vast majority of patients do not require surgical intervention, which is limited mainly to where the diagnosis is uncertain or for drainage of a pancreatic abscess or psuedocyst. Patients with gallstone-induced pancreatitis may benefit from cholecystectomy or cholecystostomy in the first 48 h in specialised centres where trained surgeons are available. The surgical treatment of severe pancreatitis is complex, generally unrewarding in the acute phase and beyond the scope of this book. Patients who undergo necrosectomy (removal of dead necrotic pancreatic fragments piecemeal) will require multiple procedures and have a long stay in ICU.

Further reading

ASTIZ ME, RACKOW EC. Septic shock. *Lancet* 1998;351:1501–5.

BOSCH J, GARCIA-PAGAN JC. Prevention of variceal rebleeding. *Lancet* 2003;361:952–4.

BRANICKI FJ, CHU KM. Multiple organ dysfunction: current concepts of aetiology and management. *Ann Coll Surg Hong Kong* 1997;1:53–61.

CHUNG SCS *et al*. Endoscopic injection of adrenaline for actively bleeding ulcers: a randomised trial. *BMJ* 1988; 296(6637):1631–1.

HUIZINGA WKJ, BAKER LW. Treatment of persistent and complicated pancreatic psuedocysts. *J R Coll Surg Edinb* 1992;37:373–6.

KHUROO MS *et al*. *Ascaris*-induced acute pancreatitis. *Br J Surg* 1992;79:1335–8.

KIIRE CF. Upper gastrointestinal bleeding in an African Setting. *J R Coll Physicians Lond* 1987;21:107.

LEVI M, TEN CATE H. Disseminated intravascular coagulation. *N Engl J Med* 1999;341:586–92.

THOMAS PG. Observations and surgical management of tropical pancreatitis in Kerala and southern India. *World J Surg* 1990;14:32–42.

3
Cardiovascular disease

The major components of the cardiovascular system are the heart and large arteries and veins. Disorders of either the heart or the main vessels may cause critical illness and cardiac failure is the commonest problem. Following discussion of cardiac failure and its causes, other common causes of critical cardiovascular disease are discussed.

Cardiac failure

Definition

Cardiac failure is a condition in which the cardiac output from one or both sides of the heart is insufficient for the needs of the body. In acute cardiac failure, cardiac output is less than the venous return, affecting either side of the heart independently or both sides together. When cardiac failure arises as a consequence of very high needs of the body (e.g. in persistent high fever) high output failure is present. When cardiac failure occurs when the needs of the body are normal or low then one speaks of low output failure.

Cardiac failure commonly arises from heart disease, which may be structural as in congenital and valvular heart disease or from ineffective pumping by the heart muscle as in cardiomyopathies, ischaemic heart disease and abnormal rhythms. Heart failure may also arise from or be aggravated by problems outside the heart such as systemic hypertension, anaemia and acute and chronic lung disease. The side of the heart predominantly affected depends on the cause of heart failure.

Recognition

It is important to recognise the different manifestations of left and right heart failure which are summarised in Table 3.1.

Table 3.1 Major features of right- and left-sided heart failure

Right-sided failure	Left-sided failure
Engorged neck veins	Dyspnoea and orthopnoea
Enlarged, tender liver	Cough with frothy bloody sputum
Dependent oedema	Cyanosis in severe cases
Ascites (sometimes)	Triple (gallop) rhythm
Right ventricular heave	Fine crepitations in the lung bases
Functional tricuspid regurgitation	Shock in severe cases
	May cause right-sided failure
	Functional mitral regurgitation

In left heart failure venous blood accumulates in the pulmonary veins and fluid enters the alveolar spaces, impairing blood gas exchange and causing dyspnoea. When severe there is acute pulmonary oedema, which is a major medical emergency. In acute pulmonary oedema the patient is very dyspnoeic and is likely to have all the signs of left-sided failure (Table 3.1). Rhonchi may also be heard in the lungs and in more severe cases (cardiogenic shock) the patient is likely to be confused and have peripheral vasoconstriction and hypotension. Acute pulmonary oedema from heart failure or over-transfusion needs to be distinguished from that due to inhalation of irritants, uraemia and the acute respiratory distress syndrome (p. 14). The history and associated clinical features usually make the diagnosis clear but in difficult cases left heart failure classically shows bilateral pulmonary mottling radiating outwards from the hila in the shape of a butterfly wing, together with cardiac enlargement on chest X-ray (Figure 3.1). Treatment of severe pulmonary oedema is urgent and is described on p. 54. Less severe forms of left-sided failure present with paroxysmal nocturnal dyspnoea, orthopnoea and exertional dyspnoea; basal crepitations are not always heard.

In right-sided heart failure there is accumulation of blood in the vena cava and this is recognised by visible engorgement of veins in the neck, oedema of the legs (or sacrum in patients in bed) and tender enlargement of the liver. Right-sided heart failure may follow prolonged left-sided failure or may arise from disease of the right side of the heart or lungs.

Less characteristic features of heart failure are due to decreased cardiac output. Depending on the side of the heart predominantly affected blood flow may be reduced to the lungs (right-sided), leading to exertional dyspnoea or through the aorta to the rest of the body (left-sided) causing tiredness, general weakness and sometimes fainting attacks. Failure of both sides of the heart is manifest by a mixture of the features already described. Severe cardiac failure causes cardiogenic shock, which can be distinguished from hypovolaemic shock (p. 22) by the presence of engorged neck veins.

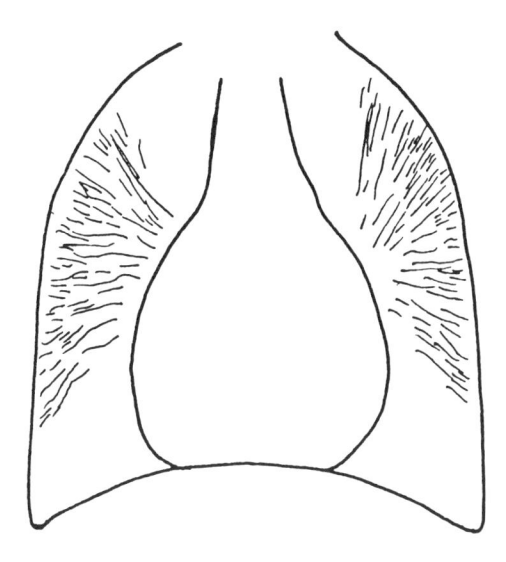

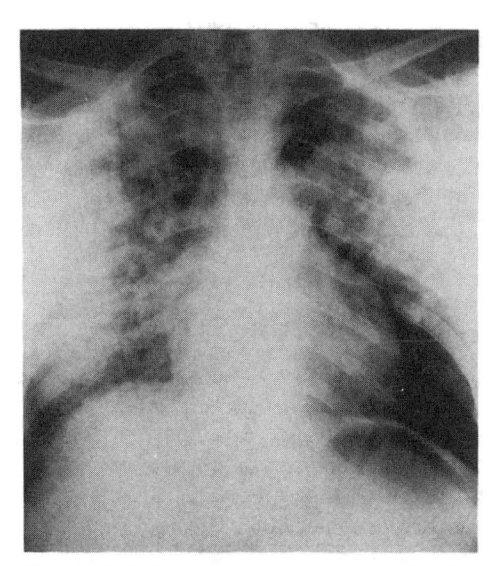

Figure 3.1 Pulmonary oedema. Note the 'butterfly wing' distribution of infiltrates.

Determining the cause

The cause of heart failure should be determined as it will influence how aggressively the patient is treated as well as the specific treatment needed. For example, in heart failure due to severe valvular disease the response to treatment (unless valve replacement is possible) will be poor and not really improved by aggressive treatment. In contrast, a patient with a minor valvular lesion may be in severe heart failure owing to a serious arrhythmia which can be corrected and this patient's prognosis is good. Cardiac failure may arise from inherited or acquired disease of the heart or may arise from problems outside the heart (Table 3.2).

In patients with normally well-compensated heart disease severe cardiac failure may be precipitated by superimposed conditions such as an arrhythmia, endocarditis, myocarditis, pregnancy, pneumonia, pulmonary embolism, septicaemia and anaemia and these precipitating factors may be relieved even if the underlying heart disease cannot be rectified.

In determining the cause of heart failure the acuteness of the illness may he helpful. Patients with structural damage to the heart, with hypertension and with cardiodiomyopathies will usually give a history of cardiac symptoms before the onset of the acute episode. In most hospitals in developing countries these conditions are not reversible. However, an acute event may be the first indication of any of these conditions and the prognosis may be quite good providing the immediate problem can be overcome. Thus patients presenting with recent onset of cardiac symptoms are more likely to benefit from aggressive management.

Recognition of the cause of cardiac failure is of prime importance because it may immediately direct the treatment (e.g. pericardiocentesis in pericardial tamponade). This will now be discussed.

Table 3.2 Common causes of right and left heart failure

Structural disorders of the heart
  Congenital abnormalities
  Acquired valvular defects
    Rheumatic heart disease
    Other infections (e.g. endocarditis, syphilis)
  Pericardial disease
    Tamponade
    Constrictive pericarditis
Disorders of cardiac function
  Abnormal heart rhythm
  Ischaemic muscle damage
  Cardiomyopathies
  Myocarditis
Causes arising outside the heart
  Hypertension
  Fluid overload
  Anaemia
  Pulmonary embolism
  Acute and chronic lung disease
  Infection
  Dissection of the aorta

Recognition of the most important causes of cardiac failure

Arrhythmias

These are described in detail later (p. 56) but should be suspected if the heart beat is irregular or abnormally slow (i.e. <50 beats per minute) or abnormally fast (>150 beats per minute). An ECG is often needed to be certain of the type of arrhythmia present.

Pericardial tamponade

Pericardial tamponade is present when there is rapid fluid accumulation in a tight fibrinous pericardium or a large pericardial effusion compresses the heart and prevents blood entering it. The cardinal signs of pericardial tamponade are engorged neck veins that do not pulsate, hypotension and shock and a pulsus paradoxus when the volume of the pulse can be felt to be greater

Cardiovascular disease 49

in expiration than in inspiration (i.e. an exaggeration of the normal). In addition, cardiac pulsations cannot be seen or felt over the front of the left chest. It is important to distinguish a large pericardial effusion that can be aspirated from pericardial constriction that requires thoracic surgery. A large pericardial effusion causes the heart sounds to be muffled, a low voltage on the ECG and an enlarged cardiac shadow on chest X-ray (Figure 3.2). By contrast, in constrictive pericarditis the ECG is often normal and on chest X-ray the heart size is usually normal or small and calcification

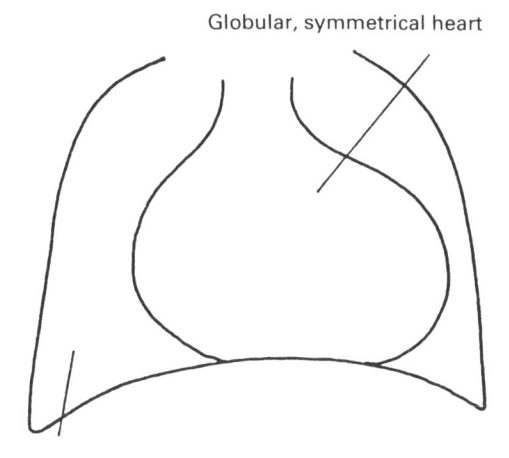

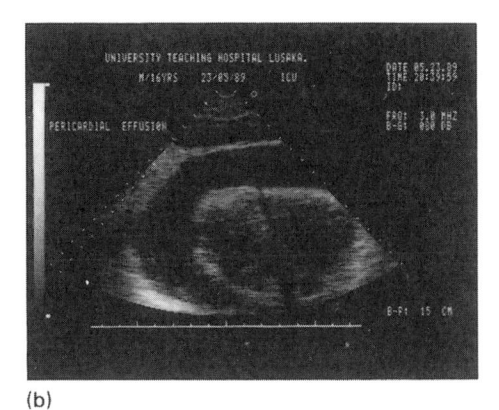

Figure 3.2 (b) Cardiac ultrasound of a large pericardial effusion. The section shows a large dark halo of pericardial fluid surrounding the lighter coloured myocardium.

may be seen around the edge of the heart shadow. If available, echocardiography is the best way of confirming the diagnosis and moreover it reveals the best site for urgent pericardiocentesis.

Ischaemic heart disease: right and left ventricular infarction

In the presence of disease of the arteries supplying the myocardium (the coronary arteries) there may be ischaemic damage to the heart muscle, which cannot pump effectively. Sudden occlusion of a major vessel commonly leads to myocardial infarction (p. 65). Myocardial ischaemia classically causes central chest pain, which is aggravated by exertion and relieved within minutes of resting, unless there has been an infarct when the pain persists. No specific signs are associated with myocardial ischaemia. Infarction is diagnosed by ECG changes (Figure 3.11) and further proved by an increase in plasma concentrations of cardiac enzymes – creatinine phosphokinase (CK – total CK and CK-MB the cardiac isoenzyme), troponins (I and T), aspartate amino transferase (AST), and lactic dehydrogenase (LDH). Troponins are raised for 7–10 days after infarction and

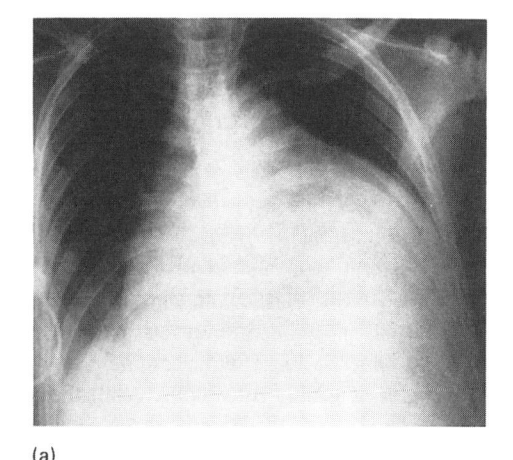

Figure 3.2 (a) Pericardial effusion.

are more specific than CK. They are useful for the late diagnosis of infarction.

In cases of acute infarction it is sometimes possible to distinguish right from left ventricular infarction and this distinction is important for therapy. Features of right heart failure (Table 3.1) but with no signs of left heart failure (Table 3.1) suggest isolated right ventricular dysfunction, more certainly present when the ECG shows an inferior infarction. The distinction can be confirmed by right and left heart pressure monitoring.

Pulmonary embolism

A pulmonary embolus is occlusion of a pulmonary artery by thrombus which has arisen in the veins of the lower limbs or pelvis. Thrombosis in these veins may follow immobilisation, myocardial infarction and conditions when blood is more viscous (e.g. dehydration) or hypercoagulable (e.g. raised platelet count). The venous thrombosis in the legs may be apparent, as in deep calf vein thrombosis, or may be silent. The effect of a pulmonary embolus is sudden occlusion of a pulmonary artery, which leads to reduced blood flow to the affected area of the lung. If the occlusion is in a large vessel then the fall in pulmonary blood flow is large and leads to a large fall in cardiac output with hypotension, as well as decreased lung function causing dyspnoea and cyanosis.

The clinical features of pulmonary embolism depend on the size of the embolus and the size of the vessel it occludes. *Massive pulmonary embolism* follows occlusion of a major pulmonary vessel by a large thrombus. The onset is abrupt and is often manifest by collapse with severe central chest pain, central cyanosis, dyspnoea, hypotension and impaired consciousness. There may be cough with bloodstained sputum and the patient may die immediately or within the first hour. Acute right heart failure may follow and the features are those of cardiogenic shock. Pain is sometimes absent. The diagnosis is difficult and classical X-ray and ECG findings of smaller embolism (see below) may or may not be present. Frequently the diagnosis is inferred from the clinical picture when it occurs in a patient at risk from pulmonary embolism. Lung scans and pulmonary arteriography are helpful if available. Echocardiography is also often helpful and tends to be underused.

Moderate pulmonary embolism occurs when the occluded artery is smaller. The onset is usually abrupt and localised pleuritic chest pain, cough and haemoptysis and moderate dyspnoea are the commonest manifestations. There may be features of deep calf vein thrombosis and the patient may be febrile. Occasionally fever or dyspnoea are the only manifestations. There may be no abnormal signs but a pleural rub and a bloodstained pleural effusion can occur. The chest X-ray may be normal or a wedge-shaped peripheral opacity may be present. In most cases the ECG is normal but suggestive changes are an S wave in lead I, a Q wave and an inverted T wave in lead III. An incomplete right bundle block or right ventricular strain may be present. As in massive pulmonary embolus treatment may need to be commenced on the basis of a suggestive clinical picture.

Valvular and congenital heart disease

These usually occur in younger patients, who often give a history of recognised heart disease. In most cases murmurs can be heard in the heart and in congenital heart disease cyanosis may be present in the absence of heart failure. The correct diagnosis is usually possible by echocardiography with Doppler but in some difficult cases cardiac catheterisation is the only way for proper diagnosis.

Heart muscle disease

This may be acute, as in myocarditis and peripartum cardiomyopathy, or chronic. Chronic heart muscle disease may be due to recognised causes such as heavy alcohol intake, and iron overload in chronic haemolytic anaemias, or be a cardiomyopathy of unknown origin (p. 70). Generally non-ischaemic heart muscle disease is not associated with significant chest pain or valvular damage but there may be cardiac murmurs. One finds the typical symptoms and signs of right- and/or left-sided failure (Table 3.1). The heart is usually enlarged on chest X-ray and the ECG changes are not specific. Arrhythmias and embolism occur commonly in many diseases of the heart muscle. Heart muscle disease may be difficult to distinguish clinically from other causes of heart failure. Again, echocardiography usually provides the diagnosis. Alternatively, cardiac function can be visualised and assessed by isotope scanning. Cardiac catheterisation with left ventriculography is a very invasive technique and the only advantage of this method is the possibility of biopsy, which sometimes influences treatment.

Non-cardiac problems

Hypertension is a major cause of heart failure in many developing countries. Prolonged elevation of the blood pressure causes enlargement and strain of the left side of the heart and left-sided heart failure ultimately occurs. Patients may present with acute pulmonary oedema. Generally the patient is known to have hypertension and the diagnosis is supported if the patient has elevated blood pressure. However, acute pulmonary oedema owing to other disorders may cause a transient rise in blood pressure and hypertensive heart failure should be diagnosed with caution unless there is also an enlarged left ventricle and changes of hypertension in the fundi, proteinuria and left ventricular hypertrophy with strain on ECG.

Lung diseases are another common cause of heart failure. They may be acute, e.g. pulmonary infarction (p. 50) and pneumonia (p. 135), or chronic as in emphysema. Heart failure due to lung disease is right-sided and is associated with right heart strain and in chronic disease with right ventricular enlargement. Evidence of these developments is often present on ECG, which together with features of lung disease such as cyanosis, signs of right heart failure and the absence of primary heart disease establishes the diagnosis.

Fluid overload, another non-cardiac cause of heart failure, generally affects both sides of the heart but the most serious consequence is acute pulmonary oedema, which has already been described. Engorgement of the neck veins, elevation of the central venous pressure and scanty fine basal crepitations precede acute pulmonary oedema and are an indication to stop infusion or reduce the infusion rate.

Severe anaemia and thyrotoxicosis (particularly if there is an associated arrhythmia) can cause heart failure. Pregnancy is associated with an increase in blood volume and cardiac output but does not normally precipitate heart failure unless there is underlying heart disease. However in pregnancy there may be some engorgement of the neck veins and peripheral oedema, which may be difficult to distinguish from mild heart failure.

Aortic dissection

Dissection of the aorta is a tear in the inner layer of the aortic wall (intima), and blood leaking from this tear can make its way in a split of the middle layer of the aortic wall (media). Rupture can occur back into the aorta or through the adventitia with sudden death by bleeding. The aortic dissection is characterised by sudden severe tearing chest pain, which often radiates to the back, abdomen or legs and there may be peripheral vascular collapse. Sometimes aortic dissection causes acute aortic incompetence and the newly formed channel can actually obliterate part of the aorta itself or its branches, which explains why there are sometimes neurological features or absent peripheral pulses. The chest X-ray may show a broadened mediastinum. Echocardiography sometimes gives the diagnosis but aortography is necessary for ultimate proof.

Cardiogenic shock

When right- or left-sided heart failure is so severe that cardiac output cannot maintain the capillary circulation to the tissues cardiogenic shock is present. It is recognised by the combination of the features of right- or left-sided heart failure (Table 3.1) with features of shock (Table 2.1). The features which help to distinguish hypovolaemic shock from cardiogenic shock are shown in Table 2.3. A fluid challenge is sometimes advocated as a therapeutic trial, but this is dangerous and will be detrimental in cardiogenic shock. It should not be considered unless it is certain that left ventricular failure is absent. In highly specialised centres, cardiac catheterisation with a Swan–Ganz catheter enables the two conditions to be distinguished.

Management of left heart failure

The objectives of management in heart failure are:
1. to rectify primary or aggravating causes whenever possible;
2. to reduce the imbalance between venous return and cardiac output:
   (a) by reducing the volume of blood in the venous side of the circulation;
   (b) by reducing the resistance against which the heart has to pump;
   (c) sometimes by an increase in the contractility of the heart.

In this section the general management of left heart failure is discussed before the more difficult specific problems of acute pulmonary oedema, resistant heart failure and cardiogenic shock.

The general management of left-sided cardiac failure is summarised in Figure 3.3. Arrhythmias (p. 56) and pericardial tamponade (p. 48) need to be recognised and corrected urgently. In critically ill patients once these are excluded the immediate crisis should be controlled before making further efforts to determine the primary cause.

After putting the patient to bed (propped up) and giving oxygen, diuretics are administered. They reduce the venous congestion and overfilling of the atrium (or atria and ventricles) thereby increasing the efficiency of the heart as a pump. Furosemide (p. 446) is a rapidly effective diuretic which can be given orally or parenterally and in an adult with moderately severe heart failure. 40 mg or 80 mg is given initially and the maintenance dose is judged according to the initial response. In critical situations and if the response to diuretics is inadequate then oral or parenteral digoxin (p. 444) may be added, but care should be taken particularly if the patient has impaired renal function and digoxin levels cannot be measured. The initial dose in a patient already taking digoxin is between 0.125 mg and 0.25 mg. In these patients intravenous digoxin is best avoided and digoxin toxicity should be excluded as a factor in their cardiac failure. In an adult patient who had not been taking digoxin recently the loading dose is 1.5 mg given over 24 to 36 h (p. 444).

Maintenance therapy with both drugs is usually necessary and aggravating factors such as chest infections, hypertension and anaemia will need to be corrected. Early measurement of haemoglobin, electrolytes

Cardiovascular disease 53

```
                        ┌─────────────────────────┐
                        │ Acute ventricular failure│
                        └─────────────────────────┘
Isolated right ventricular failure         Left ventricular failure
                    ↘                    ↙
                   Exclude specific treatable causes
```

Pericardial tamponade — Arrhythmias
Pulmonary embolism   Valvular lesions esp. with endocarditis
                         Severe hypertension
                         Aortic dissection

Observe
N.B. Diuretics are not indicated

Mild / Severe

- Mild: Furosemide 40 mg
- Severe:
  - Sit patient up
  - Give oxygen by mask
  - Furosemide 80 mg i.v.
  - Morphine 10 mg i.v.
  - Nitrates sub-lingually

If no response consider:
- Nitrates i.v.
- Sodium nitroprusside
- Hydralazine
- Captopril

If no response
↓
Mechanical ventilation → Not available
↓
Leg tourniquets
Venesection
Dobutamine

No shock normal B.P.

Shock hypotension

Plasma expanders (raise CVP to 15–20 cm)
↓
If no response
↓
Dopamine or dobutamine or beta agonists are an alternative

Dopamine or dobutamine
↓
If there is a response i.e. BP rises
↓
Diuretics
Nitrates   } can be added as necessary
Nitroprusside
Captopril

┌──────────────────────────┐
│ Chronic ventricular failure │
└──────────────────────────┘

Isolated right ventricular failure   Left ventricular failure
            ↘ Treat underlying cause if possible ↙

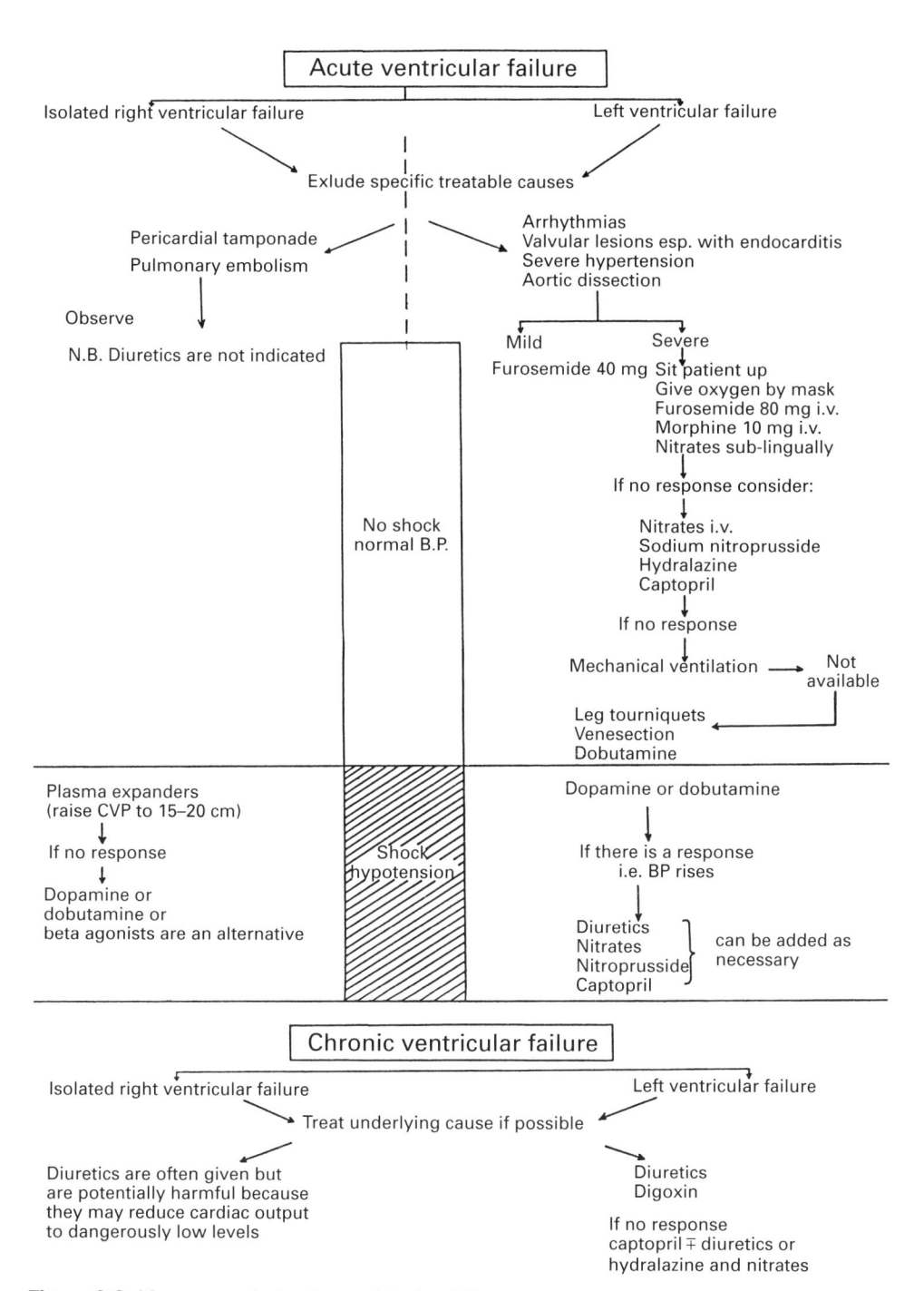

Diuretics are often given but   Diuretics
are potentially harmful because   Digoxin
they may reduce cardiac output
to dangerously low levels   If no response
                                       captopril ∓ diuretics or
                                       hydralazine and nitrates

Figure 3.3 Management plan for ventricular failure.

and blood urea is advisable if possible and any abnormality should be corrected. Intravenous fluids should be given with extreme caution in cardiac failure.

Acute pulmonary oedema

The management of acute pulmonary oedema due to heart failure or pulmonary venous congestion differs in some respects from that due to other causes and the differentiation has already been described. All patients should be sat up and given oxygen by face mask. In acute left ventricular failure intravenous furosemide 80 mg and intravenous morphine 10–15 mg are given immediately (a few doctors give simultaneous digoxin 0.5 mg by slow intravenous injection to patients who have not been taking digoxin). If the patient does not improve within the next half to one hour then furosemide can be repeated. At this stage nitrates (e.g. isosorbide dinitrate 5–10 mg sublingually or by intravenous infusion) can be tried. If not successful mechanical ventilation should be considered, especially in severely dyspnoeic or cyanosed patients. If ventilation is not available then venesection of one or two units of blood may give immediate relief but is contraindicated in the presence of anaemia. Alternatively, 'medical venesection' can be very helpful in an emergency. It is done by occluding venous return from the lower, and, if severe, the upper limbs by applying sphygmomanometer cuffs inflated to a pressure of 20 mmHg below the arterial pressure. If these measures fail then those described for resistant heart failure can be tried.

In patients with acute pulmonary oedema from causes other than cardiac failure (and if the diagnosis is in doubt cardiac catheterisation may help) morphine should be avoided because of the risk of respiratory depression. These patients are more likely to need mechanical ventilation, which should be commenced early. Diuretics are sometimes helpful and are usually tried. Dehydration should be avoided. Patients with pulmonary oedema are at increased risk of secondary pneumonia. Prophylactic antibiotics do not reduce this risk but at the first indication of an infection antibiotics are indicated.

Resistant left-sided cardiac failure

Indications that a patient is responding to treatment include a decrease in dyspnoea, improved pulse and blood pressure and improvement in the urine output. If these developments do not occur within a few hours of starting treatment then resistant cardiac failure may be present and additional measures are probably necessary. Failure to improve may be due to persistence of one or more precipitating factors (e.g. an arrhythmia) or to electrolyte or pH abnormalities. These should be corrected. Prompt correction of anaemia is seldom possible in severe cardiac failure because of the increase in venous return with blood transfusion. However, if anaemia is severe a very slow infusion of packed red cells should be considered with diuretic cover. If these measures are not required or fail to lead to improvement then additional measures may be considered. Aggressive treatment of patients with resistant heart failure or cardiogenic shock should be considered only if the underlying cause is reversible or if there is a reversible aggravating factor, in which case the prognosis for recovery may be good.

1. A further reduction of the volume of blood in the venous circulation can be beneficial by reducing atrial overfilling (preload). This can be achieved through drugs that dilate the veins, notably nitrates, sodium nitroprusside and captopril. Note the dual action of captopril and sodium nitroprusside in cardiac failure. See Figure 3.4.

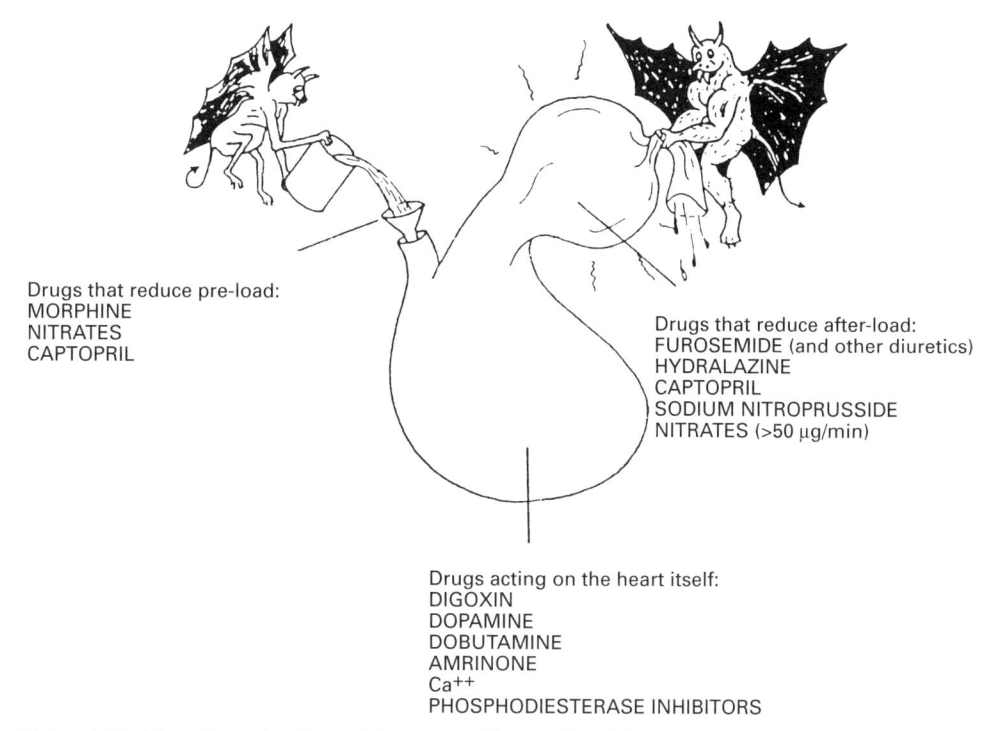

Drugs that reduce pre-load:
MORPHINE
NITRATES
CAPTOPRIL

Drugs that reduce after-load:
FUROSEMIDE (and other diuretics)
HYDRALAZINE
CAPTOPRIL
SODIUM NITROPRUSSIDE
NITRATES (>50 µg/min)

Drugs acting on the heart itself:
DIGOXIN
DOPAMINE
DOBUTAMINE
AMRINONE
Ca^{++}
PHOSPHODIESTERASE INHIBITORS

Figure 3.4 The sites of action of drugs used in cardiac failure.

2. Arteriolar resistance (after load) is the pressure against which the heart has to pump and may be reduced by giving arteriolar dilators such as hydralazine (p. 447), captopril or sodium nitroprusside. In addition this results in improved tissue perfusion and therefore reduced cellular hypoxia. See Figure 3.4.
3. In some cases the heart muscle can be stimulated to greater contraction by the use of dopamine or dobutamine (p. 444) by careful intravenous infusion. If these are not available then adrenaline (p. 439) or isoprenaline (p. 448) are possible alternatives but their use is associated with a greater risk of adverse effects. See Figure 3.4.
4. In selected centres mechanical measures such as the aortic balloon pump may be available. Centres with these facilities are usually also equipped to undertake cardiac surgery and may be able to help patients with serious structural lesions. Such centres are infrequent in developing countries but if available the opinion of a cardiologist should be obtained before transferring problem patients.

Management of right heart failure

Right heart failure can arise in three ways:
1. as a consequence of left heart failure;
2. as isolated right heart failure;
3. as mixed right and left heart failure.

Treatment of right heart failure consequent on left heart failure consists essentially of the management of left heart failure, which is the primary cause. This had been described above and no further discussion is necessary.

The best example of isolated right heart failure is that due to right ventricular infarction and the primary aim of treatment is to maximise right ventricular output. Because of the failure of the pump induced by the infarction the *right* ventricle is not able to maintain its output. The consequence of this is that the left ventricle gets *too little* blood and is often *underfilled*. This leads to a low cardiac output, which needs to be corrected by the administration of fluid. Saline or colloid solutions are given until there is an adequate left atrial filling pressure or the blood pressure improves. This then is a paradoxical situation in which one finds a high jugulo-venous pressure (JVP) caused by the right ventricular failure and yet fluid should be administered. The often-present reflex, 'high JVP means diuretics', is *not* indicated and may be detrimental, for it will increase shock. Do not give diuretics blindly unless isolated right ventricular failure has been excluded; clinically it can be suspected if there is an elevated JVP and hepatomegaly *but without* signs of pulmonary oedema or a third heart sound. If there is no improvement with a fluid load then myocardial stimulators such as dopamine or dobutamine can be given by infusion (p. 444). If there is still no improvement one should try and reduce pulmonary vascular resistance with oxygen, vasodilators (e.g. hydralazine) and beta-2-agonists (e.g. salbutamol). The results of these treatments are unpredictable and haemodynamic monitoring with a Swan–Ganz catheter helps decision making in this difficult situation.

Specific problems

Arrhythmias

Definition

Abnormal heart rhythm is known as arrhythmia and it may be manifest by an abnormal rate and/or irregularity of the

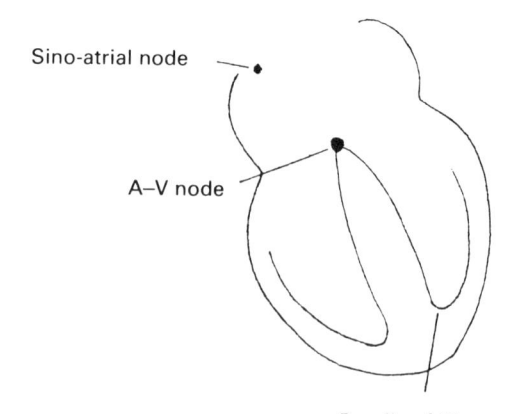

Figure 3.5 The conduction pathways in the normal heart.

heart beat. Normally the heart beats regularly and in adults the rate ranges between 60 and 100 beats per minute (sinus rhythm), increasing with exertion and anxiety. In the absence of heart disease the rate may rise to as much as 140/min in for example fever, anaemia and hypovolaemia and may be as low as 40/min in well-trained athletes or in disease such as terminal hypoxia or raised intracranial pressure.

Normal heart rate and rhythm depend on the the conducting tissue of the heart (Figure 3.5). Impulses generated in the sino-atrial (SA) node pass to the atria and then through the atrio-ventricular (AV) node to the ventricles.

Damage to the conducting fibres can lead to any arrhythmia and may be caused by ischaemia as in myocardial infarction, by inflammation as in myocarditis, by scarring and fibrosis as in cardiomyopathies and by stretching or hypertrophy of heart muscle as may occur in valvular and hypertensive heart disease and in cardiomyopathies. Arrhythmias may also arise from hypoxia and metabolic abnormalities.

Arrhythmias originate in the atria or the ventricles and may cause abnormal heart rate with or without an irregular rhythm. They can be classified according to where

Table 3.3 Clinical diagnosis of arrhythmias according to heart rate and rhythm with or without shock

In asystole or ventricular fibrillation the patient will be unconscious.

Pulse	Arrhythmia	Shock present
Slow and regular[1]	Atrioventricular block	Sometimes
Fast and regular[2]	Supraventricular tachycardia	Absent (usually)
	Ventricular tachycardia	Present (usually)
Irregular	Atrial ectopic beats	Absent
	Atrial fibrillation	Seldom
	Ventricular ectopics	Seldom
None palpable	Asystole	Circulatory arrest
	Ventricular fibrillation	Circulatory arrest

Slow = <50 beats per minute. Fast = >150 beats per minute.
1 Non-cardiac causes include drugs, terminal hypoxia and intracranial hypertension.
2 Non-cardiac causes include fever, hypovolaemia, respiratory failure, anaemia and anxiety.

they arise in the heart (supraventricular or ventricular), whether they are fast (tachyarrhythmia) or slow (bradyarrhythmia) and whether they are regular or irregular. Dangerous arrhythmias may need to be recognised clinically to allow them to be corrected quickly.

Recognition

A heart rate of less than 50/min or more than 150/min or an irregular heart beat suggests an arrhythmia. Sometimes not every heart beat is felt at the wrist pulse and it is important to listen to the heart and count the actual heart rate. The clinical features which suggest a dangerous arrhythmia are:

1. the patient is in shock;
2. intermittent loss of consciousness;
3. cardiac failure.

Patients with any of these features require urgent management. Even in the absence of these features a dangerous arrhythmia may aggravate cardiac failure and if possible should be corrected promptly in patients in cardiac failure.

Clinical recognition of the type of arrhythmia

The type of arrhythmia is often suggested by the rate and rhythm of the heart beat and by the presence or absence of severe reduction in the cardiac output (Table 3.3) and this may be important for urgent management.

Specific arrhythmias are discussed in relation to the heart rate and rhythm.

Slow regular heart beats

If due to heart disease the problem is of *complete atrioventricular (AV) block* or a *sick sinus syndrome*. Either of these conditions can be suspected if the pulse rate does not increase with exercise, particularly if there are signs of shock. The main differential diagnosis is bradycardia from drugs, particularly beta-blockers (p. 453) and this will usually be apparent from the history.

Fast regular heart beats

If due to an arrhythmia the problem is of supraventricular or ventricular tachycardia. Differentiation from sinus tachycardia is necessary, but in general an arrhythmia is likely to be present if there is no cause for a sinus tachycardia and the heart rate is above 150/min, though it may occasionally be present at rates between 120 and 150/min. If there are associated features of shock the diagnosis is usually *ventricular tachycardia*, which will require urgent correction. Faster rates (>200/min) usually occur in supraventricular tachycardia, which is seldom associated with shock and does not require such urgent correction except in the infrequent case associated with shock.

Irregular heart beats

These are always due to arrhythmia but they are often not dangerous ones. The commonest causes of an irregular heart are *atrial fibrillation* and *ectopic* or *premature* beats. In both these conditions the heart may be fast or normal but is virtually never too slow.

In atrial fibrillation the AV node is being bombarded with impulses from the atria and only some impulses are able to provoke a ventricular beat. The volume of the pulse beat varies and some are too weak to be felt at the wrist. This leads to a pulse apex deficit, which means that the heart rate by auscultation is faster than the rate judged by counting the pulse.

Premature beats occur when the impulse stimulates the ventricle earlier than usual. Following this there is a longer-than-normal pause before the next beat; this pause may not be detectable clinically if the heart is fast or there are many premature beats. Premature beats may arise from the atria or the ventricles and an ECG is needed to tell the difference.

Clinical distinction between premature beats and atrial fibrillation depends largely on recognising the pattern of irregularity. If there are runs of regular beats and then an irregular beat, the problem is of premature beats. In contrast, complete irregularity with no periods of regular rhythm is due to atrial fibrillation. However, in patients with atrial fibrillation who are controlled on digoxin the distinction may be impossible without an ECG.

Absent central pulses

Absence of the carotid and femoral pulses indicates a dying or dead heart and this is clinically recognised as a cardiac arrest (p. 396). It may be due to the heart stopping (asystole) or to ventricular fibrillation. In ventricular fibrillation the ventricles do not contract effectively and there is no cardiac output. The distinction between asystole and ventricular fibrillation requires an ECG but initial resuscitation (p. 396) is the same for both conditions.

ECG recognition of arrhythmias

The ECG indicates the electrical activity of the heart by the shape, direction and timing of the recorded waves. These waves are identified by letters (Figure 3.6). The P wave represents contraction of the atria and the QRS wave represents contraction of the ventricles. The T wave indicates recovery of the ventricles ready for the next beat.

The paper recording the ECG runs at a fixed rate (usually 25 mm/s); each small square represents 1 mm (or 0.04 of a second) and the large squares 5 mm or 0.2 of a second. This allows the rate of the regular heart to be calculated by counting the number of small squares between two complexes (using identical points in both complexes) and dividing the answer into 1500. It also allows the time between each complex to be calculated. To recognise an arrhythmia on ECG you need to note:
1. the heart rate and regularity;
2. the presence or absence of P waves;
3. the relationship of the P waves to the QRS waves;
4. the shape of the QRS waves.

Figure 3.6 is of a normal ECG and Figures 3.7 to 3.10 show different arrhythmias according to the rate and regularity of the heart.

Management

Not all arrhythmias need treatment and the decision to treat them is made after considering the risks of treatment against the

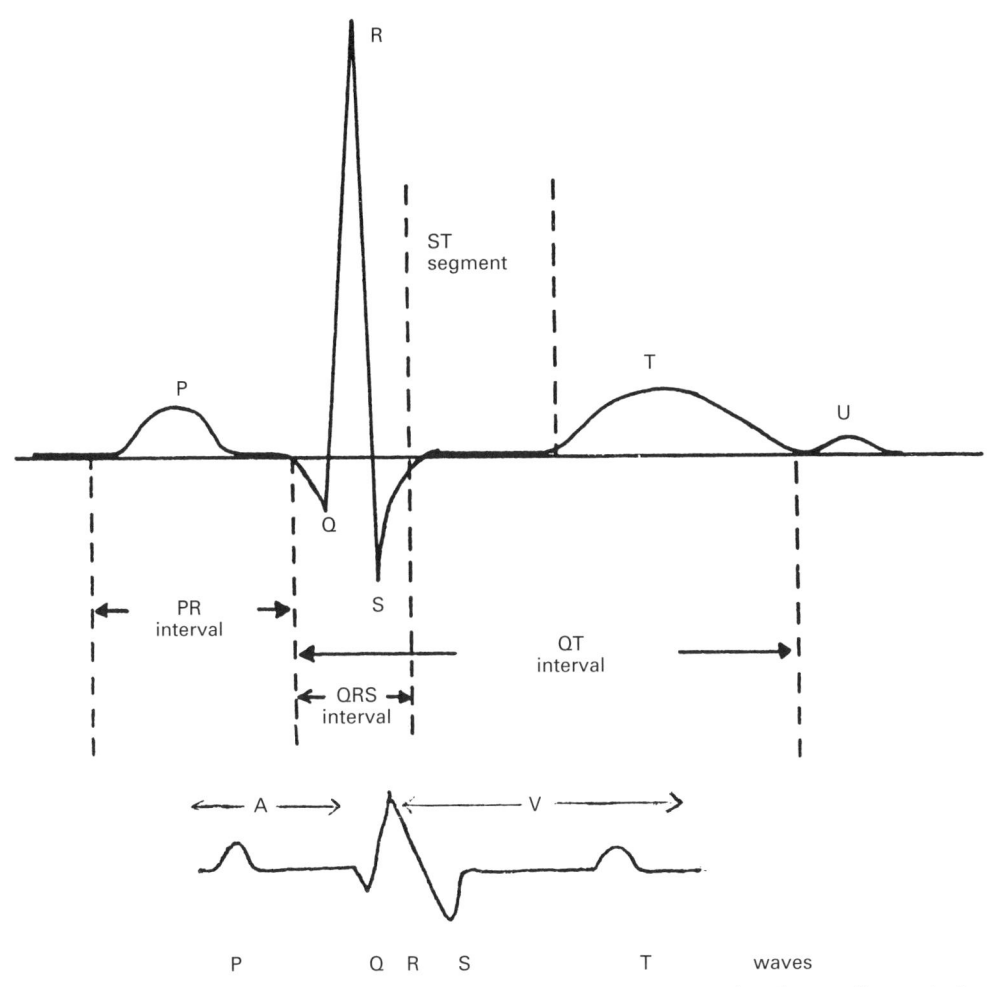

Figure 3.6 The normal ECG showing the electrical waves representing the cardiac cycle in relation to the carotid pulse. (*Note:* A = contraction of the atria and filling of the ventricles; V = contraction of the ventricles and coincides with the arterial pulse.)

risks of the arrhythmia without treatment. Those causing a significant fall in cardiac output or aggravating heart failure will require treatment. Metabolic abnormalities which may contribute to the arrhythmia (e.g. hypokalaemia, hypoxia and acidosis) should usually be corrected before giving specific anti-arrhythmia treatment. The treatment for arrhythmias may be drugs or an electric current known as d.c. counter-shock or defibrillation (p. 397). Detailed description of the management of arrhythmias in non-critical situations should be obtained from general medical textbooks. In cardiac arrest cardio-pulmonary resuscitation (CPR) takes precedence over any other. Consideration and treatment of any arrhythmia present (usually asystole or ventricular fibrillation) comes later and is described on p. 396. This section is concerned largely with immediate management of dangerous arrhythmias and refers mainly to patients in cardiogenic shock or with critical pulmonary oedema. In these cases

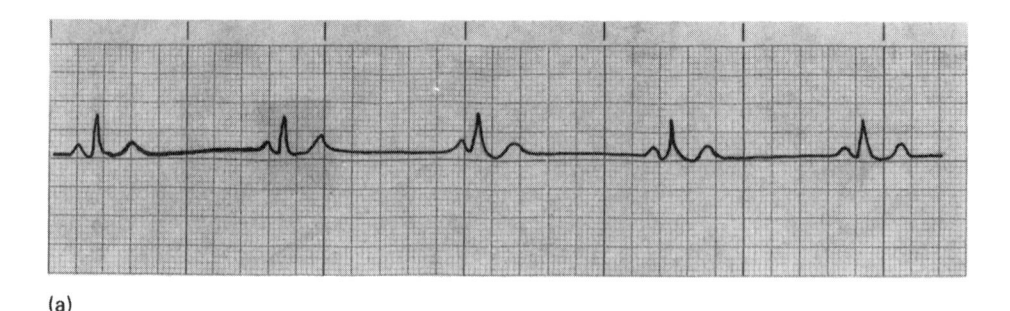

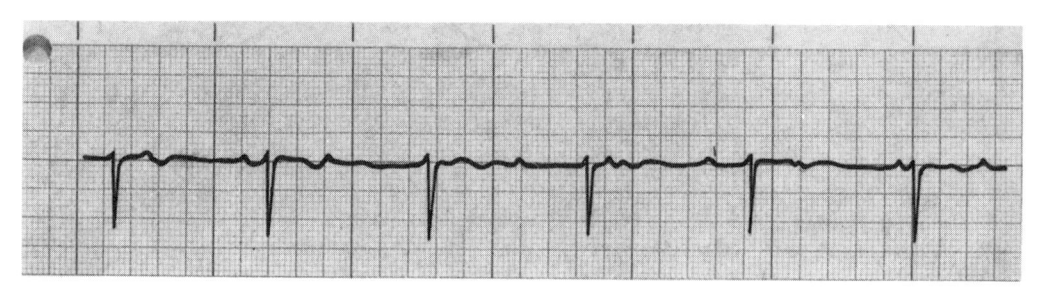

Figure 3.7 The slow regular heart.
(a) Sinus bradycardia. (*Note:* The P wave is regularly followed by a QRS complex.)
(b) Complete AV block. (*Note:* Both P waves and QRS waves are present but are completely independent of each other.)

treatment will often be given according to the clinical diagnosis of the arrhythmia. Table 3.3 (p. 57) identifies the probable diagnosis.

The slow heart

The differential diagnosis is between complete AV block and sinus bradycardia. Adequate ventilation should be confirmed and oxygen given.

Initial treatment is with atropine 0.6 mg i.v. bolus injection, which may be repeated once after a few minutes if there is no response.

If this fails isoprenaline is infused giving 0.5 µg/min (in saline or dextrose 5%) and increasing the dose by 0.5 µg/min every 5 min until there is a satisfactory response or the maximum dose of 5.0 µg/min is being given.

Should these methods fail the only other treatment is to insert a temporary pacemaker if this is available.

The fast regular heart

The differential diagnosis is between supraventricular tachycardia (SVT) and ventricular tachycardia (VT); if the patient is collapsed it is usually VT.

The patient should be given oxygen and if the cardiac output is very low CPR should be commenced.

The objectives of treatment of *ventricular tachycardia* are to convert the patient to sinus rhythm and to maintain them in sinus rhythm.

Cardiovascular disease 61

(a)

(b)

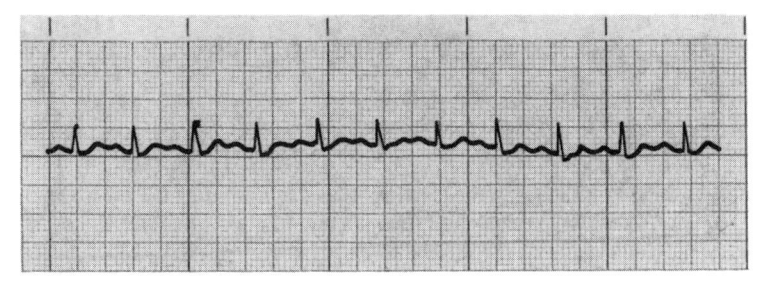

(c)

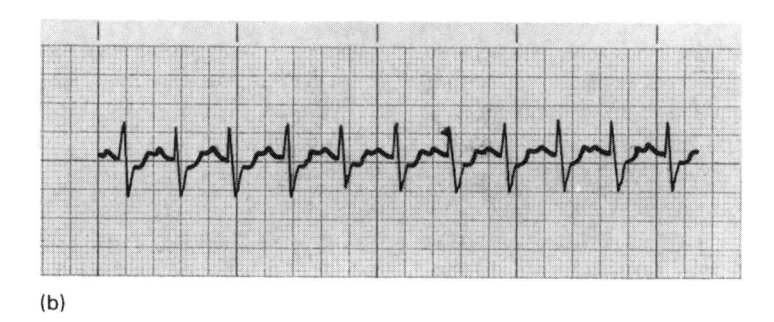

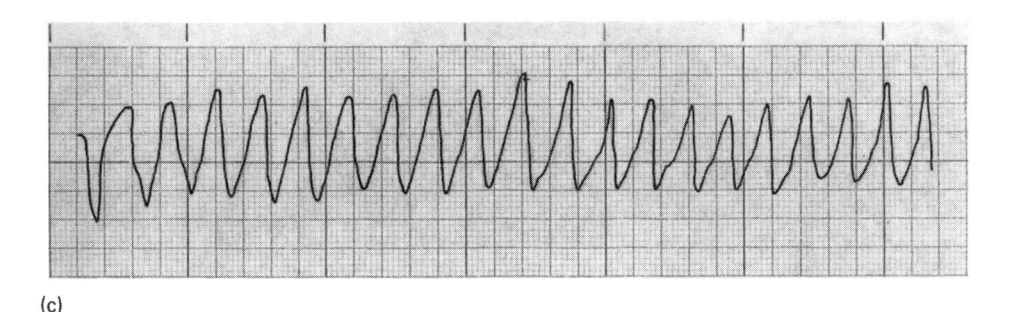

Figure 3.8 The fast regular heart.
(a) Sinus tachycardia.
(*Note:* the P wave is regularly followed by a QRS complex.)
(b) Atrial tachycardia.
(*Note:* 1. The fast atrial rate, which in this case is 160 beats per minute, usually ranges between 160 and 220 beats/minute.
2. The rhythm is usually regular.
3. The shape of the P wave is abnormal, indicating that it does not arise from the SA node.
4. A QRS complex follows each P wave; this is not always the case in patients with block.
5. The ventricular rate is usually the same as the atrial rate.
6. The T wave cannot always be identified separate from the QRS complex.)
(c) Ventricular tachycardia.
(*Note:* 1. The shape of the QRS complex is abnormal.
2. QRS beats are usually more or less regular.
3. Often there is slurring of the ST segment and inversion of T waves.)

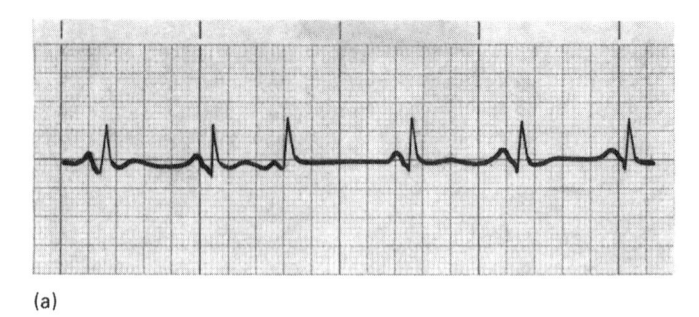

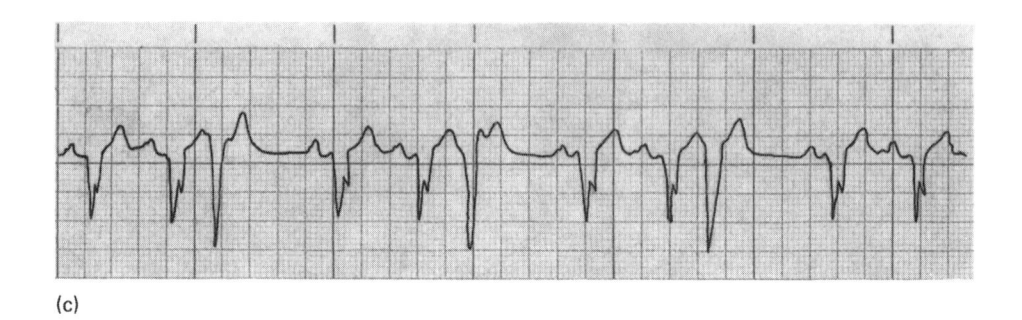

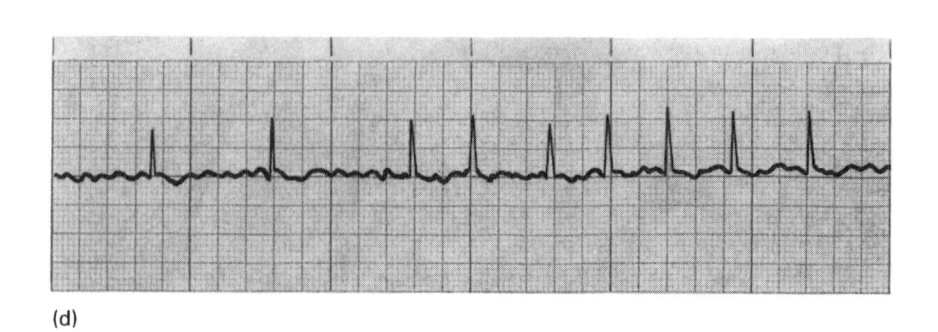

(a)

(b)

(c)

(d)

Cardiovascular disease 63

◀ **Figure 3.9** The irregular heart.
(a) Atrial ectopic beats.
(*Note:* The P wave is sometimes of abnormal shape and comes out of rhythm. The P wave is followed by a normal shaped QRS complex. Atrial ectopic beats are not dangerous.)
(b) Ventricular premature beats.
(*Note:* Runs of normal sinus rhythm with interspersed irregular beats. The irregular beats have no preceding P wave. The QRS complex is of an abnormal shape or is abnormally wide. The QRS complex is followed by an extra long pause.)
(c) Following recent myocardial infarction ventricular premature beats with the following characteristics are generally considered to be a warning of a dangerous ventricular arrhythmia and therefore they should be treated when more than 5 occur in any one minute; variation occurs in the shape of the abnormal QRS complexes, indicating that they arise from a number of different abnormal foci (multifocal); more than 3 occur together; and they occur close to a previous beat (R on T phenomenom).
(d) Atrial fibrillation.
(*Note:* There are no normal P waves and they are replaced by waves which are irregular in rate and in shape. The QRS complex is of normal shape. A QRS complex does not follow every P wave and they are completely irregular.)

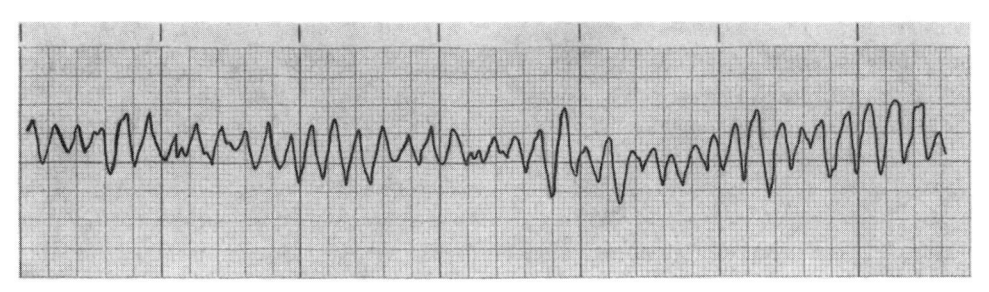

(a)

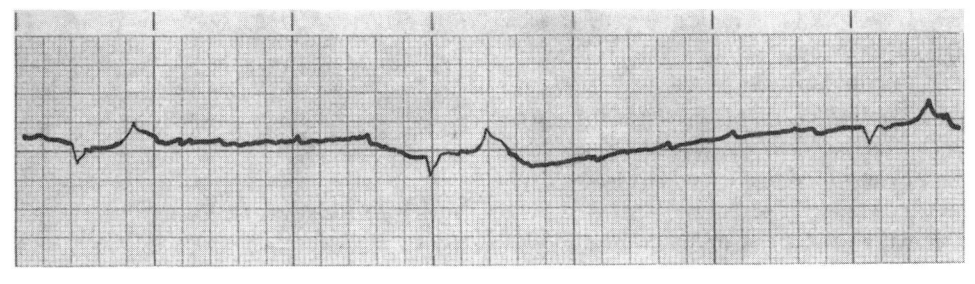

(b)

Figure 3.10 The dying heart.
(a) Ventricular fibrillation.
(*Note:* No P waves are visible. The QRS complexes are irregular in rhythm and of an abnormal shape. This heart is not contracting.)
(b) Agonal rhythm.
(*Note:* The wide slurred abnormal beats. Bradycardia is usually marked. This heart has no effective contraction.)

To convert ventricular tachycardia to sinus rhythm the optimum treatment is defibrillation commencing with 200 joules and then at 300 until a maximum shock of 400 joules is administered or sinus rhythm is restored. It is common to give sedation or light general anaesthesia for cardioversion.

If the arrhythmia persists then electrolyte or metabolic imbalance and hypoxia should be suspected. Defibrillation should be tried again after any abnormalities are corrected.

Once sinus rhythm has been re-established, maintenance therapy is given with a bolus injection of lidocaine 100 mg followed by infusion of lidocaine at 2.0 mg/min. The dose is gradually reduced over the next 48 h. If there is underlying irreversible heart disease and the risk of a recurrence is high then long-term maintenance should be considered and amiodarone, procainamide, quinidine or disopyramide can be used. These drugs can also be used for initial maintenance if lidocaine is unavailable or ineffective.

If defibrillation is not available an attempt can be made to convert ventricular tachycardia to sinus rhythm using drugs. Lidocaine 100 mg i.v. bolus is the drug of first choice and if it fails it can be repeated after a few minutes using 50 or 75 mg. Amiodarone is an alternative treatment.

Urgent treatment of *supraventricular tachycardia* (SVT) is indicated only if the patient is in heart failure or cardiogenic shock or the arrhythmia has been present for a number of hours and cardiac failure is considered likely to develop. However, the methods described below can be tried earlier.

- Carotid sinus massage rarely converts to sinus rhythm but may slow the rate and reveal the underlying rhythm. It is helpful in differentiating it from atrial flutter and fast atrial fibrillation.
- Adenosine – this slows conduction and is especially useful for terminating re-entry SVT of the Wolff–Parkinson–White type. Give 6 mg i.v. rapidly, followed by a saline flush. Further doses of 12 mg may be given at 2-min intervals if there is no response to the first dose. The effects of adenosine last only 10–15 s. It should be avoided in asthma.
- Verapamil, beta-blockers, or other drugs such as amiodarone or flecainide may control the rate or convert to sinus rhythm.
- Verapamil 5–10 mg i.v. slowly over 2 min. A further 5 mg may be given after 10 min if required. This may cause a significant fall in blood pressure. Administration together with beta-blockers may cause severe hypotension and asystole.
- Beta-blockers, e.g. propranolol 1 mg over 1 min repeated if necessary at 2-min intervals (maximum 5 mg), sotalol 100 mg over 10 min repeated 6-hourly if necessary. Esmolol is a relatively cardioselective beta-blocker with a very short duration of action and may be given by intravenous infusion at 50–200 μg/kg/min.
- Digoxin should be avoided – it facilitates conduction through the AV accessory pathway in Wolff–Parkinson–White syndrome and may worsen the tachycardia. Atrial fibrillation in the presence of an accessory pathway may allow very rapid conduction which can degenerate to ventricular fibrillation.

When the patient is in heart failure or cardiogenic shock it is our opinion that d.c. shock is the treatment of choice if it is available. Treatment can be with 50–100 joules initially increasing to 400 joules, which will almost never be necessary. Management with drugs as already described can be used for less alarming situations and this leads to the following:

General Rule **In patients in shock with supraventricular or ventricular tachycardia d.c. shock is the treatment of first choice.**

Cardiovascular disease

The irregular heart

The differential diagnosis is between fast atrial fibrillation and multiple ectopic beats (Table 3.3, p. 57).

Multiple premature ventricular beats

These seldom cause cardiogenic shock unless there is serious underlying heart disease, in which case they should be controlled. Intravenous lidocaine as described for ventricular tachycardia is the drug of choice. If this is not available the alternative drugs used for treatment of ventricular tachycardia can be used.

Atrial fibrillation

In atrial fibrillation (AF) of recent onset restoration of sinus rhythm may be considered but this is not indicated in established atrial fibrillation and can be dangerous as it may cause systemic arterial emboli. The usual objective of treatment of AF is to control the ventricular response rate.

If the patient is critical this will need to be done urgently. Amiodarone (5 mg/kg over 20 min) is the drug of choice. The alternative is digoxin in the same dose as recommended for atrial tachycardia. A smaller dose is used if the patient is already digitalised and maintenance digoxin will usually be necessary. Other alternatives are electroconversion, verapamil (5–10 mg i.v.) or beta-blockers. Here again, if the patient is in shock then defibrillation is the first choice of treatment.

In non-urgent situations digoxin is usually given in AF if the heart rate is consistently greater than 100/min at rest. (The pulse rate may be unreliable because of the pulse apex deficit.) In patients not already taking digoxin the initial dose is 0.5 mg orally and this is repeated twice at between 6- and 12-h intervals. The maintenance dose is between 0.25 and 0.125 mg daily and is judged according to the heart rate.

Pericardial tamponade

Pericardial tamponade arises from a large or rapidly accumulating pericardial effusion. Management of uncomplicated pericardial effusions is described in general medical texts and this discussion is limited to the complication of tamponade. The clinical features and diagnosis have already been described (p. 48).

Urgent pericardial paracentesis is required to reduce the pressure within the pericardial sac and allow proper cardiac filling. This will immediately correct the patient's shock. The method is described on pp. 394–395. The fluid should be analysed to determine the primary cause of the effusion and appropriate management given. The management of cardiac and chest trauma is discussed on pp. 205–210.

Ischaemic heart disease

Definition

Ischaemia of the myocardium follows a fall in blood supply to the myocardium and is usually due to disease of the coronary arteries. Atheroma is less frequent in indigenous Africans than in other races.

The degree of ischaemia relates to myocardial blood supply and to the energy requirements of the heart which are increased by physical exertion. Transient ischaemia may occur with exertion, ceasing if exertion ceases. However, persistent ischaemia with death of part of the myocardium (infarction) may follow occlusion of an artery. The major critical problems related to myocardial ischaemia are myocardial infarction and unstable or rapidly increasing angina (see p. 68), which may lead to myocardial infarction.

Recognition

The classical symptom of myocardial ischaemia is central chest pain that radiates down one or both arms and may also radiate to the jaw and through to the back. It is important to distinguish transient ischaemia from myocardial infarction and this can usually be done from the patient's history. Short-lived episodes of this pain (angina) are due to transient myocardial ischaemia and are relieved by rest and by glyceryl trinitrate. Prolonged pain and exceptionally severe pain not relieved by rest or glyceryl trinitrate is likely to be due to myocardial infarction. Vomiting, heavy sweating, collapse and dyspnoea may also occur in infarction. Anginal pain of increasing frequency or duration is described as unstable angina and may precede myocardial infarction. As many as 30% of myocardial infarctions may occur without pain and these patients may present with cardiac arrhythmias, cardiac failure or unexplained hypotension. There are no diagnostic physical signs of myocardial infarction unless complications (see below) are present and often the physical examination is normal.

The diagnosis of myocardial infarction is primarily clinical and is supported by serial ECG changes (Figure 3.11). It is important to realise that the ECG may be normal within the first few hours of an infarct. Additional evidence of an infarct is elevation of serum AST and CPK, which occurs from about 6 h after the event and persists for about 72 h. Troponins are elevated for 7–10 days. Clinically, myocardial infarction needs to be distinguished from a perforated viscus including the oesophagus, acute pancreatitis, pericarditis, pulmonary infarction and dissecting aneurysm.

In angina, the resting ECG may be normal but on exertion ST depression or T-wave inversion occurs.

(a)

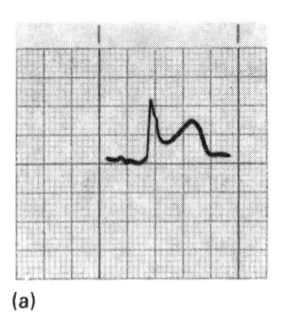

Figure 3.11 (a) Myocardial infarction at 24 h.
(*Note*: Elevated take-off and convex shape of the ST segment.)

(b)

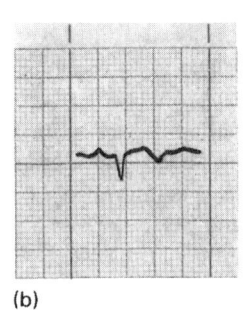

Figure 3.11 (b) Myocardial infarction at about 8 days.
(*Note*: Q wave broader than 1 mm. Symmetrical inversion of the T waves reducing ST elevation.)

(c)

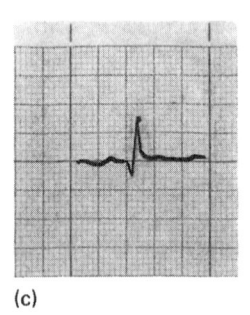

Figure 3.11 (c) Myocardial infarction after a few weeks.
(*Note*: Persistent Q wave. Normal ST segment and T wave.)

PRACTICE POINT
A stress ECG is dangerous if infarction is suspected.

Management

The objectives in management of a myocardial infarct are to minimise the area of myocardial destruction and to prevent complications.

Immediate management

The quicker management is implemented the better is the patient's prognosis. Pain and stress increase the risk to the patient; oxygen helps to minimise ischaemia an i.v. line allows immediate administration of drugs should they be necessary, and cardiac monitoring allows early recognition and treatment of life-threatening arrhythmias. The most critical time following an infarct is the first 48 hours and during this time the patient should be kept at rest.

Establish an i.v. line and give all patients with ECG evidence of myocardial infarction or typical chest pain:
1. aspirin (300 mg chewed),
2. morphine (2.5–5 mg i.v.) and
3. oxygen;
4. nitrates (GTN 600 mg) can also be given if the patient has not taken sildenafil (Viagra) in the last 24 h.

THROMBOLYTIC THERAPY
For those with pain for less than 12 h give thrombolytic agents such as streptokinase. It should be given promptly for:
- <12 h continuous chest pain with ST elevation or presumed new LBBB,
- <6 h pain with qualifying ECG criteria.

The value of giving thrombolytic therapy to patients with chest pain for 12–24 h, is of uncertain value and a matter for clinical judgement.
- Streptokinase 1.5 million units by intravenous infusion over 20–30 min.
- If systolic BP is <80 mmHg then the infusion rate should be halved.
- If systolic BP is <70 mmHg then the infusion should be stoped and restarted at half the previous rate once >70 mmHg.

OR
- Alteplase 15 mg bolus intravenously followed by an infusion of 0.75 mg/kg over 30 min up to 50 mg then 0.5 mg/kg over 60 min up to 35 mg (total dose should not exceed 100 mg).

OR
- Reteplase 10 units bolus i.v. followed by another 10 units 30 min later.

Allegic reactions are common to streptokinase. Anaphylactic shock is rare but delayed hypersensitivity reactions may also occur. Use promethazine 25 mg and/or hydrocortisone 100 mg for mild to moderate reactions. Use adrenaline 1 ml of 1 in 10 000 over 5 min if there is a severe reaction.

Aboriginals may have raised titres of anti-streptokinase antibodies so other thrombolytic agents may be more effective in some developing-world populations with high antibody titres.

MAJOR CONTRAINDICATIONS:
Active internal bleeding; recent surgery within 2 weeks or at a non-compressible site within 6 weeks; prolonged cardiopulmonary resuscitation with rib fractures; ischaemic stroke or neurosurgery within 6 months.

RELATIVE CONTRAINDICATIONS:
Peptic ulcer disease within last 3 months especially with bleeding unless healing documented by endoscopy; diabetic retinopathy; pregnancy.

The selection of cases for urgent angioplasty or coronary artery bypass surgery is beyond the scope of this book. If these facilities are not available we do not recommend transfer unless there is full coronary and intensive care support during the transfer.

The prophylactic use of anti-arrhythmic drugs is not usually recommended except for beta-blockers, which will reduce the risk of ventricular arrhythmias and may reduce the area of infarction. However they will aggravate cardiac failure and should not be used if there is a risk of AV block or if there is hypotension. Atenolol can be given intravenously (1 mg/min until the pulse rate is less than 60 min or up to a maximum of 10 mg) and if this is not available oral propranolol 80 mg twice daily is a reasonable alternative. (See A to Z of Drugs (p. 453) for contraindications and complications.)

The usual precautions should be taken to maintain fluid and electrolyte balance and measures to prevent deep vein thrombosis (p. 250).

Later management

After 48 h and providing there are no complications the patient should commence ambulation and discharge from hospital can be considered at 7–10 days. The patient should be encouraged to return gradually to normal activities. Maintenance therapy with beta-blockers reduces the risk of reinfarction and sudden death. Aspirin 150 mg daily or 300 mg on alternate days will likely prove to be beneficial in the future.

Complications

The major common complications and their management are shown in Table 3.4. Less common complications include cardiac rupture, ventricular aneurysm, mitral valve incompetence and non-infective pericarditis.

Unstable angina

Unstable angina (also known as crescendo or pre-infarction angina) is myocardial ischaemia, which is more persistent than stable angina and which may lead to myocardial infarction.

Recognition

Unstable angina can be distinguished from stable angina because episodes of pain are

Table 3.4 Common complications of myocardial infarction

Complication	Management
Cardiac failure	Diuretic therapy (p. 448). Digoxin should generally be avoided except in atrial fibrillation with a rapid ventricular response.
Cardiogenic shock	Treat as outlined on p. 52, but the prognosis is poor.
Arrhythmias	Sinus bradycardia, AV block, premature ventricular beats, ventricular tachycardia and fibrillation are the dangerous arrhythmias. Treatment is described on pp. 60–65.
Thrombo-embolic	Calf vein thrombosis and pulmonary infarction may occur 1 to 2 weeks later. Treatment is with anticoagulants and supportive measures (p. 69).

of longer duration (up to 45 min), they are often not relieved by rest or trinitrates and they usually occur spontaneously without being precipitated by, for example, exertion. It may be impossible to distinguish from myocardial infarction without ECG.

Management

The objective of management is to prevent myocardial infarction. Immediate management should include oxygen (6 1/min) by face mask and morphine for relief of pain. Treatment with a trinitrate preparation (glyceryl trinitrate ointment 1 to 2 inches (2.5–5 cm) applied 4-hourly, or isosorbide 10 mg to 20 mg three times daily) and a beta-blocker such as propranolol 80 mg twice daily and aspirin 150 mg daily should be commenced. Calcium entry blockers (e.g. nifedipine) are often administered. The patient should be kept in bed with an intravenous line in place and if possible cardiac monitoring should be done. Investigations to exclude myocardial infarction are performed (p. 65). As the symptoms improve activity can be gradually increased and maintenance therapy commenced as described in medical texts. Patients may benefit from referral for coronary angiography and consideration for coronary artery bypass surgery.

Pulmonary embolism

The effect of occlusion of a pulmonary artery by thrombus has already been described (p. 50), together with how you would establish the diagnosis. The discussion here is limited to management of pulmonary embolism. In massive pulmonary embolism morphine may be needed to control pain and in all cases oxygen should be given by face mask, cardiac arrhythmias controlled and anticoagulants commenced. Intravenous heparin 10 000 units is given as a bolus injection and followed by a continuous heparin infusion of 1000 units every hour. Alternatively, intermittent i.v. heparin 5000 units 4-hourly can be given. The heparin dose is adjusted according to the whole-blood clotting time, which should be measured every 4 h and kept at between two and three times normal. It can also be monitored using the partial thromboplastin time. Oral anticoagulants (warfarin) are commenced simultaneously, which enables heparin to be discontinued after 72 h and anticoagulation is then controlled to produce a prothrombin time which should be two to three times normal values.

It is important to emphasise that the elevated JVP in this condition should not be treated with diuretics as a high venous pressure is needed to increase right ventricular output; the rationale for this has already been explained under isolated right-sided heart failure (p. 47).

Treatment of smaller pulmonary emboli requires anticoagulation as described above and control of symptoms, which may include use of oxygen and analgesics.

If available, thrombolytic therapy can be used in massive and moderate pulmonary embolism providing the diagnosis is certain. Following 125 mg methyl prednisolone i.v., streptokinase 600 000 units in 100 ml 0.9% saline is infused intravenously over 30 min followed by 100 000 units/h for 6 h. Haemorrhage is the most important side effect of thrombolytic therapy and patients in whom it should not be used are mentioned on p. 67.

Prevention

Patients at risk of pulmonary embolism have been described (p. 50). Prevention includes regular leg movements and in unconscious patients regular turning. Leg exercises should be continued during bed rest. Subcutaneous heparin (5000 units three times daily) has been used successfully in prevention of deep vein thrombosis following major operations, e.g. pelvic surgery. Special compression stockings are used in some centres.

Valvular and congenital heart disease

Detailed description of these conditions is beyond the scope of this book. The presence of most of them is usually known to the patient (history taking is important) and ideally should have been treated surgically before reaching a critical condition. If surgery is impossible most of these conditions will progress to end-stage medically intractable disease. However, an arrhythmia may sometimes provoke acute deterioration (e.g. atrial fibrillation in mitral valve stenosis) and this should be treated appropriately.

A rapid and unexpected onset may occur in mitral and aortic regurgitation.

Acute mitral regurgitation

This is usually caused by:
1. necrosis of a papillary muscle following myocardial infarction;
2. bacterial endocarditis with cusp perforation or tear.

Recognition is usually possible on clinical grounds: the apex beat is hyperdynamic, there is a pan-systolic blowing murmur at the apex radiating to the left axilla, a third heart sound and further signs of left ventricular failure. In endocarditis there is usually fever and sometimes splinter haemorrhages, microscopic haematuria, splenomegaly and systemic embolism. Echocardiography and sometimes cardiac catheterisation are necessary for definitive diagnosis.

If acute mitral regurgitation is severe the patient does not usually survive without cardiac surgery. Pending operation, medical treatment of acute left ventricular failure (p. 52) should be instituted. In this condition the best drugs are those which are effective in reducing afterload (e.g. hydralazine, captopril and sodium nitroprusside), as they diminish the regurgitation.

If endocarditis is present or suspected blood cultures will direct the choice of antibiotic, but after collecting blood for culture, treatment can be started with crystalline penicillin 4 megaunits 6-hourly by intravenous injection or infusion pending blood culture results. If cardiac failure complicates bacterial endocarditis surgery is often the only solution.

Aortic valve regurgitation

This is caused by:
1. infective endocarditis;
2. acute dissection of the aorta (p. 51).

Again, recognition is usually easy on clinical grounds: there is a collapsing pulse and wide pulse pressure (high systolic and low diastolic pressure), a hyperdynamic left ventricular impulse and a high-pitched blowing early diastolic decrescendo murmur along the sternum. Echocardiography will usually confirm the diagnosis but sometimes cardiac catheterisation is necessary and in the case of aortic dissection aortography is necessary.

Treatment is surgical in cases with acute aortic valve regurgitation. Pending operation treatment requires control of left ventricular failure and particularly afterload reduction (e.g. sodium nitroprusside or other vasodilator). Endocarditis should be treated with appropriate antibiotics as described above.

Heart muscle disease

The most common heart muscle diseases that lead to acute cardiac failure are acute myocarditis, peripartum cardiomyopathy and acute rheumatic fever with pancarditis. Acute rheumatic fever occurs mostly in children and is the most important *acute* cardiac disease in children. Acute myocarditis may be caused by infections, drugs and systemic diseases, but commonly no clear cause is found.

Recognition

Since the myocardial muscle is damaged contractility is reduced and left and right heart failure will develop with the corresponding symptoms and signs (p. 46). The diagnosis is often made by exclusion but echocardiography can confirm it.

Management

The treatment is that of left and/or right ventricular failure. As mentioned above, treatment may be very difficult because of extensive myocardial damage and because treatments of left and right ventricular failure often require a different and even antagonistic approach (pp. 52–56). Swan–Ganz catheterisation will certainly facilitate the decisions. Arrhythmias and AV block should be treated as already described (p. 65). Since contractility is diminished inotropic agents such as dopamine or dobutamine are often needed. In acute heart muscle disease it is important to appreciate that cardiac failure may be reversible over a few days or even weeks. If it is possible to overcome this difficult period the outcome and final prognosis are sometimes excellent and full treatment should be attempted at all times.

If a specific cause can be identified appropriate treatment is indicated. Some authorities suggest a course of corticosteroids (sometimes with azathioprine) in severe myocarditis that is refractory to therapy. In acute rheumatic fever treatment with prednisolone (2 mg/kg/day) is well established and should be administered together with treatment for cardiac failure if present and penicillin.

Heart disease in pregnancy

All forms of heart disease tend to get worse in pregnancy, but with proper management the patient should return to her prepregnancy state within weeks of the delivery. It is exceedingly rare to need to advise abortion on cardiac grounds. The following points should be noted:
1. All patients with valvular disease should be given prophylactic antibiotics at the time of delivery to prevent endocarditis.
2. Adequate analgesia should be available during labour and delivery (e.g. nitrous oxide or expertly given epidural anaesthesia).
3. Prolonged labour should be avoided and assistance with the 'ventouse' should be liberal.
4. Deliver the patient sitting or propped up; avoid raising the legs as this will increase the return of blood to the heart.
5. On delivery of the baby give the mother furosemide 80 mg i.v. stat.
6. Pulmonary oedema may occur during the 24 h immediately after delivery because of the return of blood from the placenta, which increases the mother's blood volume.

Note: Peripartum cardiomyopathy is a distinctive type of heart muscle disease occurring before, during or soon after delivery. To make the diagnosis there should be no history of pre-existing heart disease or of symptoms in the first or second trimester of the pregnancy. Even this entity forms a heterogeneous group: (1) patients with high output failure with a very good prognosis and (2) patients with a low cardiac output who have a much worse prognosis. Patients should be advised against further pregnancies, as the condition tends to recur. Treatment has already been described under heart muscle disease.

Non-cardiac problems

The most important of these are hypertension, lung diseases, fluid overload, severe anaemia and thyrotoxicosis. The treatment is aimed at resolving the underlying cause. Since hypertension can by itself cause a critical illness it is further discussed here.

Hypertensive crises

This section is limited to discussion of critical illness caused by or aggravated by systemic hypertension. The main problems are acute pulmonary oedema due to hypertensive heart failure, malignant hypertension, hypertensive encephalopathy and preeclampsia. The risk of bleeding from an aortic aneurysm is increased by hypertension.

Acute pulmonary oedema

This has already been described (p. 47). If it is due to hypertension rapid lowering of the blood pressure is indicated in addition to other treatment and is described below.

Malignant hypertension

Distinguished from 'non-malignant' hypertension by the level of the diastolic blood pressure (usually >130 mmHg), the presence of retinal exudates, haemorrhages and papilloedema (which may lead to blurred vision), and gross haematuria and albuminuria, malignant hypertension can occur without symptoms and be recognised only when the blood pressure is measured.

Hypertensive encephalopathy

This complicates hypertension and may be the first indication of hypertension. It is present whenever there is altered consciousness, confusion or fits due to raised systemic arterial pressure and the diagnosis is made clinically. Severe headache is commonly present but there is no meningism. Focal neurological signs may occur. The condition develops rapidly and other causes of acute encephalopathy (e.g. poisoning, infections, alcohol and trauma) must be excluded. There may be other signs of hypertensive disease including left ventricular hypertrophy and hypertensive retinopathy and it may complicate malignant hypertension. When first seen it may be difficult to distinguish from a cerebrovascular accident but the rapid improvement within 24 h of treatment and the absence of residual neurological disability allow the diagnosis to be made within a few days.

Pre-eclampsia

Described on p. 264, pre-eclampsia may be complicated by hypertensive encephalopathy.

Less serious hypertension

A diastolic blood pressure greater than 130 mmHg without any of the above problems is a less serious medical emergency. Transient hypertension is common immediately after a cerebrovascular accident, even in patients without established hypertension, and should be lowered with caution as a precipitious fall in blood pressure will decrease perfusion of the infarcted area of the brain and increase the amount of damage.

Management

The aim of management is a smooth reduction of the blood pressure to safe levels without causing dangerous hypotension. Patients who are normally hypertensive require a higher perfusing pressure in the cerebral vessels; they are at risk of cerebral ischaemia at higher pressures than are normotensive individuals. Treatment with intravenous hypotensive agents may cause a precipitious fall in blood pressure and is recommended only for patients in whom the immediate threat to life is great. Common conditions are:
- severe hypertensive heart failure;
- hypertensive encephalopathy;
- malignant hypertension;
- severe pre-eclampsia;
- acute dissection of an aortic aneurysm.

Other patients with diastolic pressures above 130 mmHg are not at such risk and can be treated with oral therapy.

General management

Patients are usually kept in bed and may need sedation. Supportive care depends on the specific problem and is described in the appropriate section. Anticonvulsants should be given to control fits.

Specific hypotensive treatment

The usual way to lower blood pressure is by oral or intramuscular therapy except in very critical situations where intravenous agents may be used. The objective is gradually to lower the diastolic pressure to between 90 and 100 mm Hg. The drugs which may used in urgent situations are described below and their side effects should be checked in the A to Z of Drugs (p. 439) or a pharmacopoeia. Propanolol, prazosin and captopril may be also be used.

Once the diastolic blood pressure is below 120 mmHg the immediate crisis is under control and more gradual lowering of the blood pressure by substituting an oral regimen, while slowly discontinuing intravenous therapy, is commenced. The final diastolic pressure should be between 90 and 100 mmHg and efforts to further reduce blood pressure in patients who are normally hypertensive are ill advised.

LABETALOL (p. 449)
May be given by intravenous infusion (0.5–2 mg/min to a maximum of 2 mg/kg) or as a bolus 50 mg i.v. injection, which may be repeated at 5–15-min intervals up to three times. It does not lead to a reflex tachycardia.

HYDRALAZINE (p. 447)
10 mg i.m. or 50 mg orally 4-hourly until the diastolic pressure is less than 120 mmHg and then oral hydralazine 50 mg 6-hourly. Propranolol 40 to 80 mg 8- or 12-hourly should be given simultaneously to control reflex tachycardia (see above).

METHYLDOPA (p. 450)
250 to 500 mg 8- or 6-hourly orally. Intravenous methyl dopa in the same dose can be used if the drugs described above for very serious hypertensive crises are not available.

NIFEDIPINE (p. 451)
This is a potent hypotensive agent and is the only drug which can be given sublingally with a rapid (within minutes) onset of action. Occasionally produces severe hypotension and coronary ischaemia.

SODIUM NITROPRUSSIDE
This is given by infusion. The effect is immediate but of short duration. This allows fine control of the dose according to the response but requires frequent and careful observation of blood pressure. If possible, intra-arterial monitoring of blood pressure should be done. Failing that, the blood pressure must be taken with measurements at 5-min intervals until it is stable and then $\frac{1}{2}$ hourly throughout the infusion. The initial dose is 0.3 µg/kg/min in 5% dextrose. Depending on the response, the dose may be increased gradually up to a maximum of 8 µg/kg/min. As the blood pressure falls there may be a reflex tachycardia, which can be controlled by using a beta-blocker such as propanolol.

DIAZOXIDE
Given by bolus i.v. injection. The effect is seen within a few minutes of administration and may last for some hours, particularly in patients with impaired renal function. This long duration of action and the frequency of severe hypotension are serious disadvantages and the drug must be used with caution. For this reason we recommend a dose between 75 mg and 150 mg given in 30–60 mg increments at 5-min intervals, and advise against using the maximum dose of 300 mg. The drug may also cause hyperglycaemia. A beta-blocker agent may be needed to control reflex tachycardia, which can occur with diazoxide.

Magnesium sulphate is used for pregnancy-induced hypertension (p. 267).

Special considerations

RENAL FAILURE
Renal function may be impaired because of the primary disease or preceding hypertension and lowering of the blood pressure may cause further deterioration in renal function. In the management of hyperten-

sive crises urinary output must be carefully monitored and the blood urea should be determined. In critical situations the diastolic pressure needs to be lowered to less than 120 mmHg even if this leads to deterioration of renal function. In patients with renal failure a short period on peritoneal or haemodialysis may be necessary.

HEART FAILURE

This can be expected to improve once the blood pressure is brought down, but the use of beta-blockers is contraindicated because they reduce the contractility of the myocardium.

CEREBROVASCULAR ACCIDENT (CVA)

Immediately after a stroke some degree of hypertension is common and unless the diastolic pressure is over 130 mmHg no immediate treatment should be given. If treatment is necessary more than usual care must be taken to lower the pressure gradually and it should not be dropped below a diastolic pressure of 110 mmHg in the first 24 h, as there may be spontaneous lowering of the pressure, which combined with overenthusiastic drug treatment can lead to dangerous hypotension. The one exception to this is subarachnoid haemorrhage, in which the diastolic pressure should be brought to 100 mHg or less within 24 h if possible.

Stroke

Definition

Any patient who develops sudden paralysis of one side of the body (hemiplegia), with or without loss of consciousness, has had a stroke, otherwise known as a cerebrovascular accident. The cause may be haemorrhage or thrombosis complicating existing disease of the cerebral vessels and this is a common complication of hypertension. A stroke may also occur following embolism, which usually arises from the heart or a carotid artery, or following severe hypotension.

Recognition

The presence of a hemiplegia is usually obvious and to determine the cause it is necessary to exclude causes of systemic embolism by examination of the heart and carotid vessels for any abnormality. Signs of hypertensive disease suggest haemorrhage or thrombosis. Immediate onset and deep coma favour the diagnosis of cerebral haemorrhage whereas evolution of paralysis over between $\frac{1}{2}$ h and 12 h favours thrombosis. The prognosis is worse for cerebral haemorrhage.

Management

Aggressive treatment of a stroke is indicated for those in whom there is a reasonable prospect of surviving the acute episode. Death may occur because of extensive brain damage or because of complications, the most important being airway obstruction, aspiration of gastric contents, pneumonia and pressure sores. Extensive brain damage is suggested if there is deep coma (Glasgow Coma Scale <8) (see Chapter 9), coma lasting more than 24 h, inadequate respiration (in the absence of depressant drugs), bilateral small pupils or bilateral rigidity. In these patients aggressive therapy is not indicated. In other patients the amount of functional recovery cannot be predicted early in the illness and it is often surprisingly good. Complications should be prevented by proper management of coma (p. 175), and if they occur then the patient should not be denied intensive chest physiotherapy with respiratory support if necessary.

Specific management

Control of hypertension has already been described (p. 72). Anticoagulants are not indicated except for stroke due to embolism, when they should be commenced a few days after the episode when the risk of haemorrhage in the infarcted area is diminished. Aspirin (150–300 mg daily) for its effect against platelet adhesion reduces the risk of recurrent thrombosis in cerebral vessels and of embolisation from carotid artery disease. At this dose side effects are rare.

Other preventative strategies include carotid endarterectomy for patients with carotid disease, or warfarin for patients with atrial fibrillation, providing there are facilities to monitor its dosage and effect. Recently immediate CT scanning may identify a small subgroup of patients with an embolic cause and who will benefit from thrombolysis with tissue plasminogen activator (tPA) within the first few hours of presentation. The best outcomes for the majority of patients with stroke are achieved by a combination of prevention of further episodes and active rehabilitation. Clopidogrel is a newer, but more expensive, alternative antiplatelet agent with some advantages over aspirin.

Aortic dissection

Definition and recognition of aortic dissection have already been described (p. 51). Treatment consists of lowering the blood pressure with antihypertensive agents such as sodium nitroprusside if available or beta-blockers. The blood pressure should be brought to the lowest level possible while maintaining an adequate cardiac output for renal function as measured by the urinary output. Dissection of the ascending aorta usually requires surgical treatment but dissection of the descending aorta can sometimes be managed medically.

Further reading

ANON. Single bolus tenecteplase compared with front-loaded alteplase in acute myocardial infarction: The ASSENT-2 double blind randomised trial. *Lancet* 1999;354:716–22.

ANTMAN EM. Decision making with cardiac troponin tests. *N Engl J Med* 2002; 346:2079–82.

BECKER RC. Antithrombotic therapy after myocardial infarction. *N Engl J Med* 2002; 347:1019–24.

BOERSMA E, MERCADO N, POLDERMANS D, GARDIEN M, VOS J. SIMOONS ML. Acute myocardial infarction. *Lancet* 2003;361: 847–58.

GOLDHABER SZ. Thrombolysis for pulmonary embolism. *N Engl J Med* 2002;347:1131–2.

JESSUP M, BROZENA S. Heart Failure. *N Engl J Med* 2003;348:2007–18.

SZOEKE C, PARSONS MW, BUTCHER KS, et al. Acute stroke thrombolysis with intravenous tissue plasminogen activator in an Australian tertiary hospital. *Med J Aust* 2003;178:324–8.

4
Fluid and electrolytes

Definitions

The quality of fluid and electrolyte management in critically ill patients is crucial. Careful attention to fluid balance, including accurate recording of fluid losses, is essential, particularly where there are no facilities for measuring electrolytes. In the absence of reliable laboratory back-up, electrolyte requirements must be estimated from a knowledge of the normal requirements and known losses. The margin for error is greatly reduced in children and babies, where too little or too much fluid may be fatal.

Body fluid compartments

At birth the total body water comprises about 75% of the body weight. This proportion drops to about 60% by the age of 1–2 years. In adults, males have a total body water of 60% and females 55% of body weight.

- 1 litre of water weighs 1 kilogram.

In a 70 kg man there are 42 litres of water, which are distributed as follows:

- 14 litres extracellular (33%), composed of 3.5 litres plasma and 10.5 litres interstitial; and
- 28 litres intracellular (66%).

Blood volume

The blood volume of an adult is approximately 5 litres of which 3.5 litres is plasma and 1.5 litres red cells. The actual blood volume can be calculated according to the weight using the formula,

body weight (kg) × 80 = blood volume in ml.

Thus for example: a 60 kg adult has a blood volume of 4800 ml.

In neonates and infants the blood volume may constitute a greater proportion per kg body weight, so the blood volume should be calculated at 85 ml/kg. Thus for example a 2500 g neonate has a blood volume of around 215 ml.

Electrolytes

Cell function is dependent on maintaining the normal balance of electrolytes, the most important being sodium, potassium, calcium, magnesium, chloride, hydrogen ion and bicarbonate. Sodium is the principal extracellular cation while potassium is the principal intracellular one.

The following terms are used to measure the concentration of electrolytes.

Mole

The molecular weight of a substance in grams. The molecular weight of a substance is obtained from chemical tables. Thus for example,

1 mole of NaCl (sodium chloride) = 23 + 35.5 = 58.5 grams;

1 mole = 1000 mmol.

Osmole

One osmole is the molecular weight of a substance in grams divided by the number of freely moving particles each molecule liberates in solution.

e.g. 1 osmole of NaCl = 58.5/2 = 29.25 grams.

Both osmolality and osmolarity are measures of the concentration of a solute in a solvent. Thus if you dissolve NaCl in water the NaCl is the solute and the water is the solvent. NaCl dissolved in water makes a solution.

Osmolality

The number of osmoles per kilogram of solvent. NaCl when dissolved in water dissociates into an equal number of Na^+ and Cl^- ions. This solution therefore has an osmolality of 2 osmol per kg. 1 osmol = 1000 mosmol.

Plasma osmolality

This are normally 290 mosmoles per kg. The actual plasma osmolality can be calculated as

2 × sodium concentration + glucose + urea (all in mmol/litre), e.g.:

2 × 140 mmol/l = 280 + 4 mmol/l + 6 mmol/l = 290 mosmol.

Because urea is distributed freely throughout both the intracellular and the extracellular fluid compartments of the body the plasma osmolality is effectively

2 × sodium concentration + glucose concentration.

Urine osmolality

In the absence of glucose and protein this is normally between 500 and 700.

Urine specific gravity	Urine osmolality (mosmol/kg)
1010	350
1020	700
1030	1050

Osmolarity

Number of osmoles per litre of solution.

Specific gravity

This is a crude assessment of solute concentration. It depends on the mass of the solute and the concentration of the particles. Thus a few heavy particles of high density will raise the specific gravity as much as many light particles. Large molecules such as protein give a false impression of solute concentration. Urine specific gravity is therefore only likely to be helpful in assessing the concentration of the urine, proving there is no proteinuria. Glucose in the urine may also affect the specific gravity, though not as much as protein.

Clinical recognition

The recognition of dehydration and fluid overload are discussed in the sections dealing with these specific problems (pp. 82–83).

Electrolyte disorders may cause confusion, coma, arrhythmias, paralytic ileus or may arise as a complication of another critical illness.

Patients at risk from fluid and electrolyte imbalance include those with:
1. vomiting;
2. diarrhoea;
3. coma or confusion;
4. heat stroke;
5. dysphagia;
6. an acute abdomen, e.g. peritonitis or obstruction;
7. postoperative patients especially after abdominal surgery;
8. high aspirates from nasogastric tubes;
9. oliguria or renal failure;
10. bleeding requiring transfusion;
11. eclampsia;
12. shock;

13. diabetes mellitus;
14. cardiac failure or underlying cardiac disease;
15. tetanus;
16. diuretic therapy;
17. metabolic illness.

Hydration is normally best assessed clinically. This should include monitoring of the urine output and in critically ill patients this usually means catheterisation. A central venous line is valuable when there is uncertainty as to fluid status but is not necessary as a routine.

Investigations

Haematocrit

This will help to assess fluid status providing the patient was not anaemic or polycythaemic before admission. The normal range is 0.40–0.45. A haematocrit of 0.30 or 30% is approximately equal to a haemoglobin of 10 g/dl if the patient is normally hydrated. Serial recordings of haematocrit are much more valuable than an individual reading.

Urea

The level of urea in the serum depends upon the balance between its production from protein and its excretion by the kidneys. The level varies with protein intake and the amount of protein catabolism and will be raised if there is blood in the gastrointestinal tract, which leads to absorption of protein. The normal range is 2.5–6.6 mmol/l and the urea level is a crude indicator of renal function. The urea is also raised when renal perfusion is reduced in dehydration or cardiac failure and when there is outflow obstruction to the urinary tract (p. 89).

Electrolytes

It is very difficult to diagnose specific electrolyte disorders without laboratory measurement. Without this you can only make a 'best guess' treatment on the basis of the electolyte content of the fluids the patient has lost and the normal requirements.

Blood glucose

The blood glucose must be known in order to calculate osmolality. In diabetic ketoacidosis there are always major fluid and electrolyte deficits (p. 102).

Management

Fluid and electrolyte input must include both maintenance requirements and extra fluids to account for abnormal losses from nasogastric tubes, drains and fistulae.

Before prescribing fluid and electrolytes you should know the answer to the following questions:

1. What is the patient's weight? Adults can be estimated but children must be weighed.
2. What is the patient's normal circulating blood volume?
3. What are the normal maintenance fluid and electrolyte requirements (Tables 4.1a, 4.1b and 4.2)?
4. What are the abnormal losses to be replaced? Give extra fluid to replace losses in addition to the normal maintenance requirements.

Fluid losses

Good fluid balance charts that can be readily understood and that make calculations easy are essential. Nursing procedures are discussed on p. 295. The output of fluids in the urine, nasogastric tube, drains and colostomy bags should be accurately measured and recorded.

Insensible fluid loss should not be recorded on the fluid balance chart but an allowance should be made for this before

Fluid and electrolytes

Table 4.1a Maintenance fluid requirements according to weight

	Weight (kg)	ml/kg/24 h	ml/kg/h
Neonate (<3 months)	3	150	6
Infant (>3 months)	3–10	120	5
	10–20	80	3
Children	>20	60	2.5
Adults		35	1.5

Table 4.1b Alternative method to calculate maintenance fluids

Weight	ml/kg/24 h	ml/kg/h
1–10 kg	100	4
11–20 kg	50	2
>20 kg	20	1

Example: 8 kg infant needs $8 \times 100 = 800$ ml/24 h
Example: 18 kg toddler needs $(10 \times 100) + (8 \times 50) = 1400$ ml/24 h
Example: 36 kg child needs $(10 \times 100) + (10 \times 50) + (16 \times 0) = 1820$ ml/24 h
The above calculations do not take into account extra losses or deficits which also need to be replaced.

writing up the fluids. Insensible loss or unseen losses of fluid are approximately 0.5 ml/kg/h. They include fluid loss from the skin, faeces and respiratory tract. Pyrexia, tachypnoea, diarrhoea and sweating increase insensible losses.

Table 4.2 Daily electrolyte requirements

Electrolyte	Paediatric requirements (mmol/kg)	Average adult requirements (mmol)
Sodium (Na)	1–2.5	100
Potassium (K)	2	75
Chloride (Cl)	1.8–4.3	120
Calcium (Ca)	1	5–12.5
Magnesium (Mg)	0.15	8
Phosphate (PO_4)	1	30

Electrolyte losses

Gastrointestinal secretions are rich in sodium and potassium (Table 4.3). If gastrointestinal losses are high give extra sodium and potassium. Therefore patients with high aspirates from nasogastric tubes need extra sodium and potassium replacement.

1 g KCl = 13.5 mmol;
1 ampoule KCl = 1.5 g = 20 mmol.

1 litre 0.9% NaCl = 154 mmol NaCl (154 mmol Na and 154 mmol Cl) (Table 4.4).

The electrolyte content of commonly used intravenous fluids is shown in Table 4.4.

Intravenous fluid requirements = maintenance fluids + abnormal losses

Always try to use a buretrol for intravenous therapy in small children.

Table 4.3 Volume and electrolyte content of gastointestinal secretions per 24 h

		Electrolytes (mmol/l)				
	Volume (l)	H^+	Na^-	K^+	Cl^-	HCO_3^-
Saliva	0.5–1.0	0	30	20	10–35	0–15
Stomach	1.0–2.5	0–120	60	10	100–120	0
Bile	0.5	0	140	5–10	100	40–70
Pancreatic	0.75	0	140	5–10	70	40–70
Small intestine	2.0–4.0	0	110	5–10	100	25
Diarrhoea			120	25	90	40

The values in Table 4.3 are for a normal 70 kg adult. Gastrointestinal losses can be much greater in patients with intestinal obstruction because the dynamic equilibrium of absorption and secretion is reversed.

Table 4.4 Constituents of commonly used intravenous fluids

Solution	Constituents (mmol/litre)					Dextrose (g/litre)
	Na	K	Cl	HCO_3	Lactate	
Plasma	140	4	97	25	1	–
Normal saline	150	–	150	–	–	–
Ringer's lactate	131	5	109	–	29	–
Plasmalyte B	130	4	109	28	–	–
5% dextrose	–	–	–	–	–	50
5% dextrose/saline 0.9%	150	–	150	–	–	50
$\frac{1}{2}$ str. Darrow's	62	18	52	–	28	50
0.45% saline/5% dextrose	75	–	75	–	–	50
0.18% saline 4% dextrose in water[1]	30		30			40

50 g of dextrose is 200 kcal or 840 kjoules.
50% dextrose contains 500 g dextrose/litre, 2000 kcal/litre.
50 ml 50% dextrose contains 100 kcal/420 kjoules.
1 g of KCl is 13.5 mmol potassium.
1 Make 500 ml by adding 100 ml of N saline to 400 ml 5% dextrose in water.

PRACTICE POINT   Drip rate and drop rate

Normal adult i.v. giving set:
15 drops = 1 ml;
ml/h = drops/min × 4.

Paediatrol/Buretrol:
60 microdrops = 1 ml;
ml/h = drops/min.

When two intravenous lines are in place be careful that fluid regimens take into account how much is being infused in the second drip. Two intravenous lines should be avoided whenever possible in children, elderly patients and those with cardiac failure.

Intravenous fluid therapy in children

The fluid and electrolyte requirements in children vary with weight. Since the margin for error is small great care must be taken to ensure the prescribed infusion is correct.

For any child on a drip the drip rate in ml/h should be recorded
1. in the notes;
2. on the fluid chart;
3. on the bag of fluid

Whenever a bag of fluid is put up a label should be stuck on the bag with the following information:
1. Name, age and weight of the child.
2. Date and time bag started.
3. Drip rate in ml per hour.
4. Drip rate in drops per minute.
5. Date and time the bag should finish.

This makes it easy for anyone passing to ensure the drip is running correctly.

Never hang a litre bag on a baby's drip without some form of infusion control, as a rapid infusion of the whole litre by mistake may result in the child being overloaded with fluid. If no other size of bag is available it is safer to empty out 750 ml from the litre so that only a 250 ml infusion is set up.

KEYPOINT

Always check the patency of the drip and the infusion rate repeatedly in babies and children.

Intravenous fluids are given for four main reasons:
1. for resuscitation;
2. for rehydration;
3. to give maintenance fluids;
4. to keep a vein open for drug therapy.

Resuscitation (See also the treatment of hypovolaemic shock, p. 22.)

The child who is shocked can be given 20 ml/kg of normal saline or Ringer's lactate fast. Should the child fail to respond to this give 10% of the estimated blood volume as colloid. If the child is bleeding, blood transfusion may be required. If an intravenous line cannot be established consider intraosseus infusion (p. 392).

EXAMPLE
An 8 kg child is admitted with severe dehydration and shock due to gastroenteritis. How should he be resuscitated?

ANSWER His blood volume is 8 × 80 = 640 ml. Give 160 ml (20 ml/kg) normal saline fast and reassess. If he is improving continue rehydration therapy. If he still remains shocked give him 80 ml of a colloid solution such as Haemaccel and continue resuscitation as indicated by clinical response.

Rehydration

Many children with moderate degrees of dehydration can be successfully rehydrated with oral rehydration solution. (The most convenient is the WHO/Unicef ORS – the contents of one sachet being dissolved in 1 litre of water.) However, if the child is having recurrent vomiting, is severely dehydrated, or has a distended abdomen, intravenous rehydration is required. Half-strength Darrow's in 2.5% dextrose and Ringer's lactate (Hartmann's) solution are both recommended fluids for this purpose. Half-strength Darrow's has a higher concentration of potassium, while Hartmann's has a higher concentration of sodium.

Bolus amounts of 20 ml/kg are run in quickly until the signs of dehydration resolve. The drip rate is then slowed, but the rate must take account of ongoing losses. If diarrhoea persists a rate of 130–200 ml/kg/24 h may be required. Oral fluids should be encouraged, and if being taken satisfactorily, the intravenous intake can be reduced.

EXAMPLE
A 12-kg child presents with signs of severe dehydration and diarrhoea. He has persistent vomiting. How should he be treated?

ANSWER He requires i.v. half-strength Darrow's solution. Give 12 × 20 = 240 ml quickly and then reassess. If still dehydrated repeat the 240 ml quickly. He may require three or even four such 'bolus' doses of fluid before the signs of dehydration resolve. When he has improved, continue the half-strength Darrow's solution at a rate of 150 ml/kg/24 h. Encourage to drink ORS and other fluids once the vomiting has settled, and reduce the i.v. fluids accordingly.

PRACTICE POINTS

1. When ORS sachets are not available half-strength Darrow's can be used for oral rehydration – but is expensive. Hospital pharmacies can make up ORS by dissolving 3.5 g sodium chloride, 2.5 g sodium bicarbonate, 1.5 g potassium chloride and 25 g glucose in 1 litre of water. In an emergency, one level teaspoon of salt and 8 level teaspoons of sugar dissolved in 1 litre of water make a perfectly adequate ORS.
2. A child with signs of severe dehydration is likely to have lost at least 10% of his body weight in water. Giving 20 ml/kg fluid is only replacing 2% body weight. It is therefore not surprising that such children may require up to 60–80 ml/kg of fluid (6–8% body weight) before the signs of dehydration resolve.

Maintenance

Maintenance rates for children are shown in Table 4.1a and b. The best fluid is 1/5 normal saline in 4% dextrose. If the child is having no oral intake for more than 24 h, 1 g of potassium chloride should be added to 1 litre of fluid. For malnourished children and others at risk of hypoglycaemia, add extra dextrose. Adding 10 ml of 50% dextrose added to 90 ml of 1/5 normal saline in 4% dextrose results in an approximately 9% dextrose solution.

To keep vein open

Use a maintenance fluid or half-strength Darrow's at a slow rate.

Specific problems

Dehydration

Dehydration occurs due to inadequate intake of fluids or excessive losses. In critically ill patients in hospital it is usually due to salt and water loss rather than water deprivation alone.

Recognition

The first symptom is usually thirst, which is experienced once 2% of body weight is lost. Later the patient feels faint. Once 3–4 litres have been lost an adult has a dry tongue, sunken eyes and increased skin turgor. In infants with 5–10% dehydration (this percentage is of total body weight, not blood volume) the anterior fontanelle is sunken. Urine output falls and if dehydration is not corrected, blood pressure will fall. Children become quiet, limp and inactive. As dehydration worsens the patient becomes comatose and dies.

Investigation

Recognition of dehydration should not normally require investigations to be performed. However, the haematocrit and blood urea rise. The urine becomes more concentrated, so that the specific gravity and osmolality rise, while urine sodium falls as the kidneys conserve salt and water.

Management

Replace the lost fluids and electrolytes by intravenous infusion until clinical signs improve. Urine output should be at least 30–50 ml/h (0.5–1 ml/kg/h in a child). Once losses are replaced maintenance fluids can be given intravenously or by nasogastric tube. Avoid overload by repeated examination of the patient.

If there is associated renal or cardiac failure a central venous line will help guide replacement therapy.

In children with severe dehydration due to gastroenteritis intravenous fluids are necessary. However once the child is able to resume oral fluids, ORS may be substituted. The electrolyte losses in the stool in diarrhoeal diseases are shown in Table 4.5.

Fluid overload

Those at risk

Patients at risk include those with cardiac or renal disorders and those receiving large volumes of intravenous fluids, particularly infants and children. Chronic anaemia may precipitate cardiac failure.

Patients with respiratory problems do not tolerate fluid overload well because the oedematous lungs do not allow good oxygenation of the blood.

Recognition

The patient with fluid overload may be oedematous and breathless. Tissue oedema over dependent areas such as the sacrum and the legs may be evident and fine crepitations can often be heard in the bases of the lungs. The jugulo-venous pressure

Fluid and electrolytes 83

Table 4.5 Clinical signs in a dehydrated 10 kg child

Degree	Clinical signs	Amount lost
5%	Dry tongue	500 ml
	Tachycardia	0.5 kg
	Early loss of skin turgor	
	Slight depression of fontanelle	
10%	Sunken fontanelle and eyes	1000 ml
	Limp, loss of skin turgor	1 kg
	Poor peripheral blood flow	
	Low BP	
	Oliguria	
15%	Shocked, comatose	1500 ml
	Near death	1.5 kg

(JVP) will be raised. Gross pulmonary oedema (Figure 1.3) may cause respiratory failure.

Fluid overload can only be recognised clinically rather than by performing investigations. Unfortunately it is sometimes an abnormal investigation that alerts one to missed clinical signs. Whenever there is uncertainty as to fluid status a central venous pressure (CVP) line is indicated.

Investigations

Haematocrit may be low. Urea and electrolytes show few changes, although the serum sodium may be low, around 124–130 mmol/l. Chest X-ray changes occur in severe pulmonary oedema, although the volume of fluid required to cause this may be low in patients with cardiac and renal disease. CVP is usually above 10 cm.

Management

1. Stop the intravenous infusion or reduce the flow rate to a minimum. If the patient has two i.v. lines remove at least one of them.
2. Give oxygen if there is respiratory distress.
3. Providing the patient is not in acute renal failure furosemide should be given (40–80 mg). The excess fluid will then be excreted in the urine.
4. In the presence of acute renal failure peritoneal or haemodialysis should be instituted (p. 95).

   Removing 500 ml of blood if the patient is not anaemic may occasionally be of benefit in severe pulmonary oedema associated with acute renal failure.
5. A central venous line should be inserted for pressure monitoring if the patient does not rapidly improve with furosemide. Always insert a CVP line if the situation is likely to recur or if there is renal insufficiency. A CVP line will only give accurate information if the tip is in a central vein (not the right ventricle) and there is no heart failure (see p. 390).
6. Ventilation is appropriate where there is respiratory failure unresponsive to the above measures and the patient's underlying condition is remediable.
7. Discover the cause of the overload and try to prevent a recurrence by ensuring accurate fluid balance, fluid restriction when indicated and that the patient does not have too many intravenous lines. Ensure that any further intravenous infusion is regularly checked and label the bag with the correct rate.

Electrolyte disorders

Those at risk

Electrolyte disorders are most likely in patients with vomiting, high nasogastric tube aspirates, diarrhoea, intestinal obstruction, paralytic ileus, intestinal fistulae, malnutrition, and severe burns, and in those who have received substantial volumes of fluids or blood. Patients with underlying cardiac diseases or on diuretic therapy may have hypokalaemia. Patients in acute renal failure may develop hyperkalemia. Chronic renal failure may cause hyperkalaemia and disturbed calcium balance.

Recognition

Electrolyte disorders are difficult to recognise by clinical examination and there is usually an associated fluid imbalance. The presence of predisposing conditions or signs of fluid depletion or overload should alert one to the possibility of electrolyte imbalance. Unexplained convulsions, confusion or coma, paraesthesiae, muscle weakness or twitching, abnormal movements, tetany, exaggerated or absent reflexes are the most common signs. Patients with hyperkalaemia may present with cardiac arrest. Hypokalaemia may cause or prolong paralytic ileus and marked muscle weakness.

Investigations

Serum sodium and potassium should be measured and calcium and magnesium when indicated. The majority of patients have disorders of sodium or potassium. Hypocalcaemia should be suspected in patients who have had thyroid surgery and magnesium deficiency in patients with chronic diarrhoea, malabsorption, short bowel syndrome or intestinal fistula.

The T wave of the ECG is peaked by hyperkalaemia and flattened in hypokalaemia.

Management

Sodium (normal range 136–144 mmol/l)

HYPONATRAEMIA

Decide whether serum sodium is low because of water overload (too much 5% dextrose) or because of salt and water depletion. Replace accordingly using normal saline or fluid restriction. Hyponatraemia can be corrected fairly slowly unless the patient is shocked or has severe ketoacidosis. There is no need to use hypertonic saline unless the serum sodium is less than 110 mmol/l with convulsions or coma.

HYPERNATRAEMIA

This is usually due to excessive saline or Ringer's lactate infusions. Give 5% dextrose for fluid replacement until electrolytes are normal.

Potassium (normal range 3.4–5.0 mmol/l)

HYPOKALAEMIA

Severe hypokalaemia (K <3.0 mmol/l) may result in muscle weakness or twitches, and cause paralytic ileus. ECG changes of hypokalaemia are flattening of the T wave, ST depression and sometimes a U wave. Muscle paralysis and respiratory failure may occur if K is less than 2 mmol/l.

Replace potassium slowly. Rapid infusion can cause transient hyperkalaemia and cardiac arrest. If K is greater than 2.5 mmol/l replacement should not exceed 10–20 mmol/h. The concentration of the infusion solution should not exceed 40 mmol/l. If the K is below 2.0 mmol/l the infusion can be at a rate of 40 mmol/h but in 24 h no more than 400 mol should be given in total. Potassium can be added to normal saline, Ringer's lactate or 5% dextrose solutions.

If renal function is normal potassium should be given to at-risk patients to prevent hypokalaemia. 1 g KCl = 13.5 mmol.

HYPERKALAEMIA

Once serum potassium rises above 7.0 mmol/l this is an emergency, since cardiac arrest may occur. Check that the sample of blood was not haemolysed, as haemolysis causes a false high potassium. If the blood was haemolysed test another sample. A peaked T wave on a full ECG (not a cardiac monitor) may confirm hyperkalaemia. The shape of the T wave on the monitor may be used to record response to treatment in the absence of electrolyte results but should not be used for diagnosis of the condition.

Treat adults as follows:
1. Stop potassium-containing infusions including blood transfusion.
2. Give 10 ml of 10% calcium gluconate to protect the myocardium.
3. Give dextrose/insulin injection as insulin stimulates the entry of potassium into the cells from the serum along with glucose. Give 100 ml 50% dextrose with 20 units of insulin over 5 min.
4. Give 100 ml 8.4% bicarbonate which neutralises any acidosis and promotes potassium re-entry to cells and excretion in the urine.
5. Give Resonium A 15–20 g three to four times daily orally, via nasogastric tube or as a retention enema. This is an exchange resin which absorbs potassium and begins to lower the serum potassium after about 1–2 h.
6. In patients with renal failure commence peritoneal or haemodialysis as appropriate.

Calcium (normal range 2.12–2.62 mmol/l)

HYPOCALCAEMIA

This may be manifest as tetanic spasms, neuromuscular irritability and occasionally grand mal convulsions. The patient may have had a parathyroidectomy (which may be an inadvertent accompaniment to total thyroidectomy) or be hypoparathyroid from some other cause. *Tetany* may develop in the presence of alkalosis, potassium or magnesium deficiency as well as hypocalcaemia.

Early signs of tetany are the development of carpal spasm on inflating a sphygmomanometer cuff above arterial pressure to occlude the blood supply to the forearm (Trousseau's sign) and contraction of the facial musculature in response to tapping the facial nerve (Chvostek's sign).

Treatment is by giving intravenous 5–10 mmols calcium over 20 min. Calcium preparations vary from country to country. Read the number of mmols carefully on the vial (1 mmol = 2 mEq). In children use 0.5 mEq/kg (0.5 ml/kg calcium gluconate). Use calcium chloride or calcium gluconate and if hypocalcaemia is persistent and symptomatic continue with an infusion while oral calcium supplementation is started. Hypoalbuminaemia lowers the calcium level so it is better to manage calcium balance by reference to the corrected calcium (N = 2.15–2.55 mmol/l which corrects for albumin level) or the ionised calcium level. Oral calcium (e.g. calcium carbonate or Sandocal) can be given alone but some tablets are unpalatable and not necessarily well absorbed or can be combined with Vitamin D (calcitriol) to improve absorption.

HYPERCALCAEMIA

This is usually discovered in association with other disease states such as hyperparathyroidism, renal failure, renal calculus, widespread malignancy. It is often asymptomatic and treatment is that of the underlying disorder. When serum calcium is over 3 mmol/l there is frequently an associated depletion of extracellular volume and so treatment begins with rehydration with normal saline.

Magnesium (normal 0.7–1.0 mmol/l)

Abnormality is usually due to insufficiency following prolonged diarrhoea and vomiting, often associated with malnutrition. The most common signs include tremor, agitation, confusion, convulsions and hallucinations. The diagnosis is confirmed by a plasma magnesium of less than 0.75 mmol/l. Intravenous magnesium sulphate or magnesium chloride can be given. Oral magnesium trisilicate (MMT) is another possibility if the above are not available. Magnesium intoxication is usually secondary to renal disease and treatment is that of the primary disorder. Magnesium toxicity due to magnesium sulphate therapy for severe pre-eclampsia is discussed on p. 267 (Table 14.3).

Electrolyte disorders in children

Sodium

HYPONATRAEMIA IN CHILDREN
The serum sodium may be low because of water overload or because of salt depletion. Water overload is sometimes caused by too much i.v. 5% dextrose, but can also result from the Syndrome of Inappropriate ADH Secretion (SIADH) which may complicate meningitis, and other severe illness, particularly in children. Treatment obviously depends on the most likely cause of the hyponatraemia. Fluid restriction may be all that is required for water overload. Salt replacement can be accomplished fairly slowly with normal saline, unless the patient is shocked or has severe ketoacidosis. There is no need to use hypertonic saline unless the patient has a serum sodium less than 110 mmol/l with convulsions and coma.

HYPERNATRAEMIA IN CHILDREN
This may be due to excessive intravenous normal saline or lactated Ringer's solution. In infancy it may result from the use of improperly prepared infant formulae. While it is tempting to reduce the serum sodium level quickly, this may result in serious neurological disturbance. It is best to go slowly and in most instances half-strength Darrow's solution or half-strength normal saline would be appropriate. Where the serum sodium is very high, it may paradoxically be appropriate to use normal saline.

Potassium

HYPERKALAEMIA IN CHILDREN
Treat as follows:
1. Stop potassium containing infusions, including blood transfusion.
2. Give 10% calcium gluconate 0.5 ml/kg i.v. over 3–5 min in children.
3. Give dextrose/insulin injection as insulin stimulates the entry of potassium into the cells from the serum along with glucose. Give 0.1 unit soluble insulin/kg with 0.2 ml/kg 50% dextrose over 5 min in children.
4. Give 8.4% bicarbonate which neutralises any acidosis and promotes potassium re-entry to cells and excretion in the urine. Dose 1–3 mmol/kg in children.
5. Give Resonium A three or four times daily orally, via nasogastric tube or as a retention enema. This is an exchange resin which absorbs potassium and begins to lower the serum potassium after about 1–2 h. Dose 1 g/kg orally or rectally in children.
6. In patients with renal failure commence peritoneal or haemodialysis as appropriate.

Calcium

HYPOCALCAEMIA IN CHILDREN
Treatment is by giving 10% calcium gluconate 0.5 ml/kg slowly in children.

5
Renal failure

Definitions

Renal failure occurs when the kidney is unable to perform all of its functions normally. These are:
1. regulation of the water content of the body;
2. regulation of the electrolyte content of the body;
3. maintenance of acid–base balance;
4. retention of other substances vital to the body – e.g. glucose, amino acids, phosphate, bicarbonate, proteins;
5. excretion of waste metabolic products including urea, toxic substances and drugs;
6. secretion of renin, erythropoeitin and participation in vitamin D metabolism (formation of 1,25-dihydroxycholecalciferol).

Normal renal function depends on (1) an adequate blood supply to the kidneys, (2) sufficient functioning renal tissue and (3) an unobstructed outflow of urine (Figure 5.1)

Renal function is best measured by the glomerular filtration rate (GFR – 125 ml/min/1.73 m^2). However creatinine clearance is often difficult to determine because of the unavailability of tests for urine creatinine levels which require a 12–24 h collection. In practice renal function is estimated from the volume and quality of the urine (p. 77), and the serum creatinine or urea levels. Ultrasound is an effective way of measuring kidney size, detecting stones and diagnosing an obstruction to urinary outflow.

Renal failure can be classified according to the site of the primary problem, as follows:

Pre-renal renal failure

This is due to inadequate renal perfusion and usually occurs as a result of low circulating blood volume or cardiac failure. Pre-renal failure causes renal hypoxia and if untreated progresses to acute tubular necrosis.

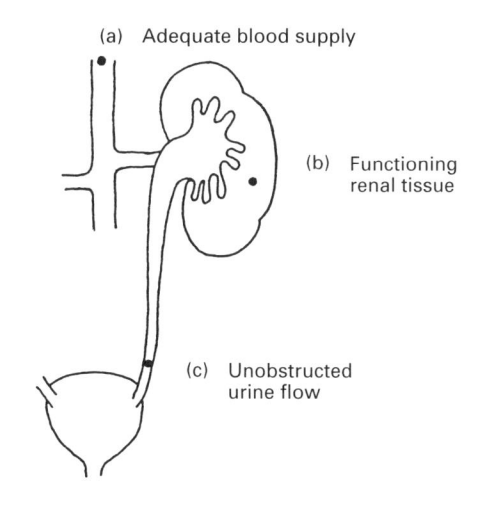

Figure 5.1 Essentials for normal renal function: (a) adequate blood supply; (b) functioning renal tissue; (c) unobstructed urine flow.

Table 5.1 Common causes of acute renal failure

Pre-renal
  Hypovolaemia from blood, fluid or plasma loss
  Cardiogenic shock

Renal
  Untreated pre-renal failure
  Glomerulonephritis
  Septicaemia
  Malaria
  Renal toxins and drugs[1]
  Snake bite
  Soft tissue trauma – myoglobin deposition
  Unrelieved post-renal failure

Post-renal
  Renal calculi
  Damage to the ureters after pelvic surgery
  Unrelieved prostatic obstruction, urethral stricture leading to chronic retention of urine

1 Renal toxins, drugs and poisons causing renal failure include pencillamine, amphotericin B, large doses of tetracyclines, streptomycin, kanamycin, gentamicin, phenacetin and aspirin, heavy metals (lead and gold).

'Renal' renal failure

Caused by impaired function of renal tissue, this may follow glomerular or tubular damage and may be primary (e.g. acute glomerulonephritis, toxicity following drugs or poisons) or secondary to delayed treatment of pre- or post-renal renal failure.

Post-renal renal failure

This occurs because of obstruction to the outflow of urine. The blockage may occur in the renal pelvis, ureters, bladder or urethra.

The main specific causes of acute renal failure are shown in Table 5.1.

Acute and chronic renal failure

Renal failure may be due to an acute process (acute renal failure) or may develop gradually from chronic renal disease (chronic renal failure). The usual problems in critically ill patients are acute renal failure and the prevention of renal damage from pre-renal failure. Patients with chronic renal failure may suffer sudden deterioration in renal function from any of the above causes, leading to acute on chronic renal failure, and they may need intensive management to tide them over the acute episode.

Acute renal failure is usually secondary to disease outside the kidneys such as shock, sepsis, disseminated intravascular coagulation, eclampsia, drugs and herbal intoxication. Occasionally it is due to primary renal damage.

Clinical recognition

The clinical features of acute and chronic renal failure differ and are described separately.

Acute renal failure

The cardinal feature of acute renal failure is a low output of urine (oliguria). Later the blood urea will rise (uraemia) and if fluid intake is in excess of fluid losses peripheral and/or pulmonary oedema develop. Electrolyte imbalance, notably hyperkalaemia, may be associated and cause cardiac arrest.

Oliguria

This is defined as an hourly urine output of less than 0.5 ml/kg/h or a 24 h urine output of less than 500 ml in an adult. In critically ill adults a urine output of less than 50 ml/h in an adult (1200 ml/24 h) should be regarded as an early indication of renal failure. Detection of renal failure depends on measuring the urine output and usually requires a urinary catheter. Before making a diagnosis of oliguria check that the catheter is not blocked or misplaced. Acute renal failure occasionally presents with a normal or increased urine output (non-oliguric renal failure), which usually indicates the diuretic phase of recovery from acute tubular necrosis.

Uraemia

Uraemia is defined as a high-serum urea (normal range 2–6 mmol/l) or creatinine (30–120 μmol/l). There may be no specific clinical features associated with moderate degrees of uraemia but as the urea rises anorexia, nausea, vomiting, diarrhoea, hiccups, a bleeding tendency and confusion progressing to coma with a flapping tremor may all occur. Uraemic frost (the presence of white urea crystals on the skin) and a pericardial friction rub are infrequent signs of uraemia.

Fluid balance

If uncontrolled fluid intake continues when renal excretion of body water is inadequate, signs of fluid overload develop with peripheral and pulmonary oedema. Pulmonary oedema is manifest by dyspnoea and crepitations at the lung bases. In fluid overload the blood pressure may be elevated. However, dehydration may be evident in patients with pre-renal renal failure.

Recognition of the type of acute renal failure

Pre-renal renal failure

This is usually associated with hypovolaemia (p. 20) or with cardiac failure (p. 46). The kidney conserves salt and water, so excretes low volumes of salt-deficient, concentrated urine (Table 5.3).

It may be difficult to recognise primary cardiac failure in patients in whom a low blood volume has been over-corrected. The clinical picture may also be unclear in patients who have developed renal damage secondary to hypovolaemia except that oliguria persists despite correcting the blood volume.

'Renal' renal failure

This follows primary damage to the kidney and may arise from loss of tubular or glomerular function. Clinically the diagnosis depends upon excluding pre- and post-renal causes and finding evidence of acute glomerulonephritis (puffy face, haematuria and hypertension) or other precipitating causes such as infection or ingestion of renal toxins. Total anuria in the absence of ureteric or bladder outlet obstruction is a sign of renal cortical necrosis. In acute tubular necrosis the kidney secretes low volumes of poorly concentrated urine (Table 5.3). Since the tubular function of conserving sodium is impaired the urinary sodium concentration is high. During the recovery phase of acute tubular necrosis large volumes (up to 10 litres per day) of dilute urine may be excreted.

Post-renal renal failure

This is recognised by detecting urinary obstruction and is probably the commonest cause of complete anuria. Physical examination may reveal bilateral renal masses in hydronephrosis or a distended bladder if there is bladder outlet obstruction. A distended bladder may be associated with

Table 5.2 Some common causes of chronic renal failure

Chronic glomerulonephritis
Diabetic nephropathy
Hypertension
Chronic pyelonephritis
Polycystic kidneys
Connective tissue diseases
Ureteric stricture from schistosomiasis
Chronic bladder outlet obstruction (prostate, urethral stricture)

overflow incontinence. Always suspect ureteric damage in any patient who develops anuria or oliguria following pelvic surgery. Plain abdominal X-ray may show enlarged renal shadows and ultrasound may show a dilated collecting system. The actual site of obstruction may be determined from cystourethroscopy, retrograde or antegrade pyelography or ultrasound as appropriate.

Investigations

Investigations may be helpful in confirming the presence of renal failure (raised blood urea and creatinine), in assessing its severity according to urea and electrolyte levels and in recognising acute tubular necrosis (Table 5.3). Other investigations may help to determine the cause and these include urine microscopy for casts, pus and red cells, culture and sensitivity for infection, plain X-ray and ultrasound for renal size and site of obstruction and biopsy for renal histology.

Chronic renal failure

In chronic renal failure the features of uraemia develop at relatively higher levels of blood urea. Other clinical signs include anaemia (due to erythropoeitin deficiency), bleeding tendency (due to malfunctioning platelets), hypertension (often with left ventricular hypertrophy or hypertensive retinopathy). Sometimes there are bone pains or pathological fractures from disordered calcium and vitamin D metabolism.

The presence of these features in a patient with oliguria strongly suggests acute on chronic renal failure, the common causes of which are listed in Table 5.2.

How to determine the cause

The common causes of acute renal failure are listed in Table 5.1 and in many instances the cause is obvious. Difficulties may arise in the following instances:

Distinguishing pre-renal renal failure from secondary 'renal' renal failure due to acute tubular necrosis

Failure to respond to volume replacement, diuretics or inotropes implies renal damage has occurred. Guidelines to adequate fluid replacement are discussed on pp. 25–29.

Acute renal failure without an obvious predisposing cause

The differential diagnosis in this situation is wide and includes primary renal disease due to drugs, toxins, infections, malaria, septicaemia, acute glomerulonephritis, post-renal failure or acute on chronic renal failure precipitated by any of the previous causes or urinary infection. A detailed history and examination may reveal the cause.

Table 5.3 Differentiation between pre-renal failure and 'renal' renal failure due to acute tubular necrosis

	Pre-renal	Renal
Specific gravity	>1020	<1010–1015
Urine sodium	<20 mol/l	>20 mmol/l
Urine urea/ plasma urea	>10:1	<10:1
Casts	Absent	Usually present
CVP	Low High (CCF)	Normal or high

Primary renal disease is suggested if the urine contains significant protein or granular casts and, in the absence of urinary tract instrumentation, red cells. Renal biopsy may be needed to determine the actual cause.

Recognising acute on chronic renal failure

Chronic renal failure is often associated with anaemia and hypertension. The patient may give a history of polyuria, prolonged symptoms of uraemia or a previous renal problem. Confirmatory investigations include a high serum potassium, low albumin, elevated uric acid, low or high serum calcium and a raised serum inorganic phosphorous. Renal size can be determined by abdominal ultrasound. Normally intravenous urogram (IVU) should be avoided in renal failure, but providing the urea is below 50 mmol/l and the patient is well hydrated to avoid renal damage from the contrast media, a high-dose IVU with tomography may demonstrate renal size. The kidneys are characteristically small in chronic glomerular nephritis and chronic pyelonephritis but enlarged in polycystic disease and hydronephrosis. The diagnosis of the cause of underlying chronic renal disease is beyond the scope of this book but diabetes should always be considered and excluded by blood glucose as urine sugar is unreliable in the presence of renal disease.

Determining the site of obstruction in post-renal failure

A history of prostatic symptoms may be obtained in a middle-aged or elderly male. A young man may have symptoms of a urethral stricture. An enlarged prostate will be palpable rectally whilst a stricture may be felt in the penis or perineum. Cystourethroscopy and/or a cystourethrogram are indicated. In hydronephrosis cystoscopy and retrograde pyelography are indicated. Alternatively, antegrade pyelography can be performed under ultrasound control.

Management

The management of renal failure depends on whether it is acute or chronic, on the probability of recovery of renal function and on the facilities available. While it is usually not difficult to distinguish acute from chronic renal failure it may be difficult to predict the prognosis, particularly when the diagnosis is uncertain. In these cases a good prognosis should be presumed until there is evidence to the contrary. The managements of acute and chronic renal failure are discussed separately.

Acute renal failure

Patients with acute renal failure are likely to die from fluid overload, hyperkalaemia, uraemia, secondary infection or the problem that precipitated the renal failure. The treatment objectives are to prevent death by controlling the above factors until there is recovery of renal function. However, renal function will continue to deteriorate unless the primary cause is corrected. The

steps in the management of acute renal failure are:
1. Treatment of the underlying cause.
2. Control of fluid balance.
3. Minimising the rate of rise of urea and other products of protein metabolism.
4. Control of electrolytes and pH.
5. Management of other problems – infection, anaemia, bleeding, hypertension.
6. Avoid if possible (or use with caution) nephrotoxic drugs and drugs excreted by the kidney.

Treatment of the underlying cause of renal failure

Pre-renal renal failure

The aim of management is to prevent progression to tubular necrosis and renal failure by restoring the circulating volume and thus renal perfusion to normal. The management of oliguria in the context of hypovolaemic shock is described on p. 29 (Figure 5.2). Restore the circulating volume to normal before considering

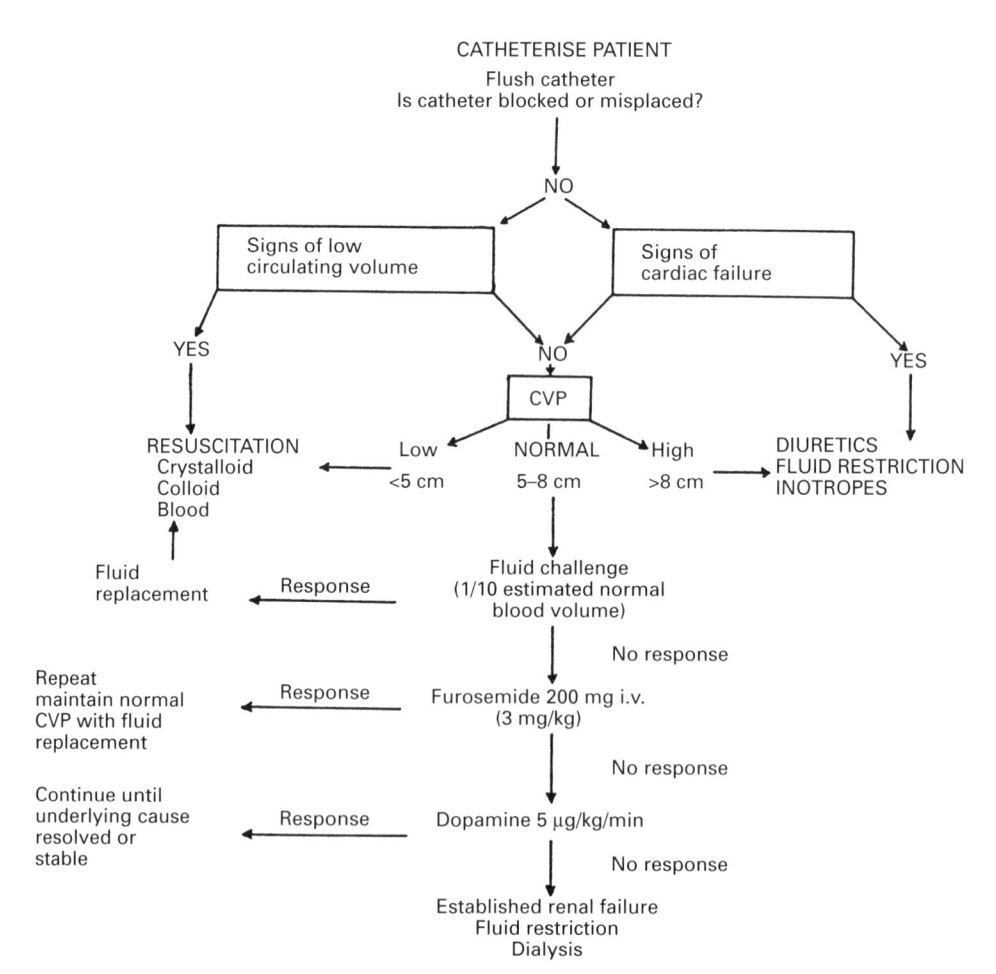

Figure 5.2 Flow chart for the management of oliguria.

diuretics. CVP measurement may be indicated to determine how much fluid the patient needs. A large dose of diuretic or inotrope infusion to restore BP may stimulate urine production should only be given once the circulating volume is normal. If the cause of pre-renal failure is cardiogenic shock the management is described on pp. 52–55.

'Renal' renal failure

Infection (malaria, septicaemia and post-streptococcal glomerulonephritis) should be controlled with appropriate drugs as soon as possible. Ingestion of nephrotoxic drugs and poisons should be stopped. If there is haemolysis this can sometimes be reduced with corticosteroids. In snake bite anti-venom therapy may prevent further renal damage.

Post-renal failure

The obstruction should be relieved and the method chosen will depend on the site of obstruction. Hydronephrosis may be relieved by percutaneous nephrostomy. Bladder outflow obstruction can be relieved by suprapubic cystotomy or urethral catheterisation. Once the kidney is relieved of the pressure its function starts to recover and definitive surgical management appropriate to the actual cause of obstruction can be planned.

Control of fluid balance

This requires accurate measurement and replacement of all fluid lost, including insensible loss. In patients who have signs of excess fluid (oedema, raised JVP or CVP, basal crepitations), fluid intake allowed should be less than daily losses and in patients who appear dehydrated (thirst, dry tongue, sunken eyes and loss of skin turgor) replacement will need to be in excess of losses. Fluid balance can be judged by daily weighing of a patient and a weight loss of 0.5 kg/day (due to catabolism) is ideal. Where fluid status is uncertain then central venous pressure monitoring is invaluable.

Patients with marked fluid overload, not responding to diuretics and fluid restriction, need urgent dialysis (p. 95).

Patients recovering from acute tubular necrosis enter a diuretic phase when large volumes of poorly concentrated dilute urine are excreted. During this phase it is important to maintain fluid balance, which may require volumes in excess of 5–6 litres to be given in addition to electrolyte monitoring and replacement.

PRACTICE POINT	
Fluid Status	*Fluid Prescription*
Hydration normal	Urine output + 30 ml/h
Dehydrated	Urine output + 50–80 ml/h
Fluid overload	Urine output per hour
Diuretic phase	Urine output + 30 ml/h
Notes: Review fluid status repeatedly during first few days of oliguria and diuresis. Measure electrolytes regularly in both blood and urine.	

Minimisation of the rate of the rise in blood urea and creatinine

This reduces the symptoms of uraemia as well as minimising the adverse effects of urea. Infection, trauma and surgery all increase protein catabolism with the production of urea and other toxic metabolites. In addition body protein will be used for energy if there are insufficient calories in the diet. The rate of rise in the blood urea may be diminished if adequate calories can be given by oral or parenteral feeding. However, dietary protein is also a source of urea and must be limited to 20–40 g/day. Below 20 g protein catabolism will be increased. A higher protein intake is possible if facilities for haemodialysis are available. A diet suitable for acute renal failure contains a minimum of 1500 kcal/day and should be 2000 kcal/day if there is infection or trauma.

Control of electrolytes and pH

In the absence of normal renal function both sodium and potassium levels depend largely on the intake of these electrolytes. Potassium accumulation is a dangerous complication with a risk of cardiac arrest. It is avoided by minimising potassium intake in foods (e.g. fruit, fruit juices and soups) and intravenous fluids (e.g. Hartmann's solution). Protein catabolism increases the potassium level due to release of potassium from cells. Blood transfusion is also a potential cause of hyperkalaemia since the red cells leak potassium during storage. Clinical recognition of hyperkalaemia is difficult and daily monitoring of potassium levels is mandatory. If the potassium rises above 6 mmol/l despite restriction of intake it can be lowered by the administration of a sodium–calcium exchange resin (e.g. Resonium A, p. 85).

Potassium

Levels greater than 7.0 mmol/l need immediate reduction because cardiac arrest may be imminent. Such high levels may be evident on ECG from a peaked (elevated) T wave. For management, see p. 85. Potassium supplements are often needed during the diuretic phase of acute tubular necrosis.

Sodium

Intake should be kept to a minimum to avoid hypernatremia. A low serum sodium (which may cause fits) is an indication for fluid restriction and not administration of sodium as it usually represents fluid overload. The only common exception is in uncorrected dehydration when a low sodium would be an indication for infusion of saline. During the diuretic phase of acute tubular necrosis, extra sodium should be given since the recovering tubules are unable to conserve sodium.

Acidosis

This is usually present in renal failure but rarely requires correction. However in the presence of severely acidotic breathing (rapid, shallow breaths without other obvious cause), a serum bicarbonate of less than 10 mmol/l or in association with dangerous hyperkalaemia the acidosis should generally be corrected by the administration of sodium bicarbonate (50–100 ml of 4.2%), providing a high serum sodium and/or fluid overload do not make this treatment unsafe.

Other problems in the management of acute renal failure

Infection

Regardless of the cause, patients in renal failure are at risk of secondary infection, which may cause further deterioration of renal function. Prompt diagnosis and effective treatment are necessary.

Anaemia

This is not a feature of acute renal failure and if present is due to some other cause. A moderately low haemoglobin (i.e. above 7 g/dl) is not known to impair recovery of renal function. The risks of transfusion in acute renal failure include pulmonary oedema and hyperkalaemia. The decision to transfuse should be made on balancing these risks against the predicted benefits. If transfusion is given packed cells are safer than whole blood and should be given by very slow infusion. If dialysis is available fluid balance can be controlled during transfusion. Anaemia may be aggravated by fluid overload and an acute fall in haemoglobin over 1–2 days without obvious blood loss may be due to fluid overload and is managed by fluid restriction.

Bleeding

Uraemia can cause spontaneous bleeding through damage to vessel walls or impaired platelet function. If present, intramuscular injections should be avoided and if blood loss is severe transfusion will be necessary. Give freshly donated blood. Spontaneous haemorrhage is a feature of the haemolytic uraemic syndrome (p. 35).

Hypertension

In acute renal failure this is usually due to fluid overload unless there is pre-existing hypertension or underlying chronic renal failure. Treat by fluid restriction. Antihypertensive drugs (e.g. methyldopa) are only indicated if hypertension persists despite normal fluid balance.

Use of drugs in acute renal failure

All drugs normally excreted by the kidneys will accumulate and cause toxic effects if used in normal doses in renal failure. Unless serum levels can be measured they are best avoided.

Dialysis

The adverse effects of renal failure can be corrected rapidly by haemodialysis and more slowly by peritoneal dialysis. The facilities for haemodialysis are extremely restricted. The technique of peritoneal dialysis is described in detail in the section on practical procedures (p. 371). The actual technique of haemodialysis and the methods used for vascular access are beyond the scope of this book but the basic principles are described at the end of the peritoneal dialysis section.

Discussion in this section is limited to describing when dialysis is indicated and when to transfer a patient to somewhere with facilities for dialysis.

In acute renal failure dialysis is used when conservative measures to control the blood urea, electrolytes and fluid balance are proving ineffective and the situation is becoming life-threatening.

Haemofiltration is an emergency alternative to haemodialysis if the renal failure is likely to soon improve or the patient is about to be transferred to a better facility. It is superior to peritoneal dialysis but requires close monitoring of fluid balance.

Indications

1. High (>40 mmol/l) or rapidly rising (>7 mmol/l/day) blood urea (or a serum creatinine greater than 1000 mmol/l). This occurs most frequently in the presence of trauma or infection.
2. Elevated serum potassium (>6 mmol/l).
3. Significant fluid overload.

The above indications may become clinically apparent from deterioration in conscious level, increasing weight, increasing peripheral oedema or the development of active bleeding, pulmonary oedema, fits, uraemic frost or a pericardial rub. It is wise to consider transferring a patient for dialysis relatively early (i.e. 2–3 days before it is expected to become necessary) but the prognosis of the patient in relation to the primary problem should be taken into account before planning transfer.

Acute on chronic renal failure

Acute on chronic renal failure should initially be managed in the same way as acute renal failure. The immediate prognosis will depend on the cause of the acute episode and if this is reversible then a return to the previous state of compensated chronic renal failure is possible. Otherwise the prognosis is poor unless there are facilities for long-term dialysis (haemodialysis or chronic ambulatory peritoneal dialysis) or renal transplant.

The management of chronic renal failure is beyond the scope of this book except to emphasise that in such patients intercurrent illness may easily cause further deterioration of renal function and that the use of nephrotoxic drugs and drugs excreted by the kidney should be avoided if possible.

Further reading

BRADY HR, SINGER GG. Acute renal failure. *Lancet* 1995;346:1533–40.

KLAHR S, MILLER SB. Acute oliguria. *N Engl J Med* 1998;338:671–5.

LEVEY AS. Nondiabetic kidney disease. *N Engl J Med* 2002;347:1505–11.

PHU NH, HIEN TT, MAI TH et al. Hemofiltration and peritoneal dialysis in infection-associated acute renal failure in Vietnam. *N Engl J Med* 2002;347:895–902.

6
Metabolic and endocrine problems

Acute liver failure

Definition

The main functions of the liver are listed in Table 6.1 together with the major clinical effects of impairment of each function.

Loss of more than about 60% of functioning liver cells leads to clinically manifest liver failure. In acute liver failure many functions fail simultaneously but altered consciousness due to hepatic encephalopathy (p. 98) is usually the dominant feature. Acute liver failure may occur *de novo* as a consequence of an acute illness – most commonly acute viral hepatitis or acute poisoning – or may complicate chronic liver disease when there is increased demand on any of the liver functions or acute deterioration of function (Table 6.2).

In liver failure the degree of disturbance of each liver function varies and the clinical picture is very variable. Some manifestations are shown in Table 6.1. The most important of these is hepatic encephalopathy, which arises from impaired detoxification of nitrogenous compounds produced by bacterial action on

Table 6.1 Main functions of the liver and effects of impairment

Function	Effect of impairment of this function
Metabolism of bilirubin	Jaundice
Glycogen metabolism and storage	Hypoglycaemia
Protein synthesis	Hypoalbuminaemia with oedema
Synthesis of clotting factors	Generalised bleeding
Metabolism of some drugs	Increased sensitivity to those drugs
Detoxification	Hepatic encephalopathy

Table 6.2 Some causes of liver failure in previously normal livers and in pre-existing liver disease

Normal liver	Diseased liver
Acute viral hepatitis	Gastrointestinal bleeding
Drug poisoning, e.g. paracetamol, isoniazid, halothane, tetracycline[1]	Infections
	Electrolyte imbalance, e.g. following excess diuretics or rapid drainage of ascitic fluid
Alcohol excess	Surgery, major trauma and anaesthesia
	Alcohol, sedatives and narcotics

1 In late pregnancy liver failure is often caused by parenteral tetracycline.

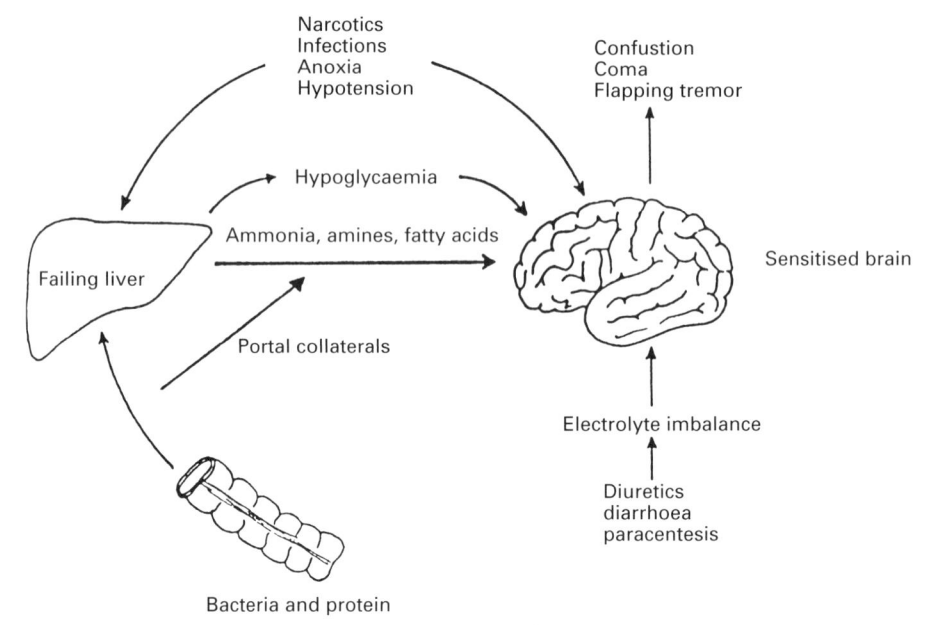

Figure 6.1 Factors altering cerebral function in liver failure.

protein in the gut. These compounds affect the central nervous system, leading to altered consciousness. Effects of chronic liver disease (such as portal hypertension and oesophageal varices) may also be present. The main factors in the development of hepatic encephalopathy are illustrated in Figure 6.1.

Recognition

Hepatic encephalopathy

The main manifestation of acute liver failure is hepatic encephalopathy. This may be mild with subtle changes in behaviour, disturbed sleep, irritability and other inappropriate behaviour or more severe with frank aggression, confusion and sometimes violence. As the encephalopathy progresses there is drowsiness followed by loss of consciousness which may proceed to deep coma. An early sign of encephalopathy is the inability to copy a pattern (drawn or made with matches) such as a five-pointed star. Later a flapping tremor becomes apparent.

This is best demonstrated by holding the arms horizontally forwards with the wrists dorsi-flexed, when coarse flexion-extension movements occur. There may be a tremor of the tongue and an ataxic gait. These signs also occur in renal failure and hypoxia. Focal neurological signs are not a feature but there may be general increase in tone with brisk reflexes and in more advanced encephalopathy general loss of tone and reflexes but extensor plantar responses. Convulsions may occur at any stage. Terminally there is respiratory depression, leading to cardiac arrest. Almost any of these features can occur in hypoglycaemia, which is a complication of acute liver failure and must be excluded. There may be rapid fluctuations in the patient's condition.

> **PRACTICE POINT**
>
> Hypoglycaemia may be mistaken for hepatic encephalopathy and failure to recognise it may lead to irreversible brain damage.

The diagnosis of hepatic encephalopathy is made on clinical grounds and it should be suspected in any patient who has liver disease and behavioural change, psychiatric symptoms or neurological features. The differential diagnosis includes hypoglycaemia, cerebral malaria (p. 140), acute alcohol withdrawal (delirium tremens or DTs (p. 116)) and septicaemia.

It may be difficult to distinguish acute liver failure arising *de novo* from liver failure complicating chronic liver disease. The presence of a low serum albumin, firm or irregular enlargement of the liver or a very shrunken liver (with reduced liver dullness) and signs of portal hypertension favour underlying chronic liver disease.

Other features of liver failure

Jaundice is common but may not be severe initially and increases as the condition worsens. Occasionally hepatic encephalopathy develops before jaundice in acute viral hepatitis. In acute liver disease the serum transaminases are usually markedly raised but terminally and in chronic liver disease they may be mildly elevated or normal.

Haemorrhage may be generalised owing to lack of clotting factors and manifest by bleeding from the gums, petechiae and skin bruising and sometimes more severe bleeding, e.g. gastrointestinal, haematuria and cerebral haemorrhage. In addition in patients with pre-existing liver disease oesophageal varices may bleed and the lack of clotting factors predisposes to this. Gastrointestinal bleeding aggravates hepatic encephalopathy.

A number of metabolic changes may occur as a result of liver failure and may precipitate or aggravate hepatic encephalopathy. Hypoglycaemia is associated with elevated insulin levels and inadequate liver glycogen and is described on p. 102. Renal failure with a falling urinary output and rising blood urea develops in nearly half of the patients with acute liver failure, leading to the hepato-renal syndrome. The cause of this complication is not well understood but infection, gastrointestinal bleeding, elevated bilirubin and endotoxaemia may contribute. Electrolyte abnormalities (p. 84) may be secondary to renal failure and may occur in its absence when hypokalaemia is common. Variable changes may occur in the acid–base balance secondary to the abnormal metabolism, electrolyte imbalance, renal insufficiency and abnormal ventilation.

Respiratory function may deteriorate because of central depression of respiration or because of pneumonia and the effects of inhalation of gastric contents, which is common. Hypoxia may be aggravated by intrapulmonary shunting and pulmonary oedema, and oxygen should be given to patients who are unconscious.

In the absence of hypovolaemia, circulatory problems develop late when central depression of brain stem function leads to a falling blood pressure, and arrhythmias, particularly bradycardia and cardiac arrest, may occur.

Management

Acute liver failure due to acute liver disease has a mortality rate of 90% in the most severe cases. Prompt treatment can sometimes prevent the deterioration to such levels of severity. However, in chronic liver disease severe hepatic encephalopathy can reverse once the precipitating factors are corrected. There is usually no specific treatment for the primary liver disease and the use of prednisolone and other corticosteroids is contraindicated. Management depends on avoiding aggravating factors and preventing avoidable complications. Management of specific problems is summarised in Table 6.3.

Table 6.3 Management of acute liver failure

Problem	Management
Encephalopathy	No oral protein
	Neomycin 1–2 g 6 hourly oral or per rectum
	Magnesium sulphate 15 ml three times daily
	OR Lactulose 15 ml three times daily
	Nasogastric drainage or aspiration
	Cimetidine 400 mg twice daily to prevent bleeding
	OR Mist. magnesium trisilicate 15 ml 2 hourly
Hypoglycaemia	Monitor blood sugar 4 hourly
	50–100 ml 50% dextrose if blood sugar <3 mmol/l
	Oral dextrose (see nutrition)
Electrolyte imbalance	Daily measurement and correction (p. 84)
Renal failure	Monitor urine output and serum creatinine
	Avoid hypovolaemia
	Control hyperkalaemia (p. 85)
	Dialysis (see text and p. 95)
Respiratory failure	Routine oxygen 4.0 l/min to comatose patients
	Airway care
	Prevent with chest physiotherapy and control of infection
	Ventilate if necessary (p. 336)
Infections	Examine and investigate to identify if present
	Antibiotics and antimalarials if indicated
	Avoid tetracycline and other hepatotoxic antibiotics
Bleeding	Avoid i.m. injections
	Apply prolonged pressure after venepuncture
	Vitamin K 10 mg i.v. daily when prothrombin time prolonged
	Infusion of clotting factors if available
Circulation	Monitor BP and if necessary CVP
	Avoid hypovolaemia and fluid overload
Nutrition	Nasogastric dextrose 50% 20 ml hourly
Convulsions	Exclude infection
	Control with oral or i.v. diazepam 2.5 to 5.0 mg 6 to 8 hourly
	OR phenytoin 100 mg twice daily orally or i.v.

Encephalopathy

In treating hepatic encephalopathy one objective is to minimise the production of nitrogenous compounds produced by the action of intestinal bacteria on intestinal protein. No protein is given by mouth and if the patient is bleeding from the gut as much blood as possible should be aspirated. Cimetidine (400 mg b.d.) or omeprazole (20 mg b.d.) and Mist. magnesium trisilicate (MMT) 15 ml 2 hourly reduces the risk of gastrointestinal bleeding (except that from varices). At the same time gut sterilisation is attempted using neomycin 1–2 g 6 hourly orally (or rectally). The addition of a laxative helps by reducing intestinal transmit time and magnesium sulphate 15 ml three times daily can be used; MMT may provoke diarrhoea. Alternatively, lactulose – a synthetic disaccharide – can be used as it has a sterilising and laxative effect.

A second objective is to reduce the sensitivity of the brain to these nitrogenous compounds by avoiding any sedative drug and by correcting factors such as infection, hypoxia and electrolyte imbalance that may contribute. All unconscious patients should receive oxygen 4 l/min by face mask, chest physiotherapy to prevent infections and respiratory support if needed. Clinical examination for signs of infection should be followed by blood cultures and malaria slides but treatment with antibiotics or antimalarials is not recommended unless there is evidence of infection. The electrolytes and haemoglobin should be checked daily and corrected if necessary.

Other measures

General supportive care is important. Patients with acute liver failure may deteriorate rapidly and are best nursed where close observation and frequent monitoring (including blood sugar) are possible. Drugs with sedative effects must be avoided or used in very small doses (say 20% of the normal). Care of the comatose patient is described on p. 166. Nutrition is maintained by administration of a high-calorie carbohydrate diet or fluids (e.g. 20 ml of 50% dextrose through the nasogastric tube hourly).

Urine output should be monitored and fluid intake adjusted according to the patient's needs, but fluid overload should be avoided as these patients are susceptible to pulmonary oedema. The serum albumin may be low from the onset in patients with chronic liver disease and will fall during acute liver failure. This will increase the tendency to peripheral and pulmonary oedema. Diuretics are not always effective in controlling oedema and may result in hypovolaemia without resolution of oedema. A falling serum albumin is a bad prognostic sign and oedema may be impossible to control; if available, albumin infusions are helpful.

The blood urea is an unreliable indicator of renal function in acute liver failure, as urea is a product of liver metabolism; serum creatinine is more reliable. Renal failure can be treated with dialysis but care should be taken to exclude hepatitis B virus infection if haemodialysis is being considered. Bleeding may create problems in both peritoneal and haemodialysis. If treatable causes of renal failure (e.g. hypovolaemia, septicaemia) are not present the prognosis of hepato-renal failure is very poor and results of aggressive treatment are disappointing.

Any bleeding tendency may be lessened by administration of vitamin K 10 mg intravenously, particularly if the prothrombin time is prolonged. If available, clotting factors can be administered if there is persistent or major haemorrhage. If blood transfusion is indicated fresh blood (<12 hours since donation) is to be preferred as it contains active clotting factors and platelets. Intramuscular injections should be avoided because of the risk of a haematoma developing.

Diabetes

Definition

Diabetes is a syndrome characterised by hyperglycaemia associated with a deficiency of insulin. Critically ill patients may present with coma or they may have another clinical problem, the treatment of which is complicated by diabetes. Diabetics are divided into those who are insulin-dependent and those who are non-insulin-dependent as regards their treatment. These categories are not mutually exclusive and patients may go from one to another depending on circumstances. For instance, a non-insulin-dependent diabetic undergoing the stress of surgery will, temporaily, become insulin-dependent.

Recognition

Diabetes may be recognised either clinically or biochemically. Clinically it presents most urgently as coma (see Chapter 9), but usually presents as weight loss, polyuria and polydipsia, or frequent infections.

Coma in diabetes may be due to the following:

Diabetic ketoacidosis

This is severe uncontrolled hyperglycaemia with increased ketones in the blood and urine, and other serious metabolic disturbances. It is precipitated by infection, trauma or omission of insulin. Coma is preceded by deteriorating health for a few days before the patient becomes confused, lethargic and finally unrousable. There is always severe dehydration and the deep sighing respiration of acidosis. The breath may smell sweet (the acetone smell of nailpolish remover) and there may be evidence of infection.

Diagnosis

The urine glucose is more than 2%, there is heavy ketonuria and a blood glucose greater than 22 mmol/l. Dextrostix will read greater than 13.9 mmol/l (dark blue on the strip). The serum sodium is usually low. Glycosuria due to a dextrose infusion in a patient with mild or moderate starvation or vomiting must not be confused with diabetic ketoacidosis.

Hypoglycaemic coma

This may occur on treatment in diabetics who take excess medication or if insulin or oral glycaemics are taken without food. It may also be seen in patients with cerebral malaria, alcohol and methanol intoxication, liver damage, widespread malignancy and unusual endocrine disorders such as insulinoma and Addison's disease. Prompt diagnosis and immediate treatment are needed to prevent irreversible brain damage.

In diabetics, the onset is rapid but will go unrecognised if the patient is already confused or comatose from one of the above conditions. Coma is preceded by a feeling of anxiety, faintness and hunger with excessive sweating, tremor, altered behaviour or confusion. The pulse is full, hydration good, the skin warm and moist. Convulsions may occur. Clinical signs may be masked in diabetics with autonomic neuropathy or patients taking beta-blockers.

Diagnosis

A blood glucose of less than 2.2 mmol/l.

Hyperglycaemic hyperosmolar non-ketotic coma

This is much rarer than ketoacidotic coma and occurs mainly in elderly non-insulin-dependent diabetics or previously undiagnosed diabetics. There will normally be a history of gradual deterioration prior to presentation. The patient will be severely dehydrated, drowsy or comatose but does not have acidotic breathing. There may be neurological signs due to altered cerebral perfusion or disseminated intravascular coagulation.

Diagnosis

1. Serum glucose is increased (>22 mmol/l).
2. Serum sodium is increased (>150 mmol/l).
3. Serum urea is increased.
4. Serum bicarbonate is normal.
5. Urine ketones are absent.

An approximation of plasma osmolality can be deduced from serum results by the formula given on p. 77.

Other causes of coma common to all patients

Examples are cerebrovascular accident, overdose etc. Since diabetics have accelerated atherosclerosis and reduced resistance to infection they are more likely to develop cerebrovascular accidents and infection.

Metabolic and endocrine problems

Table 6.4 Distinguishing features of coma in diabetes

	Ketoacidotic coma	Hypoglycaemic coma	Hyperosmolar coma
Onset	Gradual	Sudden	Gradual
Dehydration	Severe	Absent	Severe
Acidotic breathing	Present	Absent	Absent
Urine sugar	++++	Absent	+++
Blood sugar	>22 mol/l	<2.2 mmol/l	>22 mmol/l
Urine ketones	+++	Absent	Absent
Serium sodium	<130 mmol/l	Normal	>150 mmol/l

Diabetes may also present with biochemical abnormalities before any symptoms are noted. A high urine glucose (3+ to 4+) is suggestive but not diagnostic of diabetes, while a random blood sugar in excess of 14 mmol/l is diagnostic of diabetes.

Urine glucose

As a screening test urine glucose is satisfactory but its limitations preclude its use in the management of the critically ill. These limitations are as follows:

1. Urine glucose is a retrospective estimate of blood sugar. In the case of a full bladder it reflects blood glucose levels some 4–6 hours previously. This can be partially corrected by ensuring the patient empties his bladder 30 min before the estimate is made, but unfortunately this is too often neglected in practice.
2. Urine glucose may be falsely low if urine is stagnating in a full bladder and metabolised by bacteria.
3. The renal threshold for glucose varies, especially in pregnancy.

Blood glucose

Blood glucose estimation by laboratory or bedside methods is best for monitoring in the critically ill.

Dextrostix is a bedside reagent strip that records blood glucose from less than 2.2 mmol/l to greater than 13.9 mmol/l. A useful economy tip is to divide the strips into two by cutting longitudinally. This does not affect visual accuracy. Two-tone colour strips, e.g. Visidex and Haemo-Glukotest, are superior as regards accuracy but are more expensive.

To convert mmol/l to mg% multiply by 18.
e.g. a blood glucose of 10 mmol/l
  = 180 mg%;
a blood glucose of 22 mmol/l
  = 396 mg%.

Electronic bedside glucose meters

These are simple to use and maintain and are reasonably durable. Measurements are generally within 5% of laboratory values. It is important to educate staff on the operation and cleaning of these machines to ensure consistent results. As a double check we record the visual reading at the same time as the machine reading.

Management

Insulin, oral hypoglycaemics and diet are used in the treatment of diabetes, although in the management of the critically ill only insulin is used.

Insulin

Short-, medium- and long-acting insulins are available. Only short-acting insulin is used in the management of critically ill patients, as the effects of therapy can be monitored and altered if necessary. Although subcutaneous insulin is routinely used for well-controlled diabetics it is **never** used in ketoacidiotic or shocked patients as absorption is unpredictable owing to altered skin perfusion in the shocked state. Intramuscular insulin is more predictable in these patients but the best route of administration is intravenous insulin. Given as a continuous low-dose infusion, this approximates to the normal physiological secretion of insulin. Although there is variable binding of insulin to plastic giving sets (between 5 and 30%) this does not affect clinical management, as adjustments are automatically made according to blood glucose in the acute phase.

Oral hypoglycaemics

These fall into two groups, as follows:
1. Sulphonylureas: include chlorpropamide, tolbutamide, glibenclamide, and glipizide. These agents sensitise the pancreatic beta cells to glucose and also magnify the effects of available insulin. Because of their tendency to cause hypoglycaemia and hence hunger they are sometimes avoided in obese diabetics. Chlorpropamide is particularly prone to cause hypoglycaemia as it has a half-life of 36 h.
2. Biguanides: only metformin is in regular use. It may be used on its own in obese diabetics, or in combination with sulphonylureas. It may very rarely precipitate lactic acidosis.

Diabetic ketoacidosis

The management of diabetic ketoacidosis relies on rapid diagnosis, intravenous fluid replacement, insulin therapy and the treatment of precipitating infection if present.

MANAGEMENT
Give: S I P = Saline 　　　　　　Insulin 　　　　　　Potassium in that order.

SALINE

The patient is severely dehydrated and will have lost 5–10% of body weight. Therefore calculate the deficit from clinical observation:

5% – patient will be conscious but will have a dry tongue and loss of skin turgor. 10% – patient may have an altered level of consciousness, and will be severely dehydrated with sunken eyes, tachycardia and possibly hypotension.

Since 1 litre of fluid weighs approximately 1 kg, then a 60 kg woman with severe dehydration (i.e. 10%) will have lost 6 kg body weight and therefore requires 6 litres of fluid to be replaced fairly rapidly, with the first 2 litres being given in the first hour and the remainder within 6 hours. Replace with normal saline until the blood glucose is less than 13.9 mmol/l, and thereafter alternate with 5% dextrose. This prevents hypernatraemia and possible cerebral oedema.

KEYPOINT
Patients with ketoacidosis are often inadequately rehydrated and require large volumes of fluid.

INSULIN

Continuous intravenous insulin infusion by syringe pump, with regular blood sugar monitoring, is the safest and speediest method of rendering the patient normoglycaemic.

ALTERNATIVE METHOD Add to 1 litre of 5% dextrose 100 units of soluble insulin

Metabolic and endocrine problems 105

and label it carefully. Insert a second cannula for this infusion or, if this is not possible, 'piggy-back' onto an existing line. Control the drop rate of the insulin infusion by giving clear instructions to the nurses. In addition, 'fail safe' devices for the regulation of the infusion should be used if available. These include the use of a paediatric burette, a mechanical 'dial a flow' device or an electronic counter. If supervision of the drip cannot be guaranteed and there is the possibility of the patient accidentally receiving the full litre plus insulin in a short period of time then add only 32 units of soluble insulin to the drip. In this case the infusion rates below should be multiplied by a factor of 3. Check the initial Dextrostix reading against the scale below and set the drip rate accordingly. The time intervals for further Dextrostix recordings are indicated and will vary with the degree of hyperglycaemia. See Figure 6.2.

DEXTROSTIX RECORDING

INSULIN DRIP ADJUSTMENT
(100 units of insulin/litre)

13.9 mmol/l

Greater than 13.9 mmol/l run insulin drip at 8 units per hour = 80 ml/h. Monitor blood glucose every 2 h.

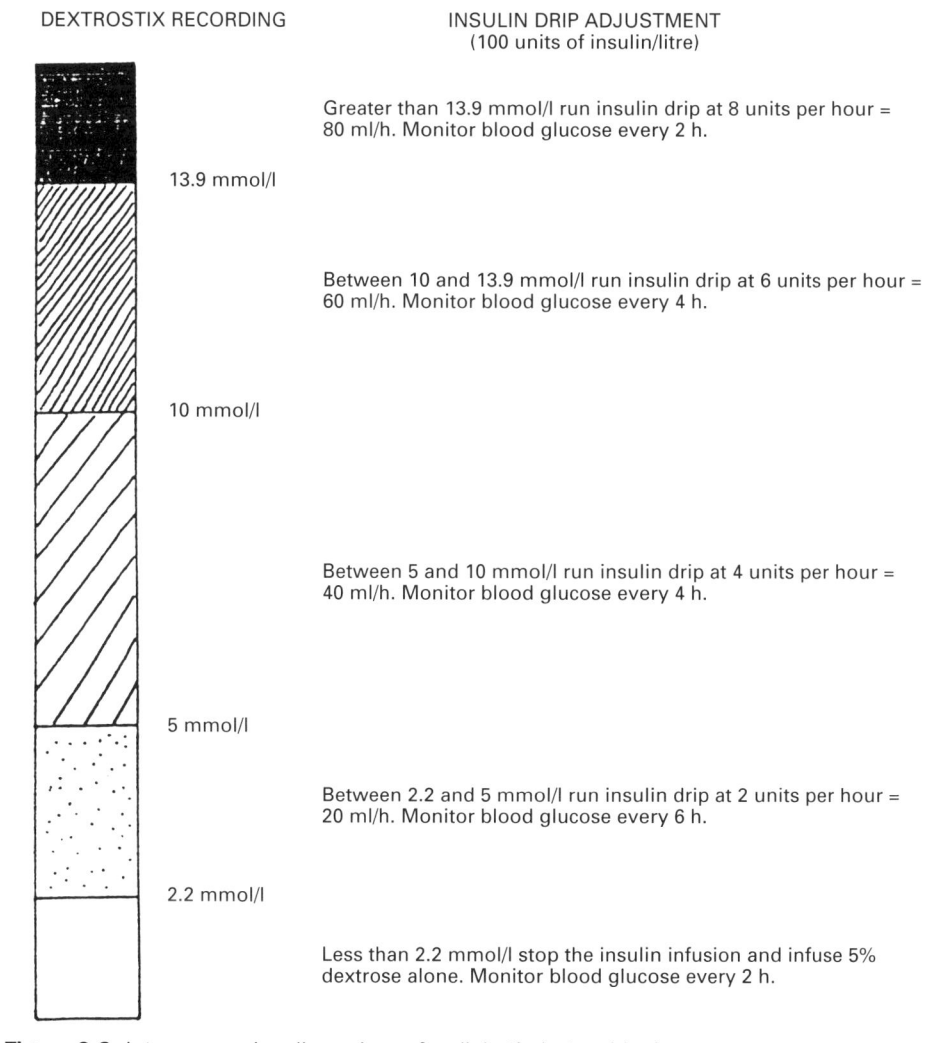

Between 10 and 13.9 mmol/l run insulin drip at 6 units per hour = 60 ml/h. Monitor blood glucose every 4 h.

10 mmol/l

Between 5 and 10 mmol/l run insulin drip at 4 units per hour = 40 ml/h. Monitor blood glucose every 4 h.

5 mmol/l

Between 2.2 and 5 mmol/l run insulin drip at 2 units per hour = 20 ml/h. Monitor blood glucose every 6 h.

2.2 mmol/l

Less than 2.2 mmol/l stop the insulin infusion and infuse 5% dextrose alone. Monitor blood glucose every 2 h.

Figure 6.2 Intravenous insulin regimen for diabetic ketoacidosis.
(*Note:* This regimen may be modified, by reducing infusion rates, for the control of diabetes in situations other than ketoacidosis.)

PRACTICE POINT
Drip rate and drop rate

Normal adult i.v. giving set:
    15 drops = 1 ml;
    ml/h = drops/min × 4.
Paediatrol/Buretrol:
    60 microdrops = 1 ml,
    ml/h = drops/min.

Once the patient is well controlled, normally hydrated, fully conscious and eating change to subcutaneous insulin. Calculate how much insulin the patient required in the preceeding 24 h, subtract 25% from this figure (this allows for the variable binding of soluble insulin to plastic giving sets) and then divide this figure by 3 to give the 8 hourly dose.

EXAMPLE

Mr K was admitted with ketoacidosis and was controlled as described above. By day 3 he was requiring 2 units of soluble insulin per hour. He was therefore changed to subcutaneous insulin and the dose was calculated thus:
   2.0 units per hour × 24 = 48 units in 24 hours;
   subtract 25% from 48 (12) = 36;
   36 divided by 3 = 12.
Therefore he required 12 units soluble insulin 8 hourly (or 18 units 12 hourly subcutaneously), given before meals.

An alternative regimen, when insulin by infusion is not possible, is to use intramuscular insulin:
On admission give 16 units soluble insulin, 8 units i.v. and 8 units i.m.
Give 8 units i.m. hourly until blood glucose is less than 15 mmol/l.
When blood glucose is 7–15 mmol/l give 8 units i.m. 2 hourly.
When blood glucose is less than 7 mmol/l give 4 units i.m. 2 hourly.

POTASSIUM

The patient with diabetic ketoacidosis almost invariably has a low total potassium, usually because of the preceding polyuria with loss of potassium. Laboratory-measured potassium values may initially be normal or high but this is due to potassium leaving the cells and does not reflect the total body potassium, which is low. Hypokalaemia will be further exaggerated by the dilutional effect of fluids infused. Therefore all patients in diabetic coma are routinely given potassium as 3 g (40 mmol) potassium chloride in every litre of fluid replaced after the first litre. Monitoring of serum potassium with electrolyte analysis or observation of T wave changes in the ECG is desirable if facilities are available.

OTHER POINTS

Alkali may occasionally be necessary. Acidosis may be marked on admission but almost always corrects with fluid replacement. We do not, therefore, routinely give alkali to patients with ketoacidosis. If however the patient remains acidotic after the fluid deficit has been replaced, or if the arterial pH is less than 7.0 then 4.2% sodium bicarbonate solution (100–200 ml) may be given. This may be repeated if the arterial pH remains below 7.0.

Pass a urinary catheter and monitor input and output.

Coma nursing procedures should be followed (see p. 291).

Pass a nasogastric tube on admission to avoid the possibility of aspiration pneumonia, as gastric stasis may be marked.

A thorough search for a possible source of infection should be performed; check the chest, abdomen, feet and legs. If there is nil apparent then test and culture the urine, check the blood for malaria parasites, take a chest X-ray and blood cultures and perform a lumbar puncture.

Hypoglycaemic coma

Management

Administration of 50 ml of 50% dextrose intravenously usually leads to dramatic recovery. If there is no response after 3 min to the first dose then repeat and follow with a dextrose drip until oral fluids and diet can be taken. Assess the cause and try to prevent a recurrence.

Hyperglycaemic hyperosmolar non-ketotic coma

Management

The aim is to correct dehydration, reduce the serum sodium and reduce the blood sugar. Follow same guidelines as for diabetic ketoacidosis with these adjustments:
1. Rehydrate with 0.45% saline (half normal strength).
2. Give heparin 5000 units subcutaneously 6 hourly in order to reduce the risk of thrombosis.

Management of diabetics undergoing surgery

Diabetics are prone to develop surgical problems. They are also more likely to develop complications of surgery. Surgery is also likely to be complicated by concurrent medical illness (Table 6.5). In Western countries 25% of diabetics on surgical wards may be newly diagnosed so that diabetes may first present to the surgeon.

Surgery and infection are diabetogenic and may temporarily convert a non-insulin-dependent diabetic into a state of insulin dependence. This is due to the action of insulin on peripheral tissues being inhibited by catecholamines, glucocorticoids, glucagon and growth hormone, all of which are secreted as part of the metabolic response to stress, infection and trauma.

Occasionally there may be an abnormal response to hypovolaemia due to autonomic neuropathy and this means that some patients fail to produce an appropriate tachycardia. Autonomic neuropathy may also result in impaired gastric motility. The increased incidence of myocardial infarction and stroke are due to underlying atherosclerosis.

Properly managed diabetics undergoing elective surgery should not normally require intensive care. The following scheme of management uses the same techniques and equipment as in the previous section.

Elective surgery

Ether and chloroform may cause hyperglycaemia in their own right, but other anaesthetic agents have a minimal effect.

Well-educated patients who monitor their own blood glucose levels effectively can be admitted on the day of elective surgery. Many patients in the tropics are unable to do this and should be admitted 24–48 h before surgery.

Patients controlled by diet alone

These patients are usually resistant to ketosis and have no risk of hypoglycaemia.
1. Check fasting blood glucose preoperatively; a level between 4 and 12 mmol/l is satisfactory.
2. No glucose infusion is needed during surgery.
3. Check blood sugar postoperatively.
4. If patient can eat normally within 6 h of operation then the usual diabetic diet is resumed and no further treatment is given.

Table 6.5 Problems of surgery in diabetics

Loss of control and ketoacidosis
Reduced resistance to infection
Increased incidence of myocardial infarction, CVA
Tendency to thromboembolism
Gastric stasis
Abnormal response to hypovolaemia

5. If the patient cannot eat normally within 6 h give an intravenous infusion:

1 litre 5% dextrose + 3 g KCl + 8 units insulin over 12 h, followed by

1 litre 5% dextrose saline + 3 g KCl + 8 units insulin over 12 h.

These two units should be infused over 24 h, giving a total of 100 g dextrose, 150 mmol sodium and 80 mmol potassium.

Patients on low-dose sulphonylureas

(e.g. 100 mg chlorpropamide/day, 5 mg glibenclamide/day)

1. Admit the day before surgery, check blood glucose and urea and electrolytes.
2. Do not give oral hypoglycaemics on the day before surgery.
3. Treat the same as those controlled by diet alone. Pre- and postoperative blood sugars should be checked.
4. Once sulphonylureas are restarted it may be necessary to give double the daily dosage for a few days to cover the stress of surgery. Biguanides should not be given until the 4th postoperative day in view of the risk of lactic acidosis.

Patients on high-dose sulphonylureas

(chlorpropamide 250 mg/day or glibenclamide 15 mg/day)

Admit the day before surgery. Half the normal dose can be given on the day before surgery and no oral drugs on the day of surgery. Treat during and after surgery as insulin-dependent diabetics since the stress of surgery makes them insulin-dependent. Oral hypoglycaemics may be recommended on the 4th postoperative day if the patient is eating normally.

Insulin-dependent diabetics

1. Admit the day before surgery and check blood glucose.
2. Ascertain diet and confirm type and dose of insulin taken by the patient. Since there are many types of insulin the patient should bring his insulin bottle with him to hospital.
3. If the patient is taking twice-daily insulin injections the evening dose of insulin should be reduced by 20% on the preoperative day. For patients on morning-only insulin no change is necessary on the preoperative day.
4. On the morning of operation, no subcutaneous insulin is given. Fasting blood glucose is checked and a drip is sited in all patients. Operate early on the list and an i.v. infusion of 5% dextrose/saline should be given. No potassium or insulin is added at this stage. If there is a long delay then insulin and potassium can be added. Once surgery is commenced 5% dextrose alone should be given. A slow infusion of dextrose removes any risk of hypoglycaemia from the previous day's insulin, while a little insulin minimises the risk of ketosis when surgery is delayed.
5. Postoperatively blood glucose is checked and an insulin–dextrose–potassium infusion is given until the patient is eating normally again. The amount of insulin added is determined by the patient's preoperative dose and then adjusted according to blood glucose results:

Normal insulin dose	Insulin infusion rate
Up to 40 units/day	2 units/h
Over 40 and up to 100 units/day	3 units/h
Over 100 units/day	4 units/h

As regards the dextrose–insulin–potassium infusion, 2 litres of 5% dextrose or 5% dextrose–saline each with 3 g KCl added should be given each day.

10% dextrose with increased insulin amounts can be given if i.v. fluids are necessary for several days. If no 10%

dextrose is available add 50 g dextrose to 1 litre of 5% dextrose.

Since fluid and electrolyte requirements can vary following surgery, additional fluid, electrolyte and blood should be given as necessary. Insulin–dextrose–potassium infusions should be in a separate infusion. Ringer's lactate should not be used since the lactate may increase acidosis.

6. Following minor procedures where the patient is able to eat normally later in the day, the drip can be taken down and subcutaneous insulin administered. If the patient is on once-daily insulin then 50% of the normal daily dose as a medium-acting insulin should be given in the evening.
7. Following major surgery, once the patient is able to eat, change from intravenous to subcutaneous insulin. Patients eating normally can go back on their normal insulin dosage while others who can at first only manage a light diet can be treated with short-acting insulin before meals as below:

Preoperative insulin dose	Postoperative dose with a light diet
Up to 20 units/day	8 units t.d.s.
Over 20 and up to 40 units/day	12 units t.d.s.
Over 40 and up to 60 units/day	16 units t.d.s.
Over 60 and up to 100 units/day	20 units t.d.s.
Over 100 units/day	32 units t.d.s.

Emergency surgery

The stress of the patient's underlying surgical problem (e.g. infection or intestinal obstructional) generally means that the patient's diabetes is out of control. They may present with ketoacidosis. (Note that ketoacidosis may also cause abdominal pain in its own right.)

The ketoacidotic patient being prepared for emergency surgery requires resuscitation with fluid, salt and potassium as described previously. Normal saline should be used for resuscitation and insulin given by i.v. infusion at a rate described on p. 105. Once the patient's blood glucose drops to 15 mmol/l, 5% dextrose infusion should be given. If there is no improvement within 2 h of commencing resuscitation then consider the use of colloid.

With good resuscitation it is usually possible to prepare the patient for emergency surgery within 6–8 h. Patients who are less severely ketoacidotic may be prepared in less time. Their losses of salt, water and potassium are less. In any case, surgery should not be delayed until complete control is achieved, as this is often not possible without first correcting the underlying surgical problem.

Once the blood glucose is below 20 mmol/l with blood pressure and urine output restored the patient should be fit for anaesthesia and surgery. Blood glucose should be checked 4–6 hourly following emergency surgery. In a few patients (e.g. those actively bleeding) surgery may be required while resuscitation is in progress.

Postoperative control of diabetes following emergency surgery

The patient will usually require an intravenous dextrose–insulin–potassium infusion as previously described. The insulin infusion rate will vary with the level of the blood sugar and the degree of sepsis. Use the same rates according to the blood sugar as for ketoacidosis (p. 105).

When maintaining diabetic control is difficult, consider the following possibilities:
1. Recurrent sepsis – this is particularly common in surgery for infected diabetic feet. Inspect the wound and remove dressings.

2. Drip tissued and not re-sited for several hours. This raises issues of nursing supervision, doctor availability and adequacy of communication.
3. Insulin infusion dose is too low.
4. Lack of resuscitation prevents peripheral utilisation of glucose due to poor perfusion of peripheral tissues.
5. Insulin resistance.
   (a) Obese diabetics – if 50% over ideal body weight consider doubling insulin dosage.
   (b) Stress of surgery or infection increases insulin requirements.
   (c) Insulin antibodies – switch to human monocomponent if available (e.g. Novo Actrapid).
   (d) Drugs such as catecholamines, steroids and beta-agonists may cause insulin resistance.

Hyperosmolar non-ketotic coma

Hyperglycaemic hyperosmolar non-ketotic coma is increasingly recognised in surgical patients (see above, p. 103). Surgical stress in association with dehydration are important precipitating factors. It may cause vascular thrombosis.

Further reading

ALBERTI KGMM. Diabetes and surgery. *Anesthesiology* 1991;74:209–11.
ALBERTI KG. Insulin dependent diabetes mellitus: a lethal disease in the developing world. *BMJ* 1994;309(6957):754–5.
BERGHE V DE, WOUTERS P, WEEKERS F *et al.* Intensive insulin therapy in critically ill patients. *N Engl J Med* 2001;345:1359–67.
MCNULTY GR, ROBERTSHAW HJ, HALL GM. Anaesthetic management of patients with diabetes mellitus. *Br J Anaesth* 2000;85:80–90.
WHITE NH. Management of diabetic ketoacidosis. *Rev Endocr Metab Disord* 2003;4:343–53.

Heat disorders

Effects of heat on the body

In a hot environment thermal receptors in the skin initiate reflex vasodilation and sweating through cholinergic sympathetic nerves. As body temperature rises, deep receptors in the heat centre, which is located in the preoptic region of the base of the brain, reinforce these responses.

Vasodilation is also produced by direct warming of the blood vessels of the skin. Vasodilation alone is able to dissipate resting metabolic heat production of the body as long as skin temperature is about 1°C or more below body core temperature.

Conduction and convection in the air can keep skin temperature low enough to allow this in slowly moving air up to about 32°C, but in warm air, or in cooler air during exercise, the heat produced can only be lost if sweat is formed and can evaporate to cool the skin. Heat acclimatisation allows sweat to be formed in large amounts and with a lower salt content.

If heat loss is insufficient the consequent rise in body temperature leads to hyperventilation, cerebral dysfunction, irritability and confusion, and ultimately to cardiovascular collapse and cessation of sweating with a rise in body temperature and death. As body temperature rises above 41°C heat denaturation of proteins causes damage first to large cells of the cerebellum and cerebral cortex, and later to vascular endothelium, hepatic and renal cells, and striated muscle. Almost all cells of the body are killed if temperature rises of 50°C for a few minutes.

Heat stroke

Definition

Heat stroke (HS) is characterised by dysfunction of the heat regulatory mechanism, with altered mental status (ranging from confusion to coma) and elevated core body temperature in excess of 41°C (105.8°F). It can be produced in normal people by several hours of physical exercise in a hot, humid environment close to or above body temperature. Exercise in hot, dry air can provoke HS if sweating is limited, whether by lack of acclimatisation to heat, by the rare condition of congenital absence of sweat glands, by dehydration, or by a failure of sweating known as tropical anhydrosis, which can follow prolonged exposure to hot climates (usually preceded by 'prickly heat' due to dysfunctioning sweat glands). Sweating may be compromised by intake of drugs: barbiturates, phenothiazines and anticholinergics. Other predisposing factors are generalised autonomic dysfunction as in diabetes mellitus, old age and alcoholism. Occasionally HS is due to damage to the heat-loss centre in the preoptic region of the brain, usually as a result of haemorrhage, encephalitis, tumour or surgery.

Recognition

Premonitory symptoms are headache, dizziness, nausea, visual disturbances, confusion and convulsions. Coma may ensue. The skin is hot, flushed (cyanosis may be present), and usually dry (although sweating may be present). Body temperature is >41°C and may be as high as 46.5°C (115.6°F). Hyperventilation may cause an initial respiratory alkalosis, which is generally followed by metabolic acidosis (accumulation of lactic acid as hepatic failure develops). Initially blood pressure is normal or elevated but falls with increasing cardiac failure.

Investigation may show signs of haemoconcentration (raised haematocrit or haemoglobin), decreased blood coagulation and sometimes evidence of disseminated intravascular coagulation (DIC). The WBC count is elevated. Hypophosphataemia and hypokalaemia are not uncommon. Hyperkalaemia is associated with acute renal failure. There is scanty concentrated urine ('machine oil urine') containing protein, tubular casts and myoglobin. Serum calcium may be low in severe cases owing to it binding to the protein of damaged cells. There is enzymatic evidence of liver and muscle damage (elevated CK, SGPT (ALT), and SGOT (AST) levels).

KEYPOINT
Never assume the patient has heat stroke until you have excluded malaria.

Management

KEYPOINT
Heat stroke is a life-threatening emergency. Act quickly to prevent further injury.

Cool immediately

Mild cooling by sponging with tepid water, which is allowed to evaporate on the skin, is often more effective than intense surface cooling by very cold water or refrigerated rubber blankets; mild cooling allows high blood flow in the skin to continue and to facilitate heat loss to the body surface. This also prevents shivering. A fan facilitates this treatment. A bed has been devised on which the patient can be sprayed with tap water at 15°C and blown with hot air at 30–35°C: it consists of a net suspended over a bath which makes the disposal of faeces and vomitus simpler. This method allows body temperature to be lowered by 2°C in 6 min. Other modifications of this method of evaporative cooling have been used at the annual pilgrimage to Mecca.

Rapidity of treatment is more important than the precise method used. In mild cases, recovery is generally rapid and complete, except in the ill and elderly when mortality is often due to coexisting conditions. Severe cases of HS may die suddenly, and if they recover may show lasting cerebellar and cerebral signs.

Cooling may also be achieved by peritoneal lavage with cold potassium-free dialysate, 2 litres every 10–15 min. When rectal temperature drops to 38°C (100.4°F) discontinue active measures to lower the temperature but continue temperature monitoring. If the temperature starts to rise again, resume the cooling process. Chlorpromazine, 10–25 mg slowly i.v., may be given as required to control shivering. Maintain an adequate airway and ensure the patient is breathing. Give supplementary oxygen, 6–10 l/min, by mask or nasal prongs.

Insert an indwelling catheter to monitor urine output and maintain adequate flow of urine (0.5 ml/kg/h).

If myoglobinuria is present (brownish urine), alkalinise the urine with i.v. administration of bicarbonate, and consider the use of mannitol 0.25 g/kg i.v. to promote a diuresis. Restore extracellular fluid volume, monitoring the central venous pressure if necessary, and correct hypokalaemia. Anticonvulsant prophylaxis is indicated if cerebral irritability persists.

Prognosis

Fits and prolonged unconsciousness indicate a poor prognosis.

Post-mortem examination shows little abnormality in case of rapid death from HS, apart from degeneration of Purkinje cells and other large cells from the cerebellar and cerebral cortex. Less rapid death shows oedema and petechial haemorrhages in the brain, and sometimes in other tissues.

Water depletion heat exhaustion

Severe cases result from deprivation of water in hot environments. They are often complicated by heat stroke. Unlike other forms of heat illness, water depletion can develop more rapidly in heat acclimatised than in unacclimatised people because of the increased ability to sweat. The diagnosis is usually obvious from history and from the presence of thirst, dehydration with sunken eyes and face, and elevated serum sodium and serum protein. Haematocrit may be normal, since water loss involves equal loss of intracellular and extracellular fluid. Death occurs when weight loss is 15–25% of body weight, and is due to hyperconcentration of salts in the body fluids. (Note: shipwreck victims cannot prolong life by drinking sea water, which contains salt in higher concentration than can be excreted by the kidneys.)

Treatment

Give up to 8 litres of water by mouth during the first 24 h, if the patient can swallow. In more severe cases give up to 5 litres 5% glucose by i.v. drip.

Salt depletion heat exhaustion

Salt depletion usually develops insidiously in people working in hot environments, particularly in unacclimatised people in whom loss of salt in sweat is relatively high. Sodium intake of up to 20 g per day in food or salt tablets may be needed to prevent it; the NaCl must be accompanied by an adequate amount of water and should not be given to people presenting with signs of dehydration due to a restricted supply of water.

Symptoms

Early cases: fatigue, weakness, headache, nausea and sometimes vomiting. One characteristic symptom is the appearance of sudden, very painful muscle cramps (e.g. 'miner's cramp'), but these develop only if the salt depletion is associated with muscular exercise.

Signs are few, apart from those of dehydration of the face and the skin generally and more often low BP with marked postural hypotension. It is important to realise that serum sodium and chloride are normal in mild cases of salt depletion, since osmotic pressure is initially maintained at normal levels at the expense of falling blood volume. However, the haematocrit, serum protein and blood urea are elevated. In severe cases water is retained at the expense of osmotic pressure, so that serum sodium and chloride then fall.

Treatment

Give 25 g salt in 5 litres of water by mouth, and then ensure daily intake of salt. Severe cases: i.v. infusion of 5 litres isotonic saline.

Heat syncope

Simple fainting may occur suddenly after exertion in the heat. Intravascular volume is redistributed to the periphery of the body. Volume loss and prolonged standing may deprive the brain of sufficient perfusion.

Clinical

The patient's skin is cool and moist, the pulse is weak and there may be transient hypotension. Temperature (core) is generally normal or mildly elevated.

Outcome

The patient generally responds well to rest in recumbent position, cooling and oral rehydration.

Note that the differential diagnosis in elderly people includes syncopal episodes due to hypoglycaemia, arrhythmias, myocardial infarction or cerebrovascular accident.

Further reading

AL-ASKA AK, ABU-AISHA H, YAQUB B et al. Simplified cooling bed for heatstroke. *Lancet*, 1987;i:381.

BOUCHAMA A, KNOCHEL JP. Heat Stroke. *N Engl J Med* 2002;342:1978–88.

MILLS J, HO MT, SALBER PA, TRUNKEY DD (eds). *Current Emergency Diagnosis and Treatment*. 2nd edn. Los Altos, California: Lange Medical, 1985.

PARRY EH (ed.) *Principles of Medicine in Africa*. 3rd edn. Cambridge University Press, 2003.

WEATHERALL DJ, LEDINGHAM JGG, WARRELL DA. *Oxford Textbook of Medicine*. 2nd edn, vol. 1. Oxford University Press, 1987: 6.92–6.93.

Malignant hyperpyrexia

Malignant hyperpyrexia (MH) is a very rare (1: 190 000 in UK), inherited abnormality of the muscles. When susceptible patients are given the drugs listed in Table 6.6 their muscles contract abnormally and fail to relax, causing a massive rise in muscle metabolism. This results in a rapid rise in body temperature, acidosis, hypercarbia, hypoxia, hyperkalaemia and cardiac arrythmias, which are associated with a high mortality.

Diagnosis

Most episodes occur under anaesthesia and the following signs and symptoms may be seen:
1. A failure to relax muscles after suxamethonium.
2. Tachycardia, arrhythmias.

Table 6.6 Drugs which trigger malignant hyperpyrexia in susceptible patients

Suxamethonium
Volatile agents (esp. halothane)
Phenothiazines
Tricyclics
Monoamine oxidase inhibitor

3. Hypertension, later hypotension.
4. Rapid rise in temperature (often >2°C/h).
5. Tachypnoeic (if breathing spontaneously)
6. Cyanosis.

Management

The only drug which reverses the condition effectively is dantrolene, which is expensive and unlikely to be available in a developing country. Overall mortality without dantrolene is of the order of 50–60%. Early recognition and management will influence the outcome.

Immediately MH is suspected change the anaesthetic technique to one using safe drugs (Table 6.7) and terminate surgery as soon as possible. If dantrolene is available give it intravenously starting at 1 mg/kg and increasing to a maximum of 10 mg/kg until an effect is seen. Start active cooling by giving bladder, gastric or peritoneal washouts with ice-cold saline. Resuscitate the circulation with cold saline. Hyperventilate the patient on 100% oxygen and maintain the urine output with fluids and mannitol (myoglobin released during the attack may cause renal failure). Measure urea and electrolytes and arterial blood gases (if available) and treat hyperkalaemia and acidosis. Monitor the patient who responds to treatment for 24–48 h in case of relapse. ECG monitoring is useful as it will detect dysrhythmias and hyperkalaemia.

Table 6.7 Drugs which may be used safely in malignant hyperpyrexia patients

Diazepam
Thiopentone, propofol
Opiates
Pancuronium
Nitrous oxide
Bupivacaine
Droperidol

Without dantrolene treatment is less effective but two drugs may be tried. Intravenous hydrocortisone 50 mg/kg and procaine up to 30–50 mg/kg have both been effective in some cases. Procaine in these doses may depress the heart.

If the patient survives the episode ensure that he has the relevant information in case he requires another anaesthetic. A history of unexpected anaesthetic deaths in a family suggests the possibility of malignant hyperpyrexia. As the disease is inherited, it is likely that close relatives of the patient (parents, brothers/sisters and children) may also be affected. This can be detected by muscle biopsy testing in some centres.

Hypothermia

Definition

Occurs when the rectal temperature falls below 35°C. Serious metabolic disturbances occur if the body temperature remains below 30°C for a protracted period.

Recognition

Should be suspected in persons exposed to low environmental temperatures, especially during the night. Those at risk include homeless people, vagrants, alcoholics, refugees in tented camps and the elderly. Some patients are particularly prone to hypothermia either because of metabolic disease (e.g. hypothyroidism) or because of extensive burns. Significant hypothermia may occur without evidence of local cold injury (frostbite). Patients with a core temperature of less than 30°C will appear lethargic, mentally slow and sometimes confused. On examination there will be increased muscle tone and bradycardia. If an ECG is taken there will be bradycardia, generalised decrease in voltages and, if the core temperature is below 27°C, there may be additional slurring of the QRS complex (J wave).

Management

Prompt treatment is required in order to reverse dangerous acidosis and avoid potentially fatal arrythmias such as ventricular fibrillation. Resuscitate the patient lying down with the legs elevated, as the blood pressure tends to fall on warming. The patient should be gently warmed in front of a heat source (avoid burns from direct heat) and wrapped in blankets. An infusion of dextran or saline may help to prevent further local cold injury. If arrythmias occur and persist then sodium bicarbonate infusion (p. 441) may be given, together with specific treatment for that arrhythmia (p. 58). Treatment of the underlying condition, where appropriate, should be given.

Other metabolic crises

Hypoadrenalism

Definition

Inadequate secretion of adrenal hormones gives rise to the clinical picture of hypoadrenalism. Secretion may be suppressed directly by disease processes in the adrenals or indirectly by the administration of corticosteroids when given in large doses for periods of greater than one month.

Recognition

Acute adrenal crisis occurs in untreated cases of hypoadrenalism when there is added stress such as a pyrexial illness, trauma or gastroenteritis. It may also occur in patients who become acutely unwell on withdrawing chronic steroid therapy (e.g. asthmatics) and in treated cases of hypoadrenalism if there is prolonged vomiting of medication or inadequate boosting of medication during an intercurrent illness. Vomiting, weakness and confusion occur together with signs of shock. There will be oliguria, pre-renal uraemia and ultimately coma. Patients in whom adrenal insufficiency is due to destruction of the adrenals (most commonly caused by TB or autoimmune disease) will present with a lengthy history of weight loss, tiredness, non-specific abdominal pain and, in women, amenorrhoea. On examination the patient will be thin, there may be postural hypotension and increased pigmentation may be seen in the buccal mucosa, in friction areas, in recent scars and along skin creases. The diagnosis of tuberculous hypoadrenalism is further supported by finding adrenal calcification on the plain abdominal X-ray. Definitive diagnosis depends on demonstrating the lack of response of the adrenals to stimulation by tetracosactide (Synacthen). Low cortisol levels must often be used in practice to make a diagnosis.

Management

Acute adrenal crisis requires immediate i.v. therapy with normal saline to replace the fluid deficit – usually 3–4 litres will be required. Hydrocortisone 100 mg i.v. 6 hourly should be given initially, changing to i.m. hydrocortisone once the blood pressure is normal. Specific treatment of the precipitating cause may be indicated, as in the case of infection. For patients presenting with hypoadrenalism, but not in crisis, then replacement therapy with oral cortisone and often fludrocortisone is required. Dosage will vary but an average adult requires 20 mg cortisone in the morning, 10 mg in the evening, and 0.05 mg fludrocortisone daily. For major surgery on such patients hydrocortisone 100 mg i.m. 6 hourly should be given, one dose before the operation then for 3 days postoperatively. In cases of intercurrent illness the patient should double their normal dose of cortisone and, if vomiting occurs, i.m. hydrocortisone 100 mg daily should be given.

Further reading

COOPER MS, STEWART P. Corticosteroid Insufficiency in acutely ill patients. *N Engl J Med* 2003;348:727–34.

Thyroid crisis

Definition

A life-threatening complication of hyperthyroidism with increase in severity of the clinical features of thyrotoxicosis. It may occur in patients with undiagnosed hyperthyroidism, in poorly controlled patients with intercurrent infection, and in surgical patients who have been inadequately prepared for thyroidectomy.

Recognition

The patient will have signs of hyperthyroidism (tachycardia, tremor, weight loss, exophthalmos) but in addition will have marked agitation, confusion, fever and even coma. There may be atrial fibrillation and cardiac failure. Diagnosis is made clinically and treatment is commenced without waiting for thyroid hormone levels (which are obviously raised).

Management

The patient requires adequate sedation, monitoring and replacement of fluids by i.v. infusion. Give propanolol 80 mg q.i.d. orally, or 1–5 mg i.v. 6 hourly. Give sodium or potassium iodide 1–2 g i.v. daily, or Lugol's solution (5% iodine with 10% potassium iodide) orally 0.1–0.3 ml t.d.s. Carbimazole 15 mg q.i.d. orally or via nasogastric tube prevents the synthesis of new thyroid hormones. The use of steroids in thyroid crisis is not of proven value.

Hypothyroidism

Definition

The clinical syndrome resulting from reduced secretion of thyroid hormones.

Recognition

Although the syndrome develops very slowly it may have gone unrecognised until the patient presents acutely to the hospital with coma, hypothermia or psychiatric problems. In the early stages the patient may complain of tiredness, weight gain, cold intolerance, hoarseness of the voice and menorrhagia in females. On examination the patient will be noted to be slow in speech and thought. There may be oedema, anaemia, dry skin and hair, bradycardia and delayed relaxation of the tendon reflexes.

Management

The clinical impression should be confirmed by measurement of thyroid hormone levels (which are low) and by finding raised plasma TSH (thyroid stimulating hormone). Treatment is by thyroid hormone replacement using thyroxine 50–100 µg daily initially, and adjusting the dose according to clinical response and thyroid function tests.

Delirium tremens

Definition

An acute confusional state with associated hyperactivity that occurs 2 to 3 days after alcohol withdrawal. It is important to recognise it for four major reasons:
1. Delirium tremens itself is associated with a significant mortality rate.
2. Its presence means that the patient has a significant alcohol problem.
3. There may be associated epileptic seizures that require treatment.
4. Alcoholics are more prone to infections because of decreased immunity.

Recognition

The patient suddenly becomes confused, restless and uncooperative. A history of alcohol abuse may be obtained from relatives. On examination there will be tachycardia, tremor, dilated pupils and in prolonged cases pyrexia. The hospitalised alcoholic will characteristically develop these symptoms and signs within 3 days of admission. The confusional state may be further complicated by grand mal convulsions (p. 177).

Management

Sedate the patient with i.v. diazepam 10–20 mg stat. Chlordiazepoxide 10 mg oral q.d.s. may be given. Check the blood glucose and if below 2.5 mmol/l give 50 ml of 50% dextrose. Commence a 5% dextrose drip. Give daily vitamin B complex, initially i.m. (e.g. Parentrovite). If convulsions are frequent and uncontrolled on the above regimen then add phenytoin 100 mg t.d.s. via nasogastric tube or orally.

Further reading

BURGER AG, PHILIPPE J. Thyroid emergencies. *Bailliere's Clin Endocrinol Metab* 1992;6(1): 77–93.

WEETMAN AP. Graves' disease. *N Engl J Med* 2000;343:1236–48.

KLEIN I, OJAMAA K. Thyroid hormone and the cardiovascular system. *N Engl J Med* 2001; 344:501–9.

7
Poisoning

Definition

Poisoning occurs when a toxic dose of harmful substance enters the body. The frequency and mortality of accidental poisoning in tropical countries is unknown but it is probably high because of informal marketing of dangerous compounds in unlabelled bottles, the low rate of literacy, use of dangerous traditional therapies and ineffective legal control of the distribution of drugs and chemicals. The commonest poison is alcohol. Children and people working with chemicals (e.g. factory and agricultural workers) are at particular risk of accidental poisoning. Suicide is a relatively infrequent cause of poisoning. After outlining the general principles of acute severe poisoning, the management of serious common causes of poisoning in tropical countries is described.

Recognition

It is seldom possible to diagnose poisoning on clinical features (organophosphate poisoning being a notable exception) and unless it is known that the patient has been exposed to a poison the diagnosis is often reached by excluding other causes. Manifestations of severe acute poisoning include coma, convulsions, respiratory failure, hypotension, dyspnoea, diarrhoea, vomiting, and hepatic or renal failure. Suspicion of poisoning may be strengthened by suggestive clinical features (see specific poisons) or suggestive circumstances.

Management

Successful management of poisoning does not usually depend on the administration of specific antidotes but on resuscitation, reduction of further absorption of the poison and supportive care. In a few instances administration of an antidote or enhancement of excretion of the poison are indicated.

Resuscitation

This takes precedence over all other problems. Before doing anything else you must confirm the airway is safe, ventilation adequate and the circulation satisfactory. Slow inadequate respiration is a feature of central respiratory depression or muscle paralysis whereas patients struggling to breathe may have an obstructed airway, inhaled gastric contents, pneumonia or pulmonary oedema.

In poisoning hypotension may be due to central depression of the vasomotor centre, peripheral vasodilatation, cardiac arrhythmias, myocardial depression or dehydration. Engorged neck veins will distingish cardiac causes of hypotension from others. The management of hypotension is described in Chapter 2.

Cardiac arrhythmias are occasionally due to the ingestion of cardiotoxic drugs but are more likely to be due to hypoxia, metabolic acidosis or electrolyte imbalance. If the arrhythmia is severe and providing metabolic abnormalities and hypoxia have been corrected then anti-arrhythmic drugs (p. 58) may be given but they should be used cautiously if cardio-toxic drug poisoning (e.g. chloroquine, tricyclic antidepressants or digoxin) is suspected.

Prevention of further absorption of poison

This helps reduce the severity of poisoning. Poisons ingested within the previous 12 h should be removed from the stomach by inducing vomiting or performing gastric lavage. Vomiting may be induced by BPC syrup of ipecacuanha given in a glass of water (10 ml for patients 6 to 18 months, 15 ml between 18 months and 14 years and 30 ml for those over 14 years). It can be repeated after 20 min. The technique of gastric lavage is described below. In unconscious patients the airway must always be protected before gastric lavage. Both these procedures are potentially harmful in patients who have taken kerosene (paraffin) or corrosive fluids. Induced vomiting is not as effective as gastric lavage, which is indicated in all potentially serious cases. Absorption of any poison remaining in the gut is prevented by giving activated charcoal (Medicoal or Carbomix, 50–100 g in water). This can be left in the stomach after gastric lavage or given orally and can be repeated 4 hourly. Many poisons bind to the charcoal and so become non-absorbable.

Poisons absorbed through skin are less common but insecticides and occasionally other chemicals can enter the body this way and are a particular risk to agricultural and factory workers. Further absorption is prevented by removing contaminated clothes and washing contaminated skin.

TECHNIQUE OF GASTRIC LAVAGE

Unconscious patients should have a cuffed endotracheal tube passed before starting gastric lavage.

1. Elevate the foot of the bed and place the patient on the left side.
2. Pass a lubricated wide-bore (Jacques gauge 30) soft rubber tube into the stomach (50 cm in an adult) and check its position (p. 374).
3. Aspirate the stomach contents – keeping a sample for analysis.
4. Pour 300–400 ml water (less for small children) down the tube through a funnel.
5. Place the end of the tube below the patient's head to siphon back the fluid.
6. Repeat the lavage until the fluid returned is clean and clear.
7. Leave activated charcoal in the stomach.

Further reading

PRESCOTT LF. The use of repeated doses of oral charcoal in acute poisoning. *Curr Med* 1988;61–71.

Supportive care and regular monitoring

These are important. Problems likely to be encountered are listed in Table 7.1. Management is described in the appropriate sections.

Antidotes

There are only a few poisons for which there are proven antidotes and these are listed in Table 7.2.

Table 7.1 Common problems in severe poisoning

Problem	Management	Page
Respiratory failure	Oxygen and ventilate	8
	Chest physiotherapy	349
Hypotension	Volume replacement	22
	Dopamine	445
Cardiac arrhythmias	Anti-arrhythmic drugs	58
Convulsions	i.v. diazepam[1]	443
	Phenytoin	453
Hypothermia	Warming the patient	114
	Warm i.v. fluids	114
Renal failure	Pre-renal – fluid load	92
	Renal – conservative, dialysis	93–96
Hepatic failure	Protein restriction	100
	Gut sterilisation	100
Acidosis	Fluids and sodium bicarbonate	357
Secondary infection	Antibiotics	436

1 May aggravate respiratory depression.

Table 7.2 Effective antidotes in poisoning

Poison	Antidote
Opiates	Naloxone, nalorphine
Organophosphate compounds	Atropine and pralidoxime (p. 123)
Iron	Desferrioxamine (p. 126)
Carbon monoxide	Oxygen (p. 345)
Methanol	Ethanol, fomepizole (p. 125)
Paracetamol	Methionine acetylcysteine
Beta-blockers	Glucagon, beta-agonists
Warfarin	Fresh frozen plasma and vitamin K
Heparin	Protamine

Increasing elimination of the poison

Although the rate of elimination of some poisons can be increased it is seldom necessary and the risks of the procedure should be weighed against any likely gain over conservative care. The methods of enhancing elimination of poisons and the poisons to which they apply are shown in Table 7.3. These procedures should only be considered if (1) there is severe poisoning, (2) supportive care alone is likely to be insufficient, (3) high blood levels of the poison are confirmed, (4) the poison will be eliminated by the proposed technique and (5) the necessary skill and equipment are available. Forced alkaline diuresis is described on p. 127 and in Table 7.6. Dialysis and haemofiltration are usually not available.

Table 7.3 Methods of enhancing excretion of poisons

Method	Substances affected
Forced alkaline diuresis	Salicylates
	Phenobarbital
Peritoneal/haemodialysis	Ethyl alcohol
	Methanol
	Salicylates
	Phenobarbital
Haemoperfusion	Barbiturates

Specific poisons

Ethanol

Ethanol is a major component of alcoholic drinks but is also used as a solvent and in industry. Most cases of acute ethanol poisoning are due to social drinking in excess. Ethanol depresses the central nervous system, giving an initial phase of excitability and abnormal behaviour followed by inco-ordination, stupor, respiratory depression, deep coma and sometimes death. Vomiting and aspiration pneumonia are common complications.

Clinical features

The clinical features of alcohol excess are well known and the smell of alcohol on the breath is often unwisely accepted as proof of the diagnosis. People who drink to excess are subject to trauma and a subdural haematoma may cause similar features; heavy drinking may be followed by hypoglycaemia and severe electrolyte disturbances; being 'dead drunk' in a ditch and vasodilated from alcohol predisposes to hypothermia; alcoholics may have liver cirrhosis, hepatic encephalopathy and peptic ulcers and are prone to infection. Thus many conditions (Table 7.4) need to be considered before a diagnosis of alcohol poisoning is made.

Management

The management of ethanol poisoning requires conscientious supportive care with attention to airway and ventilation, electrolyte and fluid balance, appropriate nursing and frequent monitoring for complications, particularly hypoglycaemia and pneumonia. There is no specific antidote to ethanol but in severe cases (blood alcohol greater than 5 g/l) haemodialysis may be helpful.

Carbon monoxide

The gas carbon monoxide is produced from wood and charcoal fires and is also present in some varieties of domestic gas and in motor vehicle exhaust. Poisoning is usually accidental, occurring at night in cold areas when people sleep with a fire burning in a room without ventilation. Carbon monoxide binds to haemoglobin, preventing the blood from carrying oxygen effectively and reducing the amount of oxygen available to the cells.

Clinical features

These are a direct result of cellular hypoxia and the main effect is on the brain. After a phase of agitation and confusion the patient becomes progressively more unconscious; convulsions may occur and respiratory failure precedes death. Despite the severity of the hypoxia there is no cyanosis because the carbon monoxide–haemoglobin complex (carboxy-haemoglobin) is pink in colour and this colour is seen in the patient's skin, mucous membranes and blood. The diagnosis is usually apparent from the history when a person or family are found comatose in their house with a fire burning and windows closed. Spectrophotometry of the blood will confirm the presence of carboxy-haemoglobin.

Management

This requires removal of the patient from the contaminated environment, oxygen therapy to reduce tissue hypoxia and increase the rate of dissociation of carboxy-haemoglobin (and the return of normal

Table 7.4 Differential diagnosis of ethanol poisoning

Hypoglycaemia	Hypothermia
Head injury	Methanol poisoning
Electrolyte imbalance	Hepatic encephalopathy
Aspiration pneumonia	Cerebral malaria
Meningitis	

oxygen carriage and release), and protection from the complications of unconsciousness. Mechanical ventilation is recommended for all comatose patients, particularly those with respiratory depression or pneumonia. Give 100% oxygen by a tight-fitting face mask for less severe cases. Hyperbaric oxygen is indicated for severe cases, if available. Intravenous diazepam may be needed to control convulsions.

Hyperbaric oxygen increases the amount of oxygen dissolved in the plasma and may be indicated for patients who are or have been unconscious, those with neurological symptoms, cardiac complications, pregnant women or patients with a carboxyhaemoglobin level above 40%. Hyperbaric chambers are often available in dive areas throughout the tropics. For some patients late referral may still be beneficial.

Further reading

THOM SR. Hyperbaric oxygen therapy for acute carbon monoxide poisoning. *N Engl J Med* 2002;347:1105–6.

Cyanide poisoning

Cyanide poisoning may develop because of cyanide gas produced by smouldering plastics such as polyurethane or nylon. The signs are those of cellular hypoxia. CNS signs include headaches, dizziness, fits and cardiovascular effects include hypertension and tachycardia leading eventually to hypotension and collapse. Heparinised blood can be taken for urgent cyanide levels (or stored for later analysis) if they can be measured. The urgent objective in cyanide poisoning is to reduce cyanide concentrations and promote detachment of cyanide from cytochrome oxidase in the tissues. These are achieved by one or more of the following three measures:

1. Conversion of haemoglobin to methaemoglobin by an antidote such as amyl nitrite, sodium nitrite and 4-dimethylaminophenol. The percentage of methaemoglobin and carboxyhaemoglobin should be measured and should not exceed a combined 40% thus avoiding excessive reduction of oxygen carrying capacity. (NB sodium nitrite may produce vasodilatation and hypotension.)
2. Augmentation of endogenous cyanide detoxification system – giving sodium thiosulphate will provide an extra source of sulphur to accelerate the normal conversion of cyanide to non-toxic thiocyanate in the bloodstream.
3. Chelation of the cyanide – dicobalt edetate forms cobalticyanide in combination with cyanide. There is the potential for cobalt toxicity and chelation is only indicated for severe cases.

Paraffin oil (Kerosene)

Children are the usual victims of accidental kerosene poisoning as it is often kept in a soft-drink bottle in the home. Kerosene does not cause serious poisoning unless it enters the lung but a small amount in the lungs will cause extensive pneumonitis. Induced vomiting or gastric lavage are avoided because of the risk of inhalation. Pneumonitis develops within one hour of inhalation and is manifest by fever, cough, tachypnoea, and generalised pulmonary crepitations. In more severe cases there is cyanosis and respiratory failure. Hepatitis and cardiac arrhythmias occasionally complicate kerosene poisoning but serious effects other than penumonitis are uncommon.

Management

For pneumonitis oxygen and chest physiotherapy are given and ventilatory support may be required. Hydrocortisone is not beneficial and antibiotics are only indicated if there is secondary bacterial pneumonia.

Table 7.5 Management of organophosphate poisoning

	Grade severity	
	Mild/moderate	Severe
Atropine therapy		
Stat. dose[1]	1.2 mg	2.4 mg
Repeat doses every 15 minutes until reversal[2]	1.2 mg	2.4 mg
Maintenance dose	1.2 mg hourly × 12	2.4 mg $\frac{1}{2}$ hourly × 12
Followed by	1.2 mg 4 hourly × 4	1.2 mg hourly until 48 h of atropine given
Reduce absorption	Gastric lavage or wash skin	Gastric lavage or wash skin
Additional therapy	Routine support Monitoring pupils and pulse	Oxygen by mask followed by ventilation for 48 h Pralidoxime

1 All doses are for intravenous administration. Continuous infusion may be used instead of bolus injections.
2 See text for signs of reversal.

Organophosphate compounds

Organophosphate compounds are present in many easily available pesticides (e.g. diazinon, dimethoate and malathion). Poisoning can follow ingestion, absorption through skin or inhalation. Agricultural workers are at particular risk if spraying crops without protective clothing, and skin absorption may occur when these insecticides are used (in powder form) against bedbugs. Accidental or intentional ingestion is common in some urban areas, particularly in East and Central Africa. All organophosphate compounds destroy cholinesterase and allow acetylcholine to accumulate in excess. The clinical features are due to the action of acetylcholine on the central nervous system, the autonomic ganglia, the parasympathetic nerve endings and neuromuscular junctions.

Clinical features

The major ones are unmistakable: intense salivation, bronchospasm, dyspnoea, constricted non-reacting pupils and profuse cold sweating. Milder cases may have only abdominal colic, diarrhoea and small pupils. In more severe cases there is confusion and coma sometimes with muscular weakness or paralysis. Death is usually from respiratory failure due to central respiratory depression, neuromuscular paralysis or secondary pneumonia. Severe poisoning is present if there is alteration in conscious level or respiratory signs (frothy sputum, generalised pulmonary crepitations, cyanosis or respiratory distress) and these patients require more vigorous management.

Management

The objectives are to reverse the effects of acetylcholine with atropine, prevent further absorption of poison, reactivate cholinesterase if possible and give full supportive care (which in severe cases includes mechanical ventilation).

Intravenous atropine should be commenced as soon as the patient is resuscitated and hypoxia corrected. It should be continued for at least 48 h because of the risk of relapse. Guidelines for the administration of atropine according to severity of poisoning are given in Table 7.5, but the dose and duration may need to be adjusted according to response. Full atropinisation is indicated when the pupil size is more than 5 mm, the pulse rate is approximately 100/min and there are no other signs of parasympathetic over-activity (salivation and excessive bronchial secretions).

Treatment with atropine may need to be continued for a number of days and occasionally for some weeks.

Gastric lavage should be carried out for ingested poison and thorough washing for poisoning through skin. In severe cases oxygen should be administered and the patient ventilated for 48 h. Atropine does not counteract the central, ganglionic or neuromuscular effects of acetylcholine and severely poisoned patients benefit from pralidoxime which reactivates the cholinesterase but only if it is given within 24 h. The dose of pralidoxime is 1.0 g intravenously over 10 min and it can be repeated once after 6 h if necessary.

Further reading

NHACHI CF. Organophosphate poisoning and management, an update. *Cent Afr J Med* 2001;47:134–6.

LUND C, MONTEAGUDO FSE. Therapeutic protocol No. 1. Early management of organophosphate poisoning. *S Afr Med J* 1986; 69:6.

TAFURI J, ROBERTS J. Organophosphate poisoning. *Ann Emerg Med* 1987;16:193–202.

Chloroquine

An overdose of chloroquine can be rapidly fatal and is usually taken intentionally. The drug is rapidly absorbed from the gastrointestinal tract, leading to transient high serum levels, which cause myocardial depression and vasodilation leading to idioventricular cardiac arrhythmias, cardiac arrest and hypotension.

Clinical recognition

This depends on the history of ingestion as there are no characteristic features. Vomiting may occur soon after ingestion and patients with chloroquine overdose are particularly likely to inhale gastric contents. Signs (if present) relate to cardiac arrhythmias and peripheral circulatory collapse and indicate severe poisoning; these patients have a disproportionate degree of tissue hypoxia and a high incidence of irreversible and unexpected cardiac arrest. The severity of poisoning alters management and may be estimated if the number of tablets taken can be ascertained. Ingestion by an adult of more than 5.0 g of chloroquine base (equivalent of approximately 33 tablets of the usual preparations of chloroquine including Nivaquine, Aralen, Resochin and Avloclor) is almost always fatal and death may follow ingestion of half that dose. The ECG is likely to show abnormalities of the ST segment and inverted T waves; prolongation of the QRS complex beyond 0.12 seconds indicates severe poisoning, as does the presence of cardiac arrhythmias or hypotension (systolic blood pressure <100 mmHg).

Management

Severe cases require prompt gastric lavage (with the airway protected), correction of hypotension and measures to prevent serious cardiac arrhythmias which include treating hypoxia. Early mechanical ventilation with added oxygen is recommended for all patients with serious poisoning. Adrenaline will oppose the myocardial depressant action of chloroquine and counteract hypotension. It is given by intravenous infusion (see A to Z of Drugs) by increments until systolic blood pressure is 100 mmHg. Alternatively, dopamine may be used. Diazepam (1–2 mg/kg/24 h by continuous intravenous infusion) reduces the effects of chloroquine on the myocardium and reduces the mortality of severe chloroquine poisoning. The mode of action of diazepam is not known. Patients judged to have mild poisoning (fewer than 10 tablets) can be treated conservatively once gastric lavage is done. They should be kept under observation with blood pressure (and if possible cardiac) monitoring for about 24 h.

Further reading

MCKENZIE AG. Intensive therapy for chloroquine poisoning. A review of 29 cases. S Afr Med J 1996;86:597–9.

Methanol

Methanol is present in solvents, paints and paint removers, varnishes and anti-freeze, but poisoning is usually from methanol put in alcoholic drinks. Infrequently, methanol poisoning follows inhalation or cutaneous absorption of methanol from one of the materials mentioned above. Methylated spirits contain only 5% methanol and their toxicity is due to ethanol. In tropical countries methanol poisoning is usually from illegally distilled alcohol consumed in bars in the poorer parts of towns and a number of victims may present within a few hours of each other; it is important to find out where they were drinking and prevent others being poisoned. Since the onset of poisoning is delayed for from 8 to 36 h after ingestion, those already poisoned can be traced and treatment begun before major symptoms appear.

Clinical features

These arise because methanol is metabolised to formic acid and formaldehyde. The major features are metabolic acidosis and impaired vision. The mortality is high and survivors may be permanently blind. After a latent interval of up to 36 h (usually 12–18 h), nausea, vomiting and abdominal pain develop and are followed by altered vision, decreasing conscious level, coma and death from respiratory or circulatory failure. The earliest signs are in the eyes, where there may be pallor of the optic disc and impairment of the pupillary response to light. Acidotic breathing develops later and the presence of acidotic breathing and dilated non-reactive pupils is virtually diagnostic of severe methanol poisoning. Complications include hypoglycaemia or hyperglycaemia, electrolyte imbalance and pulmonary oedema. Severe acidosis leads to circulatory and respiratory failure.

Management

Specific management depends on two facts. Firstly poisoning is due to the metabolites of methanol and secondly methanol is metabolised by the same enzyme (alcohol dehydrogenase) as ethanol. Therefore ethanol blocks the enzyme and reduces methanol metabolism and the severity of the effects. Metabolic abnormalities present when the patient is first seen (i.e. acidosis, electrolyte imbalance, hypoglycaemia or hyperglycaemia) must be corrected and progress monitored by clinical and biochemical parameters.

Acidosis is corrected by giving sodium bicarbonate intravenously and large amounts (up to 2 mol) may be needed. If possible the blood pH should be monitored. Ethanol can be given orally but intravenous preparations may be available and are more reliable. The initial dose is 50 g (equivalent to 125 ml whisky/gin/vodka by mouth) followed by 10–12 g/h while monitoring progress. Care should be taken to avoid fluid and sodium overload leading to pulmonary oedema but this also develops as a result of acidosis. Blood sugar monitoring is required and correction of hyperglycaemia (with insulin) or hypoglycaemia (with dextrose) may be necessary. Intravenous folinic acid (30 mg i.v. 6 hourly) may protect the retina. In severe cases dialysis should be considered.

Recently good results have been obtained with i.v. fomepizole, an inhibitor of alcohol dehydrogenase, which has fewer side effects than ethanol.

Further reading

BRENT J. Fomepizole for the treatment of methanol poisoning. *N Engl J Med* 2001; 344:424–9.

Salicylates (Aspirin)

Aspirin poisoning is usually accidental and is most common in young children. The main effects are due to direct stimulation of respiration causing a resipratory alkalosis together with metabolic changes, leading to a metabolic acidosis and sometimes hypoglycaemia. In addition, a direct action of salicylates on the brain causes nausea and vomiting, altered conscious level and respiratory depression. Effects on the auditory nerve account for tinnitus and deafness. Despite anticoagulant effects of salicylates spontaneous bleeding rarely occurs.

Clinical features

These develop soon after ingestion. Nausea, vomiting and abdominal pain are followed by general irritability, tinnitus and impaired hearing. In more severe cases breathing becomes rapid and there may be excess sweating, hyperpyrexia, dehydration, excitement, tremors, confusion and coma. Non-cardiogenic pulmonary oedema occurs but infrequently. In moderate and severe cases hypokalaemia, hyperglycaemia or hypoglycaemia, and a mixed respiratory alkalosis and metabolic acidosis are present and identified by blood tests. Blood salicylate greater than 750 mg/l indicates severe poisoning.

Management

Immediate steps to be taken are initial resuscitation followed by gastric lavage and the use of activated charcoal (p. 119). Electrolytes, blood sugar and blood pH should be measured and corrected; sodium bicarbonate is given for severe acidosis. Cooling may be necessary for hyperpyrexia. In critically ill patients or severe poisoning as judged by serum salicylate measurement, forced alkaline diuresis may be indicated (see Table 7.6).

Iron

Iron poisoning usually occurs in children who mistake brightly coloured sugar coated iron tablets for sweets.

Clinical features

These develop within 6 h of ingestion if significant amounts have been absorbed. The initial effects are irritation of the gastrointestinal tract, leading to abdominal pain, nausea, vomiting and diarrhoea; vomit and stool are characteristically grey or black. More serious effects develop 12 to 48 h after ingestion and include shock, hyperglycaemia, metabolic acidosis, coma and renal or hepatic failure. Ulceration of the small bowel may cause bleeding and heal with formation of a stricture. The diagnosis depends on the history, the grey/black colour of vomit and stool and on the level of serum iron. Iron tablets are radio-opaque and may be visible on straight abdominal X-ray.

Management

Reduce further absorption of iron from the stomach, provide supportive care and in severe cases enhance iron excretion. Following gastric lavage, 5.0 g of desferrioxamine is left in the stomach. This chelates the iron, which cannot then be absorbed. Clinically severe cases should also receive desferrioxamine 2 g i.m. followed by an infusion of desferrioxamine 15 mg/kg/h with reducing doses as

Poisoning

Table 7.6 Forced alkaline diuresis

Indications	Contraindications
Severe poisoning with	Impaired renal function
Salicylates	Hypotension not responding to volume replacement
Phenobarbital	Cardiac disease
Table 7.3 criteria fulfilled (p. 120)	No facilities to monitor electrolytes

Technique
Infuse
   Normal saline 0.5 l   In rotation at 1.5 to 2.0 l/h +   Up to total of 6.0 l
   5% dextrose water 0.5 l   potassium chloride 20 mmol/l
   1.26% (0.5 l) sodium bicarbonate

Monitor
Urine pH and maintain between 7.5 and 8.5[1]
Fluid balance
Electrolytes hourly
Lung bases and JVP at least hourly

Complications
Hypokalaemia, hypocalcaemia and hypomagnesaemia
Pulmonary oedema

---

1 Urine pH should be measured using narrow-range litmus indicator papers. If the urinary pH is outside the desired range of 7.5–8.5 the proportion of normal saline to sodium bicarbonate infused is altered. When the pH is too low correction requires more sodium bicarbonate and proportionately less saline and the converse is required if the pH is too high.

---

improvement occurs (maximum dose 80 mg/kg/24 h). Shock and coma indicate severe poisoning but even when the clinical condition is satisfactory severe poisoning is likely to develop if the serum iron is greater than the anticipated iron binding capacity (usually about 90 μmol/l), the white blood count is greater than 15×10^9/l, the blood sugar greater than 8.3 mmol/l within 6 hours of ingestion, or tablets are visible on plain abdominal X-ray. If facilities are not available to measure serum iron, severe poisoning can be recognised if after a single dose of desferrioxamine 50 mg/kg (maximum dose 2.0 g i.m.) the urine colour becomes orange or red.

Snake bite

All snakes feed on animal prey and have sharp teeth. Poisonous (venomous) snakes have fangs, which are hollow teeth through which venom is discharged during a bite. Snakes usually bite humans in self-defence out of fear when disturbed. Their victims are usually children and young adults who walk barefoot.

Snakes may be venomous or avenomous. Venom contains enzymes which may be cytotoxic, neurotoxic, haemotoxic or myotoxic. The different types of snake and their venom are classified in Table 7.7.

Snake bite is a common cause for admission to ICU and mechanical ventilation in many parts of the tropics, particularly Papua New Guinea.

Recognition

The snake has usually been seen but is unlikely to have been accurately identified merely from its appearance by startled victims or bystanders. If the snake has been

Table 7.7 Venomous snakes

Snake group	Names	Fangs (Figure 7.1)	Effects of venom
Viperidae	Russell's viper True vipers and adders	Anterior, curved, mobile, long	Cytoxotic, haemotoxic
Crotalidae	Rattlesnakes Malayan pit viper	Anterior, curved, long	Haemotoxic, cytotoxic
Elapidae	Cobras, mambas, kraits, harlequin	Anterior, short, mobile, gum covered	Neurotoxic
Colubridae	Boomslang	Back-fanged	Haemotoxic
Hydrophidae	Sea snakes	Short, fixed, erect, anterior	Myotoxic

killed then a positive identification can be made. Examine the area of the bite carefully for fang marks and local tissue effects. Non-venomous snakes do not have fangs, but teeth marks causing a small ragged wound without much local reaction may be seen with the aid of a magnifying glass.

Anyone bitten by a venomous snake may present with an anaphylactic reaction, with or without shock. The treatment of anaphylaxis is described on p. 30, and if there is upper airway obstruction with laryngeal oedema, an endotracheal intubation or a tracheostomy may be necessary (see pp. 329 and 359).

Cytotoxic venom causes local pain and swelling. Tissue necrosis may occur but may take some days to develop. Always check the circulation in a limb distal to the snake bite.

Haemotoxic venom may cause disseminated intravascular coagulation (DIC) which is manifest as petechiae and a bleeding tendency. Frank bleeding from the gums, gastrointestinal tract or urinary tract may not develop for 48 h. Intracerebral haemorrhage may cause coma or convulsions. Coagulation tests can be used to monitor the progress of the patient.

Neurotoxic venom causes myasthenia, the first sign of which may be ptosis. This is followed by bulbar palsy and intercostal muscle paralysis resulting in inadequate breathing. Excess salivation may result in aspiration. Cobra venom has a cardiotoxic effect also and mamba venom may cause convulsions. The black-necked or spitting cobra sprays venom at the face of its prey and is accurate up to 2 m. This venom causes conjunctivitis and even blindness if not washed out immediately.

Myotoxic venom causes muscular pain and in severe cases trismus, muscle weakness including blurring of vision due to weakness of the muscles of eye movement, myoglobinuria and renal failure.

Management

All snake bites will benefit from appropriate local treatment which includes cleaning, elevation of the limb unless a tourniquet is to be applied, antibiotics if local reaction is severe and anti-tetanus toxoid. However, anaphylaxis with laryngeal oedema and circulatory collapse, myasthenia and respiratory failure due to inadequate breathing, or disseminated intravascular coagulation are the critical problems which require immediate therapy. The use of antivenom is discussed under the appropriate species of snake. Antivenom should not be given for non-venomous snakes or if there is no severe reaction and the snake has not been identified. Anaphylactic reactions to antivenom may be fatal and a test dose should always be given first.

(a) Viperine fangs: anterior, curved, long and mobile.

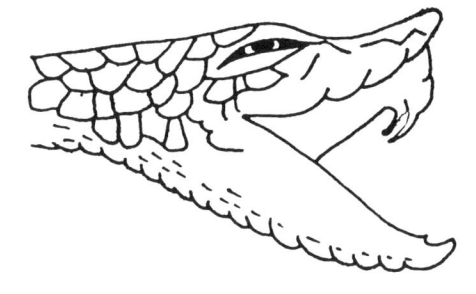

(b) Elapid fangs: anterior, short, fixed and gum-covered.

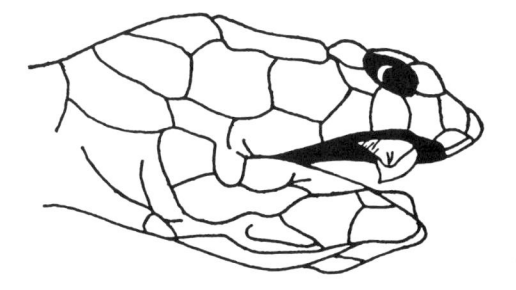

(c) Colubrid fangs: posterior and short with restricted mobility.

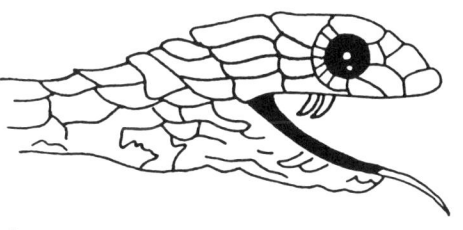

Figure 7.1 Types of fangs in venomous snakes.

KEYPOINT
Do not give antivenom when there are no systemic effects and the snake has not been identified. Do not withold antivenom, for fear of anaphylaxis when it is clearly indicated Large doses especially in children, may be required. Observe patients with snake bite carefully Systemic effects may develop slowly.

Snake identified

VIPERIDAE
(adders) – anterior, long, curved fangs
Tourniquets should not be applied as they concentrate the effects of the cytotoxic venom in one area, resulting in more extensive tissue loss. The wound should be cleaned and the limb elevated. Release incisions as for escharotomy or fasciotomy may be required if tissue tension increases to the point where the circulation is impaired. In small children bitten by Gaboon or puff adders antivenom can be given.

Russell's viper, the Malaysian pit viper (SE Asia) and the sawscaled viper (SE Asia and Southern Africa) may cause coagulation disorders. Russell's viper is a common cause of renal failure in Burma. Mild cases are treated with fresh frozen plasma and resuscitation as required. In severe cases specific (but not polyvalent) antivenom is effective and the dose should be titrated against the clotting time of the patient.

ELAPIDAE
(cobras, mambas, harlequin) – small anterior fangs covered with a fold of gum
A tourniquet should be applied and antivenom given. A test dose of 0.1 ml venom diluted 1:10 in normal saline should be given subcutaneously. If there is no reaction 2–4 ampoules (10 ml) of antivenom are given by slow intravenous infusion in 150–200 ml saline.

If ptosis is the only sign of neurotoxicity atropine, neostigmine and oxygen therapy may delay the onset of severe symptoms. Once bulbar palsy, convulsions or inadequate breathing develop the patient will require intubation and mechanical ventilation. Deterioration in the patient's condition can develop very rapidly and since snake bites usually occur in rural areas where resources are scarce ventilatory support may have to be given using an Ambu bag.

African cobras and green mambas have a neurotoxic venom which resolves after 36–40 h.

COLUBRIDAE
(boomslang) – back-fanged
A bleeding tendency may not be noticed initially. Treatment is to support the circulatory system and provide clotting factors via fresh frozen plasma and/or fresh blood. Specific antivenom should be given.

Snake not identified

1. No fang marks, no local reaction, no systemic signs – treat as a non-venomous bite with cleaning of the area and anti-tetanus toxoid.
2. Small fang marks set close together with incipient myasthenic picture and increased salivation – apply a tourniquet and give antivenom for Elapidae. If there are convulsions assume a mamba bite and ventilate.
3. Large fang marks, intense local pain, increasing swelling without myasthenia or a bleeding tendency – probably a Gaboon or puff adder bite. Give antivenom in small children. Treat associated shock.
4. Large fang marks, intense local pain and swelling but no myasthenia or bleeding – a small adder bite which requires supportive treatment only.
5. Small fang marks with slight oozing, slight local reaction and slight bleeding, no myasthenia but a delayed bleeding tendency – back-fanged Colubridae. This requires supportive treatment, correction of coagulation defects with fresh frozen plasma and fresh blood. Renal failure may complicate DIC, so the output and quality of urine should be closely monitored.

Spider bites and scorpion stings

Lactrodectus (black widow or button) spiders are found throughout the tropics. The spiders of medical importance in the Asia-Pacific region include widow and Australian funnel-web spiders, cupboard and Australian mouse spiders. They may cause a severe local reaction complicated by a neurotoxic effect which is not usually severe enough to warrant ventilatory support.

Scorpions vary in size from 1.5 to 20 cm and have a sharp curved needle-like sting at the end of the terminal segment of their jointed tail. The local reaction to the sting may be extremely painful. Although systemic effects are rare the mortality rate from scorpion stings in some areas of the tropics is high, especially in children. Scorpion venom may cause myocarditis, pulmonary oedema, renal failure, circulatory collapse, convulsions, coma or myelopathy. The sting of the scorpion *Tirtius trinitatus* from Trinidad causes acute pancreatitis, which is discussed on p. 44. Treatment of scorpion stings where there is a systemic reaction includes specific antivenom (if available) and support of failing systems.

Victims should be observed for generalised symptoms which may occur any time from a few minutes up to 24 h or more. Vomiting, sweating and hypersalivation may suggest a systemic reaction.

Oral prazosin (0.5 mg in adults, 0.125 mg in children) may be of benefit for cardiotoxicity or pulmonary oedema. Antivenom if available should be given when systemic signs are evident.

with inability to pass urine and failure of erection.

Stonefish envenomation in tropical waters around coral reefs may occasionally require cardiopulmonary resuscitation and antivenom.

Poisoning from eating puffer fish (*Lagocephalus scleratus*) has resulted in occasional death from respiratory failure. Tetrodotoxin is the responsible agent. It is found in the liver, ovaries, and intestines of the fish and the onset occurs within 6–20 hours of ingestion. Early symptoms include nausea, paraesthesia and numbness which may progress to paralysis, and respiratory failure. Eighteen of 25 cases in Thailand required ventilation usually for 12–24 h. Gastric lavage should be given to remove toxin from the stomach. Consumption of ciguatera and paralytic shellfish poisons may cause similar effects by blocking sodium channels in myelinated and non-myelinated nerves.

Venomous stings in the sea

Box jellyfish may cause severe systemic symptoms with low back pain, excruciating muscle cramps in the limbs and trunk, headache, sweating, anxiety and restlessness. The Irukandji syndrome, so named in 1952 (due to *Carukia barnesi*), may be complicated by life-threatening hypertension, pulmonary oedema and toxic global heart dilatation. First aid measures include dousing vinegar to prevent further envenomation from inactivated stinging cells on the skin. The blood pressure needs to be monitored and hypertension treated with 5 mg phentolamine i.v.

Reversible parasympathetic dysautonomia following stinging by another species of box jelly fish (*Chironex fleckeri*) has been reported. The case presented with gaseous abdominal distension, a distended bladder

Further reading

ABROUG F. Serotherapy in scorpion envenomation: a randomised controlled trial. *Lancet* 1999;354:906–9. (No benefit in routine administration of scorpion antivenom).

CHAND RP. Reversible parasympathetic dysautonomia following stinging attributed to the box jelly fish (*Chironex fleckeri*). *Aust NZ J Med* 1984 Oct;14(5):673–5.

FENNER PJ. Fatal envenomation by jellyfish causing Irukandji syndrome. *Med J Aust* 2002;177:362–3.

GOLD BS, DART RC, BARISH RA. Bites of venomous snakes. *N Engl J Med* 2002;347: 347–352.

IBISTER GK *et al*. Puffer fish poisoning: a potentially life-threatening condition. *Med J Aust* 2002;177(11–12):650–3.

KANCHANAPONGKUL J. Puffer fish poisoning: clinical features and management experience in 25 cases. *J Med Assoc Thai* 2001 Mar;84(3):385–9.

KHAN MN. Scorpion stings in the Middle East. *Postgrad Doct* 1988;12(1):25–6.

LALLOO DG et al. Severe envenomation by the taipan (*Oxyuranus scutellatus*) *Med J Aust* 1997;167(1):54–5.

MILANI JUNIOR R et al. Snake bites by the jararacucu (*Bothrops jararacussu*): clinicopathological studies of 29 proven cases in Sao Paulo State, Brazil. *Q J Med* 1997 May;90(5):323–34.

MILLS AR, PASSMORE R. Pelagic paralysis. *Lancet* 1988;1(8578):161–4.

MWINT-LWIN, WARRELL DA, PHILLIPS RE, et al. Bites by Russell's viper (*Vipera russelli siamensis*) in Burma: Haemostatic, vascular and renal disturbances and response to treatment. *Lancet* 1985;ii:1259–64.

SOLLEY GO, VANDERWOUDE C, KNIGHT G. Anaphylaxis due to red imported fire ant sting. *Med J Aust* 2002;176:521–3.

TREVETT AJ et al. The efficacy of antivenom in the treatment of bites by the Papuan taipan (*Oxyuranus scutellatus canni*). *Trans R Soc Trop Med Hyg* 1995;89(3):322–5.

TUN-PE et al. The efficacy of tourniquets as a first-aid measure for Russell's viper bites in Burma *Trans Roy Soc Trop Med Hyg* 1987;81:403–5.

WARRELL DA et al. The emerging syndrome of envenoming by the New Guinea small-eyed snake *Micropechis ikaheka*. *Q J Med* 1996 Jul;89(7):523–30.

WARRELL DA. Attacks by animals: bites, stings and other injuries. In: Ellis BW, Paterson-Brown S (eds). *Hamilton Bailey's Emergency Surgery* 13th edn. London: Arnold, New York: OUP, 2000:787–97.

WARRELL DA. An open, randomized comparative trial of two antivenoms for the treatment of envenoming by Sri Lankan Russell's viper (*Daboia russelii russelii*). *Trans R Soc Trop Med Hyg* 2001;95(1):74–80.

WARRELL DA. Taking the sting out of ant stings: venom immunotherapy to prevent anaphylaxis. *Lancet* 2003;361(9362):979–80.

General reading in poisoning

GUPTA S, TANEJA V. Poisoned child: emergency room management. *Indian J Paediatr* 2003;70:S2–8.

MOKHLESI B, LEIKEN JB, MURRAY P et al. Adult toxicology in critical care: part I: general approach to the intoxicated patient. *Chest* 2003;123:577–92.

MOKHLESI B, LEIKIN JB, MURRAY P et al. Adult toxicology in critical care: Part II: specific poisonings. *Chest* 2003;123:897–922.

See also website www.spib.axl.co.uk

8
Infections

Definition and introduction

Infection is defined as invasion and destruction of tissues by micro-organisms.

Infection may be the primary cause of a critical illness or may be a complication of another serious condition. Patients with immune deficiency are prone to develop severe or opportunistic infections. Endotracheal tubes, urinary catheters and central venous lines can provide bacteria with a route of entry to the body whereby they may cause infection. Thus critical illness is often complicated by infection because resistance to infection is reduced and because treatment involves the introduction of tubes and catheters into the patient.

The basic principles governing the prevention and control of infection are described in Chapter 16. This chapter aims to describe the recognition and management of specific life-threatening infections.

Septicaemia

Definitions

Septicaemia is defined as the presence of pathogenic bacteria in the circulation which invade and destroy cells throughout the circulation. The septicaemic process occurs in all vascular beds and so any tissue or organ of the body may be affected.

Septic shock is a term used to describe the combination of septicaemia and shock.

It is often called endotoxic shock because endotoxin release from Gram-negative bacilli is responsible for the widespread intravascular and endothelial damage throughout the microcirculation. However, septicaemia and septic shock may also be caused by Gram-positive bacteria which release exotoxins or fungal infection.

In this book septic shock is classified as a type of hypovolaemic shock because leakage of fluid from the circulation into the interstitial space causes hypovolaemia (p. 20). Initially hypotension results from a low peripheral resistance, which is caused by the shunting of blood away from the capillary beds through arteriovenous channels. Later, blood re-enters the capillaries and it is at this stage that fluid leaks out of the vascular space through the capillary endothelia. The fluid loss results in poor blood flow and thus poor oxygen delivery to the tissues. The circulatory management of septic shock is described in detail in Chapter 2.

Clinical recognition

Septicaemia presents in a variety of ways. The severity may range from a mild tachycardia and fever to unexplained confusion or frank shock. Anyone in whom deterioration is rapid or unexplained should be suspected of having developed septicaemia. The patient may complain of fever, headache, rigors or some localised infection.

However many are so confused, lethargic or comatose that no history is available.

Pyrexia, tachycardia, tachypnoea and altered mental state are common signs. A subnormal temperature is associated with a poor prognosis. Initially the circulation is hyperdynamic, as manifest by a bounding pulse and warm peripheries. Later the peripheries become cold and clammy as the state of the circulation deteriorates. Oliguria, respiratory failure, jaundice, cardiac failure, or gastrointestinal bleeding may develop as a result of microcirculatory damage and underperfusion of vital organs (p. 28). Petechiae or frank bleeding may be present if there is disseminated intravascular coagulation (DIC; see p. 34).

Shock may develop suddenly, particularly during a procedure such as laparotomy or instrumentation of the genito-urinary tract if large numbers of bacteria are dislodged into the circulation within a short space of time. Often, however, shock may develop some time after the onset of septicaemia.

Investigations

The white blood-cell count (WBC) is usually raised except in severe septic shock where a low WBC signifies a poor prognosis. Blood cultures will often identify the causative organism and, whenever possible, should be taken before antibiotic therapy is started. Thrombocytopaenia, a prolonged bleeding time and other changes consistent with DIC (p. 34) may also be present.

How to determine the cause

The cause of septicaemia is often obvious from the history and examination. When the source of sepsis is not immediately apparent re-examine the patient looking in particular for:
1. neck stiffness or a positive Kernig's sign;
2. enlarged lymph nodes;
3. infection in the ears, nose, mouth or sinuses;
4. cellulitis, abscesses, ulcers or pressure sores (examine the entire skin surface including the external genitalia);
5. signs of pneumonia or empyema;
6. peritonitis, intra-abdominal or pelvic infection (palpate the abdomen and do a rectal or vaginal examination).
7. endocarditis, murmurs, splinter haemorrhages.

Urinary catheters and central venous lines may act as a source of infection if they become contaminated by bacteria. If no other obvious source for sepsis is found remove the catheter or line and send the tip for culture.

Relevant diagnostic investigations include:
1. urine microscopy and culture;
2. blood slide for malaria and trypanosomes in endemic areas;
3. blood culture;
4. sputum or endotracheal secretion microscopy and culture;
5. lumbar puncture if unexplained fever, confusion or coma;
6. chest X-ray;
7. peritoneal aspiration using a 21-gauge needle (green) where peritonitis is suspected (in the absence of abdominal ultrasound or CT).

The following conditions are the most commonly overlooked:
1. meningitis (p. 154);
2. sinusitis leading to osteomyelitis of the skull or intracranial abscess, particularly if orbital cellulitis (p. 181);
3. septic abortion, since many patients do not admit to criminal interference;
4. urinary tract infection in children;
5. diabetes presenting with infection;
6. pelvic and peritoneal sepsis;
7. septic arthritis and osteomyelitis, particularly in children;
8. malaria;
9. abscesses, pyomyositis, injection abscess;

10. pressure sores in comatose and bed-ridden patients.

Management

Delay in management may be fatal or may result in prolonged, difficult and more expensive treatment.

Resuscitate the patient

Respiratory failure and shock should be managed as described in Chapters 1 and 2.

Antibiotics

When culture facilities are available, specimens should be taken before antibiotics are started and the specimens transported to the laboratory in the correct manner (p. 303). Use the 'best guess' antibiotics until the results of culture are available. The principles of antibiotic therapy are described on p. 436. It is prudent to reserve one or two antibiotics for use only on critically ill patients in whom other antibiotics may be ineffective (e.g. 3rd and 4th generation cephalosporins and penicillins such as cefotaxime and ticarcillim).

Treat the source of sepsis

This may involve draining abscesses, debriding wounds and excising necrotic tissue, removing sutures from infected wounds, laparotomy or relaparotomy where there is peritoneal sepsis, drilling bone in osteomyelitis, and arthrotomy in septic arthritis. Antibiotic therapy will be ineffective in combating septicaemia if the primary source of sepsis is not correctly managed. Damaged heart valves may harbour bacteria causing recurrent episodes of septicaemia or may be further destroyed by bacterial invasion during septicaemia.

Treatment of complications

Septicaemia may be complicated by shock, disseminated intravascular coagulation, respiratory or renal failure. The treatment of these complications is described in the appropriate chapters. Other complications which may cause critical illness include abscesses in the brain, lungs, spine, long bones or kidneys.

Pneumonia

Pneumonia may be acquired in the community or in hospital. It is a common cause of severe illness, respiratory failure and acute respiratory distress.

Community acquired pneumonias

The typical syndrome is usually pneumococcal. Bacterial pneumonia may be severe in young children and in the presence of malnutrition, splenectomy, chronic lung disease and in immune deficiency. In healthy adults it seldom leads to respiratory failure. If there is severe acute respiratory distress it is suggestive of viral or atypical pneumonia; alternatively aspiration or chemical pneumonitis.

Viral pneumonias

Primary viral pneumonia differs from bacterial pneumonia complicating a viral infection. In viral pneumonia the virus is responsible for lung damage which is extensive and causes patchy consolidation throughout the lung fields. Respiratory insufficiency is relatively common. Adenoviruses and the viruses of influenza, measles and chicken pox are recognised causes of viral pneumonia and in immunocompromised patients other viruses may be responsible.

In contrast to bacterial pneumonia, respiratory symptoms develop a few days after the onset of general malaise, myalgia and fever. Patients with viral pneumonia always have a cough, non-purulent sputum and dyspnoea and they may be cyanosed. Auscultation of the chest is deceptive because it may be normal or there may be generalised crepitations but no signs of consolidation. Other features of the causative virus (e.g. measles) may be present. The chest X-ray reveals multiple diffuse opacities scattered throughout the lung fields. The white blood cell count is low or normal unless there is complicating secondary bacterial infection.

No antibiotic is effective against viral pneumonias and management depends on supportive care, particularly oxygen, chest physiotherapy and if necessary ventilation. Prophylactic antibiotics do not prevent secondary bacterial infection.

Severe Acute Respiratory Syndrome (SARS) is associated with viral infection (a coronavirus) and recent contact with an infected individual or travel to/from SE Asia, particularly the Guangdong province of Southern China, Hong Kong and Singapore. Severe cases will require intensive care for respiratory support and strict isolation/barrier nursing. Anti-viral agents may be helpful if available.

Atypical pneumonias

Mycoplasma and Chlamydia pneumonias

Pneumonia due to *Mycoplasma* and *Chlamydia pneumoniae* is not often severe enough to cause respiratory failure except in immunocompromised patients and patients with sickle cell disease. The lesions are usually limited to one lower lobe where there is patchy consolidation. The clinical illness is similar to viral pneumonia but dyspnoea and cyanosis are uncommon. Headache is a feature of chlamydial pneumonia. Signs of consolidation may be absent. Approximately half the patients will have a skin rash and cold agglutinins in the blood. The diagnosis is difficult depending on sophisticated culture techniques or delayed serological responses. These pneumonias respond well to tetracycline, doxycyline or erythromycin but not to penicillin.

Legionnaires' disease pneumonia

Pneumonia due to *Legionella* bacteria was first recognised in 1976. The organism commonly contaminates air-conditioning systems and epidemics may occur. Infection is acquired by inhalation but person-to-person spread does not occur. The mortality ranges from 8% to 30% and is usually due to respiratory failure.

Fever, headache and myalgia precede respiratory symptoms for up to 5 days. The patient is likely to be tachypnoeic, ill and confused. Consolidation is detectable clinically in only one-third of cases but is always present on chest X-ray and may be patchy and involve more than one lobe. The white blood-cell count is between $10 \times 10^9/l$ and $15 \times 10^9/l$ with a marked lymphopenia (usually less than $1 \times 10^9/l$). Confirmation of the diagnosis is difficult and relies on culture and serology and the condition often has to be treated without confirmation.

Specific treatment is with erythromycin. The adult dose is 1.0 g four times daily and in severe cases it should be given parenterally. Renal failure, cardiac involvement and pleural effusions may complicate the infections.

Hospital-acquired (nosocomial) pneumonias

Serious illness is commonly complicated by pneumonia due to hospital organisms, many of which are resistant to commonly used antibiotics. In some instances it can be prevented by avoiding predisposing situations and giving chest physiotherapy in those at risk. The situations that predispose to secondary pneumonia include immobility, inadequate respiratory movement and inadequate coughing, which may arise from coma, excessive sedation, uncontrolled pain, severe weakness, muscular paralysis and splinting of the diaphragm after abdominal or chest surgery or trauma. Additional predisposing causes are the use of contaminated equipment in intubation or ventilation of patients. Old age, smoking and obesity are additional risks.

Gram-negative organisms such as *Pseudomonas*, *Klebsiella*, *Proteus* and *E. coli* together with anaerobes are responsible for more than three-quarters of cases of secondary pneumonias. Because of the wide range of organisms and the probability of a high degree of antibiotic resistance sputum should, if possible, be sent for culture before commencing specific treatment with broad-spectrum antibiotics. Treatment may need to be adjusted when the culture results are received.

Infections causing paralysis

Infections involving the central nervous system (e.g. meningitis, encephalitis and brain abscess) may lead to focal paralysis, but the emphasis in this section is on infections where the dominant problems are respiratory or bulbar (palatal and laryngeal) paralysis.

Poliomyelitis

Poliomyelitis is a viral infection that, in a few cases, involves the nervous system causing meningitis and paralysis. It is spread by the faeco-oral or respiratory route and in the absence of a vaccination programme is endemic in countries with poor sanitation. In endemic areas infection is acquired in early childhood and is followed by lifelong immunity. With improved sanitation and a decrease in faeco-oral transmission there are fewer infections and less immunity in young children. Without vaccination older children and adults are then susceptible and they are more likely than young children to develop paralytic polio.

Recognition of paralytic polio

Prior to paralysis there is a febrile illness and sometimes meningitis. The virus attacks the anterior horn cells of the spinal cord, causing a flaccid lower motor neurone paralysis. Limb paralysis is characteristically asymmetrical; the limb is floppy and the reflexes absent; sensation remains normal; paralysis does not progress after 2 or 3 days and initial muscle pain resolves; there is gradual partial recovery. Occasionally the main impact is on the nuclei of the lower cranial nerves (the bulbar nuclei) and swallowing is paralysed.

Recognition of respiratory failure

Respiratory failure may arise from paralysis of the muscles of ventilation or from bulbar paralysis. *Intercostal paralysis* is recognised by the presence of a rapid respiratory rate without obvious increase in respiratory effort but with intercostal indrawing, which may be generalised or asymmetrical. *Diaphragmatic paralysis* causes the respiratory rate to rise together with increased intercostal activity and is recognised by paradoxical abdominal movement during inspiration (i.e. during inspiration the upper abdomen is drawn inwards not pushed outwards as normal). Respiratory function may be adequate or inadequate in intercostal or diaphragmatic paralysis alone but is likely to be inadequate if both occur together or there is pneumonia. *Bulbar paralysis* is characterised by difficulty in swallowing and the tendency for fluids to regurgitate up the nose or be inhaled. Respiratory depression may be associated. Bulbar paralysis may occur without any other paralysis and if these patients can be kept alive they usually make a full recovery.

The diagnosis of paralytic poliomyelitis is largely on clinical grounds and it is virtually the only condition that causes asymmetrical lower motor neurone paralysis of the limbs. Cerebrospinal fluid (CSF) examination will reveal increased protein, normal glucose levels and usually a lymphocytosis. The virus can be isolated from pharyngeal secretions, stool or CSF, and serum antibody titres rise during acute infection. The differential diagnosis is generally limited to 'polio-like' illnesses usually due to Coxsackie and other enterovirus infections.

Management

There is no effective antiviral therapy and management is supportive. Chest physiotherapy is important to prevent pneumonia in patients with respiratory muscle paralysis. The development of respiratory failure requires mechanical ventilation. The degree of recovery of muscle power is variable but seldom complete. Many patients become independent of the ventilator but remain prone to chest infections and are vulnerable to recurrent respiratory failure.

Bulbar paralysis without respiratory failure carries an excellent prognosis but requires skilled nursing to prevent inhalation pneumonia. Patients should be nursed in a head-down position and lying prone. Nasogastric or nasojejunal feeding is mandatory.

Diphtheria

Diphtheria is due to infection with *Corynebacterium diphtheriae* and a bacterial toxin is responsible for paralysis. The infection may occur in a number of sites but serious consequences usually follow pharyngeal or tonsillar infection, which is spread by aerosol. Vaccination effectively prevents diphtheria but even without vaccination serious diphtheria is relatively uncommon in tropical countries. This is attributed to the frequency of cutaneous diphtheritic ulcers, which seldom lead to severe consequences but contribute to immunity.

Recognition

Tonsillitis or pharyngitis with an adherent white membrane is the usual presentation of the acute illness. The membrane may extend to the larynx and cause respiratory obstruction. Paralysis develops 5 to 7 weeks after the initial infection and is due to toxic demyelination of peripheral nerves. Diplopia may occur but bulbar paralysis is infrequent. When it occurs palatal paralysis allows regurgitation of fluids through the nose and laryngeal paralysis aspiration into the lungs. Paralysis of the respiratory muscles may cause respiratory failure. There may be associated limb paralysis. The clinical findings are similar to those of paralytic poliomyelitis (p. 137). Confirmation of diphtheritic paralysis depends on acquiring a history of the previous illness and on the detection of rising serum antibodies.

Management

Paralysis due to diphtheria can be expected to recover completely providing the patient does not die of respiratory failure or inhalation pneumonia. By the time the paralysis has occurred it is too late to administer specific antitoxin (which should be given during the acute illness) and although penicillin or erythromycin are usually given the organism is unlikely to still be present. The most important aspects of management are prevention of inhalation pneumonia by positioning the patient as described under bulbar polio and giving nasogastric feeds, prevention of chest infections with chest physiotherapy and prompt ventilation if respiratory failure develops.

Acute ascending polyneuropathy (Guillain–Barré Syndrome)

This is an acute peripheral nerve lesion causing symmetrical ascending paralysis and occasionally sensory neuropathy. It is due to peripheral nerve demyelination and is attributed to a form of hypersensitivity reaction. In about half the cases there is a history of an infection (usually respiratory) about 3 weeks before the onset of the paralysis.

Recognition

The usual presentation is with progressive symmetrical weakness of the legs, which may progress over a few days to complete paralysis and ascend to involve spinal and abdominal muscles, the intercostal muscles, the upper limbs and the diaphragm. Occasionally there is bulbar paralysis and involvement of other cranial nerves. The paralysis is of lower motor neurone type with flaccidity and absent reflexes. The signs of intercostal, diaphragmatic and bulbar paralysis have already been described (p. 137). Urinary retention may occur.

The diagnosis is based largely on the ascending and symmetrical paralysis together with the absence (usually) of sensory loss. White blood cells in the CSF may be slightly increased and the protein is usually raised. Other causes of generalised paralysis, such as snake bite (p. 127) and myaesthenia gravis, are unlikely to cause confusion because of the ascending pattern of paralysis in this condition.

Management

The paralysis recovers gradually and the aim of management is to prevent the patient dying of respiratory failure or pneumonia. There is no specific therapy and corticosteroids have been shown to be ineffective and possibly harmful. Treatment consists of supportive care, chest physiotherapy and mechanical ventilation for respiratory failure, which may need to be continued for some weeks. Some centres are using plasmaphoresis with effect. The use of gamma globulin may be helpful if available.

Further reading

AGGARWAL AN, GUPTA D, LAL V et al. Ventilatory management of respiratory failure in patients with severe Guillain–Barré syndrome. *Neurol India* 2003;5:203–5.

Viral haemorrhagic fevers

The viral haemorrhagic fevers are specific infections with a number of clinical features in common, notably the occurrence of generalised haemorrhage. A number of different viruses are responsible and each has a limited geographic distribution (Table 8.1). Most are zoonoses (of animal origin); some are due to arbor viruses spread by mosquitoes (e.g. yellow fever,

Table 8.1 Geographic distribution of viral haemorrhagic fevers

Yellow fever	Africa and South America
Haemorrhagic dengue	S and SE Asia, Caribbean, Pacific Islands
Chikunyunga	Africa, S and SE Asia, India
Rift Valley fever	Africa and the Arabian Peninsula
Congo-Crimean fever	Africa and parts of Russia
Kyansur Forest fever	India
Lassa fever	West and Central Africa
Bolivian haemorrhagic fever	Bolivia in South America
Argentinian haemorrhagic fever	Argentina in South America
Marburg and Ebola infections	Africa

dengue haemorrhagic fever and Rift Valley fever) or ticks (e.g. Congo–Crimea haemorrhagic fever); others are due to arena viruses (e.g. Lassa, Bolivian and Argentinian haemorrhagic fevers) and infection is acquired from wild rodents; others (Marburg and Ebola virus infections) are due to viruses as yet unclassified and the source of infection is not known. Lassa, Marburg, Ebola and Congo–Crimean haemorrhagic fevers can spread from person to person. Most reports implicate contact with blood and other body fluids or tissues but there is some evidence that Lassa fever can be transmitted by aerosol. The use of unsterile syringes was responsible for a large number of cases in an epidemic of Ebola virus infection and a doctor has died of Lassa fever after performing a post-mortem examination. However the risk to staff caring for patients and to laboratory staff is small unless basic precautions are neglected.

Recognition

In the early stages viral haemorrhagic fevers are difficult to recognise and the diagnosis is often not suspected until generalised bleeding occurs during the second week of illness. Suggestive features before there is bleeding include the absence of any clinical pointers to the site of infection, myalgia that is more severe than usual, marked prostration, conjunctival congestion, severe exudative pharyngitis, a macular skin rash and a low or normal WBC. The diagnosis should be considered in any patient with an undiagnosed febrile illness and hypotension in whom malaria and septicaemia have been excluded. Later, bleeding from the skin, gums, urinary or gastrointestinal tract may develop and lead to shock and/or anaemia. Another serious complication is secondary bacterial infection. The differential diagnosis of acute fevers without localising signs and with a low WBC include malaria, typhoid and other virus infections. The diagnosis of a viral haemorrhagic fever is confirmed by serology or virus isolation but these techniques are seldom available.

Management

The real importance of establishing a firm diagnosis is containment of the infection within both the hospital and the community. Even a suspected case should be notified to the national health authorities. If one of the viruses which can spread from person to person is suspected then barrier nursing and disinfection of linen and excreta should be implemented and the laboratory staff should be warned that samples may be infectious.

There is no specific treatment of the infection and management is limited to supportive care. Hypovolaemia or anaemia due to bleeding is best corrected with fresh blood, which contains clotting factors. Secondary bacterial infections require aggressive treatment. Serum from convalescent patients has been shown to be helpful in some infections.

Life-threatening malaria

Definition

Life-threatening malaria can be defined as malaria with any of the complications listed in Table 8.2. After initial comments on the dangers of untreated serious malaria this section will describe the individual's risk and some difficulties that may be encountered in the diagnosis before describing the major problems and their management.

Table 8.2 Causes of death in malaria

Cerebral malaria
Hypoglycaemia
Severe anaemia
Renal failure
Pulmonary oedema
Septicaemia

The hazard to the patient

Untreated cerebral malaria is nearly always fatal and other serious complications of malaria also carry a high mortality. Treatment can reduce the mortality of serious malaria to 10%. Patients who recover from life-threatening malaria rarely have any residual disability. It is one of the most rewarding and cost-effective diseases to treat.

Those at risk

Life-threatening malaria occurs in people with no immunity to malaria. People who live in areas where malaria is transmitted throughout the year acquire partial immunity to malaria following repeated attacks in early childhood. This immunity protects against the serious effects of malaria and is lost during pregnancy, if exposure to malaria ceases and if regular malaria prophylaxis is taken. Single or occasional attacks of malaria do not lead to immunity. **Therefore those at risk of life-threatening malaria are children under five, pregnant women, everyone living in areas where malaria is seasonal and visitors from non-malarious areas.** *Plasmodium falciparum* is the main type of malaria in tropical Africa. It is the only type of malaria that commonly causes death.

When to suspect life-threatening malaria

Any deterioration in a patient with malaria is likely to be due to development of one of the complications (Table 8.3). The initial

Table 8.3 Management of the complications of malaria

Problem	Causes	Recognition	Management
Cell hypoxia	Red cell clumping Hypotension Anaemia	Confusion/coma Renal failure	Antimalarials (pp. 145–148) Transfusion
General hypoxia	Pneumonia Pulmonary oedema	Chest signs	Antibiotics ? Diuretics ? Ventilate
Hypotension	Hypovolaemia Septicaemia	Cold patient Warm patient	i.v. fluids Antibiotics
Hypoglycaemia	Parasites ++ Quinine	Confusion Blood glucose < 2.2 mmol/l	i.v. 50% dextrose
Haemolysis	Parasites ++ G6PD deficiency ? Others	Anaemic ++ Jaundice Black urine	Tranfuse (p. 31)
Hyperpyrexia	Parasites ++	Rectal T >39°C	Cooling (p. 111)
Infection	Lowered immunity i.v. cannulae etc.	Remains febrile	
Pregnancy			
Maternal	Parasites ++ Hypoglycaemia + Pulmonary oedema		Adequate antimalarials +
Fetal	Placental damage Sick mother	Premature labour IU death	General measures

symptoms of malaria are non-specific. Fever and general malaise are common and may be associated with headache, diarrhoea, anorexia, vomiting or cough. There are no physical signs that are diagnostic of malaria.

How to confirm the diagnosis

To diagnose life-threatening malaria, parasites must be present on the blood slide, the patient must be a non-immune and there must have been exposure to malaria within the previous 6 weeks. Recent consumption of antimalarial drugs whether for prophylaxis or treatment does not exclude the diagnosis, particularly if the patient has been vomiting and in areas of chloroquine-resistant malaria.

The ICT rapid test is an immunochromatographic test for plasmodium antigens. A blood drop on the card shows two lines versus one for the control.

PRACTICE POINT
The diagnosis of serious malaria requires: 1. Blood slide positive; 2. Non immune patient; 3. Exposed to malaria.

Problems with blood slide diagnosis

In untreated life-threatening malaria numerous parasites are usually present on the blood slide. However a *false negative* blood slide may occur if there is faulty preparation or examination of the slide or if the patient has already received antimalarials or antibiotics. Occasionally in severe untreated malaria the parasites move to the central circulation and are undetectable in peripheral blood. **A negative blood slide does not exclude life-threatening malaria** and further slides should be carefully examined. If clinical suspicion of serious malaria is strong then antimalarial treatment should be commenced at the same time as other possible causes of the illness are being investigated. *False positive* blood slides may occur in people who have some immunity to malaria. These people do not usually get severely ill with malaria and in them a positive blood slide is not uncommon without illness. **A positive blood slide does not prove serious malaria** and in people who are partially immune to malaria a serious illness should not be attributed to malaria. If there is doubt it is reasonable to give the patient treatment for malaria, providing investigation for other causes of the illness continues.

The problems

The primary cause of life-threatening malaria is the enormous number of parasites that develop in the blood of the patient. Parasites cause the red cells to clump together in the capillaries. Even with normal blood pressure, haemoglobin and lung function the oxygen supply to cells of vital organs may be seriously diminished. In the presence of hypotension, anaemia or respiratory insufficiency tissue hypoxia is increased. These conditions are among those that may occur in complicated malaria (Table 8.3). Parasite toxins and accumulated metabolites contribute to these problems.

Cellular hypoxia

This is the major cause of cerebral malaria and renal failure and may be responsible for pulmonary oedema.

Cerebral malaria

Cerebral malaria is the commonest severe complication of malaria and accounts for up to 80% of deaths from malaria. The

Table 8.4 Conditions that must be distinguished from cerebral malaria

Hypoglycaemia
Meningitis and encephalitis
Head injury
Cerebrovascular accident
Brain abscess
Intoxication and poisoning

clinical features are varied but are all manifestations of disturbed brain function. They include confusion, delirium, abnormal and psychotic behaviour, deteriorating conscious level, focal neurological signs and epileptic fits. Fits may be the first indication of illness in children and may be focal or generalised. In addition to alteration of consciousness focal neurological signs may be present including increased tone in the limbs with hyper-reflexia, extensor plantar responses and absent abdominal reflexes. Meningism is not usually present in cerebral malaria and fever may be absent. In tropical Africa any unexplained psychiatric or neurological illness may be cerebral malaria, particularly if there is a fever. **Without a positive blood slide** the diagnosis cannot be confirmed but **in addition** the conditions listed in Table 8.4 should be excluded as far as is possible. To do this a careful history is required, blood sugar should be measured and a lumbar puncture done. Confusion in a patient with malaria may also be due to fever, hypotension, respiratory failure or septicaemia.

> KEYPOINT POINT
>
> The diagnosis of cerebral malaria is not established until hypoglycaemia and meningitis have been excluded.

In the *management* of cerebral malaria parenteral antimalarial therapy (p. 145) must be given promptly after blood slides have been taken. Blood sugar should be monitored 4 hourly until the patient recovers consciousness. Fits should be controlled by anticonvulsants (p. 179). General supportive care does not differ from that of coma of other cause (p. 175) except in the need to be aware that other complications may develop.

Renal failure

Renal failure due to severe malaria is always acute and is recognised because of oliguria or a rising blood urea and serum creatinine. Oliguria due to hypovolaemia must be distinguished from true renal failure due to acute tubular necrosis (p. 90). Cellular hypoxia affecting the kidney is largely responsible for acute tubular necrosis and the risk of this occurring is higher if the patient is hypovolaemic or hypotensive. Renal failure may also follow blackwater fever (p. 144). Apart from the administration of antimalarial therapy the treatment of renal failure in malaria is the same as from other causes and is described on p. 91.

Pulmonary oedema

Pulmonary oedema is sometimes precipitated by excess intravenous fluids but may occur in patients in normal or negative fluid balance and is then probably due to direct damage to the pulmonary capillaries. Pulmonary oedema is often a relatively late complication of malaria and is particularly likely to occur in pregnant women shortly after delivery. Dyspnoea is the cardinal feature of pulmonary oedema and fine crepitations are audible at both lung bases. If it is severe cyanosis, tachycardia, hypotension and confusion are also present. The presence of a positive fluid balance and elevated jugular or central venous pressure will distinguish acute pulmonary oedema due to fluid overload from that attributed to damage to pulmonary capillaries. Clinically it is not always possible to distinguish pulmonary oedema from aspiration pneumonia but in pulmonary oedema the chest X-ray shows widespread bilateral opacities radiating from the hilar region towards the periphery (Fig. 3.1). The *treatment* depends on the cause. In the presence of fluid overload it is the same as outlined in the management of left ventricular failure (p. 52) with oxygen and diuretics as the main therapy. In the absence of fluid overload it is the same as for acute respiratory distress syndrome (p. 14) and respiratory support may be necessary.

Hypotension

In malaria hypotension is usually due to hypovolaemia from vomiting, diarrhoea and fever and to inadequate fluid intake. In these patients the skin is cold and there is peripheral vasoconstriction and a weak pulse. Vasodilatation due to septicaemia may also cause hypotension in which case the skin is warm and the pulse full. In any patient with unexplained hypotension malaria should be considered. In a patient with confirmed malaria the presence of persistent hypotension after correction of hypovolaemia suggests septicaemia. In addition to antimalarial therapy *treatment* is with fluid replacement or is that of septicaemia (p. 135) depending on the primary cause.

Hypoglycaemia

Malaria parasites need glucose and when present in large numbers they use up the body's stores, leading to hypoglycaemia. This is a particular danger in children and in pregnant women but may occur in any patient with severe malaria. Hypoglycaemia may also be precipitated by quinine. Behavioural change or altered conscious level is characteristic of hypoglycaemia but in severe malaria other classical signs of hypoglycaemia (a bounding pulse, warm extremities, sweating and a raised systolic blood pressure) may be absent. Only frequent measurement of the blood sugar will prevent hypoglycaemia going unrecognised and the patient suffering irreversible brain damage. Confusion due to hypoglycaemia is distinguished from that due to cerebral malaria by the improved mental state which follows *treatment* of hypoglycaemia with intravenous 50% dextrose.

Haemolysis and anaemia

The main cause of anaemia in malaria is increased destruction of red blood cells (haemolysis) in the spleen. Haemolysis causes jaundice and contributes to enlargement of the spleen. Occasionally there is massive destruction of red cells within the circulation (intravascular haemolysis) and the urine contains free haemoglobin and turns dark brown or black – a condition known as blackwater fever. Blackwater fever is sometimes associated with quinine but the cause is not always clear. In inherited red cell deficiency of glucose-6-phosphate dehydrogenase (G6PD deficiency) haemolysis similar to that seen in blackwater fever may be precipitated by certain drugs. Folic acid deficiency and bone marrow supression contribute to the anaemia of severe malaria. Anaemia may develop rapidly in malaria and the haemoglobin or haematocrit should be measured at least daily. Transfusion of whole blood or packed cells is indicated if haemoglobin falls to 7.0 g/dl and if haemoglobin is falling rapidly arrangements for transfusion should be commenced at higher levels of haemoglobin.

Blackwater fever

Blackwater fever or acute haemolysis from G6PD deficiency is recognised by the passing of very dark brown or black urine. The presence of haemoglobin in the urine can be confirmed by spectrophotometric examination. If spectrophotometric examination is not possible positive chemical tests for blood in the urine (e.g. Haematest) without red cells being seen on urine microscopy is highly suggestive of haemoglobinuria. As haemolysis decreases the colour of the urine returns towards normal. During acute haemolysis the blood test for red cell G6PD deficiency is unreliable and all cases of acute intravascular haemolysis are generally treated as blackwater fever. The aim of *treatment* of blackwater fever is to stop haemolysis with steroids, and control anaemia by transfusion as described above. If the patient can take by mouth prednisolone 20 mg three times daily is given until the urine colour has returned to normal (usually 2 or 3 days). Thereafter prednisolone can be discontinued abruptly. For patients not able to take by mouth intravenous hydrocortisone 100 mg every 8 h can be given instead of prednisolone.

Hyperpyrexia

Hyperpyrexia is defined as a rectal temperature greater than 39°C and is attributed to toxins released by the parasites. It is a dangerous complication of malaria recognised by the body temperature and often associated with a hot dry skin and inadequate sweating. It is treated with cooling and antipyretic drugs (p. 111).

Secondary infection

Resistance to bacterial infection is reduced in malaria. This accounts for the frequency of secondary infection such as septicaemia and pneumonia. Persistence of fever 36 h after commencing effective antimalarial therapy is highly suggestive of secondary infection and the site should be identified by clinical examination. Antibiotic therapy should be commenced after appropriate samples have been taken for culture.

Complications specific to pregnancy

Malaria is often exceptionally severe in pregnant women and there is great risk to the mother and the child. The mother will have lost any immunity she may have had and the placenta is a fertile breeding ground for malaria parasites, particularly in primigravida. The mother may experience any of the complications described above and is at particular risk of hypoglycaemia and, in late pregnancy, of pulmonary oedema. Hypotension, hypoxia, hypoglycaemia, hyperpyrexia and septicaemia are harmful to the fetus and may precipitate premature labour or intra-uterine death. The dangers of malaria greatly exceed the risks from antimalarial drugs. In doses used to treat malaria chloroquine and quinine are safe in pregnancy and Fansidar has not been proved to cause fetal damage but tetracycline should be avoided.

How to manage life-threatening malaria

Successful management of severe malaria requires antimalarial therapy, supportive care and early recognition and treatment of additional complications.

Antimalarial therapy

The emergence of drug resistance in *P. falciparum* parasites has complicated the drug treatment of malaria. In life-threatening malaria the drug chosen must be known to be effective and quick-acting. Initial treatment should be intravenous or intramuscular and oral therapy should be commenced as soon as possible.

Artemisins

Artemisinin derivatives (artesunate 50 mg tablets or artemether injection 80 mg/ml) are preferable to quinine. Quinine may be safer in the first trimester of pregnancy. Give single daily dose as follows:

Artesunate oral daily dose
Day 1   4 mg/kg bodyweight
Days 2–7 2 mg/kg bodyweight
If unable to take oral medication use artemether i.m.

Artemether i.m. daily dose
Day 1   3.6 mg/kg bodyweight
Days 2–7 1.6 mg/kg bodyweight
Change to oral artesunate when able to take oral medication

Fansidar 25 mg/kg on day 3 (oral) with either artesunate or artemether.

Artemisins are the agents of choice with quinine the next choice.

Quinine (Tables 8.5 and 8.6)

Quinine may have serious side effects but its risks are diminished by careful attention to dose and rate of administration. These risks are fully justified because of the danger of death in severe malaria. Quinine should be given intravenously or by mouth. Intramuscular quinine should be avoided as it may lead to dangerously high serum levels. When used intravenously it is given as a slow infusion and not as a bolus injection to avoid transient toxic serum levels. Quinine may also cause hypoglycaemia and when it is used the blood sugar should be monitored at 4-hourly intervals. If quinine is not available quinidine may be used instead and is given in the same doses and by the same routes as quinine.

In patients who are receiving intravenous quinine and remain seriously ill after 48 h the dose of quinine should be reduced to 5.5 mg *base*/kg 8 hourly to prevent cumulative toxicity.

Chloroquine (Tables 8.7 and 8.8)

Chloroquine is often used for uncomplicated malaria but it is not indicated in life-threatening malaria wherever there is drug resistance. If there is doubt alternative agents such as artemesinins or quinine should be used. Intramuscular chloroquine should be avoided in children as it has been followed by sudden death. If it has to be used the dose should be divided into two injections given one hour apart.

Table 8.5 The administration of quinine

Indications
  All cases of life-threatening malaria except in areas where chloroquine-resistant malaria is uncommon.
Route
  Initial dose(s) by slow intravenous infusion changed to oral therapy as soon as possible.
Dose
  Initial dose: 16.7 mg *base*[1]/kg (omitted if given intramuscularly) (20 mg/kg salt)
Maintenance
  8.3 mg *base*[1]/kg every 8 hours for 7 days.
  Intravenous administration (10 mg/kg salt)
    Dilute in 5% dextrose water or normal saline, allowing 1.0 ml of fluid for every 1.0 mg *base* of quinine. *Infuse* the initial dose over 4 h and maintenance doses over 2 h.

1 The dose of quinine is for the base.
  Depending on the salt used the equivalents are:

	Base	Salt
Quinine sulphate	300 mg	362 mg
Quinine bisulphate	300 mg	508 mg
Quinine hydrochloride	300 mg	405 mg

Table 8.6 Side effects of quinine

Severe
  Sudden death from hypotension or cardiac arrhythmias.
  Hypoglycaemia.
  Blindness, deafness and central nervous system depression.
Moderate
  Hypersensitivity reactions – fever, skin reactions and asthma.
Mild
  The symptom complex known as cinchonism consists of tinnitus, nausea and vomiting, excess salivation and blurred vision.
Rare
  Blood dyscrasias.

Table 8.7 The administration of chloroquine

Indications
  In life-threatening malaria in areas where parasites are chloroquine-sensitive.
Route
  Initially intravenous changing to oral as soon as possible.
Dose
  5.0 mg *base*[1]/kg every 12 h for 5 doses. (*Note*: In children, it used intramuscularly give each dose as two injections of 2.5 mg *base*/kg one hour apart.)
Intravenous administration
  Dilute in 5% dextrose water or normal saline allowing 2.0 ml of fluid for every 1.0 mg *base*. *Infuse* over 2 h.

1 The dose of chloroquine is for the base.
Depending on the salt used the equivalents are:

	Base	Salt
Chloroquine sulphate	100 mg	136 mg
Chloroquine diphosphate	150 mg	250 mg

Additional antimalarial therapy

To prevent the emergence of quinine resistance a second antimalarial drug – either Fansidar (pyrimethamine 25 mg with sulfadoxine 500 mg per tablet) or tetracycline – is generally given with quinine.

FANSIDAR

The action of Fansidar is too slow to be used alone in life-threatening malaria but it is used to augment the action of quinine. The dose for adults is 3 tablets as a single dose given on the second day or when the patient can take orally. Smaller doses are used in children. Fansidar should not be given to patients with a history of any reaction to sulphonamides. The main risk of Fansidar is of hypersensitivity skin reactions (e.g. Stevens–Johnson syndrome) but severe reactions are uncommon when used in treatment (as opposed to

Table 8.8 Side effects of chloroquine

Severe
  Hypotension and sudden death.
  Abnormal movements and deafness.
Mild
  Abdominal discomfort, nausea and vomiting, headache, dizziness and weakness.
  Blurred vision.
  Itching.

In the doses used in treatment of malaria chloroquine does not damage the eye.

prophylaxis). This dose of Fansidar carries little risk of bone marrow depression.

TETRACYCLINE

Like Fansidar, tetracycline acts too slowly to be used alone in the treatment of life-threatening malaria and is used to supplement the effect of quinine. The adult dose is 250 mg four times daily for 7 days. Tetracycline should not be used in pregnant women or in children under 8 years. Tetracycline should be avoided in renal failure when doxycycline (100 mg twice daily) can be used instead. Diarrhoea is the only common side effect of tetracycline.

OTHER DRUGS IN MALARIA

Maloprim (pyrimethamine 12.5 mg and dapsone 100 mg per tablet) is only used in malaria prophylaxis and amodiaquine is not used in treatment of life-threatening malaria because no parenteral preparation is available. Mefloquine, a newer antimalarial drug effective against chloroquine-resistant parasites, is not available in a parenteral form and its value in life-threatening malaria has not been established.

Steroids have no role in the treatment of severe malaria except in the management of blackwater fever. There is no evidence that cerebral oedema contributes to death in cerebral malaria and the use of agents such as dexamethasone and intravenous mannitol has now been abandoned. Disseminated intravascular coagulation has not been shown to be a major problem in malaria and the dangers of giving heparin outweigh any theoretical benefit.

Table 8.9 Special observations required in life-threatening malaria

Blood sugar
  Monitor 4 hourly if unconscious or on quinine
Renal function
  Measure urinary output
Haemoglobin
  Measure once or twice daily
Parasites
  Daily blood slide

Supportive care and monitoring

In these respects management of the patient with life-threatening malaria differs little from that of any critically ill patient and the points specific to malaria that require regular observation are summarised in Table 8.9.

Further reading

SEATON RA *et al*. Randomized comparison of intramuscular artemether and intravenous quinine in adult, Melanesian patients with severe or complicated, *Plasmodium falciparum* malaria in Papua New Guinea. *Ann Trop Med Parasitol* 1998 Mar;92(2):133–9.

Tetanus

Definition

Tetanus is an acute, often fatal disease, caused by an exotoxin produced in wounds by *Clostridium tetani (t)*. Tetanus is a non-contagious disease. It is characterised by generalised increased rigidity and convulsive spasms of skeletal muscles (Figure 8.1). Mortality for untreated tetanus is in excess of 80%, while with good treatment this may be reduced to less than 20%. The main causes of death are secondary pneumonias, and autonomic instability.

Recognition

In one-quarter of cases no previous history of injury is obtained. Local or generalised spasms occurring after injury, burns or septic abortion should immediately bring the diagnosis to mind. 'Lockjaw' or increasing difficulty in opening the mouth is often the first symptom. Another early symptom may be stiffness at the wound site, which may be followed by general muscle pains. The temperature and con-

Infections 149

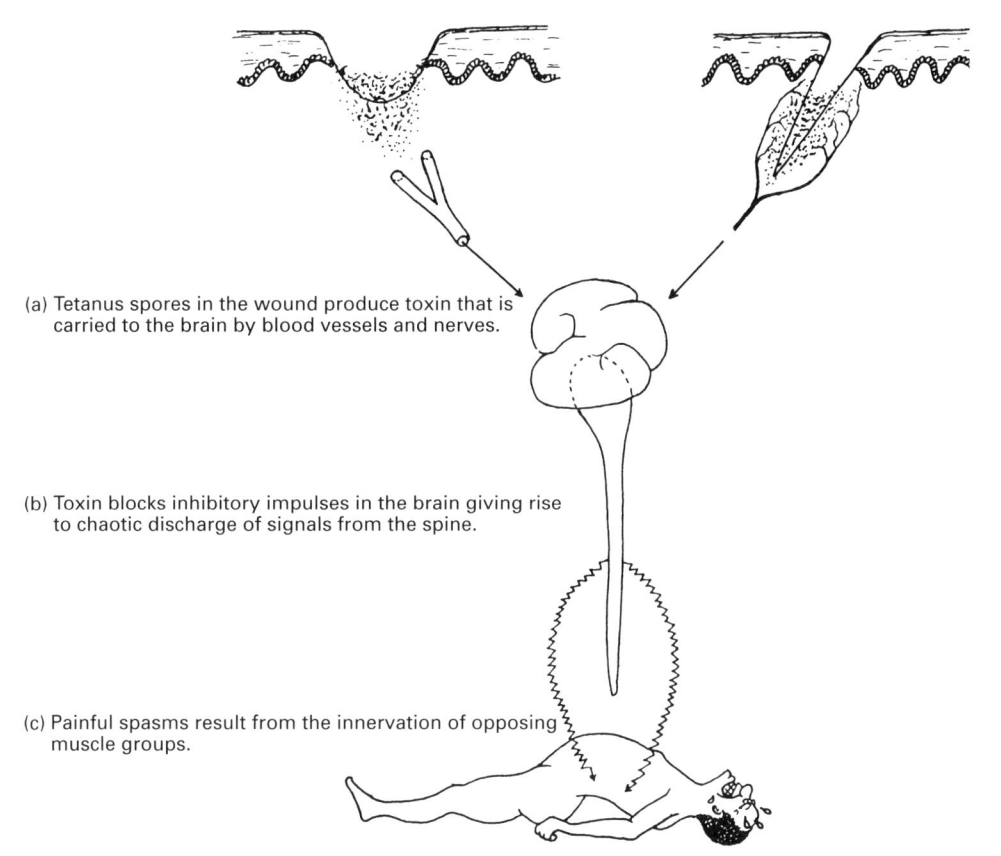

Figure 8.1 Tetanus toxin and spasm production.

(a) Tetanus spores in the wound produce toxin that is carried to the brain by blood vessels and nerves.

(b) Toxin blocks inhibitory impulses in the brain giving rise to chaotic discharge of signals from the spine.

(c) Painful spasms result from the innervation of opposing muscle groups.

scious level are normal and abdominal rigidity may be noted. *The* diagnostic feature of tetanus is muscular spasm. There are no laboratory tests for tetanus. The differential diagnosis includes epileptic fits, severe meningitis and hysteria.

Patients with the following features have a bad prognosis:

1. Spasms occurring more frequently than one every 15 min.
2. If the time interval between the development of lockjaw and the onset of spasms is less than 48 h.
3. If the incubation period is less than 7 days.

Tetanus occurring in neonates carries a high mortality.

Management

In severe cases the priority must be to control spasms. Use diazepam by infusion giving enough to control or ablate spasms. Dose: 120 mg/24 h increasing to 360 mg/24 h; if spasms are still uncontrolled add chlorpromazine 50 mg b.d. increasing to 50 mg, q.i.d.; if spasms are still uncontrolled consider paralysing with muscle relaxants, intubating and ventilating. In milder cases oral diazepam, commencing at 10 mg b.d., increasing to 20 mg t.d.s. may be effective either alone or in combination with oral chlorpromazine. Start reducing sedation after 7 days (diazepam has a cumulative effect that takes several days to wear off). Be prepared to increase sedation again should spasms increase in frequency.

Nursing

This is of paramount importance. Patients should be nursed head-down (to prevent aspiration of secretions) in a well-lit area with constant nurse attendance. Should nursing procedures provoke spasms then the patient requires more sedation. Turning should be performed hourly and secretions must be aspirated as frequently as they accumulate. Feeding, by nasogastric tube, should be commenced on admission.

Eradication of infection

Excise the wound; in the case of septic abortion perform hysterectomy. Give penicillin G 1 megaunit 6 hourly i.v. for 7 days. (Erythromycin 1 g i.v. 8 hourly is a suitable alternative drug in cases of penicillin allergy.)

Toxin neutralisation

Human immune globulin is preferable as the risk of anaphylaxis is negligible. If horse serum (10,000–15,000 units) must be used it should be given slowly i.v. or i.m. observing for anaphylaxis and always having adrenaline available. Sensitivity testing is of no use in the prevention of anaphylactic reactions. Tetanus toxoid (0.5 ml i.m.) should be given while the patient is hospitalised to promote active immunity, and this should be followed by a full course for those not recently vaccinated. Most patients can be managed satisfactorily using these methods. In a minority of patients respiratory assistance may be required. No assistance is required if spontaneous respiration is adequate and secretions can be cleared.

Indications for respiratory assistance are:
1. frequent spasms;
2. laryngospasm;
3. intercurrent pneumonia;
4. excessive secretions.

The options for assistance will depend on what is locally available but tracheostomy to facilitate aspiration of secretions is often satisfactory. Alternatively intubation with a PVC tube, paralysis, and intermittent positive pressure ventilation may be performed.

KEY POINT
Patients who are nursed in darkened side-rooms die of neglect, pneumonia and starvation.

Complications

Tachycardia and hypertension

Monitor pulse and BP closely. Should the pulse exceed 120/min or BP increase above 100 mm (diastolic) add propanolol 40–80 mg q.i.d.; labetalol is a suitable alternative drug.

Chest infection

Frequent turning of the patient prevents accumulation of bronchial secretions. Perform regular tracheal aspiration; chest physiotherapy may be combined with this. (*Note:* Avoid hypoxia during aspiration.) Examine the chest clinically daily and check the chest X-ray regularly.

Urinary problems

Catheterise and chart urine output. Examine the urine frequently for evidence of urinary tract infection.

Hyperpyrexia

Physical cooling using fans and wet sheets. Aspirin 300 mg b.d. or q.i.d. is antipyretic as is chlorpromazine 50 mg. b.d. or q.i.d. Paracetamol may also be used.

Thrombophlebitis

Avoid superficial thrombophlebitis by using long i.v. lines in central veins, especially for diazepam infusions. Alternatively change drip sites regularly. Prevent deep vein thrombosis by regular physiotherapy and adequate hydration. Treat established thrombosis with anticoagulants.

Inadequate nutrition

Pass a nasogastric tube on admission and commence feeds (3000 kcal/day) early (p. 287).

Prevention of tetanus

With simple measures tetanus is a disease which can and should be completely eradicated.

Prompt and adequate care of wounds

This is very important in prevention. Wounds should be thoroughly cleaned, foreign bodies removed and necrotic tissue excised.

It is emphasised that tetanus is not spread from person to person.

Active immunisation

In patients suffering from tetanus active immunisation is necessary because the disease does not confer natural immunity. This may wait until the recovery phase of the illness. Vaccination with anti-tetanus toxoid, repeated at three intervals confers immunity for 5–10 years. Vaccination of children at 2, 3 and 15 months protects until school age when a booster dose is recommended. Vaccination in the eighth and ninth months of pregnancy confers protection on both mother and child. Adults with a wound and a complete vaccination history within 10 years need only a booster dose of toxoid. In case of uncertain or unknown status a full course of tetanus toxoid is given.

It is recommended that a tetanus toxoid booster dose is given every 10 years as many old or middle-aged people (70% of people over 50 years) have been shown to have non-protective antibody levels (less than 0.01 i.u./ml).

Further reading

COOK TM, PROTHEROE RT, HANDEL JM. Tetanus: a review of the literature. *Br J Anaesth* 2001;87:477–87.

Neonatal tetanus

Neonatal tetanus results from contamination of the umbilical stump and is associated with a very high mortality. It is prevented by maternal immunisation with tetanus toxoid during pregnancy and by aseptic technique in cutting and caring for the umbilical cord. The earliest sign in the neonate is difficulty feeding, caused by spasm of the jaw muscles (risus sardonicus). Spasms of other muscle groups follow and generalised spasms may be mistaken for neonatal fits.

Management

- Keep the baby warm.
- Handle and disturb as little as is necessary.
- Give oxygen if spasms are severe.
- Sedate as heavily as is necessary to control spasms.

Control of spasms: an initial dose of i.m. paraldehyde 0.2 ml/kg for babies with severe spasms allows initial sedation to insert a good i.v. line. Put up a drip of 4.3% dextrose in 0.18% normal saline with 1.5 gKCl/l and run at 6 ml/kg/h. (The concentration of dextrose can be increased to 9% by adding 10 ml 50% dextrose to 90 ml.) Give successive doses of 2.5 mg i.v. diazepam slowly every 5 min until the spasms and rigidity are controlled. Run the i.v. fluid quickly while giving the diazepam and inject it as near to the cannula as possible, since diazepam is absorbed onto plastic tubing. Continuous sedation is achieved by giving nasogastric diazepam 1–2 mg/kg 12 hourly, alternating with chlorpromazine 5 mg/kg 12 hourly (i.e. sedation every 6 hours) and control 'breakthrough' spasms with additional doses of 2.5 mg i.v. diazepam. Hiccoughs can be controlled with i.v. chlorpromazine 2.5 mg. If it is available give dexamethasone 2 mg i.m. b.d. for 5 days. In babies with very severe tetanus the dose of diazepam required for control may be sufficient to stop respiration. The question of ventilation then arises. Whether or not this is attempted (or whether or not the baby is paralysed and ventilated earlier) depends on availability of equipment and expertise.

To reduce the toxin load give human tetanus immunoglobulin 375 units i.m., and infiltrate 125 units around the umbilicus. Give another 250 units the following day. (There is an i.v. preparation which is given both intravenously and intrathecally but this is very expensive and unlikely to be available. To eradicate the infection use benzyl penicillin (50–60 mg/kg i.v. 6 hourly) and gentamicin (5–7 mg/kg i.v. once daily). Clean the umbilicus thoroughly with hydrogen peroxide, and then apply gentian violet or acriflavine in spirit b.d.

Commence nasogastric feeding with expressed breast milk, starting with 3 ml/kg/h and gradually increasing to 10 ml/kg/h and then 30 ml/kg third hourly once severe spasms have been controlled (usually after 2–3 days). Reduce the i.v. fluids accordingly. The doses of sedation should be reduced gradually over a period of 2–3 weeks.

Complicated typhoid

Definition

Typhoid is an acute septicaemic illness resulting from ingestion of *Salmonella typhi*. If severe or untreated the disease may progress with a high rate of complications of which the major ones are perforation of the distal ileum and haemorrhage.

Recognition

Typhoid usually presents as fever and headache without localising signs and without diarrhoea in the early stages. It may present with complications and should be suspected, in the absence of other obvious causes, in the following circumstances:

1. The shocked patient (cold, clammy and confused).
2. The pyrexial patient with an acute abdomen.
3. The febrile patient with rectal bleeding.

There is no one group of signs which is characteristic, indeed it is often the absence of signs in a patient who has a fever for a few days and who looks ill, lies listless, speaks little, and likes to be left alone, which suggest typhoid. Mental confusion is very common and the patient may be frankly psychotic. On examination there may be splenomegaly and abdominal tenderness. A very tender abdomen is suggestive of intestinal perforation and the patient may also show signs of shock.

> **KEY POINT**
>
> A normal or low white cell count in an acute, severely ill female patient is often due to typhoid or malaria.

Table 8.10 shows the laboratory findings that may help in the diagnosis of typhoid. However, as most of these are bacteriological and take a number of days to be performed they should not influence the initial management of the critically ill patient with suspected typhoid.

Table 8.10 Diagnostic findings in typoid fever

Test	Time of disease	Comments
FBC (leucopenia)	Febrile phase	Pyogenic complications are indicated by a leucocytosis
Blood culture	1st week	70–90% positive
Bone marrow culture	—	Useful in partially treated cases 75% positive
Stool culture	2nd week onwards	75% positive
Urine culture	As stool culture	More variable
Serology (Widal)	3rd–4th week	50% show no rise in titre

Management

Fluid replacement using i.v. fluids is almost always required to replace deficits caused by prolonged anorexia and fever. Reduction of fever using tepid sponging, fans and aspirin is useful. When the illness is prolonged and there are no intestinal complications then oral or nasogastric feeding should be commenced early on.

Chloramphenicol is historically the antibiotic of choice for the treatment of typhoid. It may be used alone or, in the treatment of very toxic patients, may be used in addition to co-trimoxazole. The dose should be 50 mg/kg/day divided into three or four doses given intravenously 6 hourly. The adult dose is usually 2–3 g/day. After the patient has become afebrile, the dose may be reduced to 30 mg/kg/day. Therapy should be continued for at least 2 weeks; 3 weeks is preferable and reduces the rate of relapse.

Chloramphenicol-resistant strains have been reported from various areas of the world. Alternative drugs now sometimes preferred are:
- Ampicillin: 100 mg/kg/day in 4 divided doses for at least 2 weeks.
- Amoxycillin: 50 mg/kg/day is equivalent to ampicillin but is better absorbed.
- Third generation cephalosporins, e.g ceftriaxone (child 75 mg/kg up to 3 g i.v. daily) or cefotaxime.
- Co-trimoxazole (Single (SS) 80 mg TMP/400 mg SMX) 4–8 tablets per day in two divided doses for 2 weeks. Less effective than chloramphenicol alone but in combination with chloramphenicol, it may be useful in the initial treatment of very toxic patients.
- Ciprofloxacin (child 15 mg/kg up to 500 mg) orally 12 hourly for 14 days or i.v. 10 mg/kg up to 200 mg 12 hourly until oral can be tolerated.

Complications

The most important of these is gastrointestinal bleeding from ulcers in the ileum. These occur in the second and third weeks of the illness and require prompt resuscitation and surgical measures to stop the bleeding. The most frequently encountered complications occur because of patient neglect. These include dehydration and occasionally renal failure (due to inadequate fluid replacement), parotitis (due to poor oral hygiene), and bed sores and deep venous thrombosis (due to inanition and lack of physiotherapy). Other complications are due to the septicaemic nature of the illness and are listed in Table 8.11.

Prevention and control

In hospital the most important point in preventing spread is good personal hygiene and hand washing, although barrier nursing is not required. Prompt disposal of any excreta or, failing this, adequate

Table 8.11 Complications of typhoid fever

Complication	Time of appearance and age group
Pneumonia (empyema)	Late: in weak, elderly patients
Meningitis	Infants and neonates
Arteritis (in aorta)	Late, in patients over 50
Myocarditis	Severe cases, children
Hepatitis	Severe cases
Disseminated intravascular coagulation (DIC)	Most often sub-clinical of may complicate severe cases
Relapse	After 2–3 weeks

disinfection is mandatory. Typhoid vaccine, a suspension of killed *Salmonella typhi*, enhances resistance to infection for a maximum period of 3 years *but* the protection is only relative and cannot resist a large inoculum of the bacterium. Adults and children 10 years and older should have 0.5 ml subcutaneously on two occasions separated by 4 or more weeks, smaller doses to younger children. A booster dose every 3 years is recommended under conditions of continuous and repeated exposure.

Meningitis and encephalitis

Definitions

Meningitis is inflammation of the meninges as a result of infection with bacteria, viruses, fungi or protozoa. Secondary infection may spread to the meninges from open skull fractures, sinusitis or middle-ear infections. Among the commonest organisms are *Neisseria meningitidis*, *Haemophilus influenzae* and *Streptococcus pneumoniae*. Viral meningitis is usually due to enteroviruses, mumps and polio.

Subacute/chronic meningitis used to be mainly tuberculous, but with the advent of HIV infection, cryptococcal meningitis has become more common.

Encephalitis is diffuse inflammation of the brain itself with an altered conscious level. The commonest organisms responsible are rabies, trypanosomiasis, postinfectious (i.e. measles, mumps, chicken pox, rubella and cytomegalovirus), herpes simplex, and arboviruses often specific to a particular geographic area (e.g. Japanese B encephalitis). In HIV infection, toxoplasma encephalitis is not uncommon, although few centres have computed tomography (CT) facilities for diagnosis.

Recognition

A high index of suspicion is required so that meningitis is not missed, especially in the early, treatable stages. Any patient who has been noted to have neck stiffness or unexplained fever or altered consciousness should have a lumbar puncture to exclude meningitis. In malaria endemic areas it is very difficult to differentiate cerebral malaria from meningitis and routine lumbar puncture for all patients is advised.

Fever, headache and neck stiffness are found in most cases of acute pyogenic and viral meningitis, although difficulties may arise in recognition of acute meningitis in the very young, very old and very ill. In these patients neck stiffness may not be present and the presence of shock may mean that fever is not present. Meningism means that the signs of meningeal irritation are present but examination of the CSF shows no cells or organisms. Two clinical signs useful for recognising meningeal irritation are shown in Figure 8.2. Meningism occurs with some systemic viral illnesses

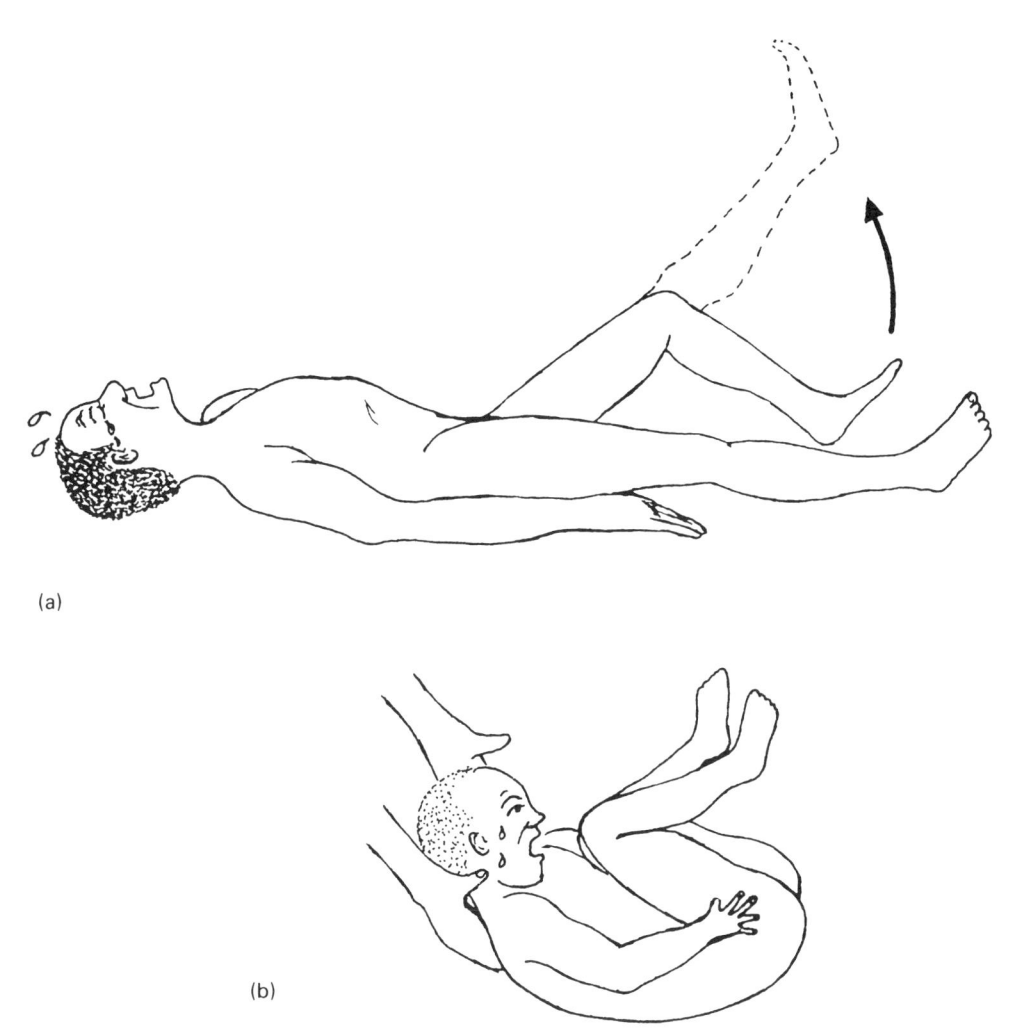

Figure 8.2 Useful clinical signs to elicit neck meningism (a) flexion of the hip and extension of the knee causes pain; (b) flexion of the neck produces reflex flexion of the hips and knees.

(e.g. influenza virus) and also with non-meningeal causes such as retropharyngeal abscess. Take care not to confuse the spasms of neck muscles in tetanus for neck stiffness in meningitis: two useful differentiating features are the absence of fever and the normal conscious level in tetanus. Subacute meningitis (tuberculous meningitis and cryptococcal meningitis) differs not only in the duration of the illness but also in the presentation. The patient may present with fever only and meningism may be absent. There may be focal neurological signs (e.g. cranial nerve lesions), ataxia, psychosis or prolonged fever and debilitation.

Encephalitis presents with global or focal brain dysfunction, e.g. focal or generalised fits, altered behaviour, confusion, focal CNS signs and altered consciousness in association with a short history and fever. Meningeal irritation is present only when there is associated meningitis. In the absence of meningitis, the CSF may not be abnormal or show only elevated protein. The glucose is usually normal. In rabies, there may be a history of animal bite and this is followed by fever, abnormal behaviour, and, latterly, by laryngospasm. The diagnosis can be confirmed from corneal scrapings and sometimes from saliva. Trypanosomal encephalitis should be considered in endemic areas and can be confirmed by identifying the organism on a blood slide or in the CSF.

Toxoplasma encephalitis complicates HIV infection and causes a characteristic appearance on CT scan. Brain biopsy is sometimes used to diagnose herpes simplex encephalitis.

Encephalitis should be suspected if there is a local clustering of cases with similar symptoms and occasionally haemorrhagic phenomena (e.g. Congo–Crimea haemorrhagic fever).

KEY POINT
Any patient who has been noted to have neck stiffness, unexplained fever or altered consciousness should have a lumbar puncture.

Management

Difficulties in management arise in the differentiation of meningism from meningitis, the specific diagnosis and subsequent therapy. Follow the flow diagram in Figure 8.3.

It is the speed of commencement of appropriate therapy that will determine the patient's outcome in non-viral meningitis. Laboratory investigations will be dependent upon local resources but CSF analysis for cells, protein and sugar are basic to differentiating the cause of meningitis. Turbid CSF in a sick patient must always be treated as pyogenic meningitis before results are known. More detailed laboratory tests and their significance are shown in Table 8.12.

Treatment

Cloudy CSF/pyogenic meningitis

Start therapy with benzyl penicillin and chloramphenicol before the organism is known. Should the organism be identified as meningococcus (or in an epidemic situation) benzyl penicillin alone may be given.

Table 8.12 Laboratory diagnosis of meningitis

Investigation	Pyogenic	Viral	Other
Blood			
Culture	Polymorphs	Lymphocytes	Lymphocytes in TB
Culture	Useful	No	No
Antigens	Useful	May be useful	No
CSF			
Appearances	Turbid or purulent	Clear	Clear
Cells	Polymorphs	Lymphocytes	Lymphocytes in TB
Organisms	Gram stain or culture	Special culture	India ink stain for cryptococcus
			Special culture for TB
Antigens	For meningococcus	No	Yes for cryptococcus
Biochemistry			
Glucose	Low	Normal	Low in TB
Chloride	Normal	Normal	Low
Protein	Raised	Raised	Raised

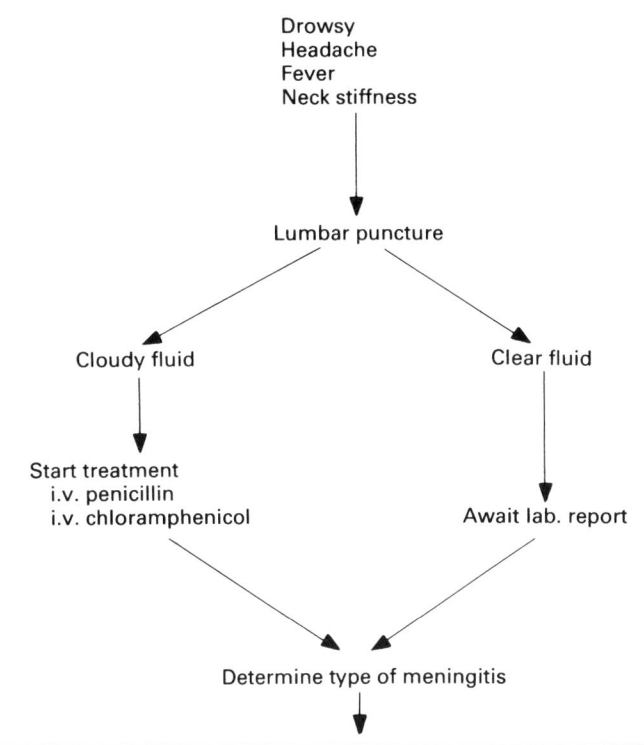

```
                    Drowsy
                    Headache
                    Fever
                    Neck stiffness
                         │
                         ▼
                   Lumbar puncture
                    ╱         ╲
                   ▼           ▼
            Cloudy fluid     Clear fluid
                 │                │
                 ▼                ▼
           Start treatment   Await lab. report
           i.v. penicillin
           i.v. chloramphenicol
                    ╲         ╱
                     ▼       ▼
               Determine type of meningitis
```

	Bacterial	Viral	TB, fungal
Cells	Polymorphs	Lymphocytes	Lymphocytes
Protein	Increased	Increased	Increased
Glucose	Decreased	Normal	Usually low
Organisms	Yes	No	Variable

Figure 8.3 Management of the patient with neck stiffness. CSF findings in different types of meningitis. Blood-stained CSF or xanthochromia suggests sub-arachnoid haemorrhage (p. 182).

- Benzyl penicillin adults 180–300 mg/kg/day (max 14 g/day) in divided doses 4 hourly. Children 50–100 mg/kg/day in divided doses 6 hourly.
- Chloramphenicol 75–100 mg/kg/day i.v. or i.m. (initially); give divided doses until 5 days after the temperature has settled.

TB meningitis

Use a double dose of isoniazid (10 mg/kg), with standard dosages of rifampicin and pyrazinamide (good CSF penetration) continuing for a total 12 months.

Corticosteroids (prednisolone 1 mg/kg) are commonly used for the first 4–6 weeks depending on symptoms and gradually weaned.

Viral meningitis

No specific treatment.

Cryptococcal meningitis

Fluconazole 800 mg i.v. or oral stat followed by 400 mg daily is as effective as amphotericin B (0.3–0.6 mg/kg/day) and much less toxic. Treatment must be continued for at least 6 weeks.

Encephalitis

With the exception of herpes simplex encephalitis (aciclovir 10 mg/kg i.v. 8 hourly for 14 days) there is no specific treatment for viral encephalitis and management is symptomatic with attention to care of the comatose patient (p. 175). Trypanosomal encephalitis is treated with melarsoprol 0.5 ml in 3.6% solution i.v., the dose being increased by 0.5 ml daily until the maximum single daily dose of 5 ml is reached. The first three daily dosages are followed by a 7-day rest period and then treatment is continued until a total of 37.5 ml have been given over 1 month. Rabies encephalitis is almost always fatal.

Failure to improve

The patient with meningitis should be reviewed daily, looking for:
1. deterioration in consciousness level: this may indicate development of a cerebral abscess;
2. persistent pyrexia – may indicate a secondary infection or undiagnosed malaria.

No improvement within 48 h should prompt re-examination of the CSF for other organisms.

Peritonitis

Definitions

Peritonitis is inflammation of the peritoneal cavity. The inflammation may be caused by bacterial contamination or chemical irritation from gastrointestinal secretions or blood.

Peritonitis may be localised or generalised. Localised peritonitis occurs when the peritoneal inflammation is confined to one area of the peritoneal cavity, as happens in acute appendicitis. Once the appendix perforates pus spreads throughout the peritoneal cavity and the signs of peritonitis are found throughout the abdomen.

The commonest causes of peritonitis in the tropics are:
1. Sepsis arising from the female genital tract:
   - tubo-ovarian sepsis;
   - perforated uterus due to criminal abortion;
   - puerperal sepsis.
2. Sepsis arising from the gastrointestinal tract:
   - perforated appendix;
   - ischaemic bowel in intestinal obstruction (sigmoid volvulus or hernia);
   - intestinal fistula;
   - perforated typhoid ulcer (ileum);
   - amoebic colitis;
   - stab and bullet wounds of the bowel.
3. Inflammation due to gastrointestinal secretions or blood:
   - perforated duodenal or gastric ulcer (bile and gastric secretions are very irritant);
   - pancreatitis;
   - blood from any cause of intra-abdominal bleeding such as ruptured liver or spleen, ruptured ectopic pregnancy.

If peritonitis due to a perforated duodenal ulcer or haemoperitoneum is not treated promptly then secondary bacterial peritonitis will supervene, worsening the prognosis.

4. Postoperative peritonitis may complicate any operation but particularly when there was open bowel or peritonitis at the previous laparatomy.
5. Primary peritonitis is usually due to bloodborne organisms and occurs without any other definable cause. It is particularly life-threatening in the elderly, the infant or those with underlying liver or renal impairment with ascites.

Clinical recognition

Peritonitis is diagnosed from the history and clinical examination. X-rays are sometimes helpful but not as important as careful examination. It is more important to diagnose peritonitis than to determine the cause, which will become clear at laparotomy. There is no substitute for clinical experience in the diagnosis and treatment of peritonitis.

Symptoms

1. *Pain* is usually severe at the start and only in the late stages does the pain lessen. Sometimes when a tense organ such as the appendix or fallopian tube ruptures the pain may subside, although the general condition of the patient will deteriorate.
2. *Vomiting* is usually present. The onset of vomiting in relation to other symptoms may help to diagnose the likely cause.
3. *Flatus and stool* – usually the patient fails to pass flatus and stool due to paralytic ileus; sometimes diarrhoea may be present in patients with intra-abdominal or pelvic abscesses or where the bowel is in direct contact with an inflamed structure.
4. Headache is usually absent unless the patient has typhoid.
5. Invariably the patient complains of fever.

> **KEY POINT**
>
> If peritonitis is not considered the patient may be wrongly diagnosed as having malaria or some other systemic illness. Always examine the abdomen in a patient with fever and generalised pains.

Ask a female patient with suspected peritonitis about vaginal discharge, pregnancy and/or criminal interference with pregnancy.

Ask about recent alcohol ingestion in regions where pancreatitis is common.

Signs

General

The patient lies anxious and immobile afraid of movement or abdominal examination. In the late stages, the patient is quieter and disinterested in his surroundings.

There is tachycardia, and rapid, shallow breathing. Signs of septicaemia and/or shock (p. 20) may be present.

Abdominal

1. *Failure of the abdomen to move with respiration* – this sign is frequently present but not invariable.
2. *Distension* – initially this is minimal but as paralytic ileus progresses distension increases.
3. *Rigidity* – the abdomen is held rigid and immobile. After some days of peritonitis the abdomen may become softer and feel thicker like dough.
4. *Tenderness* – may be localised or generalised, depending on the origin and distribution of sepsis within the peritoneal cavity. Rebound tenderness will be present but it is not always necessary to inflict the demonstration of this sign on the patient.
5. *Bowel sounds* – these disappear early and only resume once the inflammation is settling.

Relevant investigations

X-Rays – erect chest radiograph

This is the most important X-ray as it may show gas or a fluid level under the diaphragm, or pathology in the chest which is causing abdominal symptoms or signs.

Abdominal radiographs

The supine film may show gaseous distension or free fluid in the peritoneal cavity. The erect film may show fluid levels which may be in a stepladder pattern suggestive of intestinal obstruction or all at a similar level suggestive of ileus.

Paracentesis

Using a green needle (21 gauge) and syringe aspirate the peritoneal cavity in the iliac fossa or flanks. If you aspirate pus or free blood you will know laparotomy is necessary. A negative paracentesis should not alter any decision based on the clinical signs.

Ultrasound

This may assist in making a diagnosis of free fluid, intra-abdominal abscess and enable solitary abscesses to be aspirated under antibiotic cover. Abdominal CT scanning is very accurate but is available only in a few selected centres.

Serum amylase or urine amylase

This should be raised in early acute pancreatitis. Other causes of acute abdomen may also raise the amylase, so that a serum level of below 1000 i.u./l is not diagnostic of pancreatitis. Likewise, the serum lipase should be >3 times the normal value.

Unusual presentations

1. Patients with underlying hepatic or renal disease may present with spontaneous bacterial peritonitis, resulting in infected ascites. Abdominal signs are often absent and deterioration in the patient's general condition, renal or hepatic function may be the only indicator of peritonitis. The mortality is high in this group of patients.
2. Peritonitis or intra-abdominal abscess may present in critically ill patients as unexplained circulatory, respiratory or renal failure. Abdominal signs may be absent. It is important to consider peritonitis as a potential cause of unexplained organ failure, particularly after surgery, since laparotomy or drainage of an abscess may be life-saving.

Management

First resuscitate the patient. Treat shock by restoring circulating volume (p. 22) and give oxygen. If there is ventilatory failure, intubate and ventilate.

At least 2 litres of fluid will be needed to resuscitate someone presenting within a few hours with a perforated duodenal ulcer. At least 3–4 litres will be needed, including some colloid or blood, in a patient who has suffered with peritonitis for some days.

Check urea and electrolyte levels. Correct electrolyte abnormalities before surgery.

Insert a nasogastric tube and a urinary catheter.

Urine may not be produced until the peritoneal cavity has been cleaned.

Once the patient has been properly resuscitated laparotomy is indicated. The key to success is a good first operation. Surgery should be thorough through a long midline incision extending both above and below the umbilicus. The blood or pus should be sucked out of the peritoneal cavity, then lavage should be carried out and the source of the contamination dealth with. The abdomen should be closed by the mass closure technique and if peritoneal sepsis was gross (or there was faecal contamination) the skin should not be sutured but left open. The practice of leaving the skin open aims to avoid wound abscesses, which may cause necrosis of the abdominal wall as well as confusing the postoperative clinical picture. Drains will be inserted at the discretion of the surgeon.

The actual operative procedures for different causes of peritonitis are described in surgical textbooks. Sepsis arising from the female reproductive organs is described on p. 276.

Systemic antibiotics covering both anaerobic and aerobic organisms should be given. Gentamicin 80 mg 8 hourly and metronidazole 500 mg i.v. or 1 g p.r. 8 hourly is one effective combination.

The patient may require postoperative ventilation. If ventilators are available and you are uncertain as to whether to ventilate or not it is probably better to ventilate the patient overnight. One cause of the patient failing to be weaned off the ventilator is recurrent intra-abdominal infection.

The patient must be carefully observed in the postoperative period for signs of recurrent peritonitis and intra-abdominal or subphrenic abscess, which may necessitate relaparotomy.

Subphrenic abscess

This is an abscess under the diaphragm which usually arises as a complication of a laparatomy for peritonitis, or for uterine, biliary or appendicular sepsis, but may complicate any abdominal operation. The patient is usually febrile, and may complain of pain on breathing or pain around the lower ribs. Examination may reveal basal crepitations or a pleural rub and tenderness over the lower ribs. The key to making a diagnosis is to suspect it, particularly when no cause can be found for fever and/or deterioration. There is an old surgical saying, 'pus somewhere, pus nowhere to be found, pus under the diaphragm'. This aphorism reminds us that subphrenic abscess is sometimes difficult to diagnose.

A chest radiograph may show a fluid level under the diaphragm (Figure 8.4). There may also be some basal lung collapse or a pleural effusion in association with the subdiaphragmatic inflammation. In about 10% of cases an empyema may develop simultaneously or subsequently. The WBC is raised, often markedly so above 15 000. Needle aspiration of the area of maximum tenderness may yield pus.

Other investigations that may detect the abscess are a chest radiograph taken on inspiration and expiration. Failure of the diaphragm to move on the affected side suggests a subphrenic abscess.

Radiological screening of diaphragmatic movement is more reliable but requires special screening equipment. Ultrasound is now replacing screening as a method of detecting subprhenic abscesses and the abscess may sometimes be aspirated under ultrasound guidance. In specialised centres CT scanning is also used.

The surgical management of subphrenic abscess is beyond the scope of this book. The surgeon will decide whether to drain the abscess extraperitoneally or to perform a full laparotomy. Radiological drainage is also an option if there is no peritonitis.

Recurrent intra-abdominal abscess

This section is not concerned with appendicular abscesses or pelvic abscess presenting the first time. The latter are discussed on p. 276. Subphrenic abscesses are discussed in the preceding section.

The diagnosis of a recurrent intra-abdominal abscess should be suspected in a patient who has had a previous abdominal operation for peritonitis or localised sepsis and who shows unexpected deterioration in condition. The severity of presentation may range from fever and leucocytosis to unexplained organ failure or septicaemic shock. The commonest findings are fever, localised tenderness and absent bowel sounds. Distension is sometimes present, and the patient may have diarrhoea if there is marked irritation of the bowel. In the case of a pelvic abscess, rectal or vaginal

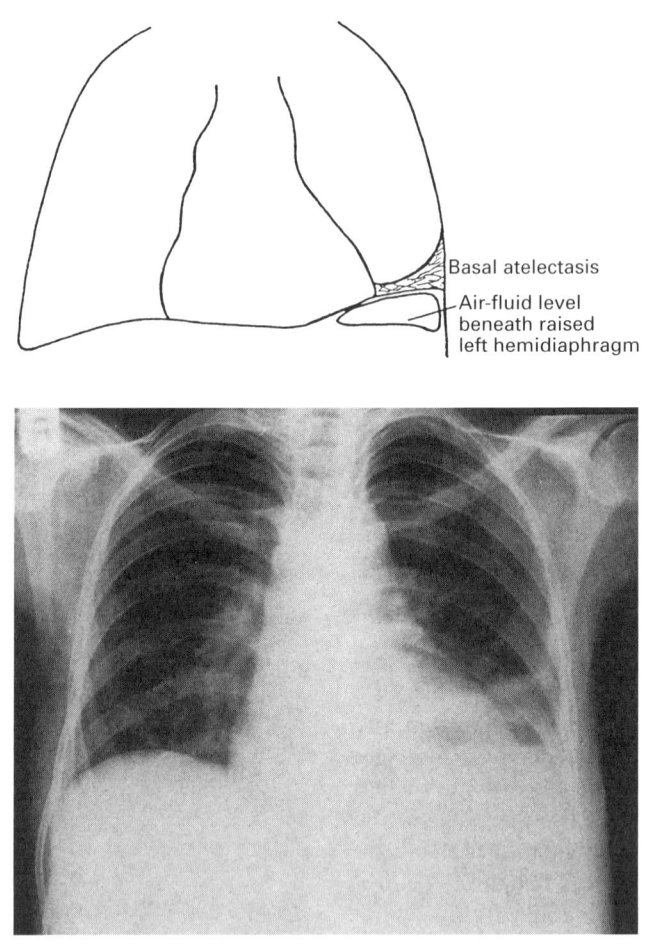

Basal atelectasis
Air-fluid level beneath raised left hemidiaphragm

Figure 8.4 Chest X-ray of a patient with subphrenic abscess.

examination may reveal a fluctuant or indurated mass in the pelvis.

Without special investigations the most accurate means of diagnosis is relaparotomy. If the patient is deteriorating or failing to improve after a previous laparatomy do not delay in re-exploring the abdomen. In referral centres the most accurate means of diagnosis is using ultrasound or CT scanning.

Recurrent intra-abdominal sepsis is difficult to treat and is best managed by a trained surgeon.

The management is drainage of the abscess at laparotomy. The abdomen should be thoroughly lavaged with tetracycline in saline (1 g/l) and areas of leaking bowel repaired and/or exteriorised. There are usually multiple abscesses, so it is advisable to explore the whole abdomen and to divide all the adhesions. If any residual abscesses are left in the abdomen the patient is likely to continue deteriorating. The patient should be given broad-spectrum antibiotics, preferably different from those he has already received.

The postoperative course is usually stormy. Septicaemic shock may complicate the laparotomy and postoperative ventilation is often required. The management of renal failure, respiratory failure and shock are discussed in the appropriate sections.

Further reading

WATTERS DAK. Severe peritoneal sepsis. *Baillière's Clin Trop Med Commun Dis* 1988; 3:275-300.

Necrotising fasciitis

Necrotising fasciitis is caused by the Group A streptococci (*Streptococcus pyogenes*), *Clostridium welchii* or a mixed anaerobic infection consisting of bacteroides and fusiform bacteria. The infection spreads in the subcutaneous tissues causing necrosis of fascia and subcutaneous fat. The skin becomes oedematous, indurated and later gangrenous as it is deprived of its blood supply by necrosis in the subcutaneous and fascial layers. Gas can be palpated in the tissues.

In men necrotising fasciitis usually originates from a perianal or periurethral abscess and spreads in the perineum and scrotum (Fournier's gangrene). Although infection may be limited to the perineum and scrotum it may also spread onto the anterior abdominal wall or down the thigh. In women it may spread into the abdominal wall, pelvis or upper thigh from a vulval infection or ulcer or a septic uterus. There is an association with poorly controlled diabetes mellitus and other immune deficiencies, including HIV infection.

The patient is usually severely ill with septicaemic shock. Aggressive resuscitation is required but excision of the necrotic tissue should not be delayed for long. Antibiotics such as imipenem, clindamycin and metronidazole must be given, the latter to deal with concomitant aerobic infection.

Definitive treatment entails wide excision of all necrotic tissue which entails excision of skin, subcutaneous fat and fascia beyond the spread of infection. The edges of the excision (which can sometimes extend from the costal margin to the upper thigh) must be vertical, not undermined, since undermining the edge would enable further growth of anaerobic organisms beneath the margin of the wound.

The wound should be cleaned, irrigated, reinspected and dressed 3-4 times daily. Further excision of the edges of the wound is normally required on the second or third day as the fasciitis usually spreads further despite aggressive excision.

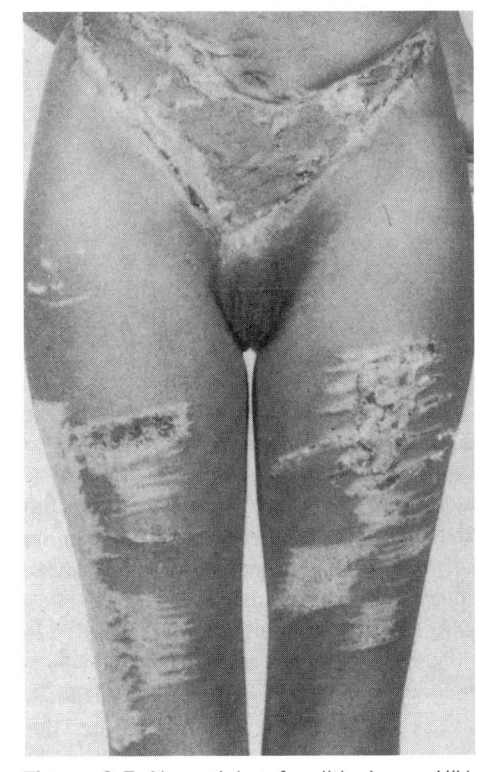

Figure 8.5 Necrotising fasciitis in an HIV-positive young woman. Initially the skin and superficial fascia were widely excised. The patient is shown here 6 weeks after skin grafting.

Providing the extent of spread of infection is appreciated and aggressive excision is performed with further excision as required the prognosis is often good. The large defect is eventually covered with a split skin graft once the bed of the wound is clean and granulating (Figure 8.5). When necrotising fasciitis or gas gangrene complicates uterine sepsis the prognosis is poor.

HIV infection and AIDS

Since the early 1980s HIV has spread rapidly in all parts of the world resulting in a pandemic. Currently about 40 million people are HIV positive and most are unaware of the diagnosis. In some countries such as much of sub-Saharan Africa prevalence rates are over 30%. Transmission occurs by sexual contact (this is further enhanced by the presence of genital ulcers or discharge) as well as perinatal and blood exposure.

HIV is a lymphotrophic retrovirus that infects and kills T lymphocytes (CD4 cells) eventually resulting in profound immune deficiency. Infection may be asymptomatic but up to 50% of individuals experience some seroconversion illness. There is a wide spectrum of symptoms from fever and generalised lymphadenopathy (infectious mononucleosis like illness) through to profound immune deficiency associated with opportunistic infections. The latency between HIV infection and full-blown AIDS is variable but ranges between 5 and 7 years in most people not receiving antiviral therapy.

In early stages of disease (CD4 count between 200 and 500/μl) there is a dramatic increase in risk of active tuberculosis, especially extrapulmonary disease, and bacterial infections such as Salmonella and pneumococcal disease. In later stages (CD4 count below 200/μl) there is further increase in other opportunistic infections (*Pneumocystis carinii* pneumonia, toxoplasmosis encephalitis, mucosal candidiasis, cryptococcal meningitis), neurologic involvement, gastrointestinal disease and malignancies such as non-Hodgkin's lymphoma and Kaposi's sarcoma.

Diagnosis is based on positive antibody by enzyme immunoassay and can be confirmed by Western blot. HIV antibody is usually detectable within a few weeks but a delay of up to 3 months has been reported. Plasma HIV RNA can be quantitatively measured by PCR and correlates with disease progression.

Testing must be performed with consent and appropriate pre- and post-test counselling.

Treatment

Treatment will be dependent on the availability of appropriate drugs. In the advanced stages of AIDS with severe wasting it may not be appropriate to treat actively and the aim should be to palliate and minimise suffering. It is also important to provide adequate explanation to family members and offer HIV testing when appropriate.
1. Treatment of opportunistic infections:
   - Tuberculosis should be managed as in the non-HIV infected host.
   - *Pneumocystis carinii* pneumonia with co-trimoxazole 20 mg TMP/ 100 mg SMX per kg daily in 2–4 divided doses for 14 days.
   - *Toxoplasmosis gondii* encephalitis with sulfadiazine 1–1.5 g oral/i.v. 6 hourly and pyrimethamine 50–100 mg stat then 25–50 mg daily.
   - Cryptococcal meningitis as per page 157.

Note: 480 mg of co-trimoxazole consists of 80 mg trimethoprim (TMP) and 400 mg sulfamethoxazole (SMX).

2. Prophylaxis against opportunistic infections:
   When CD4<200/μl
   Co-trimoxazole (Double (DS) 160 mg TMP/800 mg SMX) oral daily effective for *Pneumocystis carinii* pneumonia, toxoplasmosis and reduces other invasive bacterial infections.
3. Highly active antiretroviral therapy in the form of combination treatment suppresses viral replication, reconstitutes the host immune response prolonging life and preventing opportunistic infections.

The three main groups of antiretrovirals are: nucleoside reverse transcriptase inhibitors (AZT or zidovudine), non-nucleoside reverse transcriptase inhibitors (nevirapine) and protease inhibitors. All agents are most effective when used in combination but have significant potential toxicity. Availabilty in most countries is very limited but with the development of generic drugs they are becoming much more affordable.

Prevention

The most important means of controlling the spread of HIV is through public education and health promotion; the promotion of safe sex practices and the use of condoms; the early empiric treatment of other STDs; and the screening of donors of blood products. A successful programme requires support and commitment across all levels of health service and government.

The risk of occupational transmission of HIV following a single percutaneous exposure is about 0.3%, and 0.09% following blood and skin or mucous membrane exposures. Factors that increase the risk include hollow needle, visible blood, deep injury and a donor with advanced HIV disease.

It is recommended that all patients be managed as potentially infected (Universal Precautions) by taking appropriate protective measures to prevent exposure. These include wearing gloves and protective eyewear when in contact with bodily fluids or performing an invasive procedure and the safe disposal of sharps.

Post-exposure prophylaxis with antiretrovirals can reduce transmission if started immediately.

Recommendations for post exposure prophylaxis:
1. For lower risk exposures:
   AZT (zidovudine) 300 mg oral adult (10 mg/kg in child); plus 3TC (lamivudine) 150 mg oral adult (4 mg/kg in child); both 12 hourly for 4 weeks
2. For higher risk exposure:
   Add indinavir 800 mg orally 8 hourly to the above.

Further reading

CHAMBERS AJ, LORD RSA. Incidence of acquired immune deficiency syndrome (AIDS)-related disorders at laparotomy in patients with AIDS. *BJS* 2001;88:294–7.

DE COCK KM *et al*. Shadow on the continent: public health and HIV? AIDS in Africa in the 21st century. *Lancet* 2002;360:67–72.

GERBERDING JL. Occupational exposure to HIV in health care settings. *N Engl J Med* 2003;348;826–33.

MARSEILLE E *et al*. HIV before HAART in sub-Saharan Africa. *Lancet* 2002;359:1851–6.

MOORE A *et al*. Estimated risk of HIV transmission by blood transfusion in Kenya. *Lancet* 2001;358:657–60.

SEPKOWITZ KA. AIDS – the first 20 years. *N Engl J Med* 2001;344:1764–72.

STEINBROOK R. Providing antiretroviral therapy for HIV infection. *N Engl J Med* 2001; 344:844–6.

WATTERS DAK, SINCLAIR JR, VERMA R, LUO N. HIV sero-prevalence in critically ill patients in Zambia. *AIDS* 1988;2:142–3.

9
Coma

This chapter outlines a clinical approach to the diagnosis and management of the patient in coma.

A wide range of conditions may cause coma and specific treatment cannot be commenced until the actual cause is determined. The recognition and management of different causes of coma is described on the pages listed below:

Head injury	Chapter 10 *passim*
Cerebrovascular accident	p. 74
Subarachnoid haemorrhage	p. 182
Cerebral malaria	pp. 142–143
Meningitis and encephalitis	pp. 154–158
Brain abscess	p. 181
Poisoning and drug overdose	Chapter 7 *passim*
Diabetic comas and hypoglycaemia	pp. 101–107
Hepatic encephalopathy	pp. 98–101
Electrolyte imbalance	pp. 84–86
Renal failure and uraemia	Chapter 5 *passim*
Hypothyroidism	p. 116

Definitions

Coma is a state of altered consciousness, the severity of which is best assessed using the Glasgow Coma Scale (see under Clinical Recognition below). The terms 'comatose', 'semicomatose', 'unrousable', and 'unconscious' are imprecise and should not be used to describe coma in the critically ill.

For normal function brain cells need oxygen, a stable intracranial pressure and glucose. Electrolyte balance must be maintained and the bloodstream must be free of toxic substances such as drugs, poisons, urea, ammonia and excess alcohol.

Coma may develop when there is:
1. inadequate oxygen supply from impaired cerebral blood flow or respiratory failure;
2. hypo- or hyperglycaemia;
3. circulating poisons, toxic metabolites, drugs or alcohol;
4. brain compression from raised intracranial pressure;
5. infection of the meninges or the brain;
6. vascular damage due to thrombosis or haemorrhage;
7. trauma; or
8. electrolyte imbalance.

Clinical recognition

Coma is recognised by a depressed Glasgow Coma Scale (GCS). The GCS (Figure 9.1) is based on eye opening, best verbal response and best motor response. Coma is graded according to the numerical value obtained.

KEY POINT
Conscious level is described by 1. eye opening; 2. best verbal response; 3. best motor response.

Figure 9.1: The Glasgow Coma Scale

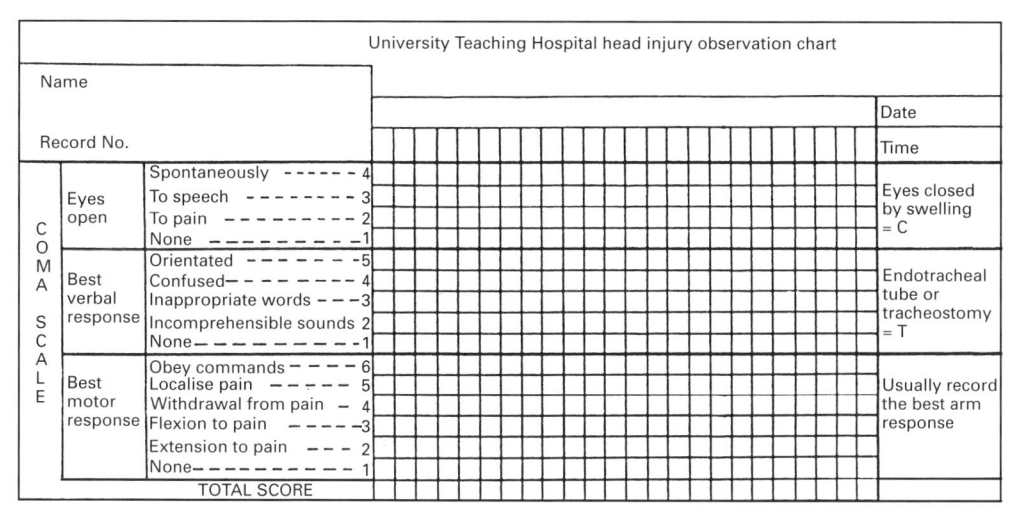

		University Teaching Hospital head injury observation chart	
Name			Date
Record No.			Time
C O M A S C A L E	Eyes open	Spontaneously ------ 4 To speech -------- 3 To pain --------- 2 None --------- 1	Eyes closed by swelling = C
	Best verbal response	Orientated ------ 5 Confused -------- 4 Inappropriate words --- 3 Incomprehensible sounds 2 None --------- 1	Endotracheal tube or tracheostomy = T
	Best motor response	Obey commands ---- 6 Localise pain ----- 5 Withdrawal from pain - 4 Flexion to pain ---- 3 Extension to pain --- 2 None --------- 1	Usually record the best arm response
		TOTAL SCORE	

Figure 9.1 The Glasgow Coma Scale. The Glasgow Coma Scale shown in the figure is but part of an observation chart which should also include pulse, respiratory rate, blood pressure and pupillary response as shown on the chart on p. 320. The GCS needs to be modified for infants and young children under 4 years (best verbal response is words 4, vocal sounds 3, cries 2, none 1).

Study Figure 9.1: a patient who does not open his eyes, makes no sounds and has no response to painful stimuli has the worst possible GCS of 3; a patient who opens his eyes to his name being called, groans with incoherent mumbles and tries to pull away your hands when you are testing for painful stimuli has a GCS of 9. The GCS allows an accurate record to be made of the change in conscious level and helps to predict outcome in both head injuries and non-traumatic coma.

When the GCS is low determine the response to pain by squeezing the patient's ear lobe, grinding your knuckles into his sternum or compressing the nail bed with the shaft of a pen. If the patient is quadriplegic from a cervical spine injury test the response to pain using the ear lobe. Difficulties arise when recording the GCS if the eyes are closed due to oedema or bruising or if the patient is intubated. A 'C' should be put after the GCS when the eyes are closed and a 'T' if an endotracheal or tracheostomy tube prevents a verbal response.

Anaesthesia, muscle relaxants and sedative drugs all influence the level of consciousness. Allow the effect of these to wear off before assessing the GCS. Do not record the GCS during or immediately after an epileptic fit. Wait until the patient has recovered from the post-ictal state. Protect the airway during a fit. If you have stopped a fit with 10 mg diazepam i.v. it is best to wait until the effects of the diazepam have worn off before reassessing the GCS.

Predicting prognosis

The two most important factors affecting the outcome from coma are the actual diagnosis and the GCS. The trend of change in the GCS is better than a single recording. For example, a patient admitted with a GCS of 5 but who then improves within 24 h to 11 has a reasonably good chance of full recovery. A patient admitted with a GCS of 5 but who fails to improve in the first 72 h is much less likely to recover.

Other clinical signs

In addition to examination of the conscious level a full neurological examination must be carried out, looking in particular for signs of raised intracranial pressure, pupillary changes, localising and false localising signs.

Coning (Figure 9.2)

A rapid increase in intracranial pressure due to an enlarging haematoma, cerebral oedema or brain abscess causes the conscious level to deteriorate. If pressure is not relieved by evacuating the haematoma or abscess or reducing cerebral oedema then the medial part of the temporal lobe may be squeezed out of the supratentorial intracranial compartment, resulting in pressure on the 3rd cranial nerve and compression of the midbrain (Figure 9.2). This is called *coning* and the signs are bradycardia, hypertension and sometimes irregular breathing. The pupils become fixed and dilated and once coning has occurred the patient is unlikely to survive long. Raised pressure in the subtentorial compartment may lead to coning of the cerebellar tonsil and apnoea.

Pupillary changes

As intracranial pressure increases the 3rd cranial nerve becomes compressed. Initially the pupil may constrict, but as pressure on the nerve increases the pupil progressively dilates and becomes unreactive to light.

False localising signs

These are due to stretching or pressure on the 3rd, 4th or 6th cranial nerves. In an oculomotor (3rd nerve) palsy the affected eye fails to look upwards and outwards, the pupil is dilated and there is ptosis. The

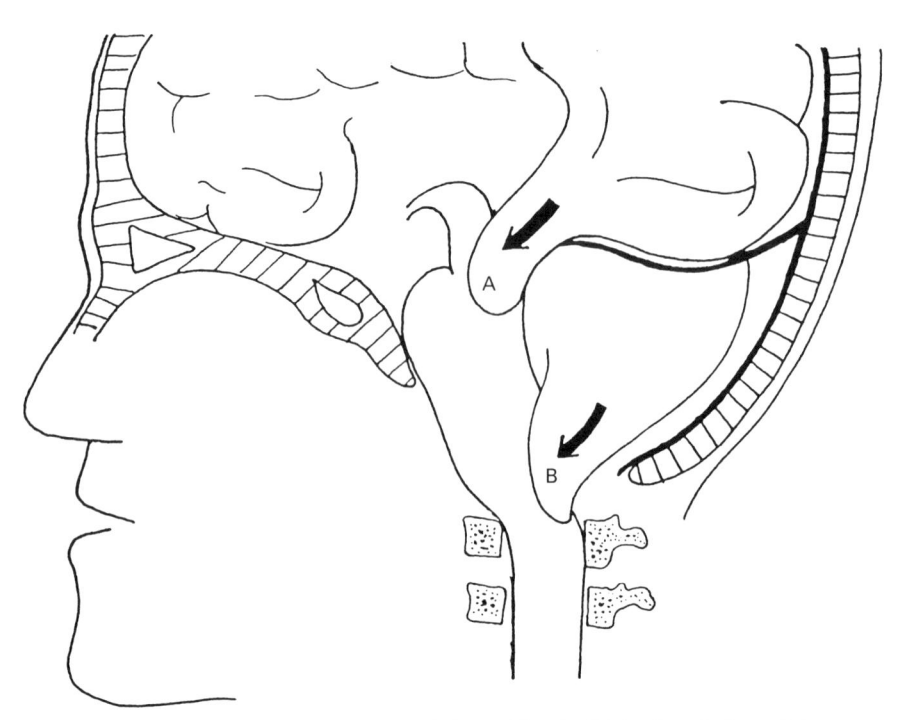

Figure 9.2 Coning: showing compression of the midbrain (A) by herniation of the temporal lobe and compression of the hind brain, or medulla, (B) by the cerebellar tonsil.

brain lesion is on the same side as the affected eye. In an abducens (6th nerve palsy) the affected eye cannot gaze laterally and may turn medially.

Localising signs

These localise the site of a lesion according to the abnormality found. Thus a right hemiplegia suggests a left-sided brain lesion. They are described in detail in texts on neurology and neurosurgery.

Papilloedema

This is due to raised intracranial pressure on the affected side (Figure 9.3). It may be present when there is raised intracranial

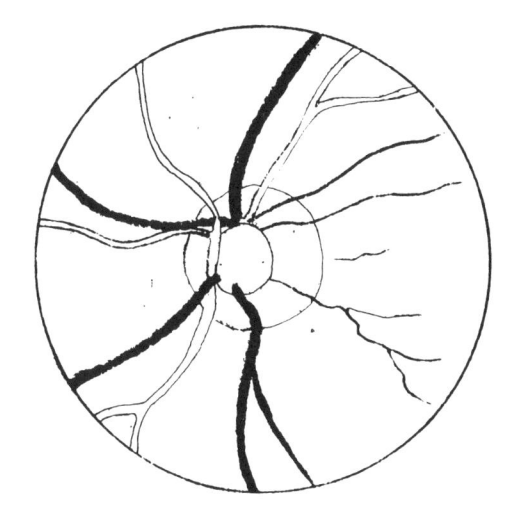

Normal fundus

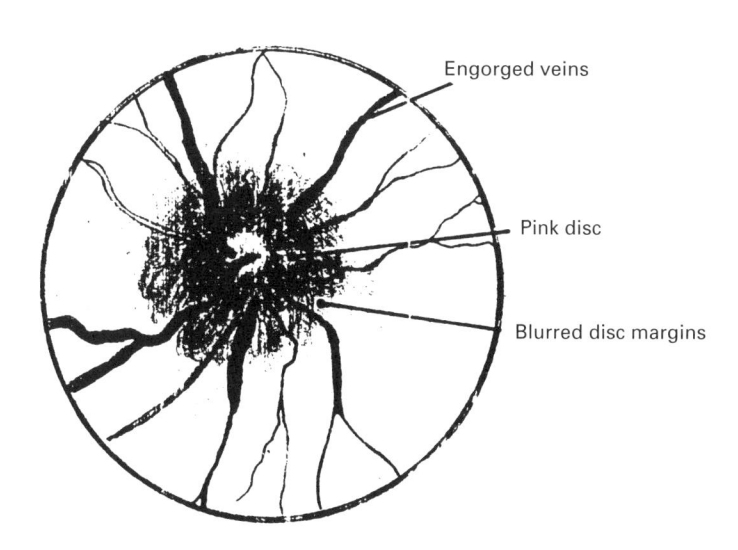

Papilloedema

Figure 9.3 The normal fundus and papilloedema.

pressure which has been present for at least a few days.

How to determine the cause

Correct treatment depends upon correct diagnosis. This involves obtaining whatever history is available and performing a full clinical examination including fundoscopy.

KEY POINT
Before assessing a patient in coma make sure the airway is secure.

The patient's history will need to be obtained from those who brought the patient to hospital. Important pointers to diagnosis are shown in Table 9.1. In particular ask about previous accidents and head injury, ingestion of alcohol, poisons or drugs and if there is a history of epilepsy, hypertension or diabetes. Determine whether the onset of coma was sudden or gradual and whether there is a history of fever.

Examination has two aims. The first is to make a diagnosis and the second to grade the severity of coma using the Glasgow Coma Scale (GCS). The change in GCS, whether deteriorating, stable or improving, is crucial to management decisions.

Look for signs of head injury; feel for fractures. Swelling in the region of the frontal sinus or orbital cellulitis may suggest brain abscess secondary to frontal sinusitis. Pus discharging from the ear or mastoid swelling may suggest temporal lobe abscess. Neurological signs such as hemiplegia or facial asymmetry may suggest a localised brain lesion. Examine for neck stiffness. Check the tone, reflexes, movements and sensation of all four limbs. Examine the pupils for their reaction to light, including the consensual reflex (light shone in one eye causes the other pupil to constrict). Look at the direction of gaze and for nystagmus. Check the optic fundus looking particularly for papilloedema, which might be a contraindication to performing a lumbar puncture. Normally you do not need to dilate the pupils to see the optic disc. If you cannot see the disc then dilate the pupils with atropine or homatropine eye drops but accept that this will affect subsequent examination of the pupils. If you still fail to see the optic disc and a lumbar puncture (LP) is indicated, weigh up the risks of coning against the benefits of the information to be obtained from LP. Usually it is in the patient's interests to proceed with an LP unless carotid angiography or CT scanning is available.

A diagnostic approach to coma is shown in Figure 9.4. The common causes of coma and appropriate investigations are shown in Table 9.1. District hospitals should be capable of diagnosing and treating most cases of non-traumatic coma.

KEY POINT
Common and often fatal errors in diagnosis are: 1. Missing hypoglycaemia. 2. Diagnosing cerebral malaria without excluding meningitis or other pathologies (in malaria endemic areas malaria parasites may be present when another pathology is responsible for coma). 3. Missing cerebral malaria in the apyrexial patient. 4. Failure to perform immediate gastric lavage in suspected poisoning (except suspected paraffin poisoning – see p. 122). 5. Failure to consider chronic subdural haematoma as a possible diagnosis (50% of cases do not give a history of recent head injury).

Table 9.1 Clinical and laboratory features of the major causes of coma

Cause	Clinical features	Laboratory findings
Cerebral malaria	Short history of illness Fever or history of fever Abnormal behaviour or coma No meningism or focal signs	Positive blood slide Normal blood glucose Normal CSF
Meningitis		
Bacterial	Short history of illness Fever and neck stiffness Sometimes purpuric rash Sometimes pneumonia	Cloudy CSF Low CSF glucose High protein Polymorphs
Viral	Short history of illness Fever and neck stiffness	CSF often clear High protein Normal CSF glucose Lymphocytes in CSF No organisms on Gram stain
TB	History over 2 weeks Fever and neck stiffness Chest may be clear or pulmonary TB present Cranial nerve lesions may occur	CSF clear High CSF protein Low CSF glucose Lymphocytes in CSF Ziehl–Neelsen stain sometimes positive
Cryptococcal	History over 2 weeks Fever and neck stiffness Cranial nerve lesions may occur	As for TB meningitis Indian ink stain positive Ziehl–Neelsen negative
Viral encephalitis	Short history, fever Neck stiffness often absent Focal signs may be present	Similar to viral meningitis but may be normal

Table 9.1 Clinical and laboratory features of the major causes of coma (*continued*)

Cause	Clinical features	Laboratory findings
Brain abscess	History at least some days Fever, periorbital cellulitis Discharging ear or septic focus (e.g. osteomyelitis) elsewhere Focal signs Confusion, coma, fits and papilloedema	LP contraindicated if papilloedema Carotid angiogram or CT reveals space-occupying lesion CSF may be normal or show increased cells and protein
Subarachnoid haemorrhage	Sudden onset, neck stiffness Initial severity ranges from headache to deep coma Hypertension may be present Neurological signs may or may not be present	CSF blood stained or xanthochromic
Cerebrovascular accident	Sudden onset, hemiplegia May be hypertensive Usually elderly	Diagnosis made clinically
Hypertensive encephalopathy	Hypertension, confusion, coma Retinopathy Focal signs usually absent	Unhelpful
Poisoning or drug overdose	History of ingestion/exposure Container beside patient Specific features of individual poisons (pp. 121–127)	Inspection and analysis of gastric lavage Serum drug levels
Alcohol	Smell on breath	Normal or low blood glucose
Diabetic comas		
Hypoglycaemia	History of diabetes History of hypoglycaemia Rapid onset, warm peripheries Bounding pulse, normal BP Sweating	Low blood glucose

Table 9.1 Clinical and laboratory features of the major causes of coma (*continued*)

Cause	Clinical features	Laboratory findings
Hyperglycaemia	Onset over a few days, may not be a known diabetic. If known diabetic may have had infection or stopped taking medication. Cold peripheries, low-volume pulse, rapid pulse, low BP, deep slow respiration, ketones on breath	Urine glucose ++++ Ketones +++ High blood glucose above 20 mmol/l
Non-ketoic hyperosmolar hyperglycaemic coma	Diabetic patient, onset over a few days, no acetone on breath	Hyperglycaemia No ketones High serum Na High serum osmolality
Post-convulsion	History of epilepsy Previous burns scars Focal signs transient or absent Afebrile, normal BP	None helpful
Sodium derangement	Exposure to heat, or history of diarrhoea, vomiting, intravenous fluids, abdominal emergency	High or low serum Na
Hypothyroidism	Coarse hair and features, pale, puffy, cold	Low T3/T4 Raised TSH

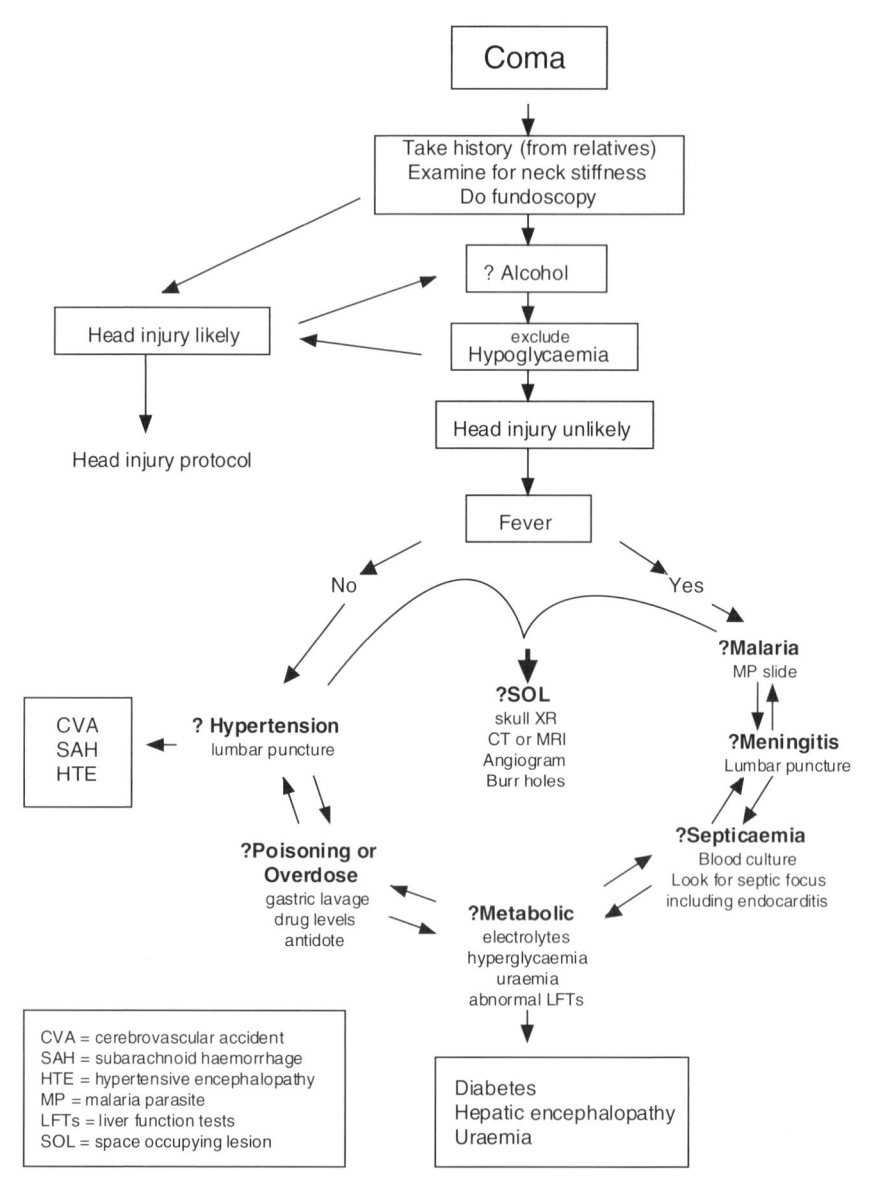

174 Care of the Critically Ill Patient in the Tropics

Figure 9.4 A diagnostic approach to coma. A diagnostic approach to coma: the presence of fever determines which order to consider different diagnoses and investigations.
Adapted from Sinclair JR, Watters DAK and Bagshawe A.
Reproduced with permission from *Neurosurgery in the tropics*,
Rosenfeld JV and Watters DAK (eds), Macmillan, Basingstoke, 2000.

Relevant investigations include blood slide, urea and electrolytes, lumbar puncture, blood glucose, drug/poison analysis, skull radiographs and microbiological culture.

Advanced investigations include carotid angiography (p. 403–406), isotope brain scan and computerised tomography (CT).

Management

General care

The management of specific conditions is described under the appropriate sections. All comatose patients need intensive nursing to prevent secondary pathology occurring due to pressure sores, malnutrition and pneumonia. Nursing techniques are described in more detail in Chapter 16.

Position

The aim of correct positioning is to protect the airway and prevent pressure sores. The coma position is shown in Figure 9.5. The head should not be twisted to the side, which obstructs venous drainage from the cranium. The neck should be in line with the trunk. Correct positioning of the patient is achieved by moving the hips, pelvis and legs, not the head and neck.

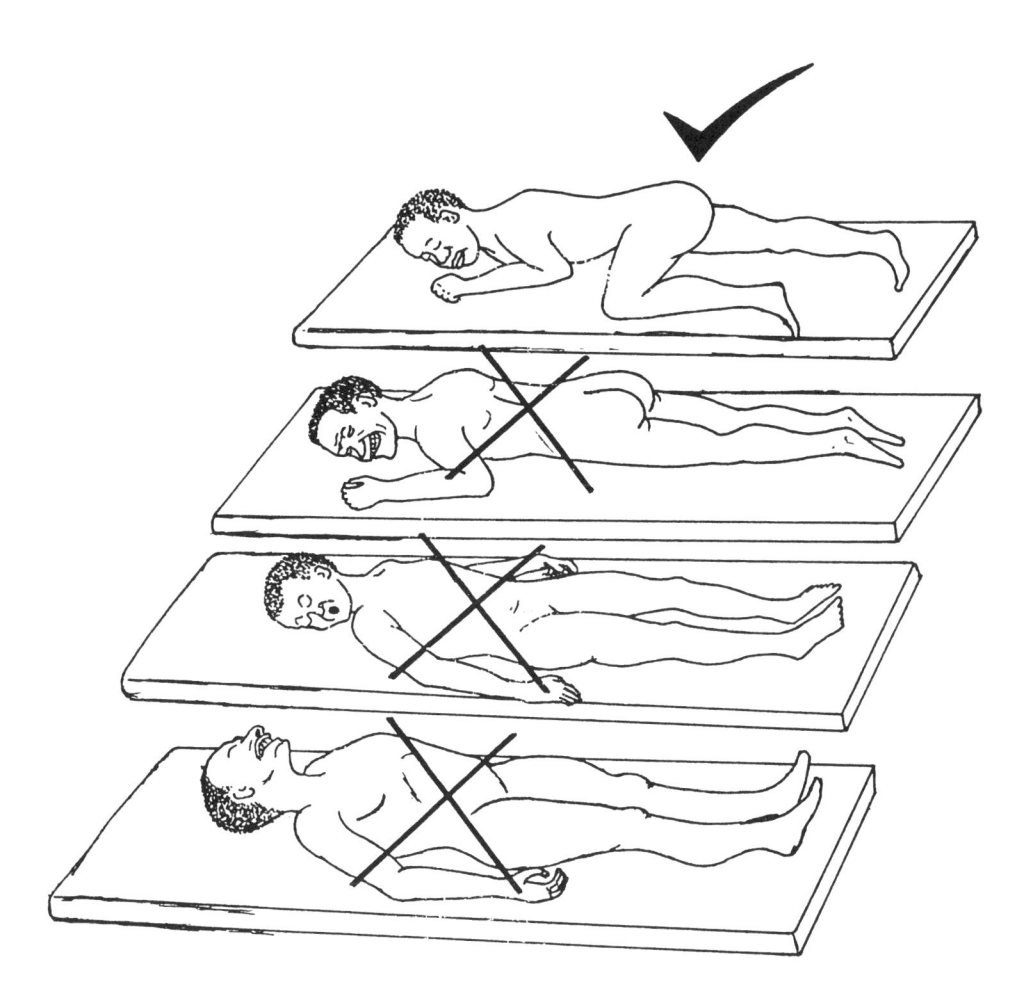

Figure 9.5 The coma position: the correct position is three-quarters prone, as shown. (*Note*: The coughing, straining, head-down tilt and jugulovenous pressure also increase intracranial pressure by reducing venous drainage from the brain.)

Comatose patients should not lie on their backs. In this position they will aspirate their secretions, their tongues will occlude their airway and they will develop pneumonia and die.

> **KEY POINT**
>
> Comatose patients must be nursed semi- or three-quarters prone.

If the airway is protected by an endotracheal tube or tracheostomy the patient can be nursed on his back as well as on his side.

Unless the patient is in shock the head of the bed should normally be elevated by 15–30° to reduce intracranial pressure.

Sometimes the patient will be nursed head down for postural drainage of the chest or to encourage expansion of the brain after evacuation of a chronic subdural haematoma.

Turning

Turn the patient 2 hourly to prevent pressure sores. The patients must be lifted when they are being turned, not pulled or dragged on the sheets. Dragging produces shearing and friction forces which cause pressure sores. Make sure there are enough people to lift rather than drag the patient to change position.

> **KEY POINT**
>
> Comatose patients must be turned 2 hourly.

Inspect the common pressure points 2 hourly (Figure 16.2) and record findings on a special chart.

Protect pressure points with sheepskin, surgical gloves filled with water, or pillows. Special ripple mattresses are available in specialised centres.

Avoid damp sheets and mattresses. Use powder to keep skin dry. Dry skin with towels after bed-baths by dabbing, not rubbing.

Fluid balance

All comatose patients should be catheterised unless there is a specific contraindication.

Catheterisation helps keep sheets dry as well as allowing accurate fluid balance.

Patients will need intravenous fluids to maintain fluid and electrolyte balance until the patient is established on enteral feeding.

Physiotherapy

Comatose patients frequently die of pneumonia. If the patient has a lot of secretions, cannot cough or protect his airway then he will need intubation until his conscious level improves. It is easier to prevent pneumonia than to treat it.

The chest must be kept clear by correct positioning, percussion and, in intubated patients, bagging and sucking.

Passive movements aim to prevent joint stiffness and deep venous thrombosis, while splintage will prevent contractures if there is peripheral nerve damage.

Nutrition

If the patient remains incapable of taking fluids orally after 48 h begin nutritional support via a nasogastric tube (p. 287).

Oral hygiene

This is described on p. 293.

Raised intracranial pressure

The brain is protected by the skull. Since bone cannot expand any increase of volume or pressure within the skull soon leads to brain cell damage from pressure. A small increase in volume within the skull (for

Table 9.2 Treatment of raised intracranial pressure

Problems	Treatment
Cerebral oedema	Head-up position
	Mannitol
Hypoxia (PaO_2 <60 mmHg)	Maintain airway
	Oxygen therapy, ventilation
Hypercarbia (any degree)	Hyperventilation (16–20 breaths per minute)
Jugular venous obstruction	Avoid twisting head
Pyrexia	Fan, tepid sponge
Ketamine	Avoid, induce with thiopentone
Anaesthestic gases	Avoid unnecessary GA
Hydrocephalus	Shunt
Space-occupying lesion (e.g. haematoma, tumour, abscess or granuloma)	Evacuate or excise

example an extradural haemorrhage) leads to a large increase in intracranial pressure (ICP).

The brain has a limited ability to compensate for raised intracranial pressure (ICP). In order to maintain the supply of oxygenated blood to the brain the blood pressure is raised in response to increased ICP. Severe hypoxaemia (PaO_2 <8 kPa (60 mmHg)) and any degree of hypercarbia result in dilatation of the cerebral blood vessels. Although this increases blood flow and oxygen supply to the brain it also increases the volume of blood within the skull so that ICP is increased. Thus if a patient with raised ICP from a head injury develops airway obstruction and hypoxia, reflex cerebral vasodilatation occurs, which further raises intracranial pressure.

The ability of the brain to compensate for space-occupying lesions also depends on the speed with which they develop. In the case of a head injury with an extradural or subdural haematoma there is no time for compensation and unless burr holes are made quickly the brain will be compressed, permanently damaged and the patient will most probably die. If there is a cerebral tumour or slowly developing hydrocephalus then some compensation is possible.

Some factors responsible for raising intracranial pressure are listed in Table 9.2 and shown in Figure 9.6. Treatment aims to keep intracranial pressure normal and prevent further brain damage.

Further reading

KIRKHAM FJ. Non-traumatic coma in children. *Arch Dis Child* 2001;85:303–12.

LIAO YJ, SO YT. An approach to critically ill patients in coma. *West J Med* 2002;176:184–7.

RWIZA HT, McLARTY DG. Assessment of prognosis in non-traumatic coma in a tropical environment. *Trop Doct*, 1987;17:52–6.

SINCLAIR JR, WATTERS DAK, BAGSHAWE A. Non-traumatic coma in Zambia. *Trop Doct* 1989;19:6–10.

Specific problems

Convulsions

Definitions

Convulsions are due to spontaneous and abnormal electrical discharge in the brain, which may remain localised, giving a focal or Jacksonian fit, or spread over a wider area, causing a generalised convulsion with loss of consciousness. All fits can be

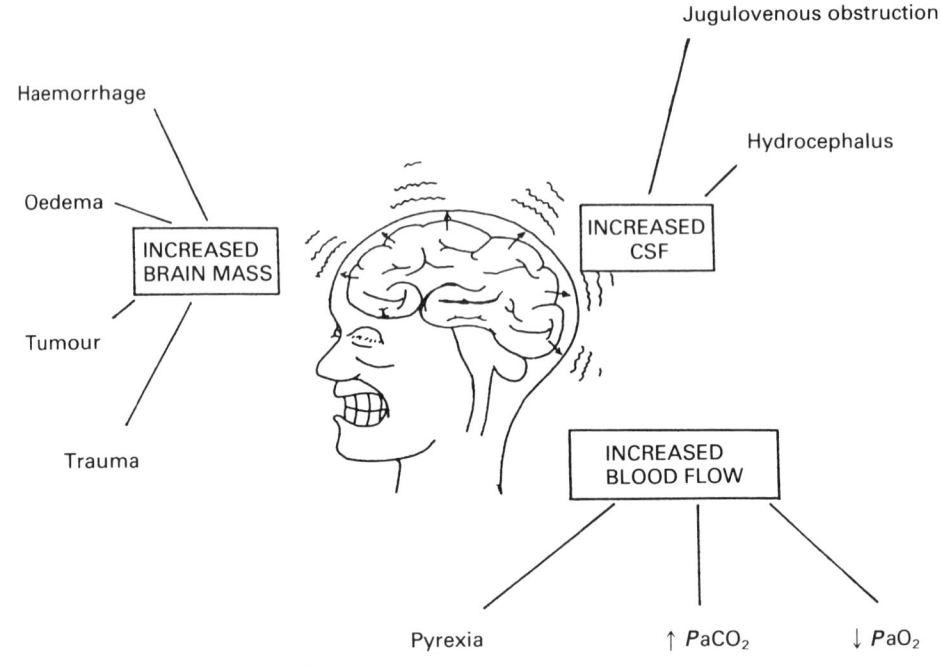

Figure 9.6 Factors responsible for increasing intracranial pressure.

Diagram labels: Haemorrhage, Oedema, Tumour, Trauma → INCREASED BRAIN MASS; Jugulovenous obstruction, Hydrocephalus → INCREASED CSF; Pyrexia, ↑ $PaCO_2$, ↓ PaO_2 → INCREASED BLOOD FLOW.

described as epileptic but the diagnosis of epilepsy implies recurrent fits.

Recognition

If the patient is not fitting when you attend to him always try to obtain an accurate account of what actually took place. Sometimes a faint or the hyperextended rigidity associated with tetanus may be mistaken for a fit.

Grand-mal convulsions may be preceded by an aura. This is followed by coma, an increase in tone (tonic phase), which proceeds to symmetrical jerkings, and contractions (clonic phase). Focal fits can also occur, only one side of the body or one limb being affected by the jerking and contraction.

After a fit a patient is said to be postictal. He will be unrousable, possibly with dilated pupils, flaccid limbs with an extensor plantar response. Frequently there will be soiling with faeces and urine. Providing the airway is patent he will wake up within 2–3 h. Sometimes patients are confused or violent during the post-ictal phase and following a focal fit there may be transient paralysis of a limb or a hemiplegia which reverses within 24 h.

Status epilepticus is said to occur when the patient is having a succession of generalised fits without the return of consciousness between them. It may cause permanent brain damage due to hypoxia. Status epilepticus may sometimes occur in a localised form, affecting the face, fingers or foot, and may continue for hours or days without loss of consciousness and is not in itself a serious threat to life.

How to determine the cause

There are numerous causes of convulsions, but in the context of a critically ill patient primary acute brain lesions (e.g. trauma, intracranial haematoma, infection or local ischaemia) and generalised metabolic disturbances (e.g. hypoglycaemia, hypoxia, hypernatraemia, hyperpyrexia or poisoning) are important, as many of these causes are remediable. Furthermore, fits may increase in an epileptic with intercurrent illness, children may have febrile fits and abrupt withdrawal of alcohol may precipitate fits which are also common in hypertensive encephalopathy and pregnancy-induced hypertension.

The likely cause of a fit also depends upon the age of the patient. Table 9.3 shows the commonest causes in children and babies according to age.

A single febrile fit in a child under five is unlikely to be complicated by further fits and usually no further investigation is necessary.

A fit in an adult who is not a known epileptic demands investigation as this may be the first sign of a cerebral tumour.

The causes of fits in an adult include:
1. idiopathic (no cause found);
2. cerebral tumour, abscess or vascular malformation;
3. sequel of severe head injury;
4. hypoglycaemia;
5. cerebral malaria;
6. cerebral atherosclerosis or hypertensive encephalopathy;
7. toxoplasmosis, cysticerosis, syphilis, tuberculoma;
8. meningitis, encephalitis;
9. hypoxia;
10. systemic lupus;
11. HIV encephalopathy;
12. other encephalopathies, including heavy metal poisoning.

Look for predisposing causes in the history and examination such as malaria, meningitis, toxoplasmosis, metabolic disturbance (uraemia, liver disease), hypertension. Always perform *fundoscopy* on a patient who presents with fits and do a full neurological examination.

Investigations

The most helpful simple investigations are lumbar puncture, blood film, skull radiographs, urea and electrolytes and blood glucose. Special investigations which may be indicated are electro-encephalogram (EEG), CT scan, isotope brain scan and carotid angiography.

Management

First aid

The first aim during a fit is to protect the patient's airway and prevent them biting their tongue. But do not force spoons blindly between clenched teeth as teeth may be broken. Keep the patient who is epileptic away from open fires. Epilepsy is a common cause of severe burns in Africa. Keep the patient on his side in the coma position after a fit.

Control of the convulsion

Fits can be controlled using diazepam. A dose of 10 mg will stop most fits in adults. In children, 0.2–0.3 mg/kg can be used i.v. or rectally. Paraldehyde 0.3 mg/kg rectally is also effective. Frequent fits or status epilepticus may need to be treated by infusion of diazepam or phenytoin. Oxygen should be given by mask. If it is impossible to stop the fits with anticonvulsants then paralyse the patient and ventilate.

Prevention of further fits

Phenytoin (at a dose discussed on p. 453) is helpful in patients considered to be at risk of further fits during their acute illness. Diazepam 40–80 mg/8 hourly by infusion can also be used but this has a more sedative effect than phenytoin and may render assessment of conscious level difficult.

Alternatively, phenobarbital (90–180 mg/day; for children see Table 9.3) or phenytoin (100 mg 1–3 times daily; for children see Table 9.3) can be given orally or by nasogastric tube.

Table 9.3 Diagnosis and treatment of convulsions in children

Age	Causes	Diagnosis	Treatment
<1 month	Birth trauma	History, CSF bloodstained	Sedate and tube feed.
	Cerebral anoxia	Difficult resuscitation	Sedate and tube feed.
	Hypoglycaemia	Low birth weight	2–3 ml 50% dextrose.
		Dextrostix below 2.5 mmol/l	Oral glucose 10% and breast milk.
	Hypocalcaemia	Bottle-fed baby	2 ml 10% calcium gluconate i.v.
		Towards end of first week	Oral Ca gluconate 300 mg 4 hourly for 3–4 days.
	Infection	LP for meningitis	Appropriate antibiotics.
		Check urine, blood cultures	
	Kernicterus	History of jaundice	Phototherapy, sedate.
	Tetanus	Spasms not fits	See pp. 148–150.
1–3 months	Brain damage	History	Phenytoin 5–9 mg/kg/day in two doses, or phenobarbital 3.5 mg/kg/day in 2–3 doses.
	Meningitis	LP	Antibiotics if bacterial.
3 months – 4 years	Febrile fit	Fever	Stop fit with diazepam 0.2–0.7 mg/kg i.v. or paraldehyde 0.3 ml/kg rectally.
			Reduce temperature with sponging and fanning.
			Paracetamol to lower temperature
			Search for cause of fever.
	Meningitis, encephalitis	LP	Antibiotics if bacterial.
	Malaria	Blood film	Antimalarial.
	Tumours	CT scan	Neurosurgery.
	HIV encephalopathy	Clinical	Treat opportunistic infections.
Over 4 years	Idiopathic epilepsy	No other cause	Phenytoin 5–9 mg/kg/day in two doses or phenobarbital 3.5 mg/kg/day in 2–3 doses.
		Recurrence without treatment	
	Brain abscess	Underlying sinusitis/mastoiditis	Drain sinus and cerebral abscess

Aggravating factors should be minimised. The temperature should be lowered in children with febrile fits. Eclamptic fits in pregnancy-induced hypertension means the baby should be quickly delivered and the blood pressure controlled (p. 268).

Further reading

CHAPMAN MG, SMITH M, HIRSCH NP. Status epilepticus. *Anaesthesia* 2001;56:648-59.

Intracranial abscess
Introduction

About 80% of intracranial abscesses are situated within the brain substance, the remaining 20% are in the epidural or subdural space. Sinusitis and mastoiditis are the commonest causes. Orbital cellulitis should alert one to the diagnosis of frontal sinusitis and when it is present there is at least a 30% chance of an intracranial abscess having already developed. Spread from infection elsewhere in the body (e.g. osteomyelitis or empyema) is another common cause. AIDS is likely to become an important predisposing factor for the development of intracranial abscess due to bacteraemia.

A brain abscess begins as an area of cerebral infection which is walled off by a glial reaction that eventually matures over a period of 2–3 weeks into a capsule of variable thickness (if the patient survives). Around the capsule is a zone of oedematous brain, which adds to the mass effect. Death occurs either from cerebral compression or from rupture into the subarachnoid space or ventricles.

Recognition

EPIDURAL
Early features are intense local pain, oedema of the overlying scalp and toxaemia with a high fever. Untreated it will cause compression of the underlying brain, focal signs, raised intracranial pressure and altered consciousness. It usually develops owing to direct spread into the epidural space from frontal sinusitis and there is often associated osteomyelitis of the skull.

SUBDURAL
A subdural abscess usually complicates sinusitis and infection is spread from the sinus to the subdural space via the diploic veins. Once pus begins to form it may spread rapidly across the surface of the brain and cause a cortical thrombophlebitis. The patient has a high fever, the conscious level deteriorates rapidly and there may be convulsions.

CEREBRAL OR BRAIN ABSCESS
About half develop as a complication of otitis media, mastoiditis or sinusitis. Others develop from bloodborne infection from distant sites (osteomyelitis, empyema, endocarditis, dental or perianal sepsis) but in about 20% of cases no cause is found. The patient usually presents with a space-occupying lesion (SOL) with coma, neurological signs and fever. Meningeal irritation is rare and the development of neck stiffness indicates herniation of the cerebellar tonsils (Figure 9.2) into the foramen magnum with compression of the medulla rather than inflammation of the meninges.

Investigations

The white cell count is usually raised. The CSF is not always turbid and if a diagnosis of brain abscess is suspected lumbar puncture carries the risk of coning and death.

RADIOISOTOPE SCANNING
Carotid angiography can be performed even at the bedside using a portable X-ray machine (p. 403). An SOL will be seen distorting the vessels on AP film of the skull. When available, CT scanning is the most reliable way of making a diagnosis.

Management

The site of the abscess must be localised by assuming localised spread from the ear or frontal sinus or else by carotid angiography or brain scan.

The objectives are to
1. eradicate the intracranial sepsis;
2. remove the mass effect of the abscess and
3. treat the primary cause.

Antibiotics

These should be given in large doses as soon as the diagnosis is suspected. Penicillin, chloramphenicol and metronidazole should be given initially until the results of culture (if available) are known.

Steroids

High doses of dexamethasone (4 mg 6 hourly) will reduce the surrounding brain oedema and mass effect of an intracranial abscess.

Surgery

Surgical treatment should not be delayed as conservative treatment is hazardous. The abscess must be drained and any infected bone excised. Mastoidectomy or frontal ethmoidectomy should be performed if infection in these cavities is the cause. When there is a brain abscess either pus is repeatedly aspirated through a burr hole until the abscess resolves or open drainage of the abscess is performed under direct vision. Whenever possible transfer the patient to a neurosurgeon.

Subarachnoid haemorrhage

This is due to bleeding into the CSF usually from a small aneurysm (called a berry aneurysm) or arteriovenous malformation. Rare causes are intracranial tumours and coagulation abnormalities. Hypertension is sometimes a predisposing factor. Angiography fails to reveal any abnormality in about 30% of cases.

Recognition

The presentation ranges in severity from neck pain and headache to severe coma. In conscious patients vomiting and photophobia are common.

The diagnosis is made by lumbar puncture. The CSF will be initially bloodstained and later will show xanthochromia (a yellow appearance due to pigment from old blood). The bloodstained CSF can be differentiated from a traumatic tap because the CSF does not clear by the time the second and third bottles are being filled.

Management

The patient who is fully conscious or who has a high grade of coma with minimal neurological deficit should be considered for neurosurgical ligation of a microaneurysm or arteriovenous malformation if such facilities are available. Those patients in whom no abnormality can be demonstrated have a better prognosis than patients with a ruptured aneurysm.

Carotid angiography should be performed between the third and fifth days and definitive surgery can be carried out before the tenth day, after which there is an increased risk of further haemorrhage.

Nimodipine (60 mg orally or by NGT), a calcium channel drug, may improve the outcome of subarachnoid haemorrhage, probably through a neuronal protective rather than anti-vasospastic effect. Tranexamic acid and epsilon aminocaprioic acid (the anti-fibrinolytic agents) are no longer used they have the potential to cause ischaemic complications.

In all parts of the world a diagnosis of subarachnoid haemorrhage in association with a GCS of less than 8 carries a very poor prognosis. Each district hospital should consult its central hospital for advice about which patients to refer for definitive investigation and treatment.

Diagnosis of brain stem death

The need to diagnose brain stem death only arises when mechanical ventilators are in use. Because the vasomotor centre is low in the brain stem it is possible for the circulation (heart beat, pulse and blood pressure) to be maintained in a ventilated patient when there is no chance of recovery of spontaneous breathing or of consciousness.

Strict criteria for diagnosis must be adhered to because no one should discontinue ventilation when there is still hope of survival. Patients who are brain stem dead and have no possibility of recovery should be certified dead and ventilation stopped, otherwise limited resources will be wasted and other patients may die because no ventilators are available. There may be legal criteria for the diagnosis of brain stem death in your country. If so follow these criteria. Some countries insist on an EEG being done but this is not the practice in many developed countries. The following is a guide if there are no established criteria for your hospital.

Brain stem death should be established by two senior doctors on two separate occasions.

Preconditions

1. Glasgow Coma Scale is 3.
2. Patient is on ventilator with no spontaneous breathing.

BRAIN STEM REFLEXES – HOW TO DO IT

Pupillary response to light

Corneal reflex Firm touch with cotton wool on cornea; reflex is present if the patient blinks.

Oculovestibular reflex 20 ml of ice-cold water is injected into both ears after ensuring the ears are not full of wax; reflex is present if there are any eye movements or nystagmus.

Pain reflex for cranial nerves Press over supraorbital nerve, which is located medially near the bridge of the nose on the orbital margin. Test bilaterally; any facial grimace disproves brain stem death.

Gag reflex Suction tube passed down endotracheal tube or tracheostomy tube into trachea; reflex is present if there is any effort to cough or gag.

Apnoea test This test is conducted in such a way that brain damage due to hypoxia is prevented while the carbon dioxide tension in the blood rises above 6.7 kPa (50 mmHg) which is an adequate level to stimulate respiration.

1. If blood gases are available then the minute volume of the ventilator can be reduced to cause a measured rise in CO_2 while preventing hypoxia. Alternatively, ventilate with 5% CO_2 in oxygen for 10 min before the test.
2. If no blood gases are available then turn the ventilator rate to one-third of normal and ventilate with 100% oxygen for 10 min. Observe for cyanosis during this preparatory period.

Carry out the test as follows:

(a) Discontinue ventilation.

(b) Oxygenate the patient with a suction catheter in the trachea connected to the oxygen supply at a flow rate of 8 l/min.

(c) Observe for spontaneous breathing over a period of 10 min. Respiratory effort disproves brain stem death.

(d) If the patient shows respiratory effort immediately reconnect him to the ventilator.

If the patient has a positive response to any of the above tests brain stem death cannot be diagnosed.

3. Pupils fixed and dilated.
4. Suffering from a condition known to cause irrecoverable brain damage.

Exclusions

1. History of poisoning or drug intoxication within previous 3 days.
2. Hypothermia <35°C.
3. Abnormal blood glucose, electrolytes or other metabolic derangement.
4. Sedation or muscle relaxants given within 24 h (72 h for muscle relaxant in renal failure). If a nerve stimulator is available, it may be used to confirm that muscle relaxants are not present.

Spinal reflexes may be present when a patient is brain stem dead. Their presence is not an exclusion.

Brain stem reflexes

These should be proven to be absent on two separate occasions.
1. Pupillary response to light.
2. Corneal reflex.
3. Oculovestibular reflex.
4. Cranial nerve response to pressure over supraorbital nerves.
5. Gag reflex.
6. Spontaneous breathing (see apnoea test).

10
Head injuries

Introduction

The commonest causes of head injury are assault, road traffic accidents and falls. Head injuries account for around 15% of admissions to many critical care units.

At the moment of impact the brain is injured. This may be at the site of impact or on the opposite side of the brain. High-velocity deceleration may cause severe diffuse brain damage due to shearing and rotational forces, especially around the base of the brain and the brain stem. Brain cells destroyed at the time of injury cannot be replaced. The aim of observation and treatment in head injuries is to prevent further brain damage due to hypoxia, shock, hypoglycaemia, compression of brain tissue by blood clot or oedema, and infection.

> **KEY POINT**
>
> The aim of management is to prevent secondary brain damage from hypoxia, shock, hypoglycaemia, cerebral oedema, intracranial haematoma, convulsions or infection.

Clinical recognition

The patient with a head injury may present with a laceration, a fracture, a history of loss of consciousness, altered consciousness or amnesia. Some patients are simply found lying unconscious due to the severity of the injury, though the effects of alcohol or hypothermia may obscure the clinical picture.

Initial assessment

Try to obtain an accurate history of what happened and in particular ask whether the unconscious patient was conscious at any time after his head injury. If there was a period of consciousness this is called a *lucid interval*.

Examine the patient carefully for other injuries, particularly when he cannot give a history. Patients with head injuries may also have a fracture or dislocation of the cervical spine.

A significant number of patients suffer unnecessary secondary brain damage due to hypoxia *en route* to hospital. The first priority is to ensure the airway is clear and that the breathing is satisfactory.

> **KEY POINT**
>
> After head injury many patients suffer further brain damage from hypoxia; ensure the airway is clear.

Vital signs

Although a patient may bleed heavily from a scalp wound, over 80% of head-injured patients who develop hypotension have another injury causing hypovolaemia. Such injuries are usually in the abdomen or thorax or from blood loss associated with fractures.

Brain stem compression causes hypertension and bradycardia, often with irregular and Cheyne–Stokes respiration.

Conscious level

After ensuring a patent airway, adequate breathing and stable circulation the GCS should be recorded. Subsequent deterioration or the history of a lucid interval in a now unconscious patient suggests that burr holes, angiography or scanning should be urgently performed.

Examine the face and head carefully. Look for blood or CSF draining from the nose or ears which would suggest a fractured base of skull.

Examination of the eyes

The pupillary response to light should be recorded. Grade the size of the pupil according to the Glasgow Coma Scale chart (Figure 17.5).

A unilateral fixed and dilated pupil may be due to a space-occupying lesion such as a haematoma on the same side. The combination of a dilated or dilating pupil with unconsciousness suggests further investigation or burr holes is necessary. Other causes of a unilateral fixed and dilated pupil include the following:
1. optic nerve injury (pupil will still constrict in response to light shone in the other eye);
2. atropine given locally to the affected eye;
3. traumatic dilation of the pupil due to eye injury (rare).

Irregularity of the pupil occurs in penetrating injury of the eye with iris prolapse.

Bilateral fixed and dilated pupils are usually a sign of severe brain damage and tentorial herniation and suggest a poor prognosis. However, other causes are as follows:
1. atropine having been given systemically or locally to both eyes;
2. an epileptic fit (bilateral dilation of pupils will soon resolve after a fit);
3. massive CVA with cerebral oedema;
4. severe encephalitis.

Ask the conscious patient if he can see. Blurred or double vision suggests an eye injury or blow-out fracture of the orbit.

If the patient is conscious check eye movements. Both eyes should move freely in all directions. Inability to move one eye laterally suggests abducens nerve palsy (6th cranial nerve). This is due to raised intracranial pressure on the side of the palsy, which causes pressure damage to the cranial nerve – a *false localising sign*. Pressure damage to the 3rd (oculomotor) and 4th (trochlear) cranial nerves may also occur.

When there is a subconjunctival haematoma and you cannot see the posterior margin of the haematoma suspect a fractured base of skull.

Associated injuries

At least a third of patients with severe head injuries have other injuries and these are often more urgent and life-threatening than the head injury itself. Thus a full assessment of injuries sustained must be made (pp. 198–201).

> **KEY POINT**
>
> Many patients with head trauma have severe associated injuries. Shock is more commonly due to an associated injury than to blood loss from the scalp.

Investigations

A lateral view of the cervical spine, which should show all seven cervical vertebrae, is the most important X-ray in an unconscious patient with a head injury. Skull X-rays rays (AP, lateral and Towne's view) are of value for documentation and detecting patients more likely to have an intracranial haematoma. However those with skull fractures usually have other criteria for admission such as a history of loss of consciousness. Thus skull X-rays do not normally affect the decision about admission and most head injuries can be correctly managed even when X-rays are unavailable or in short supply. If there is a scalp laceration, palpation or exploration of the wound is a reliable means of detecting an underlying fracture.

> **KEY POINT**
>
> The most important radiograph in an unconscious patient with a head injury is a lateral view of the cervical spine.

The role of special investigations such as ultrasound, carotid angiography, diagnostic burr holes and CT scanning is discussed under management.

Management

Immediate management

Ensure the patient's airway is clear and protected, the breathing is satisfactory, active bleeding controlled and resuscitation commenced. Exclude the possibility of a fracture or dislocation of the spine or else move the patient with due regard for the spinal cord (p. 203) and stabilise the cervical spine in a collar designed for the purpose.

Who should be admitted?

Even an apparently trivial injury may be complicated by intracranial haematoma. It is therefore wise to admit patients with the following complaints for 24 hours' observation:

1. history of loss of consciousness;
2. unconscious on arrival in hospital;
3. focal neurological signs;
4. post-traumatic amnesia;
5. significant drowsiness;
6. severe headache or vomiting;
7. blurred vision;
8. associated injuries;
9. skull fracture or CSF leak.

Most of those admitted need only be kept in hospital overnight.

Observation

After admission the patient should be closely observed, noting the GCS, pattern of breathing, vital signs and pupil reaction at hourly intervals. The decision as to what treatment is necessary is more often determined by changes in GCS or other parameters rather than by the initial findings on admission.

This chapter now deals with the management of the 15% or so of head injury admissions that are severe.

The aim is to prevent secondary brain injury. The causes and treatment of this are summarised in Table 10.1.

General measures
Position

The airway must be safe (Figure 9.5). Head-injured patients should be nursed with a 15° head-up tilt unless there is hypovolaemia. This position aims to reduce cerebral oedema by gravity. The general care of a comatose patient is discussed on p. 175.

> **KEY POINT**
>
> Head injuries should be nursed with the head of the bed elevated 15° and on their side in the coma position if they are unconscious and the airway is not protected by an endotracheal tube.

Table 10.1 Causes and management of secondary brain injury

Cause	Management
Hypoxia	Secure airway and breathing
Shock	Stop bleeding, resuscitate, treat associated injuries
Hypoglycaemia	50% dextrose
Brain compression	Head-up tilt 15°, keep temperature below 38°C
1. Haematoma	Evacuate by burr holes
2. Oedema	Mannitol, hyperventilation
Infection	Debridement, antibiotics
Fits	Secure airway, anticonvulsants

Fluid therapy

Head-injured patients who are not hypovolaemic from blood loss should be kept a little dehydrated to minimise cerebral oedema. Give sufficient fluid just to maintain a urine output of 0.5–1 ml/kg/h (around two-thirds of usual maintenance fluids).

Use of diuretics

These are used to shrink the brain and reduce intracranial pressure. They are indicated when a deteriorating patient is being taken to theatre or transferred for further investigations. They may also be given when deterioration is known or suspected to be due to cerebral oedema.

Mannitol is an osmotic diuretic which may be used to buy time when transferring the patient to theatre or another hospital. A single large dose of 0.5–0.75 g/kg will reduce intracranial pressure by shrinking the brain and also reducing the volume of CSF. Subsequent doses of 0.25 g/kg can be given. The initial effect of an osmotic diuretic such as mannitol is to increase intravascular volume which may precipitate heart failure in elderly patients with underlying cardiac disease. In contused brain where breakdown of capillary walls occurs mannitol will leak into the extravascular space and ultimately increase the bulk of brain in this area.

Furosemide (0.5–1 mg/kg i.v.) is just as effective and also reduces CSF production.

Steroids are not indicated for reducing cerebral oedema in acute head injuries.

Indications for further investigation or burr holes

Many patients with low coma scales on admission do not have blood clots which can be evacuated, but rather diffuse cerebral damage. Equally, some patients who deteriorate in the first 48 h do so because of rising intracranial pressure due to cerebral oedema. In children the most common pathology is diffuse cerebral oedema and haematomas are found in less than 10% of severe head injuries.

It is better to obtain objective evidence of intracranial haematoma before doing burr holes. In practice, further investigations depend on what facilities are available.

1. Cranial ultrasound (echoencephalography) may demonstrate shift of the midline but will not diagnose the cause.
2. Carotid angiography does not need a radiologist nor sophisticated equipment. A bedside method which can be performed with a portable X-ray machine under either local or general anaesthetic is described as a practical procedure (p. 403).
3. Computerised tomography (CT) is only available in specialised centres in tropical countries. It is the most accurate investigation for the diagnosis of intracranial haematoma. However, reasonable man-

agement of head-injured patients can usually be achieved without it.
4. Diagnostic burr holes may be the only form of specific investigation available in many district hospitals.

The indications for performing diagnostic burr holes are as follows:
1. a deteriorating level of consciousness;
2. an unconscious patient with focal neurological signs;
3. hemiplegia which is becoming more extensive;
4. failure to improve with a GCS less than 9; and
5. the development of fits or focal signs some days after injury.

The technique of performing burr holes is described on pp. 407–414. Before commencing burr holes you must decide what you hope to achieve and how you will cope with the possible findings:
1. Extradural haematoma has a good prognosis if promptly evacuated, but probably occurs in less than 5% of severe head injuries. Usually it is not possible to control the bleeding from the middle meningeal artery (or branch of it) through the initial burr hole. Either a bone flap will need to be raised or else bone nibblers used to obtain access to the middle meningeal vessels. These are the most rewarding patients to operate on. If you find one but are unable to stop the bleeding then you will have to pack or preferably clip the bleeder and transfer the patient.
2. Acute subdural haematoma is more common but has a mortality of around 70% even in specialised centres. It is sometimes difficult to completely drain a subdural haematoma without raising a flap. Bleeding from a venous sinus is found infrequently but may be extremely persistent and hard to stop.
3. Drainage of an intracerebral haematoma is beyond the capabilities of those without neurosurgical training and should be attempted only in a specialised centre.

Transfer to a neurosurgical centre

The ease with which transfer of a head-injured patient can be effected will often determine whether or not carotid angiography and/or burr holes are performed locally. If communications with senior staff at a referral centre are good it may be possible to obtain advice.

Assuming the journey will take less than 3 hours either by road or air, the indications for transfer are similar to those listed above for performing burr holes.

Patients with a poor prognosis should not generally be transferred: i.e. those with GCS 3–5 despite good oxygenation, blood pressure and having excluded hypoglycaemia, alcohol or hypothermia. Such patients would not normally have burr holes performed unless a haematoma was diagnosed by scan. The likelihood is that most have diffuse brain damage and the prognosis is poor. In the tropics over 90% of such patients will have an unfavourable outcome. Those patients who improve can continue to be observed and subsequently be transferred if improvement is not maintained.

Patients with an admission GCS 6–8 deserve investigation and aggressive therapy, particularly if they deteriorate or fail to improve. If they improve after admission they will probably not require intervention unless there are focal signs.

The patient with a deteriorating GCS having been admitted with or having at some time a GCS of 6 or more deserves intervention, investigation or transfer as appropriate.

Before transfer ensure the following:
1. Scalp wounds have been debrided and sutured even if there is an underlying depressed fracture.

2. Associated injuries have been treated. Do not transfer a head-injured patient who needs a laparotomy unless your institution is incapable of performing the procedure. Ensure fractures are properly splinted.
3. An experienced doctor, paramedic or nurse capable of suctioning and intubation accompanies the patient. The patient must not become hypoxic or hypotensive during transfer. His airway must be safe. Most patients should be transferred intubated.
4. The patient is given mannitol or furosemide when appropriate.
5. Prophylactic antibiotics and antitetanus toxoid have been given when appropriate.
6. You have informed the receiving centre when communications allow.
7. Good documentation is sent of the condition of the patient and what treatment has been carried out, also the patient's X-rays.

> **KEY POINT**
>
> Before transferring a patient with head injury ensure wounds and associated injuries have been correctly treated, that the airway is safe and that someone experienced accompanies the patient.

Ventilation for head injuries

Ventilatory support for severe head injuries avoids hypoxia and reduces intracranial pressure if $PaCO_2$ is kept in the range of 3.3–4 kPa (25–30 mmHg) by hyperventilation. The rationale for hyperventilation is that cerebral blood flow increases linearly with $PaCO_2$ and that increased cerebral blood flow is one of the determinants of intracranial pressure.

Ventilation for patients with irregular breathing owing to brain stem injury is unlikely to save life and is often inappropriate. Elective hyperventilation to reduce intracranial pressure is widely practised where resources are abundant but the evidence that it improves the eventual outcome is marginal. This author does not advise the use of ventilatory support for head injuries where resources are limited, nor should patients be transferred merely in the hope that ventilation may be of benefit. This is in contrast to cases with severe associated chest problems where ventilation is most rewarding.

Further advice

Further advice about the management of severe head injuries with a GCS <9 is given in the practical procedure on intracranial pressure monitoring p. 415.

Specific problems

Scalp laceration

This should be treated as other wounds with debridement and cleaning followed by suturing. Primary closure can be done up to 24 h for wounds of the scalp and face. Good haemostasis avoids haematoma collection, which can subsequently become infected. The deep fascia (galea) should be sutured if torn with 0 to 2/0 chromic catgut and the skin sutured with 2/0 silk or nylon. Alternatively the galea can be included in the skin suture. Skin sutures should be removed after 5–7 days. Always try to cover the exposed cranium as it may dessicate and necrose if left exposed to the atmosphere. A flap of galea can be used to protect the cranium if the skin should be left open. If the cranium cannot be covered due to extensive degloving or scalp loss dress the wound, keeping exposed bone moist, and refer the patient for a rotation flap once his condition is stable.

Scalp lacerations and open skull fractures are a common cause of tetanus so it is always important to clean and debride the wound well.

> **KEY POINT**
>
> Immunise the patient with a scalp laceration against tetanus.

Skull fracture

This may be diagnosed by palpation of the wound before closure or by X-ray. The standard views of AP and lateral of the skull may not show an occipital fracture. A Towne's view should be taken if occipital fracture is suspected.

The significance of a skull fracture is that it indicates a severe head injury. Patients with skull fractures are three timer more likely to have intracranial haematoma than those without. All patients with skull fractures should be admitted for head injury observations.

Open fractures and those which pass through the sinuses, the ear or nose cavities should be treated with prophylactic antibiotics to reduce the risk of osteomyelitis, subdural, brain or meningeal infection. Whenever there is a CSF leak there is an open fracture. Give penicillin and sulphonamide for 5 days.

Open depressed fractures should be elevated as part of the exercise of debridement. If no tools are available to make a burr hole then the patient should have the wound cleaned, debrided and closed after removing all foreign matter. Closed depressed fractures may not need to be elevated at all. There is no urgency to operate unless there are neurological signs and/or a deteriorating level of consciousness. The stable patient with a large closed depressed fracture should be observed for 24 h before referral. The term 'large' refers to those in whom the depression is greater than the thickness of the cranium or those in whom there is an unsightly depression.

Fractures of the base of skull are usually associated with severe brain injury and have a mortality rate over 80%. The fracture is often not seen on X-ray. Bleeding and watery discharge (CSF) from the nose or ear suggests a fractured base of skull. Direct injuries to the ear or nose can also cause bleeding in their own right.

CSF leak

A CSF leak means the dura is torn. Usually this dries up within a few days of the injury. The indications for referral to a neurosurgeon for exploration are:
- a persistent leak over 7 days;
- the development of meningitis;
- an angulated spicule of bone in the roof of one of the air sinuses; and
- a broad fracture line.

All patients with CSF leak need prophylactic antibiotics.

Fits

These indicate brain injury. Secondary brain damage due to hypoxia can occur during fits.

Fits should be controlled with diazepam and the patient put on anticonvulsants. A phenytoin infusion is best to prevent further fits. Phenytoin 100 mg t.d.s. by nasogastric tube is a reasonable alternative when parenteral phenytoin is not available. Phenobarbital 60 mg t.d.s. can be used if phenytoin is not available (paediatric dosage, see Table 9.3). Phenobarbital may also be given i.m. 50–200 mg, repeated after 6 h if necessary (max. 600 mg daily).

Fits are not in themselves an indication for burr holes. Focal fits suggest localised damage and should be treated as under focal signs after controlling the fit. Fits developing after 24 h may be due to the development of a subacute subdural haematoma, although increasing cerebral oedema is more likely and further investigations as described above are indicated.

Focal neurological signs

Hemiplegia or monoplegia suggest localised brain damage. A depressed fracture with focal signs should be elevated. Focal signs in association with a GCS below 12 or deterioration in GCS suggests burr holes should be done promptly. Increasing hemiplegia, perhaps associated with extensor posture, usually indicates brain stem distortion due to an expanding hemisphere lesion (clot, bleeding or oedema).

Aerocoele

If air is seen within the cranium on skull X-ray it suggests an open fracture or fracture line extending into a sinus. Prophylactic antibiotics should be given. Very occasionally aerocoeles can be tense and cause compression, in which case a burr hole must be done to relieve the tension.

Other problems

1. Neurogenic pulmonary oedema may develop rapidly and is thought to be due to the release of vasoactive amines which temporarily raise intravascular pressures. The pulmonary endothelium leaks fluid and even when pressures return to normal there is a permeability defect in pulmonary capillaries. The management of pulmonary oedema is discussed on p. 54, but since the underlying cause may be raised intracranial pressure this should also be controlled (p. 176).
2. Disseminated intravascular coagulation may occur owing to release of thromboplastin from the injured brain. If DIC is confirmed treatment should commence with fresh frozen plasma or fresh blood. Coagulopathies are discussed further on pp. 34–35.
3. Diabetes insipidus is a sign of hypothalamic compression. The secretion of antidiuretic hormone (ADH) from the posterior pituitary is impaired owing to pressure on the hypothalamic–pituitary axis. The patient is found to be passing large volumes of urine each hour. The treatment is to ensure accurate fluid balance and give vasopressin, but the prognosis is poor.

The patient who does not improve

Primary brain damage may be so severe that full recovery is not possible. Some patients deteriorate despite correct treatment because cerebral oedema inevitably increases in the first 48 h after brain injury. Treatment is directed at reducing intracranial pressure (p. 176) and excluding haematoma or other causes of secondary brain damage.

A distinction needs to be made between deterioration in conscious level and failure to improve. The deteriorating patient requires investigation, burr holes or transfer to exclude an intracranial haematoma. For those who fail to improve, the decision must be whether to continue observation and wait or proceed to further investigations. Further management also depends on the prognosis. Intracranial pressure monitoring is discussed on p. 415.

Assessment of prognosis

Assessment of prognosis is necessary to determine which patients will benefit from treatment, investigation, operations or transfer.

Severity and outcome are related to the following:
1. Best Glasgow Coma Scale on admission or in the first 24 h:

GCS	Unfavourable outcome
3–5	90%
6–8	30%
9–10	20%
11–15	10%

Most deaths in patients with a GCS of greater than 8 are due to associated injuries. A small proportion of patients in this group (9–15) still die because of haematoma or oedema.

Patients with a GCS of 6–8 one week after the injury have only about a 10% chance of making a good recovery.

2. Duration of post-traumatic amnesia – the longer this is the more brain has been damaged.
3. Skull fracture – those with a fractured base of skull do worst. A fractured base of skull in association with a GCS of 3–5 makes survival unlikely. Patients with skull fractures are the most likely to have intracranial haematomas.
4. Head injury pathology:

Pathology	Mortality
Extradural	20–30%
Acute subdural	60–90%
Brain contusion	80–90%
Chronic subdural	5–20%

5. Age: children have a better prognosis than adults and this is particularly so for diffuse cerebral oedema associated with road accidents and a low GCS.
6. Associated injuries: about one-third of head-injured patients have significant associated injuries which may also influence the prognosis.
7. Proximity to neurosurgical services, intensive care and CT scanner. The results of head injury management in developed countries are better if neurosurgeons rather than general surgeons look after head injuries. However figures from Leicester, England, which has CT scanning, and Lusaka, Zambia, which does not (Table 10.2), suggest only a small difference. In both centres head injuries are managed by general surgeons, although Leicester can refer head injuries to a neurosurgical centre if necessary. These are compared with neurosurgical centres in Glasgow (Scotland), Rotterdam (Holland) and Los Angeles (USA) in Table 10.2.

The outcome from head injury is ultimately assessed according to the Glasgow Outcome Scale (GOS). It is unwise to grade a patient before 3 months and the GOS can be expected to improve for at least a year.

Glasgow Outcome Scale	
Good recovery:	any disability is minor.
Moderate disability:	disabled but independent.
Severely dependent:	disabled and incapable of living independently.
Vegetative:	dependent on others for most functions (bladder, bowels, nutrition, etc.)
Dead	

Favourable outcome includes those patients with good recovery or moderate disability. They are able to live independently.

Unfavourable outcome comprises the severely dependent, vegetative and dead. The survival of vegetative patients is a

Table 10.2 Outcome of head injuries in different centres

Centre	% favourable outcome		
	GCS 3–5	GCS 6–8	GCS ≥ 9
Lusaka	9	75	80 (GCS on admission)
Leicester	15	46	70 (GCS on admission)
Glasgow Rotterdam Los Angeles	20	52	80 (best GCS in first 24 h)

disaster for the family and for society, who must then provide support. Such patients may subsequently die from poor nutrition, pressure sores or pneumonia.

A Glasgow Assessment Schedule (GAS) has been devised to study the psychological, emotional and social impact of head injury. Head injuries may be complicated by behavioural changes which can lead to aggressive tendencies. The rate of divorce rises after severe head injury.

Prevention

The poor outcome associated with a significant proportion of severe head injuries makes prevention of head injuries an important issue. Road safety, the wearing of seat belts and crash helmets, protection of workers from industrial accidents and control of crime are issues for politicians and the general public to tackle as well as health workers. It is cheaper and more effective to prevent a head injury than to treat it.

THE SEVEN DEADLY SINS OF HEAD INJURY MANAGEMENT

1. **Hypotension and inadequate resuscitation in the shocked patient.** Hypotension worsens the prognosis whether it occurs prehospital, in the emergency room or during surgery for associated injuries. A systolic blood pressure of less than 90 mmHg is associated with a worse prognosis.

2. **Late establishment of an adequate airway:** Hypoxia causes brain injury. It must be prevented. If endotracheal intubation is not possible make a surgical airway.

3. **Delay in the diagnosis and treatment of an intracranial haematoma often due to inadequate observation.** The purpose of observation is to detect deterioration and act. The patient should be nursed somewhere where deterioration will be recognised and immediately reported. When a haematoma is diagnosed or suspected give the patient mannitol to temporarily reduce intracranial pressure and take the patient to theatre. In deeply unconscious patients who are deteriorating rapidly local or no anaesthetic may be required. Do not delay evacuating a haematoma.

4. **Lack of cervical spine immobilisation following severe head injury:** Always consider the diagnosis of cervical spine injury. Safeguard the spine when managing the airway and always insist on seeing seven cervical vertebrae and the top of T1 on the lateral X-ray view. Cervical spine X-rays are more important than skull X-rays in an unconscious patient.

5. **Sedation of a restless head-injured patient.** Restlessness or agitation following head injury may be due to raised ICP and the administration of sedatives to the patient may mask any further deterioration which is due to changing pathology in the head. Restless patients may be hypotensive or hypoxic. They might also have a distended bladder or be reacting to a blood transfusion. Never assume that aggressive or restless behaviour is due to alcohol intoxication.

6. **Lack of epilepsy prophylaxis when indicated.** Phenytoin is a good prophylactic agent but diazepam or phenobarbital (or paradehyde in young children) should be used to stop fits. Fits cause hypoxia and a rise in ICP.

7. **Sending a patient home without observation when there is an indication to admit:** In every series of trauma mortalities there are patients who are discharged from an emergency department without an adequate period of observation. The period of deterioration is then missed and the patient is readmitted when coning has already occurred.

Further reading

GENNARELLI TA, SPIELMAN GM, LANGFITT TW et al. Influence of the type of intracranial lesion on outcome from severe head injury. *J Neurosurg* 1982;56:26–32.

LEVY LF. Care of the head-injured patient with minimal resources. *Baillieres Clin Trop Med Commun Dis* 1988;3:233–56.

LIKO O, CHALAU P, ROSENFELD JV, WATTERS DAK. Head injuries in Papua New Guinea. *PNG Med J* 1996;39:100–4.

MILLER ES, NEOPTOLEMOS JP, AITKENHEAD AR, FOSSARD DP. Management of severe head injuries in a non-neurological centre. *J R Coll Surg Edinb* 1985;30:82–7.

PASCUCCI RC. Head trauma in the child. *Intensive Care Med* 1988;14:185–95.

ROSENFELD JV and WATTERS DAK. Head injury In: *Neurosurgery in the tropics*. Basingstoke: Macmillan, 2000:52–89.

TEASDALE G, JENNETT B. Assessment of coma and impaired consciousness. *Lancet* 1974;ii: 81–4.

WATTERS DAK. Clinical practice: management of severe head injuries. *PNG Med J* 2001;44:63–5.

WATTERS DAK, SINCLAIR JR. Outcome of severe head injuries in Central Africa. *J R Coll Surg Edinb* 1988;33:35–38.

11
Trauma

Introduction

This chapter deals with the overall management of patients with multiple injuries. The immediate priorities of ensuring a clear airway and adequate breathing and maintaining the circulation are described first. The patient then requires resuscitation and a full assessment of the nature and severity of the injuries. The management of respiratory failure and hypovolaemic shock are described in Chapters 1 and 2. This chapter is concerned with priorities in the traumatised patient whose life is at risk and outlines the basic management of only a few important specific injuries. However, the management of major problems should not be accompanied by complete neglect of other less urgent ones which may result in unnecessary disability later. It is anticipated that the reader may wish to refer to texts on traumatology and fractures for a more detailed account of the management of certain injuries.

A short outline of the management of mass disasters is included. All hospitals need a disaster plan so that everyone knows *who* must do *what* in the event of a disaster. When large numbers of casualties are received, rapid grouping of patients according to the severity of their injuries is necessary to ensure that the severely injured, but salvageable, patients are treated first. Those whose lives and limbs are in danger must receive priority. Those with less urgent problems can be dealt with later and patients too severely injured to survive should not distract attention from the rescuable. Prior planning is necessary to ensure that materials, drugs and personnel can be rapidly obtained to meet the needs.

Multiple injuries: immediate management

This section is written with a view to explaining how to do it when the patient is actually in front of you. It follows the same principles as Advanced Trauma Life Support (ATLS) courses.

There are three phases to emergency management of the patient with multiple injuries:
1. Primary survey of airway, breathing and circulation – any problems encountered should be managed as they are found.
2. Resuscitation and secondary survey (full assessment of the injuries).
3. Definitive treatment of specific injuries.

The initial treatment in hospital often determines the outcome. Many deaths from trauma occur within a few hours of admission due to hypoxia or haemorrhage. Some deaths occur later due to complications of poor early management.

Primary survey

A Airway with cervical spine control

The immediate aim is to clear and maintain the airway, at the same time protecting the cervical spine from further potential injury. A Stiffneck or similar collar (Figure 11.5) can be applied to minimise risk to the spine.

Potential airway problems are recognised by:
1. listening for noisy breathing suggestive of upper airway obstruction,
2. looking in the mouth for blood, vomit or broken teeth which may occlude the airway or be aspirated.

Action which may be required includes:
1. clear debris with fingers, handkerchief or suction;
2. maintain airway using chin lift and jaw thrust manoeuvres;
3. insert oral airway if unconscious;
4. intubate if the airway is not clear, or there is aspiration or bleeding into the pharynx;
5. perform a cricothyroid stab (Figure 11.1) if there is no time for tracheostomy;
6. perform a tracheostomy if the upper airway is damaged and intubation is impossible (see Tracheostomy on pp. 359–364).

B Breathing

The immediate aim is to maintain adequate ventilation and oxygenation of the blood Potential problems are recognised by:
1. cyanosis,
2. tachypnoea,
3. insufficient breathing,
4. poor respiratory pattern (one side moving better than the other),
5. paradoxical movement (flail chest),
6. tachycardia and shock.

The action that may be required includes:
1. oxygen therapy,
2. Ambu bag ventilation by mask,
3. intubation and ventilation,
4. pleural release for tension pneumothorax (14 gauge cannula in 2nd interspace mid clavicular line),

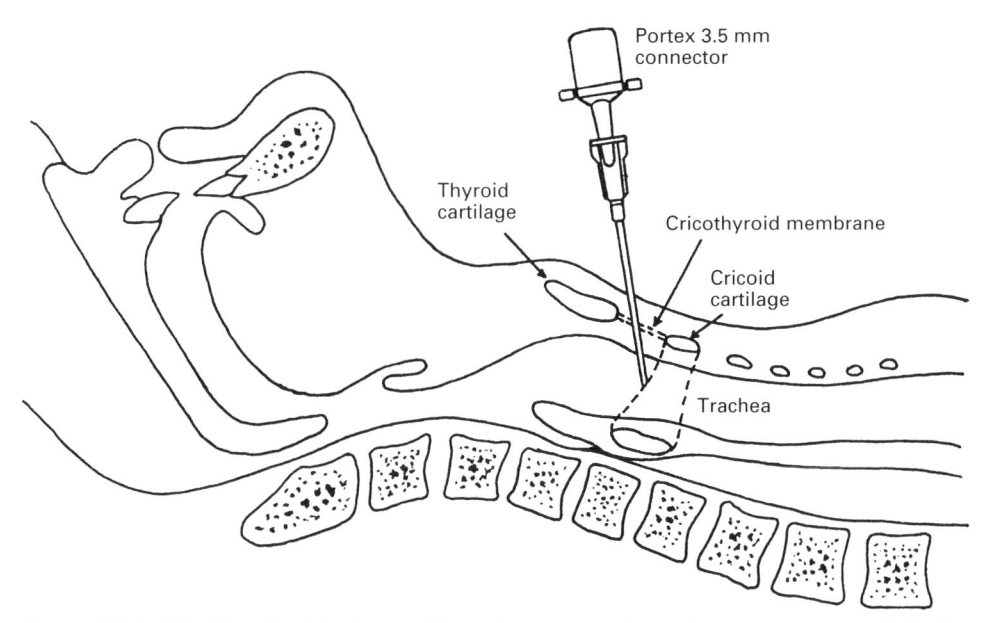

Figure 11.1 Cricothyroid stab: to provide a temporary airway in an emergency. A Portex 3.5 mm connection is pushed into the cannula and an Ambu bag may be connected to this to provide controlled ventilation.

Table 11.1 Initial assessment of the circulation in trauma

Findings	Interpretation
Active bleeding	Stop by pressure or suture
Pale tongue/conjunctivae	Blood loss
Poor peripheral, good central pulse	Peripheral shutdown
No peripheral, no central pulse	Cardiac arrest present or imminent
	Start external massage
	Cardiac arrest drill
Poor peripheral and central pulse, bulging neck veins, raised JVP	Suspect cardiac tamponade or tension pneumothorax
Good peripheral and central pulse	Circulation satisfactory

5. insert intercostal drain (5th interspace mid-axillary line).

C Circulation

The immediate aim is to: prevent further blood loss and determine degree of circulatory impairment (shock); recognise potential problems (Table 11.1).

1. Look for sites of active bleeding and stop active bleeding.
2. Assess circulation by feeling central (carotid) and peripheral (radial) pulses.

Perfusion can also be quickly assessed by the capillary refill time (normally less than 2 sec) and the temperature and moistness of the hands and feet.

The interventions that are likely to be required in shocked patients with multiple injuries include:

1. Use the largest cannulae possible (preferably 14 gauge in adults).
2. Insert two i.v. lines in appropriate sites (Figure 2.1) (if i.v. access is difficult do a cut down on the long saphenous vein at the ankle – see Figure P23 page 381).
3. Give 2 litres normal saline fast (in children give 20% estimated blood volume).
4. Cross match.
5. Give uncrossmatched blood (group-specific or O-negative) if there has been massive bleeding and little or no response to crystalloid/colloid resuscitation.

6. Insert urinary catheter to monitor response to resuscitation. Record initial volume drained from bladder. Unless there is more than one doctor, catherisation is normally performed after full assessment of the patient's injuries – always after considering the possibility of urethral injury (p. 213).

D Disability

Make a rapid assessment of the patients conscious level using either the Glasgow Coma Scale (p. 167) or grade the patient as Alert, responding to Verbal commands, responding to Pain or Unresponsive (AVPU).

E Environment, Exposure

Ensure the patient is removed from any dangerous environment (e.g. chemical waste or risk of explosion).

Whether or not the patient is conscious remove the patient's clothes so a comprehensive secondary survey can be performed. Cut them off where necessary.

Secondary survey

If the patient is conscious ask where he has pain. Ask whether he/she has sensation, tingling, numbness in his limbs and whether he can move his limbs in case there is any injury to the spine. Any collar should be temporarily removed to allow the cervical spine to be palpated.

Wear gloves and examine systematically from head to toe. Do not forget to log roll the patient to examine the back during the secondary survey. Figure 11.2 shows some common injuries and external signs not to miss.

> **KEY POINT**
>
> Always do a complete physical examination.

Conscious level

Enquire if there is a history of loss of consciousness or lucid interval? Did the patient walk or talk after the accident?

Determine the conscious level using the Glasgow Coma Scale (p. 167), which is based on eye opening, the best verbal response and best motor response.

If the patient is comatose assume there may be a cervical spine injury until proven otherwise by X-ray.

Consider the possibility of hypoglycaemia, particularly if the patient smells of alcohol and is unconscious – check Dextrostix or give 20 ml 50% dextrose.

Look for blood or CSF leaking from the nose or ear, which suggests a fractured base of skull, often associated with severe brain damage.

Feel the bony points of the head and face for fractures. Palpate scalp lacerations for depressed fractures, which will need to be debrided and elevated after the patient has been fully assessed. (If you do not feel confident to elevate a skull fracture then debride the wound as well as you can; suture it and transfer when stable.)

Pupils

Record the size and reaction to light – fixed and dilated pupils suggests severe brain damage.

Always ask the conscious patient if he can see with both eyes. Look specifically for an eye injury in the unconscious patient.

Examine the conjunctivae and tongue for pallor and cyanosis. You are not looking for signs of anaemia but rather the pale white tongue of massive haemorrhage or a discoloured purplish tongue suggestive of hypoxia.

Mouth

Can the conscious patient open and close his mouth? Do the teeth occlude properly? Failure to do either of these suggest a fracture or dislocation of the mandible. Is the mandible stable? Make sure there are no loose teeth.

Chest

The important points to consider are listed below:
1. Is there pain on breathing?
2. Watch the breathing; is there paradoxical movement or inequality between the sides of the chest?
3. Assess the depth of breathing; does the patient use accessory muscles?
4. Are there bruises or penetrating wounds?
5. Palpate for fractures and surgical emphysema.
6. Is the trachea central?
7. Percuss the chest – are both sides equal? Is there any hyper-resonance suggestive of a pneumothorax?
8. Auscultate for reduced air entry and added sounds. Coarse crepitations may suggest aspiration of blood or vomit.

Abdomen

The following may suggest intra-abdominal injury:
- abdominal or shoulder tip pain,
- reduced movement with respiration,
- distension,
- bruising,

Examination of the injured patient with multiple injuries
look specifically for common and / or serious injuries

Superficial appearances of injury
- Scalp lacerations
- Blood stained CSF
- Malocclusion of teeth / Broken or missing teeth
- Surgical emphysema / Air entry
- Bruising
- Abdominal distension
- Blood at external urethral meatus
- Swelling + Deformity
- Open wound
- Absent foot pulses or poor superficial circulation

Common skeletal injuries/fractures
- (Depressed) Skull
- Zygoma
- Mandible
- Humerus
- Ribs
- Dislocated hip
- Pelvis
- Thumb
- Femur
- Tibia

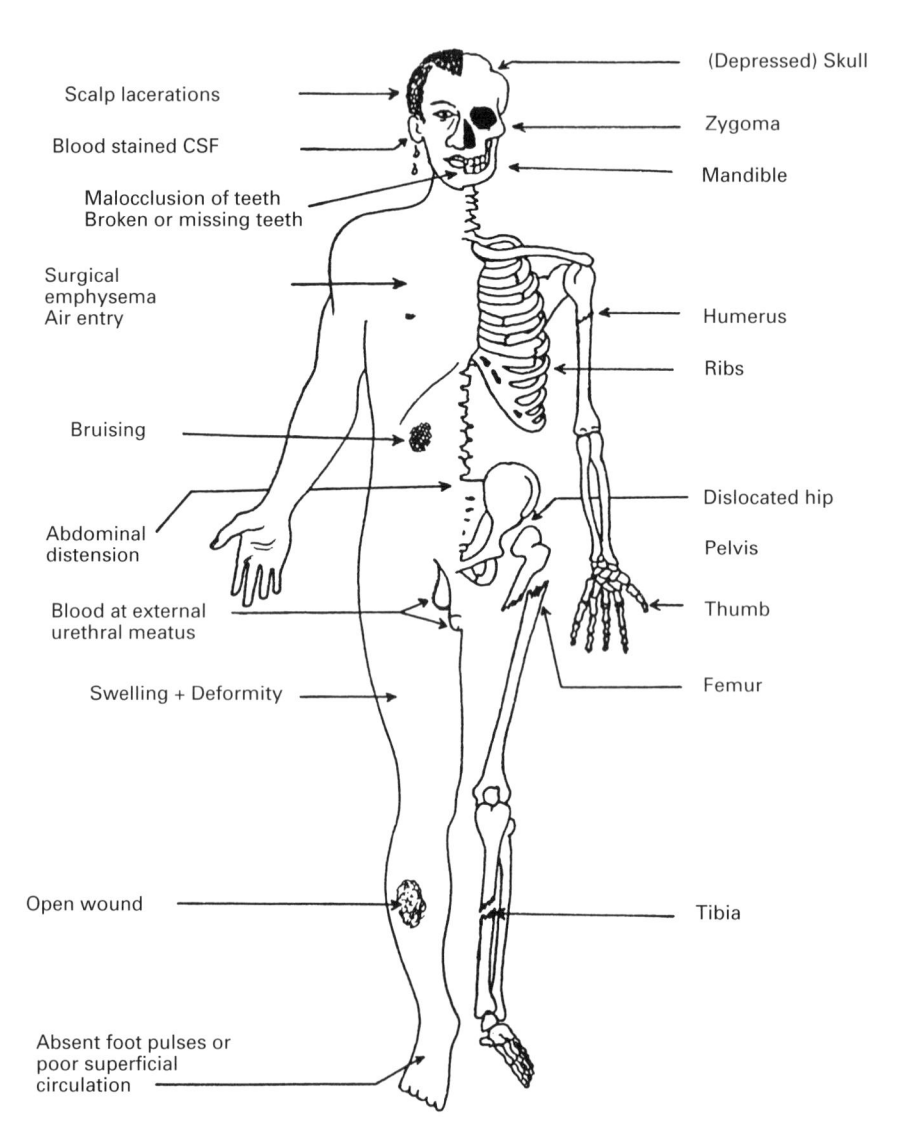

Figure 11.2 Systematic examination of the patient with multiple injuries.

- rigidity,
- tenderness,
- absent bowel sounds.

If there is major haemorrhage within the abdomen signs of hypovolaemic shock will be present (Table 2.1, p. 20).

Pelvis

1. Compress the iliac bones and spring the pubis to determine whether there is a fracture.
2. Look for blood at external meatus of urethra, which would suggest a urethral injury.
3. Is the bladder full, empty or ruptured?

Limbs

1. Look for swelling, bruising, rotation or deformity.
2. Feel distal pulses, for example the dorsalis pedis and radials.
3. Test sensation.
4. Palpate all bones unless there is severe pain or obvious injury.
5. Move all joints unless painful.

KEY POINT
Always examine the distal pulses when there is a fracture or soft-tissue injury to a limb.

KEY POINT
Record all injuries and wounds carefully in the patient's notes.

A trauma form with a two figures of a body, one front and one back view, will help to record injuries and it is quicker to draw the site of a laceration than to describe it.

In the amnesic or unconscious patient obtain accident details from relatives or attendants; e.g. front or back seat, driver or passenger, seat-belts, iron bar or brick, knife or gunshot?

Obtain any drug or allergic history.

Are there underlying chronic medical diseases which may complicate management and recovery?

Estimate blood loss

Decide how much fluid and blood to give. Peripheral perfusion, pulse, blood pressure and urine output will help guide therapy. Estimate blood loss from fractures.

If the patient is shocked he will have lost over 25% of his blood volume.

Fracture	*Adult blood loss*
Pelvis	2–4 litres
Femur	1–2 litres
Tibia	0.5–1 litre
Humerus	200–300 ml

Always replace blood in children according to their actual or estimated weight (Figure 2.2, p. 24). Blood volume can be estimated to be 80 ml/kg.

If there is shock replace 20% of estimated blood volume with crystalloid (normal saline) rapidly and then 10% aliquots of colloid (blood or dextran), reassessing progress of resuscitation after each aliquot.

Decide what urgent surgery is required and ask when the patient's last meal or drink was.

Decide if there is time for X-rays and which ones are necessary at this stage. Never leave a seriously ill or unconscious patient unattended in the X-ray department (Figure 11.3).

The most important X-rays will be chest, cervical spine, pelvis. X-rays of fractured limbs can be done when convenient. Supervise moving of the patient. Resuscitation is more important than X-ray.

A repeat secondary (or tertiary) survey should be carried out within 24 h when the patient is in the ward, as despite a careful secondary survey sometimes injuries are overlooked.

Further management of specific problems in trauma

KEY POINT
Do not forget tetanus prophylaxis. Do not assume immunity.

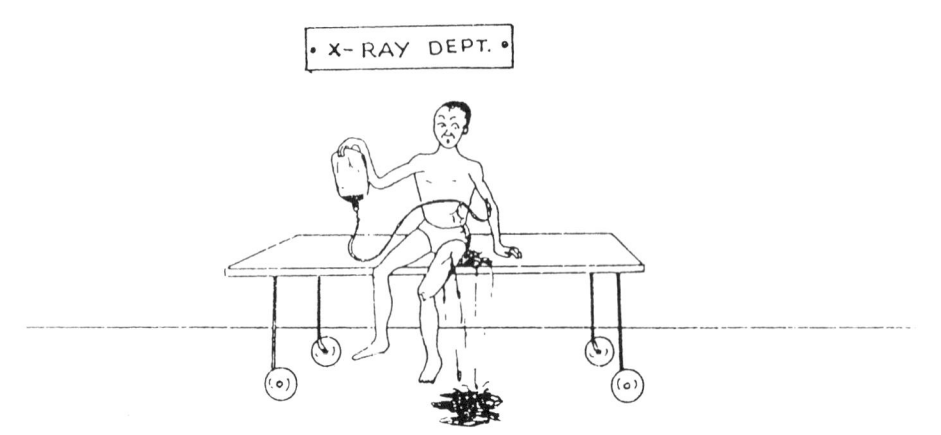

Figure 11.3 Never leave a seriously injured or unconscious patient unattended in the X-ray department.

Head injuries

These are discussed in Chapter 10.

Facial injuries

The immediate aim is maintenance of the airway. Swelling may be severe and should be anticipated. If there are any signs of airway problems intubation or tracheostomy should be performed early. It is better to perform an emergency tracheostomy that may subsequently prove to be unnecessary than to lose control of the airway. Prophylactic antibiotics should be given for facial fractures as the fracture line enters bacterial lined cavities such as the nose, mouth and sinus. Functional and cosmetic problems can be managed once the critical phase is over.

Spinal injuries

A cervical spine injury should always be suspected in a patient with a head injury or multiple trauma. The unconscious traumatised patient should be assumed to have a cervical spine injury until proved otherwise. If the patient is conscious he may complain of pain radiating down a limb, numbness, parasthesia, or weakness in the limbs. Lack of chest wall movement with respiration and marked abdominal breathing using the diaphragm suggests an injury of the cervical spine.

Move a patient with a suspected cervical spine injury carefully. Avoid rotation and extremes of flexion and extension. One person, usually the most senior attendant, should assume responsibility for the neck. He should stand at the top of the patient, hold the head, placing the fingers under the angle of the mandible with the palms over the ears and parietal region and maintain gentle traction to keep the neck straight and in line with the body (Figure 11.4). When the patient is not being moved the neck can be splinted by a sandbag placed on each side or a cervical collar (e.g. Stiffneck collar) (Figure 11.5).

The diagnosis is made by lateral X-ray of the cervical spine. All seven cervical vertebral bodies and the disc space between C7 and T1 should be seen (Figure 11.6). Someone may need to pull on the arms while the X-ray is being taken in order the lower the shoulders. A swimmer's view can also be taken to view the C7/T1 part of the cervical spine. An open mouth view will be required to view the odontoid peg.

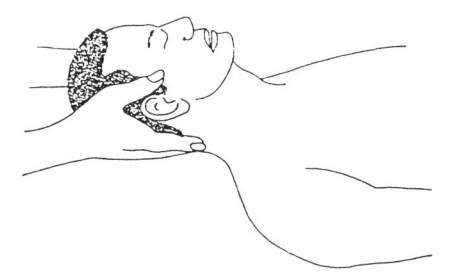

Figure 11.4 Moving an unconscious patient who may have a spinal injury: the head and neck should be controlled by the most experienced attendant.

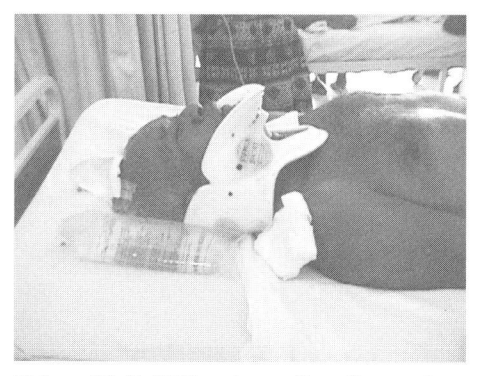

Figure 11.5 Stiffneck or other firm collars will minimise risk to the cervical spine while the patient's injuries are being assessed and managed.

KEY POINT

Do not assume the cervical spine is normal until all seven vertebral bodies have been seen on X-ray.

If there is an unstable fracture or dislocation of the cervical spine, skeletal traction should be instituted. The most effective method is using Gardiner–Wells tongs, the pins of which are screwed into the outer table of the skull (Figure 11.7a). An alternative measure is to use stainless steel wire and four burr holes to apply skeletal traction (Figure 11.7b). Initially 6 kg of weight should be applied (two bricks); increase the weight over a few hours up to 12 kg until the fracture/dislocation is reduced. In an emergency and during transfer sandbags can be used. If the patient must be transferred, send someone senior with the patient. If there is paraplegia or quadriplegia then catheterise the patient before transfer.

Manipulation or surgical reduction should not be attempted except by those with considerable experience.

Fractures of the thoracic spine usually require bed rest. They are often stable. Immediate spinal decompression of the narrow spinal canal in cases with paraplegia is often not possible in tropical countries but, if available, a neurosurgeon should be consulted.

Unstable fractures of the lumbar spine and those with neurological involvement require skin traction and bed rest for about 6 weeks. Stable fractures without neurological impairment require bed rest until pain or other injuries allow the patient to be mobilised.

Spinal injuries with neurological impairment

Shock may occur owing to loss of peripheral vascular tone so that blood becomes pooled in the peripheries rather than supporting the central circulation to vital organs. In this instance the treatment is volume replacement to support the central circulation. If bradycardia develops atropine may be given. Other principles of management are:

1. Stabilise the spine by traction. Supervise all movement of the patient.
2. Turn 2 hourly to avoid pressure sores from the first day. Wedge the mattress by placing 30–40° wedges between the mattress and base of the bed. Alternatively, a Stryker frame bed makes turning from front to back safe and easy.
3. Catheterise the patient. Clamp and release 3–4 hourly to maintain bladder

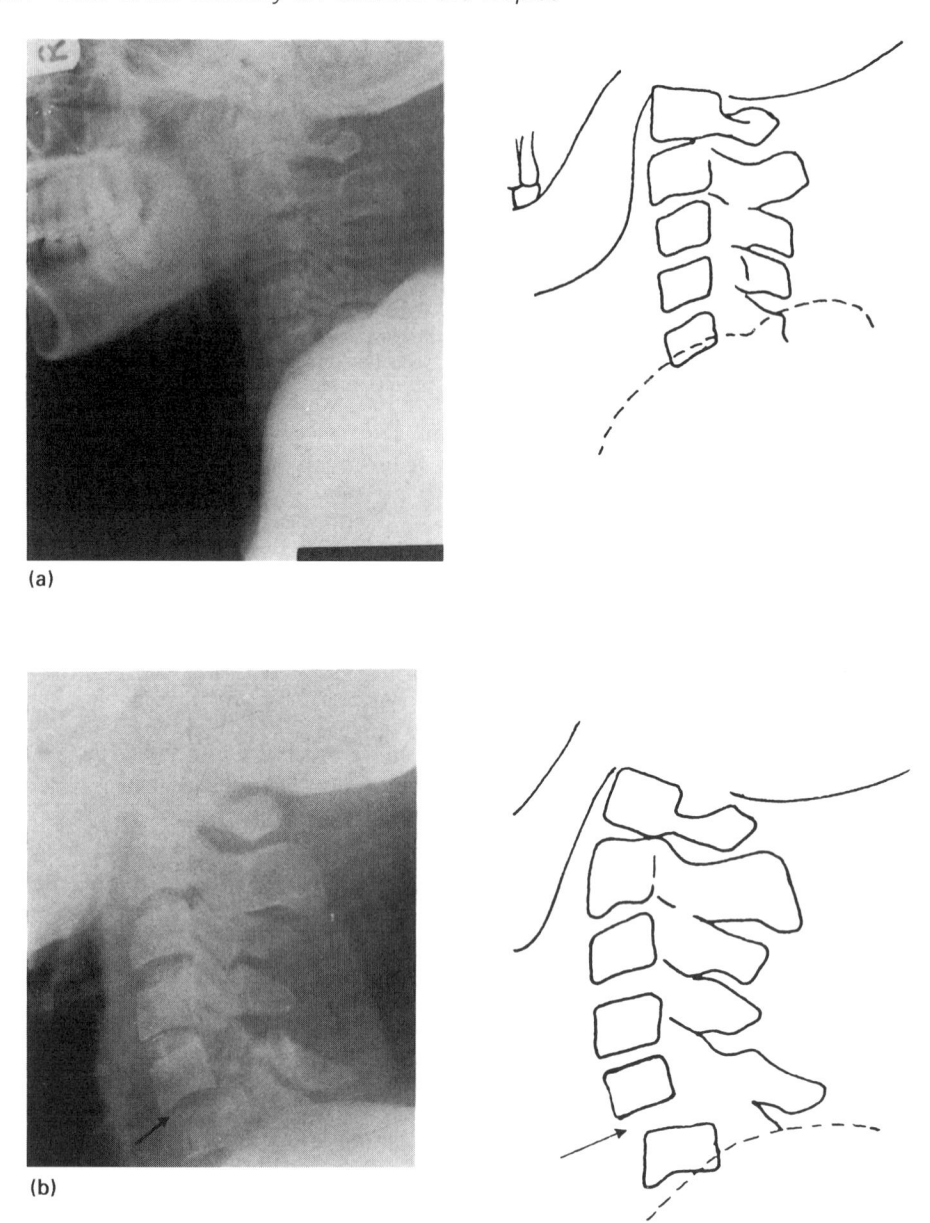

Figure 11.6 The importance of adequate cervical spine X-rays. (a) An inadequate view that failed to show dislocation of C5/6 because only five vertebrae are seen. (b) A repeat film showing the dislocation of C5/6. Note that this film is *still* inadequate as the seventh cervical vertebra is not seen.

tone. A better alternative is intermittent catheterisation if feasible with available nursing resources.
4. Give prophylactic steroids to reduce any cord oedema: dexamethasone 10 mg stat 4 mg 6 hourly.
5. Give antibiotics (chloramphenicol ± sulfadimidine) if there is a penetrating

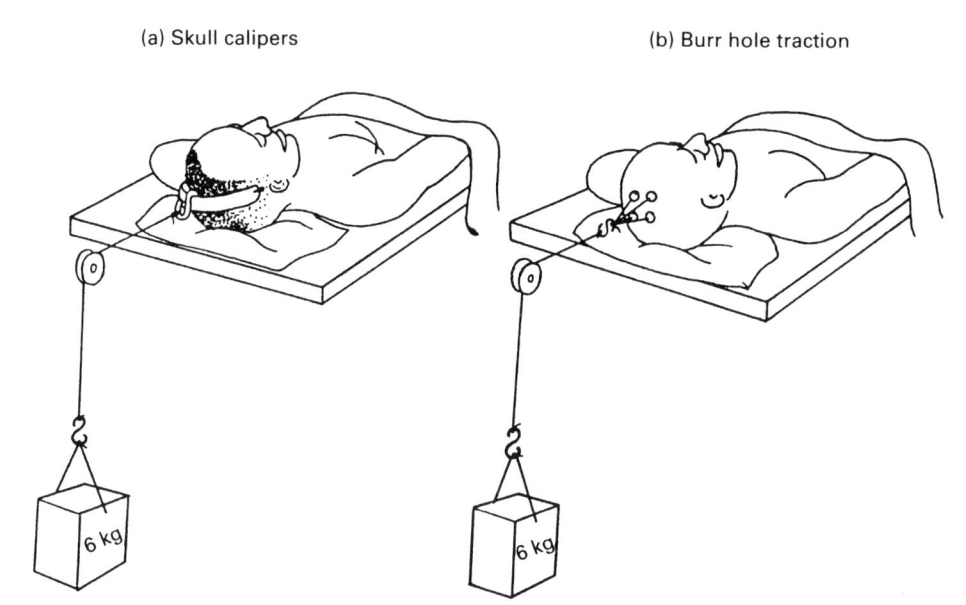

Figure 11.7 Methods of applying skeletal traction for fracture/dislocations of the cervical spine.

injury to the spinal cord.
6. Transfer to a spinal unit as early as possible if such a unit exists and other injuries allow.
7. Discuss the situation with the patient and his relatives as they will need considerable social, psychological and spiritual support.

Eye injuries

The management of eye injuries is beyond the scope of this book. Refer to a specialised text. The flow diagram in Figure 11.8 gives an outline of the pathways of management.

Chest trauma

If conscious, the patient may complain of pain on breathing. There are non-specific and specific signs of chest injury (Table 11.2).

Bruising

If there is bruising over the lower left ribs and upper abdomen consider the possibility of a ruptured spleen. Bruising over the right lower ribs may be associated with a ruptured liver.

Rib fractures

These do not require any specific treatment other than analgesia. Their importance is to prompt the doctor to look for more severe associated chest injuries such as pneumothorax, haemothorax and flail chest. If pain restricts the patient's breathing the lung may partially collapse, so ensure the patient can breathe comfortably by giving generous and frequent analgesia.

Patients undergoing general anaesthesia with fractured ribs may develop a pneumothorax due to positive pressure ventilation during anaesthesia. This is due either to the pleura being punctured on the sharp end of rib as the lung is inflated or else to the inflation pressure bursting an already sealed perforation of lung tissue. An intercostal drain should be inserted before anaesthesia is induced. If a traumatised patient under anaesthetic develops hypoxia,

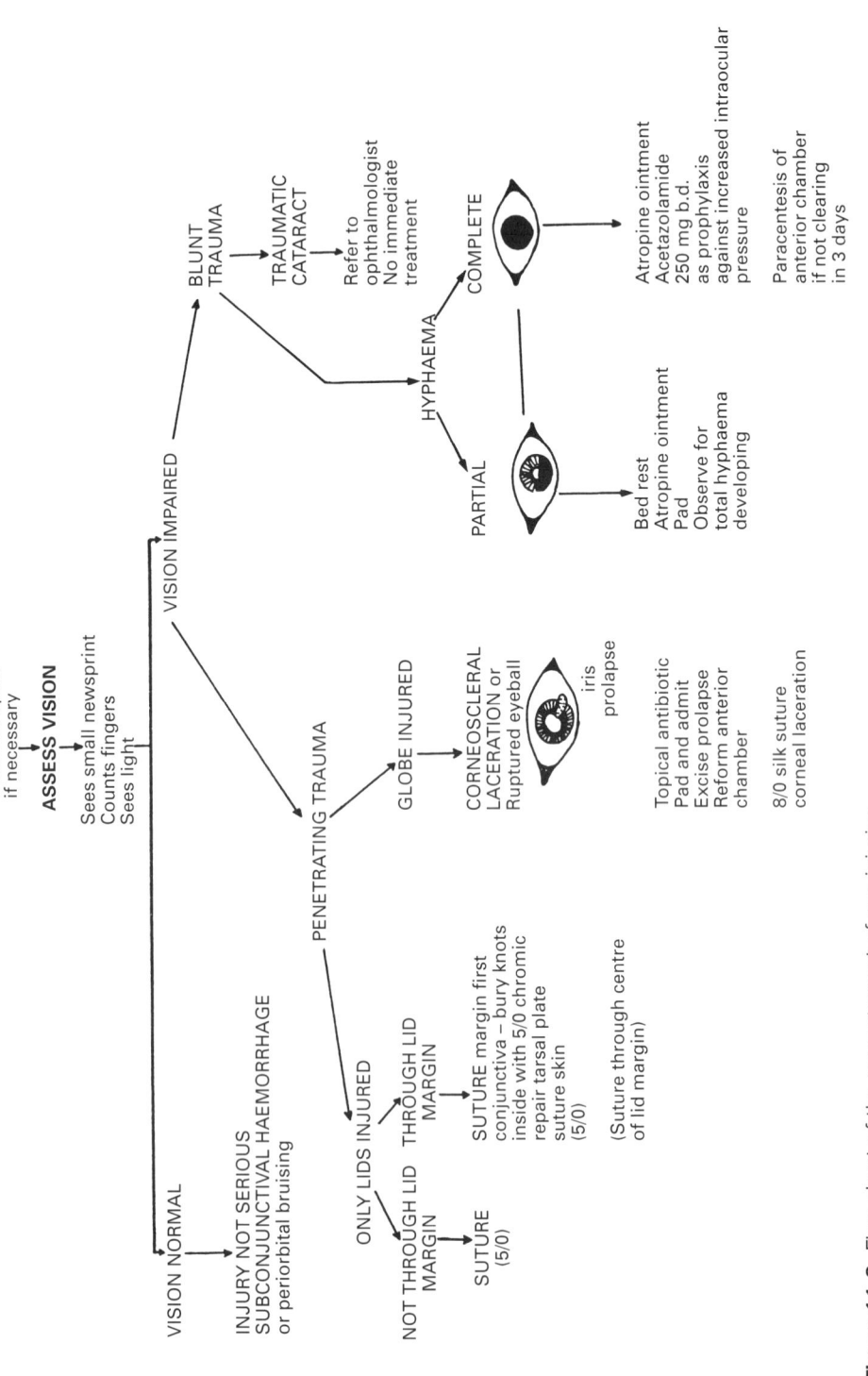

Figure 11.8 Flow chart of the management of eye injuries.

Table 11.2 Non-specific and specific signs of chest injury

Non-specific	Specific
Dyspnoea	Unequal movement
Restlessness	Paradoxical movement of chest wall
Central cyanosis	Surgical emphysema of neck and chest
Tachycardia	Palpable rib fractures
Hypotension	Bruising
Sweating	Tracheal deviation

hypotension or difficulty in ventilation then check the air entry in the chest by auscultation and consider the possibility of a tension pneumothorax.

> **KEY POINT**
>
> Always insert a chest drain if a patient with fractured ribs is to have a general anaesthetic.

Flail chest and paradoxical movement

Normally the chest wall moves out on inspiration. If there are multiple fractures of the chest wall so that one part is isolated there will be inward movement on inspiration. The inward moving part of the chest wall is called a flail segment. There is usually associated lung contusion and often a pneumothorax or haemothorax (Figure 11.9).

The patient with a flail chest has a severe injury. A chest drain should usually be inserted, as underlying injury to the lungs is expected regardless of the X-ray appearances. If the patient is young or the flail segment is small it may be possible to treat the patient with analgesia, oxygen and physiotherapy. Good analgesia is necessary to enable the patient to co-operate with physiotherapy. Older patients, patients with underlying lung disease or those with large flail segments often require mechanical ventilation for 10–14 days until the ribs start to heal and the flail segment stabilises.

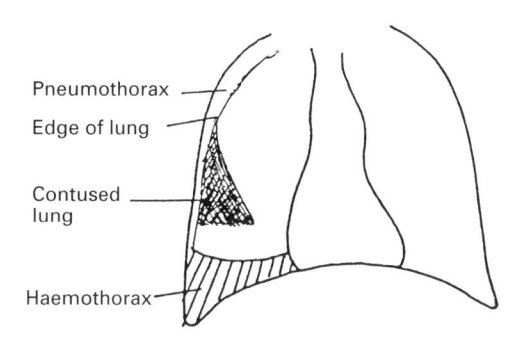

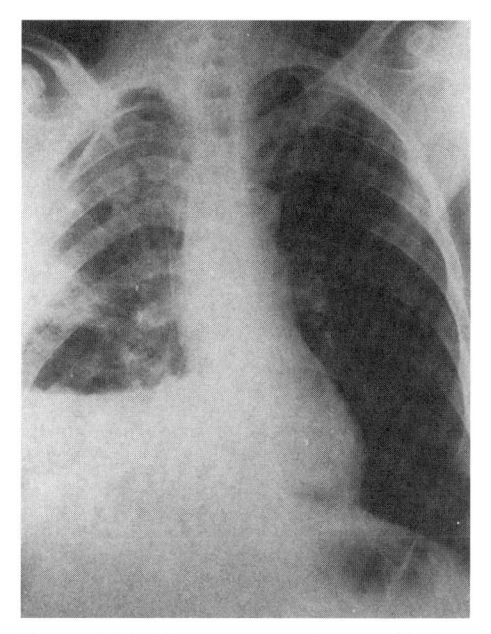

Figure 11.9 Haemo-pneumothorax with lung contusion.

The best analgesia is provided by an epidural block, intercostal nerve block intrapleural analgesia or opiate infusion according to the facilities and expertise available. Good analgesia may improve the patient's own ventilatory efforts. If there are no facilities for ventilation, the rib fractures can be fixed under anaesthesia using stainless steel wire. The problem of limited ventilatory efforts due to pain and lung contusion are not cured by fixation, so ventilation is the better form of management.

Patients with a flail segment often get

worse on the second or third day after injury owing to the blockage of small airways with retained secretions and lung tissue oedema, which both lead to alveolar collapse. The pain in moving the chest wall in breathing reduces the patient's ability to compensate by increasing his ventilatory effort.

Penetrating chest injuries

In any penetrating wound of the upper abdomen, chest, back or lower neck there may be damage to the lung, heart or great vessels. Examine the patient for signs of respiratory failure, shock and look in particular at the neck veins. Distended neck veins associated with shock suggests cardiac tamponade or tension pneumothorax.

Open wounds of the chest are often associated with pneumothorax or haemothorax. If the patient's condition is stable, a chest X-ray should be taken. If the condition is unstable insert a chest drain in the 6th intercostal space in the mid or anterior axillary line on the affected side. Do not insert a chest drain through the wound itself as this predisposes to infection. The wound should be cleaned and debrided and closed. The rule of not closing a wound after 12 h may have to be broken in the case of an open chest wound as communication between the pleural cavity and the atmosphere will prevent the lung expanding for adequate ventilation. An alternative would be to debride and dress the wound with an airtight dressing. Full exploration of a chest wound involves thoracotomy and should only be undertaken as an emergency for rapid or continuing bleeding, cardiac tamponade, diaphragmatic rupture or a large bronchopleural fistula rendering ventilation ineffective. The vast majority of patients with penenetrating injuries of the chest and underlying lung injury do very well with intercostal drainage, debridement and suturing of the chest wound. Prophylactic antibiotics are not indicated.

Surgical emphysema

Surgical emphysema is a term used to describe the presence of air in the tissues. There is a crackling, bubbly feeling on palpating the skin due to air in the subcutaneous tissues. The commonest cause is a pneumothorax. Occasionally a ruptured trachea or oesophagus may cause surgical emphysema in the neck. Surgical emphysema means that the patient needs a chest X-ray. An intercostal drain should be inserted only if there is radiological evidence of a pneumothorax or if the patient's general condition is poor. If the patient is to have a general anaesthetic, an intercostal drain should be inserted in the patient with surgical emphysema.

Pneumothorax

A pneumothorax is due to air in the pleural cavity, which causes collapse of the lung (Figure 1.4).

The patient may be breathless or complain of pain on breathing, but this is not invariable. On examination, there is hyperresonance and often reduced air entry. There are two types of pneumothorax, as follows:

Simple pneumothorax

The air in the pleural cavity causes partial or complete collapse of the lung, but the amount of air in the pleural cavity thereafter remains static because the tear in the lung becomes sealed. If the distance between the edge of the chest wall and the edge of the lung is more than the width of two ribs, insert a chest drain. A simple pneumothorax may sometimes enlarge so that the patient should be observed closely and X-rayed again the next day if a decision is made not to insert an intercostal drain. If the condition of the patient is poor, or the patient is to undergo general anaesthesia, insert a chest drain whatever the size of the pneumothorax. Antibiotics are not necessary as a routine.

Tension pneumothorax

This is a rapidly expanding pneumothorax. Not only does the lung collapse but the pressure of air pushes the mediastinum across the thoracic cavity to compress the opposite lung (Figure 1.7). The patient becomes progressively hypoxic as more and more lung is compressed. The high intrathoracic pressure reduces venous return to the heart and compromises the circulation. The patient will be hypoxic, dyspneoic, hypotensive and the neck veins may be distended. The central venous pressure is raised. A tension pneumothorax is an emergency requiring relief of the mounting pressure and tension in the pleural cavity or else the patient will die.

There may be no time to X-ray the patient. If you suspect a tension pneumothorax clinically, insert a wide-bore needle or i.v. cannula into the chest in the midclavicular line. If tension is present you will hear the escape of air. If you fill a syringe with water and remove the plunger there will be a bubbling of air through the water when you attach the syringe to the needle or cannula. Once the tension is relieved an intercostal drain can be inserted in the 5th or 6th interspace in the mid-axillary line.

Bronchopleural fistula (Figure 1.4)

In bronchopleural fistula there is a communication between the airway and the pleural cavity. If the communication is based on peripheral lung tissue (i.e. a small bronchiole or alveolus) then the air leak will seal rapidly. When there is a large leak from the lung the chest drain bottle may bubble with each expired breath for a few days. The fistula usually settles spontaneously.

However, if a major bronchus is torn the lung will remain collapsed despite intercostal drainage (Figure 1.4). The bubbling through the intercostal drainage bottle will be gross and mechanical ventilation only makes the patient worse. Ventilation may be ineffective because a large proportion of the tidal volume is lost. In this dangerous situation it is best to use a double lumen endotracheal tube (if available). Another tactic is to twist a standard ETT so that the end of the tube passes down the main bronchus of the healthy side. This may enable effective ventilation to be achieved until emergency thoracotomy is carried out to repair the bronchus or perform a lobectomy or pneumonectomy. Transfer a patient with a suspected major bronchus injury breathing spontaneously with an intercostal drain after resuscitation.

Haemothorax

This is a collection of blood in the pleural cavity. It is recognised by reduced air entry on auscultation and a typical X-ray appearance of fluid in the pleural cavity (Figure 1.5) associated with fractured ribs or penetrating trauma. Treatment involves inserting an intercostal drain in the 6th or 7th intercostal space in the mid- or anterior axillary line.

Most haemothoraces are adequately treated by drainage. However, if two chest drain bottles are filled up and the patient continues to bleed then emergency thoracotomy is required to tie the bleeding vessel. Usually it is an intercostal or internal mammary artery which is bleeding. If the chest X-ray shows a white-out (complete opacification of one lung field) and the patient is shocked, the pleural cavity is probably full of clot and thoracotomy should be performed to evacuate the clot and stop the bleeding. When there is a large clot in the pleural cavity, blood drains out through the chest drain only intermittently. This may tempt the attendants to believe that the bleeding is stopping. Do thoracotomy early in this situation.

Cardiac tamponade

Cardiac tamponade occurs when the pumping action of the heart is imparied by blood or fluid in the pericardium. The classical signs are a weak and feeble pulse, hypotension, distended neck veins and CVP above 30 cm. The patient is often restless and confused. The signs of pulsus paradoxus and quiet heart sounds are rarely detected in traumatised patients. There is often no abnormality on the chest X-ray.

Cardiac tamponade in trauma is usually due to a stab or bullet wound to the heart. Suspect cardiac damage whenever there is a penetrating wound to the chest or upper abdomen. Some patients present without shock and some on the point of cardiac arrest. If the patient has a cardiac arrest on arrival at hospital there is still a 20% chance of survival if immediate thoracotomy is performed.

Pericardiocentesis (Figure P32) may buy time on transfer to theatre but thoracotomy should not be delayed by attempts to do this.

Injury to the thoracic aorta

Injury to the arch of the aorta usually presents with either absent pulses depending on the actual site of injury or with a widened superior mediastinum on erect chest X-ray (Figure 11.10). When this is suspected the patient's best chance is to be transferred for angiographic assessment and aortic surgery.

Abdominal trauma

Penetrating trauma

Penetrating trauma to the abdomen is usually due to stab and bullet wounds. The

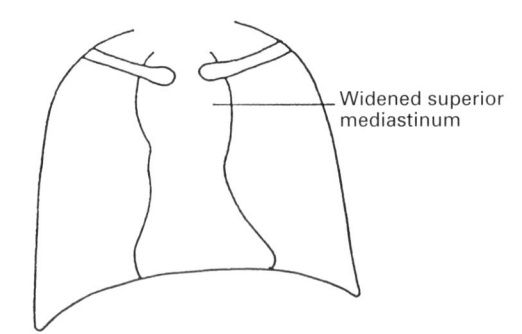

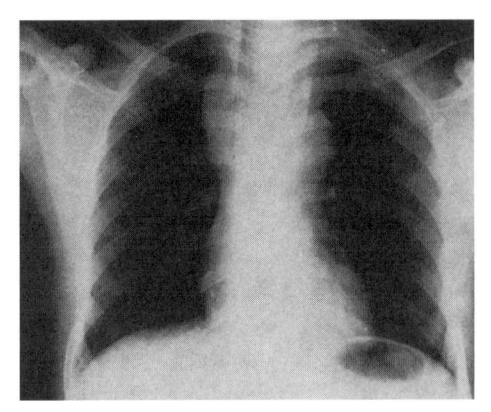

Figure 11.10 Widening of the superior mediastinum due to blunt chest trauma.

patient presents with a stab or bullet wound, an omental protrusion or disembowelment.

Bullet wounds

Find out what sort of gun was used. The higher the velocity of bullet the more damage is caused. High-velocity bullet wounds usually have an exit wound. Low-velocity bullets may remain in the patient.

All abdominal bullet wounds should be explored by laparotomy.

Stab wounds

All stab wounds should be explored. This can be done under local anaesthesia if there are no signs of intra-abdominal injury. If the posterior rectus sheath has been penetrated perform a laparotomy. Intact peritoneum may be misleading as the perforated peritoneum retracts with abdominal rigidity. If in doubt perform a laparotomy. The size of the stab wound bears no relation to the size of the blade or the damage caused within the abdomen. The victim is rarely accurate in his description of the depth or direction of the stab. Any abdominal wound may penetrate the diaphragm or damage a major vessel. Any wound over the chest may enter the abdomen or heart. **Do not guess: explore**. Only experienced surgeons should treat a stab abdomen without exploration if there are no abdominal signs.

Omental protrusion through the stab wound means a laparotomy should be performed. If bowel herniates through the wound (disembowelment) laparotomy is urgent. Check the colour of the bowel: if it is blue widen the stab wound with a scalpel either with or without anaesthetic. Support the protruding bowel manually or with a pack to minimise traction on the mesentery.

KEY POINT

Always look for diaphragmatic injury at laparotomy and check limb pulsation before surgery.

A urinary catheter should be inserted. Macroscopic haematuria suggests renal injury.

Untreated pneumothorax or haemothorax may cause upper abdominal pain and rigidity. If in doubt re-examine the patient an hour after intercostal drainage of the chest.

Blunt abdominal trauma

The conscious patient with haemoperitoneum complains of pain. There will be abdominal distension, rigidity and tenderness. Bowel sounds are usually absent and the abdomen moves poorly with respiration.

Abdominal girth measurements have been shown to be misleading and inaccurate. Do not use them.

Tachycardia, hypotension and other signs of shock are often present. These are as important in the decision to perform laparotomy as the local signs on abdominal examination.

Investigations

These should be limited to peritoneal aspiration (paracentesis) and peritoneal lavage.

PERITONEAL ASPIRATION
Perform a four-quadrant tap using a green 21 gauge needle. The chances of damaging intra-abdominal organs is minimal. Failure to aspirate blood does not exclude intra-abdominal injury. If blood is aspirated perform laparotomy.

PERITONEAL LAVAGE (p. 373)
This is the most accurate method of diagnosing haemoperitoneum. An unconscious patient with a suspected intra-abdominal injury should have a peritoneal lavage where there is uncertainty if the decision to perform laparotomy has not already been made on other criteria. Peritoneal lavage will save some unnecessary laparotomies as a negative result is normally correct (see practical procedure p. 373). If one can be confident that the spleen is the only organ injured, a blunt splenic injury can be managed non-operatively in over 50% of cases. Therefore a positive lavage does not always mean a laparotomy should be performed in the tropics.

KEY POINT

The patient with suspected abdominal injury should always be examined at frequent intervals.

X-RAYS

The most important X-ray in the traumatised abdomen is a chest X-ray. Abdominal X-rays are unlikely to influence management and normal X-rays may give a false sense of security. A plain X-ray may show a soft-tissue shadow in the renal area suggestive of renal haematoma.

Ruptured diaphragm

This occurs occasionally and may be associated with a fractured pelvis. The stomach, spleen, and large or small bowel may be in the left chest, which is the commonest side for the rupture. Bowel sounds may be heard in the chest. Frequently the chest X-ray of a ruptured diaphragm is misinterpreted as a haemothorax with lung contusion (Figure 11.11). Insertion of an intercostal drain may result in perforation of the stomach, spleen or bowel.

Suspected renal injury

In blunt abdominal trauma a renal injury may be due to a direct blow or to the mobile kidney rotating on its pedicle or being torn from its supporting capsule with deceleration.

Recognition

The abdominal signs may be the same as those of intraperitoneal injury. There is usually macroscopic haematuria. Rarely the kidney is completely avulsed from the renal pedicle and haematuria may be absent.

Catheterise the patient. Macroscopic haematuria suggests renal injury. If blood is present at the external urethral meatus see below under 'Fractured pelvis'.

A plain abdominal X-ray may show a soft tissue mass due to haematoma in the region of the kidney.

High-dose intravenous urography (IVU) is indicated for blunt abdominal injury, particularly in the unconscious patient. 100 ml of urografin should be given intravenously (1–1.5 ml/kg) and a plain abdominal film taken at 1, 2, 5, and 20 min. A full IVU is not necessary. The 20 min film can be omitted if the condition of the patient is poor. Contrast will be seen leaking from the kidney at 1, 2 and 5 min if the kidney is burst. If there is renal avulsion no contrast will be seen on the affected side.

Blunt renal injuries should be observed unless the patient is exsanguinating or the whole kidney is avulsed. In avulsion the kidney must be removed. Occasionally avulsion injuries detected early have been treated by reanastomosis of the renal vessels but only in major centres.

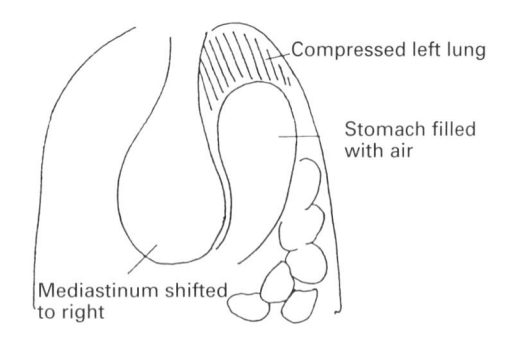

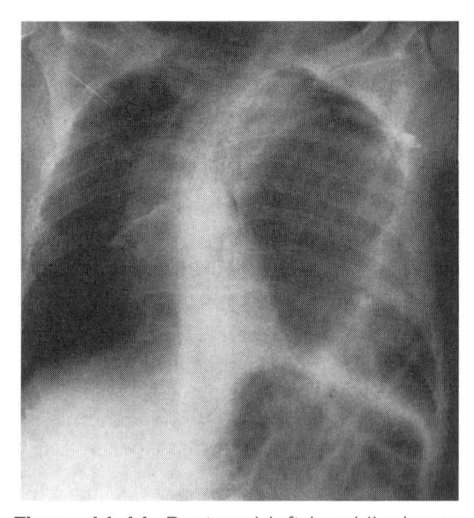

Figure 11.11 Ruptured left hemidiaphragm showing stomach in the left chest. Bowel sounds were heard on auscultation of the chest.

Penetrating trauma

Exploration of the kidney is advised if laparotomy is indicated and there is a large retroperitoneal haematoma or haematuria is severe. If the bleeding cannot be stopped by repair then nephrectomy should be done.

When available in major centres, arteriography is the best investigation for penetrating trauma leading to severe haematuria. A bleeding vessel can sometimes be embolised during arteriography so that nephrectomy will not be necessary.

Fractured pelvis

This may be detected by examining and springing the public rami by backward pressure on the pubis and compressing the iliac bones towards the midline. The patient will complain of pain and is unable to walk.

A fractured pelvis is associated with large volumes of blood loss (3–4 litres). Transfusion is usually necessary and sometimes bleeding continues for some days, necessitating massive transfusion.

A fractured pelvis may be associated with urethral injury, usually in the male patient. If there is no blood at the external meatus of the urethra pass a catheter gently into the bladder. A good flow of clear urine is an encouraging sign and means that a ruptured urethra is unlikely.

If blood is present at the external meatus you must decide whether to do a urethrogram, pass a diagnostic catheter or perform a suprapubic cystotomy once the bladder distends.

The urologist or surgeon to whom you normally refer difficult cases will advise how he wants this problem to be tackled as it is he who must later attempt repair and reconstruction.

Ruptured urethra

This is suspected if there is blood at the external urethral meatus or failure to pass a diagnostic catheter. An ascending urethrogram may show the rupture (see below). If there is a ruptured urethra perform an open cystotomy and try to railroad a catheter from the urethra into the bladder under direct vision. If you fail to do this or do not feel competent to try then simply perform an open or puncture suprapubic cystotomy (pp. 376–378). This will drain urine and save the patient's life. A urethral injury can be repaired later in a referral hospital. If the bladder does not distend then either the bladder is ruptured or the patient is inadequately resuscitated.

Ruptured bladder

A fractured pelvis may also be associated with a ruptured bladder, particularly after being run over by a car or lorry. Urine draining through the urethral catheter may be in the peritoneal cavity, not in the bladder. Usually the patient has severe lower abdominal pain and tenderness and progressive abdominal distension and loss of bowel sounds. An ascending urethrogram may not detect a ruptured bladder.

ASCENDING URETHROGRAM

1. Pass a small Foley catheter (size 12 or 14) into the fossa navicularis of the urethra and blow up the balloon with 2–3 ml saline. No anaesthetic is necessary although lignocaine gel, if available, does make the procedure more comfortable for the patient.
2. Inject water-soluble radiological contrast (Conray 280) into the urethra (5–10 ml) and as the injection is finishing take an oblique film. Contrast should be seen passing up the urethra into the bladder.
3. Contrast may be seen extravasating, suggesting there is a rupture of the urethra.

Bladder rupture may be intraperitoneal or extraperitoneal. Laparotomy may miss extraperitoneal rupture of the bladder unless this injury is specifically looked for. A cystogram will demonstrate a ruptured bladder and is simple to perform with a catheter *in situ*.

Wounds and lacerations

Detailed descriptions of wound management are given in surgical texts. This section is restricted to an outline of the principles of wound care so that critically ill patients do not develop unnecessary complications from wounds which in themselves may not be life-threatening problems at the outset. However, mismanagement of a wound in a traumatised patient may give rise to serious morbidity, loss of function of a limb or even mortality.

A wound is a break in the continuity of the surface of a structure (usually the skin) caused by a sharp or blunt object which either penetrates or bursts open the structure concerned.

Penetrating wounds are caused by a sharp object such as a blade, bullet or exploding piece of metal (shrapnel). The skin may be torn or burst open by blunt objects with high momentum such as a car tyre, stone or iron bar. The force required to wound is greater for a blunt than a sharp object. Blunt trauma is therefore associated with greater bruising and contusion of tissues.

The size, sharpness, direction and velocity of a wounding agent will determine its effects on the injured person. The depth and direction of a wound and the potential damage to underlying structures such as major vessels, nerves, tendons or vital organs can rarely be appreciated by simply looking at the wound. Wounds must be explored after careful clinical assessment of the likely underlying injuries. The greater the velocity of the penetrating agent the

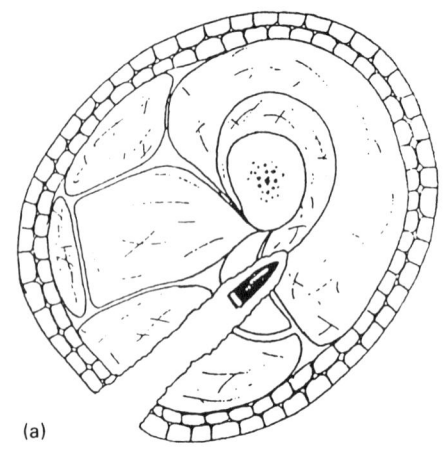

Figure 11.12 (a) Low-velocity gunshot wound. Tissue damage is restricted to the track of the bullet.

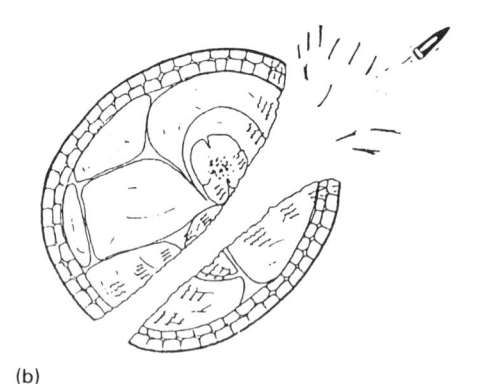

Figure 11.12 (b) High-velocity gunshot wound. The exit wound is larger than the entry wound and tissue damage extends beyond the track of the bullet owing to shock waves emanating from the bullet as it passes through the tissue.

further from the track of penetration will tissue damage extend (Figure 11.12a and b). Thus in a stab or low-velocity bullet wound injury is confined to the track of the wound whereas in a high-velocity bullet wound (e.g. automatic weapon) shock waves emanating from the bullet pass through the tissues, traumatising around and outside the track.

Wound management will be discussed under the following headings:
1. Assessment of underlying injuries:
   (a) clinical examination;
   (b) wound exploration.
2. Cleaning, debridement, excision, and removal of foreign bodies.
3. Wound closure.
4. Dressings.
5. Antibiotics and prevention of tetanus.
6. Other factors, influencing healing.
7. Special problems.

Assessment of underlying injuries
Clinical examination
Always check distal pulsation, sensation and motor function before exploring a wound. Major vessels, nerves and tendons and vital organs may be injured even under small, innocent-looking lacerations. Look for signs of major organ injury (including spinal cord injury) in wounds over the abdomen, chest and back. Radiographs taken in two planes will help to localise foreign bodies such as bullets or shrapnel. Record the site and size of wounds in the patient's notes.

VASCULAR INJURY

Loss of pulsation distal to the site of a wound or fracture is an indication for arteriography (if available) or surgical exploration. In an emergency lacerated major vessels can usually be safely ligated in young people. However, most major vessels can be repaired by those with experience, which usually results in better recovery.

INJURY TO VESSELS AND NERVES

If you do not know how to repair tendons or nerves simply debride and clean the wound. The ends of nerves and tendons can be trimmed. Then suture or leave the wound open as appropriate and refer once the patient's condition is stable.

WOUNDS IN THE NECK

Consider oesophageal, tracheal, spinal cord and major vessel injury. Feel the carotid pulses. The absence of a carotid pulse is an indication for arteriography (when available) or at least exploration by a trained surgeon. If the patient cannot swallow freely oesophagoscopy is indicated. If you can hear air coming out of the wound on expiration, the wound extends into the airway and a tracheostomy is likely to be required.

Wound exploration
A wound should be explored whenever there is uncertainty about which underlying structures are injured and providing exploration does not increase the risks to the patient's life or limb. Adequate anaesthesia is required in conscious patients and the choice of anaesthesia (local, regional or general) will depend on the site and size of the wound and the condition of the patient.

Exploration of a wound normally involves extending it to two or three times its original size.

Wounds on distal parts of a limb are best explored using a pneumatic tourniquet. When clinical assessment has revealed no evidence of injury to underlying vessels, tendons or nerves, proceed to cleaning, debridement and wound excision.

Cleaning, debridement, excision and removal of foreign bodies
Cleaning
Clean all wounds with soap and water or Savlon (cetrimide + chlorhexidine). If dirt and foreign matter cannot easily be removed by irrigation and rinsing then scrub the wound under local anaesthetic.

Pour the cleaning fluid onto the wound and scrubbing brush from above rather than dipping the same dirty brush back into the same basin. The choice of cleaning fluid is less important than a meticulous cleaning and removal of dirt and necrotic fluid. Savlon is an example of a suitable wound disinfectant but at this stage ordinary water from a tap is cheap and generally available in large quantities. A large volume of water of saline which can be poured on from above is preferable to a basin of Savlon into which the scrubbing brush is dipped again and again!

Debridement and excision

Wounds should be debrided after cleaning. Debridement (literally, unbridling or breaking down) involves excision of all dead and devitalised tissue. The wound edges should also be excised for a distance of 2–3 mm. Grossly contaminated wounds (including most war and battle wounds) should be more widely excised. On the face excision is often unnecessary or can be minimal.

Gunshot wounds, particularly those due to high-velocity bullets, will need wide excision of the entry and exist sites in order to gain access to the track. Loose bone fragments not attached to periosteum should be removed. Excision will have to be limited if it is likely to cause exsanguination or where important structures could be damaged.

Removal of foreign bodies

This should be done whenever the patient's life or limb is not jeopardised by the incision required to remove them. If it is not possible to remove a foreign body take comfort in the fact that objects such as bullets and shrapnel are usually minimally contaminated. Many patients have lived happily ever after with bullets or shrapnel in the skull, chest, abdomen or pelvis! Ensure the track is able to drain adequately. It is rarely possible to remove the majority of pellets in a patient with multiple shotgun injuries.

Wound closure

Decide whether the wound is suitable for immediate primary, delayed primary or secondary closure.

Primary closure

This is achieved by direct suture and can be performed immediately (within 6–12 h for most clean wounds and up to 12–24 h for the scalp and face) or delayed for 2–3 days. Primary closure aims to achieve primary healing. The following conditions must be met before performing primary closure:
1. the wound must be clean – this can be decided immediately or after dressing the wound and reinspecting it at 2–3 days;
2. the wound must be able to be closed without tension.

IMMEDIATE PRIMARY CLOSURE
The indications for this are:
1. scalp, facial or eyelid wounds;
2. all clean, incised wounds of recent origin where the patient does not have to be transferred, except perineal, foot and open femoral and tibial fractures.

Use appropriate sizes of sutures with sharp cutting needles. Do not pull the edges too tight as this will cause tissue oedema and necrosis predisposing to pain and infection.

DELAYED PRIMARY CLOSURE
This can be achieved by suturing on day 2 or 3 after injury. The edges may need to be undermined to avoid tension otherwise closure can be achieved by skin grafting. The main indications are:
1. crushed or contaminated wounds that have had cleaning and debridement;
2. wounds presenting after 6–12 h;
3. wounds that cannot be closed without tension (the exception is the scalp which can tolerate some tension);
4. potentially infected wounds (following laparotomy for peritonitis or a colonic injury).

Between wound toilet (day 0) and wound inspection for possible delayed primary closure (day 2–3) the wound should be dressed with a sterile gauze and left alone unless fever or concern about gangrene makes earlier inspection mandatory.

Secondary closure

This can be achieved by allowing spontaneous closure to occur (this involves granulation and contraction to effect healing) or the wound can be sutured, grafted or covered by a myocutaneous flap once it is clean and no longer infected. The indications are:
1. wounds originally selected for delayed primary closure which became infected;
2. already infected wounds,
3. wounds where it is usually safer to allow granulation to occur before closure such as an open fracture of the tibia or perineal laceration.

Dressings

Wounds that have been sutured only require dressing for 1–2 days if at all. After skin graft, dressings' are normally left untouched for 4–7 days. Myocutaneous flaps will need to be inspected regularly to ensure the flap remains viable.

Open wounds should be dressed and initially the dressing should be left for 2–3 days until the wound is inspected. Before removal of the dressing moisten the dressing material with saline to allow the dressing to be removed without damage to the bed of the wound. Analgesia or anaesthesia may be required to enable the wound to be inspected and dressed. A decision will then be made about whether the wound is to undergo delayed primary or secondary closure. If the wound is dirty then dressings should be performed three times a day, cleaning the wound with Savlon or saline and removing slough, dead tissue and loose scab before redressing. Trauma to the wound and the ingrowing granulation tissue must be avoided each time the dressing is changed. If the wound is heavily infected, irrigating with hydrogen peroxide and packing the wound with gauze may help to decontaminate the wound faster. Honey, yoghurt or Betadine (povidone–iodine) mixed with granulated sugar (the main purpose of the Betadine is to act as a paste to hold the sugar in the wound) have also been shown to be effective in persistently infected wounds. The wound should be kept covered to avoid desiccation until it either is closed by secondary suture/skin graft or heals by secondary intention. (Desiccation is the process of drying out of tissue by evaporation.)

Antibiotics and prevention of tetanus

Antibiotics are not necessary for uncomplicated lacerations. Give prophylactic antibiotics for open fractures including skull fractures. When there is a deep penetrating dirty wound this should be cleaned, debrided and excised as far as possible and in addition to tetanus toxoid, penicillin therapy should be given.

Patients with dirty and heavily contaminated wounds who are not fully immunised against tetanus should be given anti-tetanus serum in addition to anti-tetanus toxoid and penicillin.

Other factors influencing healing

Wounded limbs are best elevated to reduce oedema, which restricts blood flow in and out of the wound. The haemoglobin should be above 10 g/dl and the patient should have an adequate nutritional intake.

Underlying fractures must be stabilised, if necessary by external fixation.

Special problems

Penetrating wounds through the skull

It is rarely feasible to achieve more than adequate cleaning, debridement and removal of foreign matter. Burr holes may need to be made around the site of entry through the skull in order to remove dead bone, foreign matter and necrotic brain.

The track of entry into the brain can be gently suctioned to remove necrotic brain. If a bullet is inaccessible do not attempt to remove it but rather make sure the track is clean and will drain. Many patients do well despite having a retained bullet within their brain. Exposed cranium must be covered by soft tissue or else it will dessicate and die.

Penetrating abdominal wounds

These are discussed on p. 210. If the posterior rectus sheath has been penetrated adequate exploration will involve laparotomy.

Penetrating chest wounds

These are discussed on p. 208.

Bomb explosions and blast lung

Injury is caused by both flying objects such as glass, metal, etc. and by the shock waves emanating from the blast. Penetrating injuries are treated as described above. In the lung shock waves disrupt air–fluid interfaces and air in the alveoli is compressed and expanded leading to tearing of the alveolar walls. This leads to bleeding and bruising of lung tissue resulting in inadequate gas exchange across the alveolar –capillary membrane. Blast injury to the lungs is recognised by the signs of respiratory failure (Table 1.1) and the chest X-ray will develop the signs of ARDS (Figure 1.3). Treatment includes oxygen therapy, ventilation and PEEP. If the patient can be supported until the damaged lung tissue recovers he will survive.

Traumatic amputation

This may occur in road, rail or machine accidents or in a landmine explosion. In a landmine injury involving loss of the foot or leg, damaged tissue and earth may be driven by the explosion deep into the fascial compartments so that the site of amputation may need to be at a higher level and the amputation stump should resemble an excised wound.

Degloving injuries

These occur when skin and soft tissue are stripped off the underlying muscle or bone. The degloving many not be immediately apparent if skin and subcutaneous tissue are only separated by a haematoma (Figure 11.13). Proximally based flaps are more likely to survive than distally based ones. Survival depends on the length of the flap, the width of the base of the flap, the degree of blunt trauma to the flap initially and whether or not the flap can be re-sutured with a minimum of tension. Obvious devascularised, ischaemic skin (blue, purple or dusky in appearance) should be excised and if some or all of the degloved flap is to be sutured back after meticulous debridement, the undersurface of the skin-flap should be cleaned of subcutaneous fat. If the flap has a narrow base it is probably better to excise it, clean its

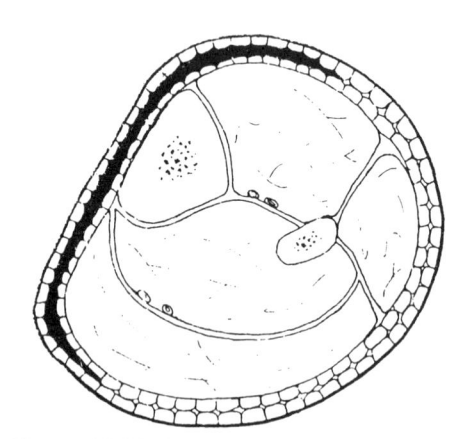

Figure 11.13 Degloving injury: blood in the subutaneous tissues between skin and fascia or bone is a sign that the skin is separated from its blood supply. Degloving may also occur when the skin is stripped off the limb with or without a proximally or distally based attachment.

Crush injuries

Crush injury to a limb results in extensive muscle trauma with release of myoglobin and other toxic products of dead muscle into the bloodstream. The patient may develop renal failure from deposition of myoglobin in the kidney.

Tourniquet damage

When the patient arrives in hospital with a tourniquet around the limb the decision is between removal of the tourniquet and amputation of the limb above the tourniquet. If the tourniquet has been in place for more than 6 h amputate as removal of the tourniquet if likely to cause death from release of myoglobin and other toxic metabolites from the limb once it is revascularised. Severe toxaemia and renal failure may still follow removal of a tourniquet in place for more than 2–3 h and the decision whether or not to amputate will also be influenced by the state of the injured limb.

Compartment syndrome

This is due to tension building up within the fascial compartments of the limb which leads to further muscle death by pressure necrosis. The limb will appear swollen, with loss of distal pulsation and superficial circulation as determined by lack of blanching of the nailbeds. Urgent and extensive fasciotomy will be required to save the limb (Figures 11.14 to 11.16). Compartment syndrome can also be caused by a tight-fitting plaster cast (Figure 11.17a, b).

Animal bites

These are heavily contaminated with both aerobic and anaerobic bacteria. Wounds due to bites should be cleaned, debrided and excised. Wound excision can be minimal on the face. The wound should be left open for delayed primary or secondary suture and prophylactic antibiotics (e.g. penicillin and metronidazole) should be given. Each wound will have to be treated on its own merits according to the principles described above, particularly in large animal bites with associated fractures or amputations due to crocodiles, hippopotamuses, or lions.

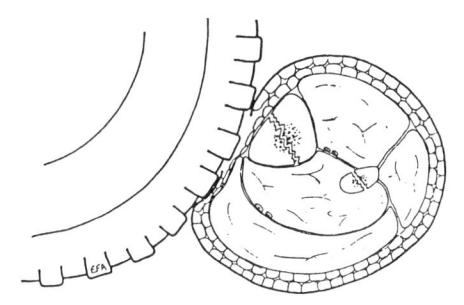

Figure 11.14 Where the limb has been run over there will be massive soft tissue injury in addition to the fractures. Management of the wound and soft tissues takes priority over the bony injury.

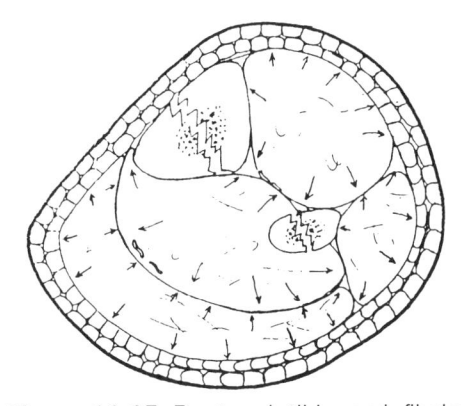

Figure 11.15 Fractured tibia and fibula leading to compartment syndrome. Pressure within the fascial compartments of the leg rises and compresses the vessels. If this pressure is not relieved there will be muscle necrosis and the leg may be lost.

Gas gangrene

This complication of wounds is caused by clostridial organisms. It is recognised by rapidly spreading oedema and gangrene with gas formation which can be felt in the tissues. The infection will have spread well proximal to the site of gangrene. Gas gangrene spreads quickly (within hours) so that the patient's general condition deteriorates rapidly due to septicaemic shock. On diagnosis the patient should be treated with high doses of penicillin and sent immediately to theatre for amputation. Amputation of the limb well above the most proximal site where gas can be felt in the tissues offers the patient his only hope of survival. Gas gangrene can be prevented by proper wound management at the outset.

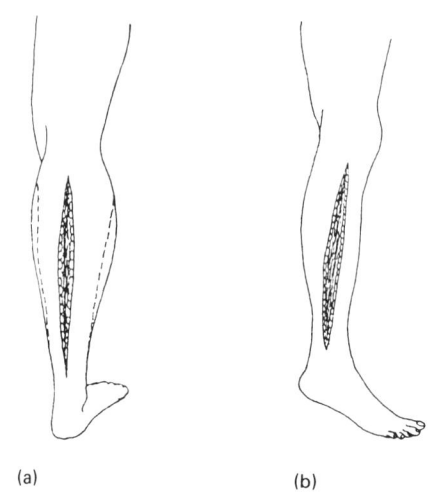

Figure 11.16 Fasciotomy incisions. (a) Posterior fasciotomy incision in calf (the dotted lines indicate the other two incisions to be made. (b) The lateral fasciotomy incision.

Further reading

COUPLAND RM. Technical aspects of war wound excision. *Br J Surg* 1989;76:663–7.

KING M. Chapters 54–56. In: *Trauma*. Primary Surgery series, Vol. 2. Oxford: Oxford Medical Publications, 1987.

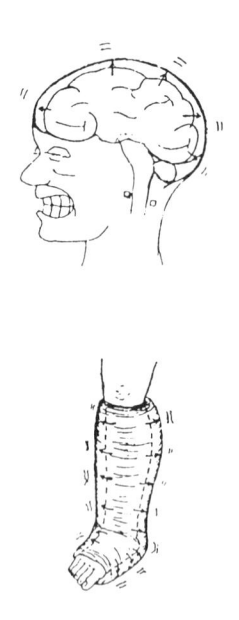

Figure 11.17 (a) A plaster cast that is too tight on a fractured limb causes the pressure within the limb to rise rapidly as soft tissue swelling occurs. This is similar to the situation within the cranium after a head injury. If a plaster is to be applied it should be split as shown in (b).

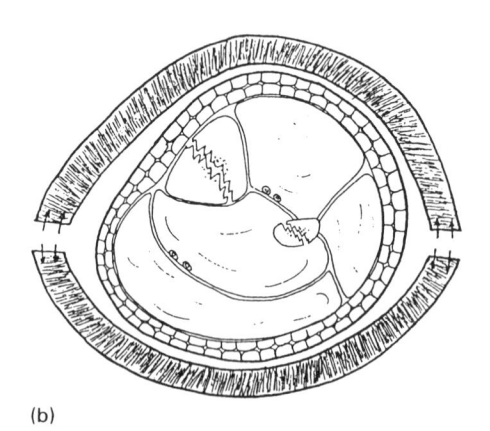

Figure 11.17 (b) Split plaster of Paris cast around a fractured leg. The cast should be split medially *and* laterally to allow it to expand as the leg swells. The limb should also be elevated and the circulation checked repeatedly.

Limb fractures and dislocations

The precise management of specific fractures and dislocations is fully described in appropriate texts on trauma and fractures. The following points are emphasised in order that the critically ill patient with such injuries will receive reasonable management (in the absence of an orthopaedic surgeon) so that during the critical phase the healing of fractures and dislocations will not be compromised by neglect or mismanagement.

Dislocation of the hip

The hip may be dislocated posteriorly, anteriorly or centrally. Posterior dislocation is the most common. A dislocated hip may not be recognised unless specifically looked for on examination.

The leg will be shortened and held in flexion, adduction and internal rotation in a posterior dislocation or extended and externally rotated in the uncommon anterior dislocation. There will be restricted hip movement and there may be sciatic nerve damage in posterior dislocation or femoral nerve damage in anterior dislocation.

An AP X-ray of the pelvis may not show a dislocation clearly to the untrained eye. Take a lateral view if in doubt. Treatment of posterior and anterior dislocation is by reduction under anaesthesia and traction to rest the joint. In central dislocation skeletal traction using a tibial pin and 9 kg is advised.

Fractured femur

The blood loss from a fractured femur is in the order of 1–2 litres, so that the patient may be shocked. Movement increases blood loss and the chance of developing fat embolism.

The fracture should be suspected by swelling and deformity. X-rays are diagnostic. Supracondylar fractures may be associated with vascular damage. Always examine the pulses and superficial circulation distal to a limb fracture.

First-aid treatment is by splintage. Skeletal traction using a Denham or Steinman pin is best during the first few days. These pins can be inserted under local anaesthesia using a hand drill (Figure 11.18). Insert 2–3 cm below and behind the tibial tuberosity at right angles to the tibia

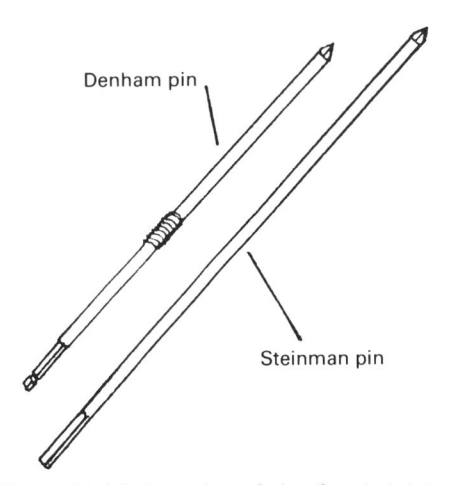

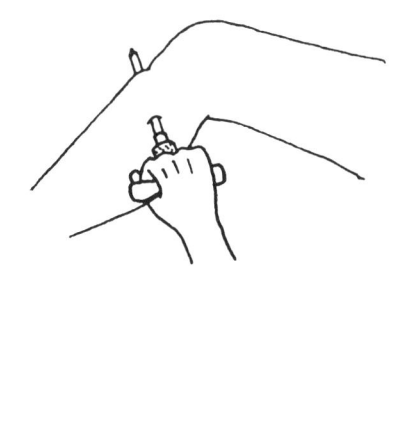

Figure 11.18 Insertion of pins for skeletal traction in fractures of the femur. Insert the pin at right angles to the tibia, 2–3 cm below and 2–3 cm behind the tibial tuberosity.

in adults. Children can be treated with skin traction.

Initial femoral traction should be 10 kg (1–3 bricks) which are attached to the pins. Subsequent treatment is by Perkin's traction or internal fixation, depending on the type of fracture and the facilities available.

Tibial fracture

Closed tibial fractures can be treated by elevation and splinting initially. Check distal pulsation carefully. If the distal circulation is impaired perform fasciotomy. This can be done under local anaesthesia. Time should not be wasted transferring the patient to theatre once the decision has been made to do fasciotomy.

All open and unstable tibial fractures are prone to develop non-union. They require aggressive and early treatment. They can be treated initially by skeletal traction via a calcaneal pin and 6 kg (2 bricks) weight. The treatment of the soft-tissue injury is most important and is outlined below.

Wounds less than 1 cm diameter: debride, irrigate, dress, leave wound open, treat like a closed fracture with elevation. They do well with prophylactic antibiotics and immobilisation, using calcaneal pin skeletal traction for 1–3 weeks. Later a plaster can be applied once the swelling has subsided.

Wounds larger than 1 cm diameter: debride, irrigate, dress, leave wound open. Elevate and check distal pulsation. External fixation or calcaneal traction may be applied.

KEY POINT
Do not suture open tibial wounds as an immediate primary procedure.

Open tibial wounds should be reinspected at 2–3 days and at this stage may suitable for delayed primary suture (p. 216) or split skingrafting providing it is clean and closure can be achieved without tension.

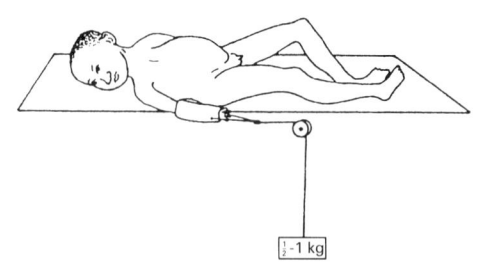

Figure 11.19 Straight-arm lateral traction for supracondylar fractures of the humerus in children. Note that the weight can be suspended over a pulley or, alternatively, a bedside locker.

Fractured humerus

This fracture poses a problem in the critically ill, who are usually recumbent so that gravity does not help to align the fracture. A fractured shaft of humerus can be splinted for the first few days with the arm bound to the chest if there is no associated chest injury. Traction via an olecranon pin with the elbow kept at right angles may be necessary if the period of recumbency if likely to be prolonged.

Use straight lateral traction (Fig 11.19) for severely displaced supracondylar fractures in children. This position safeguards the circulation. It is difficult to manipulate these fractures in the first few days as they often present late and are very swollen. Other alternative methods include traction using an olecranon pin. After one week a collar and cuff can be applied and good functional results can be achieved after a few months with remodelling. An orthopaedic surgeon may prefer to achieve an accurate anatomical reduction with K-wires by open operation, or percutaneously using an image intensifier.

Mass accidents and disasters

Disasters occur unexpectedly, except in wartime. All hospitals need to have a disaster plan to cope with large numbers of casualties.

Disaster plans should be devised for coping with 25, 50, 100 and 200+ casualties. There needs to be a disaster team or committee who ensure that each department in the hospital knows what to do in the event of mass casualties.

The team will need to include members of the following departments:

1.	Administration	Co-ordinate efforts, communication, press releases
2.	Ministry of health	Political implications, outside help
3.	Pharmacist	Drug supply
4.	Catering	Food for staff and victims
5.	Stores	Supplies of surgical sundries
6.	Blood bank	Organisation of donors
7.	Medical team	Surgery, anaesthesia, casualty, critical care
8.	Nursing	Theatres, casualty, surgical wards, critical care
9.	Heads of clinical departments	Care of other patients, allocation of junior staff

A disaster file should be kept in each department of the hospital stating what each department's responsibility is. The file should provide a clear, stepwise approach to the action required by the head of department.

Rehearsals should be held at specified intervals. Emergency equipment throughout the hospital should be checked on a daily basis. Batteries and bulbs should be functional. A disaster store of essential items such as drugs, giving sets, intravenous fluids and dressings should be kept and regularly inspected to make sure that the contents are not beyond their expiry dates.

- Disaster plan.
- Disaster file in each department.
- Check emergency equipment daily.
- Rehearse disaster plan.
- Disaster stock cupboard.

The size of the hospital, the number of staff and number of casualties will determine the impact of the disaster on normal hospital function.

Each hospital will need to determine its own strategy. The following shows the levels of impact.

1. Small number of casualties: normal on-call surgical team copes with all cases.
2. In order to cope, other surgical teams need to help.
3. Department of surgery unable to cope. Junior- and middle-grade staff required from other departments and surgical subspecialities. At this stage, clinics will need to be closed and clinics will be required as wards.

Doctors, clinical officers and nurses should work 12-hour shifts and should go home to rest when off duty. Good food and refreshments should be freely available to them during shifts. The same is true for porters, cleaners, ward clerks and the catering department.

Triage

Triage means division of patients into groups according to whether they require immediate, delayed, palliative or minor treatment. Triage should be performed by a senior doctor, and is made on the basis of the following:

- airway,
- breathing,
- circulation,
- conscious level,
- actual injuries,
- urgency of treatment required.

Management proceeds as follows:
1. Those dead should be sent to the mortuary. Those so severely injured that

they are not going to survive should be transferred to the receiving or emergency ward for palliative treatment.
2. Those who are rescuable but need immediate airway management, urgent resuscitation and urgent surgery should be sent to a resuscitation area close to the theatre. There should be a senior doctor and, if possible, an anaesthetist present, who assess the immediate problems and instruct and guide junior doctors and clinical officers who resuscitate the patients.
3. Those with severe but currently non-life-threatening injuries who require early but not immediate surgery should be transferred to an emergency ward. Radiological assessment may be indicated. This group includes those who need vigilant head-injury observation. The emergency ward will probably be manned by middle-grade doctors.
4. Those with minor injuries including the walking wounded who do not require major or immediate surgery should be transferred to a clinic equipped for wound management manned by clinical officers and nurses, supervised by a junior doctor. After treatment they are likely to be discharged home.

In addition, theatre should be geared for round-the-clock operating. Senior surgeons should commence operating according to priorities. Junior- or middle-grade surgeons can operate in a separate theatre under the supervision of a senior. The surgery performed needs to be fast, simple and straightforward.

On hearing of the disaster, the ICU staff should discharge those patients who could reasonably be treated in a general ward. Equipment and procedure trays should be prepared in readiness for patients being transferred from the resuscitation ward, emergency ward or the operating theatre.

Further reading

The references listed below are not intended to be comprehensive but rather to provide further reading for the management of trauma in a tropical setting.

MATTHEW PK, KAPUA F, SOAKI PJ, WATTERS DAK. Trauma in the Southern Highlands of Papua New Guinea. *Aust NZ J Surg* 1996;66: 659–63.
SMITH GS, BARSS P. Unintentional injuries in developing countries: the epidemiology of a neglected problem. *Epidemiol Rev* 1991;13: 228–30.
WATTERS DAK, DYKE T. Trauma in Papua New Guinea: What do we know and where do we go? *PNG Med J* 1996;39:121–5.
WATTERS DAK, LOURIE JA. (Editorial) Trauma in Papua New Guinea – an epidemic out of control. *PNG Med J* 1996;39:91–2.
WATTERS DAK, DYKE T, MAIHUA J. Trauma admissions in Port Moresby. *PNG Med J* 1996;39:93–9.
ZWI A. Injury control in developing countries. *Health Policy Plann* 1993;8:173–9.

Penetrating injuries

BARSS P. Penetrating wounds caused by needlefish in Oceania. *Med J Aust* 1985;143: 617–22.35
FINGLETON LJ. Arrow wounds to the heart and mediastinum. *Br J Surg* 1987;74:126–28.
JACOB OJ. Penetrating thoracoabdominal injuries with arrows: experience with 63 patients. *Aust NZ J Surg* 1995;65:394–6.
VANGURP G, HUTCHISON TJ, ALTO WA. Arrow wound management in Papua New Guinea. *J Trauma* 1990;30:183–88.

Abdomen and spleen

BOONE K, WATTERS DAK. The incidence of malaria after splenectomy in Papua New Guinea. *BMJ* 1995;311:1273.
HAMILTON DR, PIKACHA D. Ruptured spleen in a malarious area: with particular emphasis on conservative management in both adults

and children. *Aust NZ J Surg* 1982;52: 310–13.

PONIFASIO P, POKI O, WATTERS DAK. Abdominal trauma in Papua New Guinea. *PNG Med J* 2001;44:36–42.

Splenic injury study group. Ruptured spleen in the adult: an account of 205 cases with particular reference to non-operative management. *Aust NZ J Surgery* 1987;57:549–53.

Cardiovascular injuries

BARSS P. Injuries caused by Garfish in Papua New Guinea, *BMJ* 1982;284:77–9.

GOLPAK V. Post traumatic false aneurysm – a frequently missed condition in penetrating injuries. *PNG Med J* 1995;38(1):57–61.

HENDERSON VJ, SMITH S, FRY WR, et al. Cardiac injuries: analysis of an unselected series of 251 cases. *J Trauma* 1994;36:341–8.

JACOB OJ, ROSENFELD MS, TAYLOR RH and WATTERS DAK. Late complications of arrow and spear wounds to the head and neck. *J Trauma* 1999;47(4):1–6.

MATHEW PK, KAINGE T, KAPUA F, BARUA R. Management of vascular trauma in a provincial hospital. *PNG Med J* 1996;39(2):126–8.

ROBBS JV, BAKER LW. Major arterial trauma: review of experience with 267 injuries. *Br J Surg* 1978;65:532–8.

ROBBS JV, BAKER LW. Subclavian and axillary artery injuries. *S Afr Med J* 1977;51:227–31.

Fractures

BONE LB, JOHNSON KD, WEIGELT J et al. Early versus delayed stabilization of femoral fractures: a prospective, randomised, controlled study. *J Bone Joint Surg Am* 1989;71A:336–40.

DALAL SA, BURGESS AR, SEIGEL JH et al. Pelvic fracture in multiple trauma; classification by mechanism is key to pattern of organ injury, resuscitative requirements and outcome. *J Trauma* 1989;29:991.

GUSTILO RB, MENDOZA RM, WILLIAMS DN. Problems in the management of type III (severe) open fractures; a new classification of type III open fractures. *J Trauma* 1985; 24:272.

KEVAU I, WATTERS DAK. Conservative management of femoral shaft fractures in adults. Clinical practice. *PNG Med J* 1996;39: 143–51.

Trees and falling coconuts

BARSS P, DAKULALA P, DOOLAN, M. Fall from trees and tree associated injuries in rural Melanesians. *BMJ* 1984;289:1717–20.

BARSS P. Injuries due to falling coconuts. *J Trauma* 1984;24:990–1.

Primary trauma care

See website: www.nda.ox.ac.uk/wfsa

12

Burns

Introduction

The early management of severe burns follows the principles of all resuscitation: Airway (with cervical spine control), Breathing and Circulation. There is an opportunity early on to prevent deaths from hypoxia and shock and also ensure that later problems are minimised by good tissue perfusion with oxygenated blood. Early deaths may be due to airway burns or smoke inhalation. Next the patient is at risk from circulatory failure due to burns shock. Later infection of the burn occurs and infected burns are the most common reason for potentially preventable deaths in the tropics. The prevention and treatment of burn shock and infection are the main objectives of acute care once the airway and breathing are secure.

An upper airway burn may compromise the airway. Tell-tale signs are singed eyelashes and eyebrows, and burns or soot around the nose and mouth (pp. 229, 232, 234–5) and the type of burn (e.g. an explosion or being trapped in a burning building). If the patient has signs suggestive of an airway burn it is often safer to intubate the patient before deterioration. It may be difficult or impossible to intubate once the airway swells. Noisy breathing is an indication to immediately intubate and secure the airway. The possibility of a cervical spine injury should always be considered in a patient who has been in an explosion (water heater explosions, propane gas, bombs) as the patient may have been thrown some distance by the explosion.

Smoke inhalation into the lungs may cause breathing problems either early or late (pp. 229, 232, 234–5). The type of burn and the environment of the burn (e.g. escaping from a burning building) and soot particles around the nares should alert the attending doctor to the possibility of these complications developing. The respiratory rate, respiratory pattern, pulse and oxygenation saturation should be monitored. The airway should be maintained and secured. Later respiratory problems may develop due to lung injury and oedema or secondary infection and require ventilatory support. Carbon monoxide poisoning may complicate some types of burn, especially where there is a lot of smoke inhalation (p. 121). Cyanide poisoning may complicate burning plastics. Removal of a burned victim from a burning scene is an important aspect of early management.

Shock may develop due to the fluid exudate from burns. The longer the patient takes to reach hospital the greater will be the circulatory deficit. Fluid therapy in burns is calculated from the time of the burn (p. 233). The poorer the tissue perfusion the greater will be the burn injury. If sepsis later develops septic shock is another cause of circulatory failure.

Other injuries may occur in patients who are thrown by an explosion (e.g.

head, spine or torso injuries) and all patients should have a full secondary survey performed to exclude other injuries which should be managed as discussed in Chapters 10 and 11. The conscious level of patients involved in an explosion should be monitored. An altered or deteriorating conscious level could be due to airway, breathing, circulatory or intracranial causes in the early phase. Later sepsis may also cause confusion and deterioration in conscious level.

The hypermetabolic state that develops in response to a major burn consumes the patient's ability to heal and resist infection. The hypermetabolic response and its ill effects can be minimised by adequate nutritional support (Chapter 15). Pain also increases the acute stress response and the outpouring of catecholamines and other stress-related hormones. Adequate analgesia is required.

The care of the burn wound and prevention of infection will be optimal if there are specially trained nursing staff and doctors dedicated to the management of burns who see decision making on burned patients as a priority. A team approach involving physiotherapists and occupational therapists, particularly for burns of the limbs, combined with adequate psychological support and rehabilitation after the acute phase will result in the best possible outcomes.

There is a valuable Early Management of Severe Burns (EMSB) course developed since the first edition of this book by the Australia and New Zealand Burn Association and also adopted by the British Burn Association since 1997. The principles taught in this course are applicable in any country although the resources for treatment of severe burns will be limited.

The following are the major changes which occur or (in the case of infections) may develop as a consequence of a burn:

Damage and healing

Extreme heat or cold kills cells. **Depth of damage depends on temperature and time.** For example, splashing hot water on the skin causes less damage than putting the skin into hot water (a longer time), or burning it with fire (much hotter).

Damage to the skin may be partial thickness or full thickness (Figure 12.1). In *partial-thickness* burns some of the dermis remains alive, and the hair follicles, sebaceous glands, and sweat glands in the dermis contain epithelial cells from which a new epithelium can generate. It is useful to consider two grades of partial-thickness burn; superficial partial thickness, which will heal in 10–14 days without scarring, and deep partial thickness (often called deep dermal), which may heal in 21 days or more, but is likely to leave bad scars.

Full-thickness burns destroy the whole dermis and all epithelial cells, so they cannot heal unless they are very small. Severe burns can go deeper, destroying fat, muscle, bone, and all other tissues.

Initially it may be difficult or impossible to tell how deep a burn is (depth uncertain), especially to tell whether it is superficial partial thickness or deep partial thickness, and the depth may be different in different parts of the wound (a mixed burn). **Any area that has not healed by 21 days after burning is a full-thickness burn.**

Full-thickness burns, if not treated by skin grafting, cause severe and permanent scarring, deformity, and disability.

Body fluid changes

After a burn there is an increase in capillary permeability, especially in the region of the burn, but in large burns this affects the whole body. Plasma leaks out of the blood into the tissues. The leak is maximum during the first 8 h after the burn,

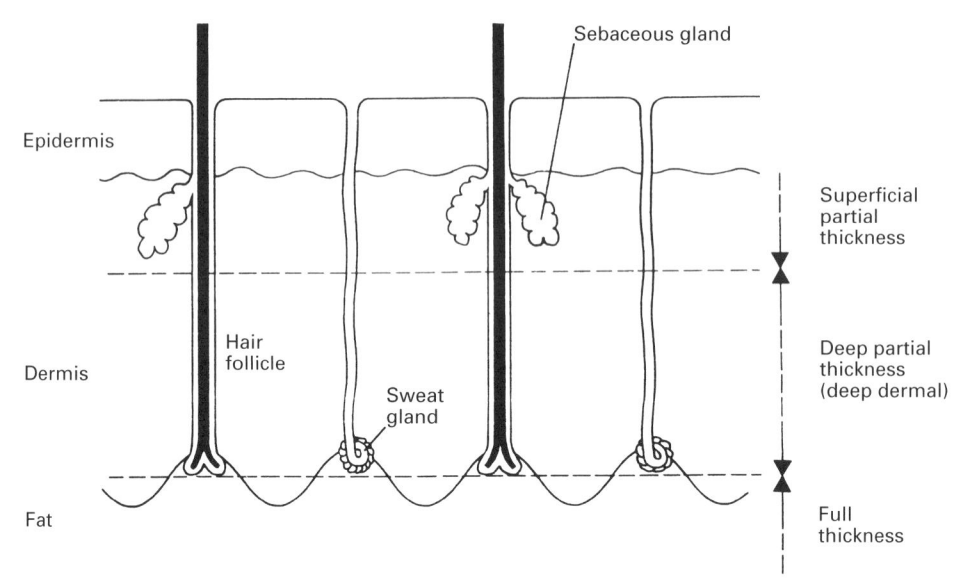

Figure 12.1 Cross-section of skin to show areas affected by differing depths of burns.

and then gets less, so that capillary permeability returns to normal between 36 and 48 h after injury.

The amount of fluid lost from the blood is proportional to the size of the burn. Burn size is measured as a percentage of total body surface area. Using this percentage and the patient's body weight, it is possible to calculate the amount of fluid lost, and therefore how much fluid will be required to replace it.

The lost fluid must be replaced to prevent hypovolaemic shock (burn shock). The fluid used to replace it must contain sodium in at least the same concentration as in the plasma.

Metabolic changes

Burned patients have an increased metabolic rate (hypermetabolism), which continues until the wound is healed. The increase is proportional to the size of the burn up to about 50% body surface area, and may be up to twice the normal metabolic rate. Hypermetabolism reaches a maximum at this point and does not increase further in burns of more than 50%.

Total body protein synthesis and breakdown are increased, but overall there is a breakdown of tissues (catabolism), particularly loss of muscle protein, which is broken down to form glucose and also for the synthesis of new proteins (e.g. for wound repair and to replace losses from the wound). The underlying reasons for this are not completely understood, but seem to depend upon a central nervous control mechanism and the actions of catabolic hormones such as catecholamines, glucagon, and corticosteroids. Cold, pain, infection, and other forms of stress all increase metabolic demands.

The clinical signs of this hypermetabolic state, which are always present in patients with large burns, are increased temperature, increased respiration, increased heart rate, and weight loss. Without proper nutrition there is severe weight loss, failure of wound healing, failure of skin grafts, anaemia, hypoproteinaemia, and a major decrease in resistance to infection, from which the patient is likely to die.

Weight loss cannot be completely prevented by nutritional support, but it can be minimised, and **it is vital that burns patients are adequately fed.** The exact effects of pre-existing malnutrition on this process, and on the patient's ability to use the nutritional support given in hospital, have not been studied in detail, but the effects of malnutrition certainly worsen the prognosis.

Infection

The burn itself is sterile immediately after injury. **The wound is soon colonised by bacteria,** the commonest of which are Gram positives such as *Staphylococcus aureus* and *Streptococcus pyogenes*, and Gram negatives such as *Escherichia coli*, *Pseudomonas*, *Proteus*, and *Klebsiella*. Culture of swabs from the surface of a burn will nearly always grow bacteria, but **colonisation does not make the patient ill,** and antibiotics are not indicated just because a swab result is positive.

If bacteria invade the living tissue beneath the burn wound (*invasive infection*) the patient becomes ill and needs aggressive treatment.

Although the wound is the commonest site for serious infection, **burns patients can develop infections at any site in the body.** The second commonest site is the respiratory tract.

Respiratory complications

These are **respiratory injuries and infections.** Most respiratory injuries happen when a patient inhales smoke in a burning building.

Injury to the upper respiratory tract causes oedema and obstruction of the pharynx and larynx. Injury to the lungs causes pulmonary oedema and respiratory failure. These effects can occur at any time during the first 48 h, and sometimes later.

Respiratory infections, especially pneumonia, are common and serious. They can occur at any time but most often develop after 48 h.

Clinical assessment

Vital functions and pain relief

Make sure the patient is breathing and the heart is beating. If not, treat as on p. 396.

The next priority is **intravenous analgesia.** An opiate such as pethidine or morphine (e.g. pethidine 1–1.5 mg/kg) is diluted in a syringe and given slowly until the patient is completely pain free. Oral, intramuscular, and subcutaneous analgesics are inadequate and dangerous, and should never be used when a patient with burns or any other major injury first comes to hospital.

History (Table 12.1)

If the patient cannot tell you, ask the family or other witnesses. The most important information is the **date and time of the burn and the nature of the burning agent** (e.g. boiling water, hot water, hot food, cooking oil, fire, etc.), and any first aid given. All the other information which normally makes a full clinical history (family and social history and direct questions about chest symptoms, gastrointestinal symptoms, etc.) is also important but can be obtained later.

Examination (Figure 12.2)

The two most important points are **the patient's weight and the size of the burn.** These must be measured accurately, especially in children. Draw the burns areas carefully on a diagram. This needs to be repeated after 24 h, when you can often

Table 12.1 Case history sheet for burns patients

HISTORY

Name

Age – *ESTIMATE* this if unknown

Sex

Date and Time of burn

Date and time of being seen by medical officer

Burning Agent, e.g. hot water or food, fire, burning kerosene, chemicals, electricity, etc.

Circumstances of Burn, e.g. water spilled from cooking pot, clothes caught fire, epilepsy, burning house, suicide, etc.

Pre-hospital Treatment, e.g. first aid, treatment at other hospital or clinic, etc.

Past Medical History including serious illness or operation, drugs taken, allergies, and a specific enquiry about epileptic fits.

---

see that the wound is larger (and sometimes deeper) than it looked at first. After calculating the burn size by whichever method is chosen, stand back and look at the patient as a whole. Does the burn size you have calculated seem about right? Small inaccuracies are unimportant, but to estimate a 30% burn as 10%, or the other way round, may result in the patient's death. Always examine the front and back of a patient.

Burn size

In adults this can be estimated by the 'rule of nines', in which the following body areas are taken to be 9% or 18%:

whole of each upper limb = 9%;
whole of each lower limb = 18%;
front of trunk = 18%;
back of trunk = 18%;
whole of head and neck = 9%;
perineum = 1%.

Children have different body proportions and this rule is inaccurate. Therefore use the burn charts shown on the left of Figure 12.2. The table underneath shows that percentage of surface area is represented by the different areas A, B and C, at different ages.

For any age, the area of the whole of one palmar surface of the patient's hand can be taken as 1% of body surface area, and this is particularly useful for scattered burns.

Burn depth

This can be difficult to determine. The history helps. Definite partial-thickness burns are pink, wet, and blistered, and pressing with a finger (wearing a sterile glove) produces a pale patch due to emptying of blood, which when released goes pink again. Definite full-thickness burns are white or grey, dry, and stiff when pressed, do not go paler when pressed, and sometimes thrombosed blood vessels are visible through the dead skin. Burns that are sensitive to pin-pricks are partial thickness. However the sensation to pin-prick is often difficult to assess, particularly in children, and this author believes the appearance of the burn and the response to pressure are more important in determining

Weight

Nutritional status (children)

Burn 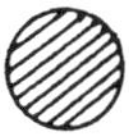 = Partial thickness/Uncertain 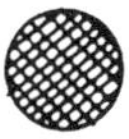 = Full thickness

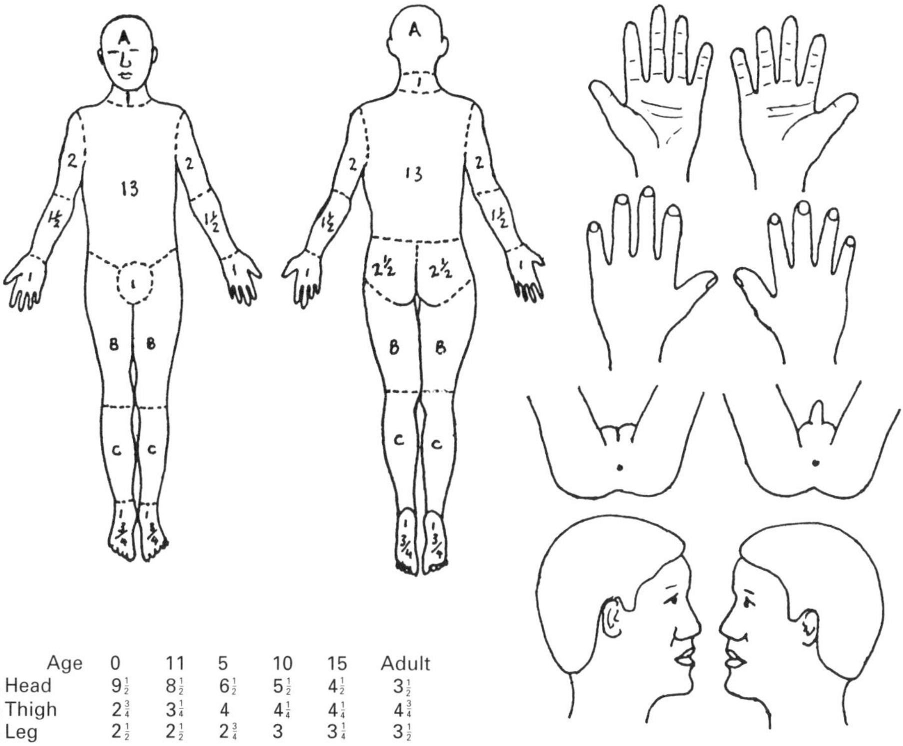

Age	0	11	5	10	15	Adult
A = ½ Head	9½	8½	6½	5½	4½	3½
B = ½ Thigh	2¾	3¼	4	4¼	4¼	4¾
C = ½ Leg	2½	2½	2¾	3	3¼	3½

OR Rule of nines for adults

OR 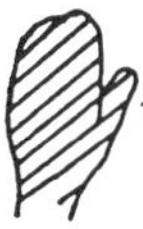 1% Surface area for any age

Total surface area of burn = __________%

Figure 12.2 Examination and calculation of percentage area burned.

the depth. In severe flame or electrical burns the tissues can be turned to charcoal.

Between these extremes is a range of uncertain appearances, which includes the appearance of deep partial thickness (deep dermal) burns. The appearances which suggest deep dermal burns are paleness without the signs of full-thickness burn described above, and sometimes mottled red areas which do not disappear when pressed. These appearances sometimes take several hours to develop.

In general, when burns management is 'conservative' (that is, waiting to see which areas heal and grafting the ones which don't), depth assessment is of limited importance on admission, but an estimate of depth may influence the initial treatment of some burns.

Respiratory system

Examine this carefully. In patients injured by fire, look for burns and soot around the nose and mouth and burned nasal hair and beard. These are signs that the patient might have a respiratory injury. Even if the patient is breathing normally and the chest sounds clear, there is a danger they may develop problems in the next 48 h, so monitor respiration frequently. The signs of obstruction due to oedema are respiratory distress and stridor. The signs of lung damage are rapid breathing, rhonchi, and crepitations.

Planning and starting treatment

The different aspects are considered in the order in which they are most likely to arise in clinical practice, rather than in order of importance, but these problems may occur in any order.

Severe burns

In modern Burns Units most burns of up to 60% would be expected to survive. Even some 60–90% burns will be saved. However, in many parts of the tropics it is very rare for patients with burns of more than 50% to survive, and such large burns are nearly always mostly full-thickness. Although they are very rare, patients with superficial partial-thickness burns of any size should be given all possible treatment, because survivors can heal fully without disability.

Full-thickness burns of more than 50% have a very bad prognosis. It is more humane to treat a patient with definitive full-thickness burns of more then 50% with enough intravenous analgesics to stop all pain and do nothing more. A patient who has no chance of survival should not be treated in the critical care area because this will divert resources from and worsen the treatment of other patients who can survive.

Analgesia

This should have been given already when the patient was first seen.

Circumferential burns

Full thickness burns all around a limb or all around the neck or chest act like a tourniquet. **They can impair the blood supply to a limb or interfere with respiration.**

These two complications must be treated urgently by escharotomy. This means cutting with a scalpel through the burned dead tissue (eschar) until living bleeding tissue appears in the bottom of the wound. The sites to make these cuts for burns in different areas are shown in Figure 12.3. No anaesthetic is required. The wound should gape widely once the constriction is relieved. Large escharotomies can cause a lot of bleeding and the patient will need a blood transfusion, but do not delay the operation while waiting for blood.

If the circulation does not rapidly return to an arm or leg, then also do *fasciotomies*, cutting through the deep fascia over the muscles at the same sites as the escharotomies. This will require an anaesthetic. If a limb becomes very painful a few hours after a successful escharotomy, or the circulation disappears again, then fasciotomies should also be done.

Fluids

Every patient needs normal maintenance fluid requirements plus extra

Burns

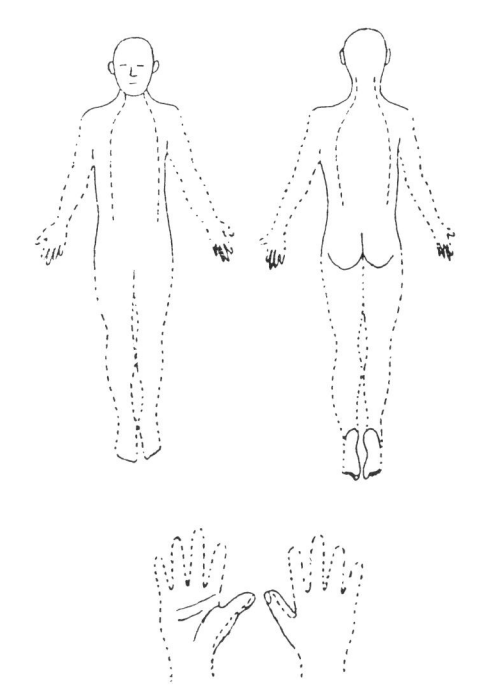

Figure 12.3 Escharotomy sites. The sites for escharotomy incision are shown as dotted lines.

fluid to compensate for that lost due to the burn. These are both calculated using the instruction in Table 12.2. All children (under 15) with burns of 10% or more, and all adults (15 and over) with burns of 15% or more, should always be given intravenous fluid. Patients with smaller burns can have their fluids by mouth but need a drip if their intake is too low.

Do not delay fluid therapy and resuscitation. Half or more of the fluid requirements in the first 24 h must be administered in the first 8 h to achieve the best outcomes.

Administered fluids must contain sodium. For oral fluids make a mixture of one teaspoon of salt, one teaspoon of sodium bicarbonate, and 2 teaspoons of sugar in 1 litre of water (you can also give oral rehydration solution).

Intravenous fluids which can be given are *isotonic* (*normal* or 0.9%) *saline*, or

Table 12.2 Fluid therapy in burns

Fluid requirements
Maintenance Requirement (as given in Table 4.1, p. 79)

Extra Requirement
Age under 6   one ration = 2 × burn size × weight
Age 6 or over one ration = 1 × burn size × weight

On top of the maintenance fluid requirement, which is given at a constant rate, one ration of extra fluid is given during the first 8 h after the time of the burn, a second ration during the next 16 h, and a third ration during the next 24 h.

Example
An 8-year-old weighing 25 kg has a 20% burn, which occurred at 04.00, and arrives in hospital at 08.00.

Maintenance = 2.5 ml/kg/h = 63 ml/h

Extra: One ration = 1 × 20% × 25 kg = 500 ml
500 ml in 8 h = 62 ml/h
500 ml in 16 h = 31 ml/h
500 ml in 24 h = 21 ml/h

Total: Rate for first 8 h = 63 + 62
  = 125 ml/h
Rate for next 16 h = 63 + 31
  = 94 ml/h
Rate for next 24 h = 63 + 21
  = 84 ml/h

The patient is admitted at 08.00, 4 h after the burn, and therefore should have a bolus of (4 × 125) ml = 500 ml, after which the infusion continues at 125 ml/h for another 4 h (until 12.00), at which time the rate is reduced to 94 ml/h.

Ringer's lactate, or *Hartmann's solution*. Add sugar (50 ml of 50% dextrose per litre) to both of these. You can also give dextrose saline solution but only if it has the same sodium content as normal saline.

Never give 5% dextrose alone. Colloids are not usually necessary unless the patient is shocked and not responding to crystalloid resuscitation.

Calculate the fluids as shown in Table 12.2. **All calculations are made from the time of injury.** Note that by the time the drip is started the patient is already several hours behind. The best way to catch up is to calculate the amount that the patient should have had by the time the drip starts and give this volume immediately as a bolus (see example in Table 12.2.) This helps the patient to catch up quickly, and also makes it easier to plan the rest of the fluids. It is not usually dangerous, but be careful when giving very large volumes rapidly because it is possible to overload the patient's circulation, and very large volumes should be given more slowly.

A useful routine, especially with children, is to put a cannula, or butterfly cannula, or even a hypodermic needle (an assistant needs to hold them in place) into the femoral vein. Start the drip, and while it is running immediately start to inject an analgesic (e.g. pethidine 1 mg/kg body weight). Continue the analgesic slowly until the patient is relaxed and drowsy. This provides analgesia, lessens the risk of a restless patient dislodging the drip, and makes other procedures easier. When about half the 'catchup' volume has been given (and the veins have partly filled), start another drip somewhere else, either an ordinary drip or a cutdown (see p. 379).

After catching up, continue the drip at the calculated rate. This is only a guide, and might later need changing. This depends on how the patient responds to treatment, and the best way of deciding this is by measuring the hourly urine output. Therefore catheterise all patients receiving intravenous fluids. Even very small children can be catheterised with a small, soft feeding tube with a blunt end. Other signs are also important in assessing whether the patient is being adequately resuscitated (see later under 'Monitoring and further treatment', p. 241).

An important early cause of renal failure may be diagnosed at this stage. This is severe haemoglobinuria or myoglobinuria due to destruction of red cells or muscle, usually by large full-thickness burns. The diagnosis is obvious; the urine is dark red. This should be treated by an immediate rapid infusion of mannitol (1 g/kg body weight), which should produce a diuresis and clear the urine. Yet more extra fluid will then have to be given to replace that lost as urine, and for several hours afterwards urine output is not a useful guide to adequate resuscitation, and other signs must be relied upon such as pulse rate, peripheral perfusion, blood pressure and jugulovenous pressure.

Consider who can be given enteral fluids if there are multiple casualties (e.g. oral rehydration solutions similar to those used for cholera). Use enteral solutions for patients who are able to swallow and are not vomiting even in those who have more than 10% body surface burns. Enteral resuscitation may also improve gut blood flow and minimise the risk of endotoxaemia due to loss of gut barrier integrity and stress ulceration. A trial of oral therapy should not be an excuse for failing to establish an i.v. line for resuscitation in individual burned patients.

Respiratory injuries

The patient can start to suffer from the effects of respiratory injury **at any time during the first 48 h.**

The sign of *upper respiratory tract obstruction* (due to oedema) is stridor. The patient may be in distress because he or she is struggling to breathe through a narrow airway.

Any sign of obstruction is treated by immediate endotracheal intubation. The tube is left in place until the oedema has settled (3–5 days). Give **chest physio-**

therapy. If intubation fails, perform immediate tracheostomy.

The signs of *lower respiratory tract damage* are first an increased breathing rate and later respiratory distress. There may be wheezing (indicating narrowed airways due to oedema and bronchospasm) and crepitations (indicating pulmonary oedema). The chest X-ray may show irregular white patches in all or part of the lungs (a 'snowstorm' appearance similar to Figure 1.3), but is usually normal in the early stages.

Mild cases are treated with **humidified oxygen, chest physiotherapy**, and **bronchodilators**.

> If the patient deteriorates with respiratory distress intubate and ventilate.

In the event of a large burn (requiring large volumes of fluid), and pulmonary oedema (theoretically requiring fluid restriction), there is a conflict of interests. In this situation give the minimum of fluid required to maintain the circulating volume and a urine flow of 0.5 ml/kg/h. Avoid diuretics except as a last resort if ventilation fails to overcome the problem.

There is no evidence that either prophylactic antibiotics or steroids are of any help for respiratory burns, and antibiotics should only be given if the patient develops signs of a respiratory infection.

The burn wound

The method of treating the burn wound itself is decided on admission. **The objectives are to prevent infection of the wound and to keep all joints fully mobile**, so that after healing there is no stiffness, deformity, or disability. The special problems of burns at certain sites are also discussed in this section.

The possible methods of management are also discussed, but many of these were developed in the West and may not be appropriate in the tropics. The author believes that a major reduction in burns mortality would most likely follow (as it did in the West some years ago) the use of topical antibacterial agents and the training of specialised nurses.

Dressings or exposure

Dressings are best avoided for most hospital in-patients. When used properly they are expensive, require large amounts of dressing materials and demand a high standard of asepsis. **Exposure is at present the general treatment of choice.** The exposed wound is drier and cooler than a dressed one, discouraging infection. It also permits frequent inspection and early detection of signs of infection.

Exposure treatment needs simple arrangements: clean (or better sterile) sheets, a bed cradle to allow free circulation of air, and a warm room. If flies are a problem use a mosquito net. Burns on both sides of the body are difficult to manage and are treated by changing the patient's position every 2 h.

There are several treatments which can be used in addition to exposure:

1. Washing every 4 or 6 h with half-strength saline (isotonic saline is painful), which can be done in bed using a waterproof sheet for protection. This solution can be made by dissolving salt in clean water, one teaspoonful of salt to every litre. The objectives are to prevent excessive drying, which may cause pain, cracking, bleeding and more damage to the wound, and to clean the wound.
2. Washing with a shower for the same reasons. Avoid baths because they may allow cross-infection from one patient to another.
3. Thick slough, which encourages infection, can be removed using 'wet to dry'

dressings; gauze soaked in saline is placed on the wound until it starts to dry but is removed before it gets dry. When it is removed it takes with it some slough which has soaked into it. Repeating this over and over again will get most wounds clean very rapidly. Dressings should never be allowed to dry and stick to a partial-thickness wound because removing them pulls off the regenerating epithelium.

Topical antibacterial agents

Although exposure should create an environment which discourages infection, many patients still die from burn infections. Large full-thickness burns get badly infected very quickly and the patient dies. This is not surprising, but what is surprising, when comparing some tropical countries with the rest of the world, is the high rate of infection and mortality which affects patients with partial-thickness burns of only moderate size, particularly children.

These patients might benefit from the use of topical agents. The agents are expensive, which is a serious disadvantage, and should not be used routinely for any burn of less than 10%. When used for large full- and mixed-thickness burns they have been shown to reduce the rate of infection and mortality. If they were used for partial thickness burns of more than 10% in children, the mortality rate in this group of patients might be reduced. By limiting the number of patients treated to those with burns of more than 10%, the overall cost could be kept to a minimum.

Agents which are effective are 0.5% silver nitrate, mafenide (Sulfamylon), and silver sulphadiazine cream. Other agents that are used include antiseptics such as povidone iodine and chlorhexidine. Of the first three, silver nitrate is the cheapest but is very messy, staining patient, staff and surroundings, has to be applied with dress-

---

MAKING SILVER SULPHADIAZINE

Reagents
Sulphadiazine (or sulphadimidine) 146 500-mg tablets. Silver nitrate crystals 48.5 g. Sodium hydroxide pellets 11.5 g. Glycerine 1440 ml. Liquid paraffin 560 ml. Non-ionic emulsifying wax 1100 g. Hibitane (chlorhexidine gluconate) solution, 5% 320 ml. Sterile distilled water as required.

Instruments
A 10 litre bucket, a mixer, a mixing rod, a beaker, and a heater.

Method
Dissolve the sodium hydroxide in about 100 ml of water. Dissolve the silver nitrate in 4000 ml of water.

Suspend the sulphadiazine tablets in 1000 ml water and stir. Heat to boiling point and add to the suspension the solution of sodium hydroxide while stirring.

Slowly add the solution of silver nitrate to the suspension of sulphadimidine and sodium hydroxide. A white precipitate of silver sulphadiazine will form.

Stop adding silver nitrate when a brown precipitate of silver oxide shows that the formation of silver sulphadiazine is complete. Boil for some minutes to make the precipitate finer and more easily filterable.

Separate the precipitate: (1) by centrifugation, or (2) with an old glass filter, or (3) by letting it stand overnight, and pouring off the supernatant. Wash the precipitate many times with water until you can detect no more silver ions in the supernatant.

Mix together the glycerine, the liquid paraffin and the emulsifying wax, and sterilise at 150°C for an hour. Let them cool and add the Hibitane solution warmed to 80°C.

Mix the two preparations and stir vigorously to obtain a fine pink cream. Put the bucket into cold water and mix until cold. Meanwhile add enough distilled water to bring the volume up to 8 litres before the preparation becomes cold.

ings, and may cause metabolic and electrolyte imbalances. Mafenide is expensive, may cause metabolic problems, and can be painful, but is the only one which penetrates eschar and is suitable for treatment of infected wounds and not just for prevention. Silver sulphadiazine is expensive but has fewer problems. It can be used with or without dressings, but some of it may get rubbed off when the patient moves. A method of making silver sulphadiazine in the hospital pharmacy is described in the panel on the left.

Topical agents need to be applied under aseptic conditions and washed off before reapplication. This has to be done by trained nurses.

Other antibacterial agents such as honey and yoghurt as topical antibacterial agents are potentially worthwhile in places where they are cheaper than conventional applications. This should only be done as part of a planned study.

Biological dressings

With major burns where the supply of split skin (autograft) is limited biological dressings reduce the septic complications and ameliorate the hypermetabolic response to burn injury. Skin cultures, cadaver skin, synthetic dressings, pigskin and amnion enable earlier tangential excision and coverage. In many tropical countries these are not available. A planned approach to burn care will be required to enable biological dressings to be used. The use of cadaveric skin or amnion may be impossible in countries with a high incidence of HIV infection. Synthetic agents are too expensive to be practical and the use of pigs also poses logistic and financial problems to be overcome. Electric dermatomes make the harvesting of pigskin a much easier process but as these are expensive they are rarely available except in a major centre.

Surgery

The surgical management of burns is beyond the scope of this book. Apart from escharotomy, described earlier, there is no situation where the burn wound must be treated by surgery soon after admission. Early tangential excision of full-thickness burns and early coverage of the burn wound requires considerable resources for patient care including a generous availability of blood transfusion. It may be beyond the resources of many tropical hospitals but is often the preferred management in major centres. However, all full-thickness burns and many deep dermal burns will require surgery at some time. In most cases this will involve skin grafting of areas that have not healed by 21 days. Surgery is also indicated where a burn wound is becoming obviously infected or the general condition of the patient is deteriorating and the cause is presumed to be sepsis.

The use of a skin graft mesher will enable a greater area of coverage of skin taken from donor sites. They are essential for the management of extensive burns and major centres in the tropics should endeavour to solve the logistic problems in obtaining an appropriate mesher.

Pharmacotherapy

The hypermetabolic response to burns is mediated by hugely increased levels of catecholeamines, prostaglandins, glucagon and cortisol. It results in profound catabolism and thus reduced resistance to infection and poor burn wound healing. It can be minimised by ensuring there is adequate oxygenation, tissue perfusion, nutritional intake and appropriate management of the burn wound as described above. Good analgesia and psychological support will also minimise the acute stress response, and thus metabolic demands and catabolism. The use of topical and systemic antibiotics is discussed throughout the chapter. Prophylactic systemic antibiotics are not recommended. DVT prophylaxis should be considered. Any co-morbid medical conditions in the burned patient will need to be managed. The use of anabolic agents such as growth hormone, insulin and immune stimulating drugs is beyond the scope of this book and the resources of most hospitals managing major burns in the tropics.

Asscociated poisoning

Carbon monoxide poisoning – see p. 121).
Cyanide poisoning – see p. 122.

Burns of special areas

Certain parts of the body are prone to special problems when burned and will be discussed individually. In general, a burn of the flexor surface at any joint is at risk of developing a contracture, and this should be prevented by physiotherapy, splintage if necessary, and skin grafting as soon as the wound is ready.

Eyes and eyelids

The eyes are protected by the speed and power of the blink reflex and may survive intact despite almost complete destruction of the eyelids. If they do not, then the injury to the eye is likely to be severe. If the cornea is burned right through, the eye must be removed.

Superficial corneal burns most often result from sudden flash burns. They usually heal if protected from infection by antibiotic eyedrops or ointment.

If the eye is exposed by eyelid burns it must be protected from drying and other damage. The best protection is a very thick layer of antibiotic ointment, although permanently wet saline dressings are also effective. As soon as possible refer the patient to a surgeon. If this involves transfer to another hospital, wait until the patient's condition is stable.

Ears

If the cartilage is exposed and becomes infected, the infection may spread rapidly through the whole cartilage and destroy it. Make great efforts to keep the wound clean. For this purpose topical antibacterial agents or frequent 'wet to dry' saline dressings may be used.

Perineum

Because the anus opens on the perineum and the area is difficult to keep exposed and dry, the burn is easily infected. Keep it as clean as possible by frequent washing. Topical agents are useful and so is traction if the legs are not burned, especially for children; it is used to raise and abduct the legs to expose the area.

Hands

Hands are very important. There is a big risk of stiffness, deformity, and permanent disability. **Start prevention early.** The best method is to put the hand in a clean plastic bag held on with a bandage round the wrist or forearm. This keeps the wound moist and comfortable and allows the patient to exercise it.

If the patient does not move the hand, and especially if you notice it being held in the bad position shown in Figure 12.4, splint it in the good position until healed. The hand is much more likely to regain full movement after being held in the good position than the bad one. Make a removable plaster slab (Figure 12.4), and continue to use a plastic bag, which protects the hand, keeps the slab dry, and can be changed easily.

If you think any part of a hand burn is full-thickness or deep dermal, refer the patient to a surgeon as soon as he or she is

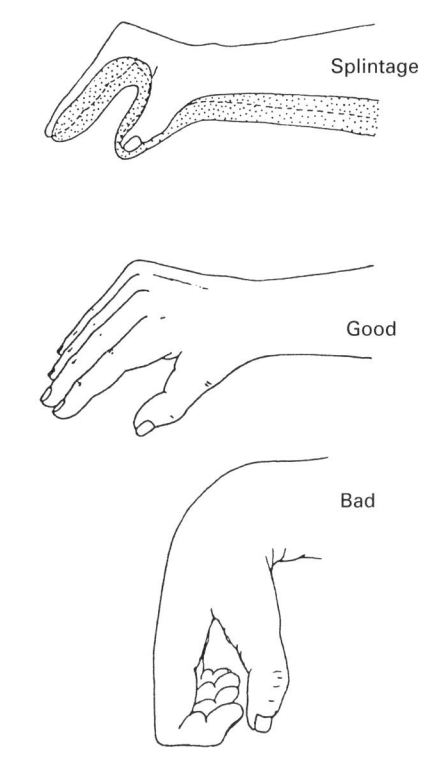

Figure 12.4 Position of splintage burns: position of immobilisation with the metacarpo-phalangeal joints flexed to 90° and the interphalangeal joints straight. **Good:** The metacarpo-phalangeal joints are flexed to 135° and the interphalangeal joints are straight. **Bad:** The metacarpo-phalangeal joints are straight and the interphalangeal joints are flexed.

well enough. Do the same for any hand burn which is not fully healed with a full range of motion 3 weeks after the injury. The hands are one site where early excision and grafting of deep dermal and full-thickness burns is strongly indicated.

Blood transfusion

Burns patients do not need emergency transfusion within 24 h of admission unless they are bleeding from some other injury or have an escharotomy which bleeds heavily. During the second 24 h after injury, blood should be given to any patient who has a full-thickness burn involving more than 10% of body surface area.

The amount given should be 1% of the patient's estimated total blood volume for every 1% of full-thickness burn, and it should be given instead of the same volume of resuscitation fluid during the second 24 h. Total blood volume can be estimated by the formula 80 ml/kg. For example, a 50 kg patient has a blood volume of 4000 ml. If the same patient has full-thickness burns of 20% they should receive 20% of their blood volume, which is 800 ml.

Burn injury shortens the life of red blood cells, so most patients will gradually develop anaemia. Haemoglobin should be checked once a week at least, and transfusion should ideally be given in large burns if the haemoglobin falls below 10 g/dl. In many developing countries this may prove difficult, but relatives should be asked to donate blood.

Gastrointestinal tract and nutrition

The two most important gastrointestinal complications of large burns during the first few days are *acute peptic ulcers* (Curling's ulcers), which may bleed or perforate, and *paralytic ileus*.

Magnesium trisilicate (15 ml 2 hourly for adults either by mouth or via a nasogastric tube), or cimetidine (400 mg b.d. oral or i.v.), or sucralfate, should be given to prevent stress ulceration in regions where this is a common complication.

Paralytic ileus may occur during the resuscitation phase and is treated by continuing intravenous fluids, making sure that serum electrolytes are normal, drainage by nasogastric tube, and waiting for the bowels to start working. Even if a nasogastric tube is used for drainage, antacids can still be given. A paralytic ileus occurring after the resuscitation phase is often associated with infection, and has a bad prognosis.

Patients with burns need a high-calorie, high-protein diet, either by mouth or by nasogastric tube. If the patient is able to drink or eat during the resuscitation phase this should be allowed providing vomiting does not occur, but it is rare for a patient to want to eat at this stage, and dextrose in the intravenous solution as described earlier will suffice. **Breast feeding should continue** if possible from the time of admission. If necessary give expressed breast milk via a nasogastric tube.

Feeding should be started 2 or 3 days after injury at the latest, provided bowel sounds are present and there is no abdominal distension. If oral intake is inadequate, then nasogastric feeding must be used, beginning with quarter-strength feeds and building up to full-strength feeds and a full calorie and protein intake over the next 4 or 5 days. Patients with large burns rarely take enough food by mouth, and in general **it is best to use nasogastric feeding as a routine.**

Adults and children have different nutritional requirements. Adults require an intake of calories and protein greater than normal, and while it used to be thought that the same was true of children, more recent evidence suggests it is better to give children an intake similar to that of a normal healthy child of the same weight. Excessive feeding in children may cause impaired glucose tolerance, fatty degeneration of the liver, and uraemia.

Guidelines for calculating nutritional requirements are shown in Table 12.3, together with examples. Monitoring of nutrition, complications, and their treatment are described in the section 'Monitoring and further treatment', below.

Some recent evidence suggests that it may be possible to start feeding within a few hours of a major burn by placing a feeding tube in the duodenum, meanwhile continuing to drain the stomach, which is more liable to ileus than the more distal parts of the gastrointestinal tract. If this is confirmed it may prove to be an extremely valuable technique in the tropics.

Give supplements of iron, multivitamins, and vitamin C to all burns patients as a routine.

Prevention of infection

Give a course of **anti-tetanus toxoid** to all burns patients unless you are sure they are already immunised.

Prevention of infection of the burn wound is discussed in the section on treatment of the burn wound. The routine use of antibiotics does not prevent infection and they should not be given at any time unless there is clinical evidence of infection.

Physiotherapy

The importance of chest physiotherapy is described in the sections on respiratory burns and infections.

Burns in the region of any joint, especially the hands, can cause permanent deformity and disability. The best way of preventing this is to keep the part mobile by active and passive exercises, starting at the time of admission. It is very important that the patient has proper analgesia for this. Anybody can do these exercises with the patient, although a trained physiotherapist is best.

When physiotherapy is not working and there is loss of movement, especially if a limb is being held flexed, splint the joint. Splint all joints straight, except the shoulder, which should be abducted, and the hand, which should be in the position

Table 12.3 Daily nutritional requirements in burns

	Energy (kcal)	Protein (g)
Adults	(25 × wt in kg) + (40 × % burn)	(wt in kg) + (3 × % burn)
Children		
Age 1	120 per kg	3 per kg
4	100 per kg	2.5 per kg
11	70 per kg	2 per kg

Energy values

   Protein   = 4 kcal per g;
   Carbohydrate = 4 kcal per g;
   Fat   = 9 kcal per g.

For all age groups give 40–50% of non-protein calories as fat and 50–60% as carbohydrate.

Examples

1. Adult weighing 50 kg with a 20% burn
    Energy requirement = (25 × 50) + (40 × 20) = 2050 kcal
    Protein requirement = 50 + (3 × 20) = 110 g

    110 g protein   = 4 × 110   = 440 kcal
    Non-protein calories   = 2050 – 440 = 1610 kcal
    50% of 1610 kcal   = 805 kcal
    Fat required   = 805/9   = 89 g
    Carbohydrate required = 805/4   = 201 g

    Approx. daily requirement = Protein 110 g
                                       Carbohydrate 200 g
                                       Fat 90 g

2. Child age 5, weight 15 kg, with 20% burn

    Energy requirement = 100 × 15 = 1500 kcal
    Protein requirement = 2.5 × 15 = 37.5 g

    37.5 g protein   = 4 × 37.5   = 150 kcal
    Non-protein calories   = 1500 – 150 = 1350 kcal
    50% of 1350 kcal   = 675 kcal
    Fat required   = 675/9   = 75 g
    Carbohydrate required = 675/4   = 169 g

    Approximate daily requirement = Protein 38 g
                                              Carbohydrate 170 g
                                              Fat 75 g

shown in Figure 12.4, and the ankle which should be at 90°. Splintage will often require dressing of the part involved to prevent friction between the splint and the wound.

Monitoring and further treatment

Simple clinical observations, made frequently and accurately, are usually all that is required to guide good management of the resuscitation phase. The same is true for management of the recovery phase (from 48 h until the burn is fully healed), although certain laboratory investigations such as regular haemoglobin measurements are very useful during this period.

Observations and recordings

The observations and recordings which should be made hourly during the resuscitation phase by nursing staff are listed in Table 12.4. Medical staff should also make a general examination as often as possible, paying special attention to the state of the circulation, the chest, and the abdomen.

During the recovery phase all the same observations should be made, but less frequently. The emphasis during ward rounds should be on correct treatment of the burn wound, prevention of contractures, nutritional intake, and prompt investigation and treatment of any sign of infection (see below). Any areas which have not healed after 3 weeks must be grafted as soon as possible.

Accurate observation is very important. Pulse, respiration and temperature are frequently abnormal, even in patients whose condition and progress is perfectly satisfactory and uncomplicated, especially during the first few days. **Rapid changes in observations mean that something is wrong.** Accurate observation is the only way to notice these changes early.

Analgesia

Complete pain relief is important at all times. During the resuscitation phase and any other time of critical illness, the best method is to give diluted intravenous opiates by slow injection until the patient is comfortable, then maintaining analgesia either with a continuous infusion or with frequent small intravenous boluses (pethidine 1 mg/kg bolus, then 0.1–0.2 mg/kg/h). Do not set limits on either the dose or on frequency; the amount of analgesic required is the amount needed to keep the patient comfortable. Continue this for as long as the patient needs it; there is little danger of overdose or addiction.

Monitoring resuscitation (Table 12.5)

The object of resuscitation is to maintain an adequate volume of circulat-

Table 12.4 Monitoring of patients with burns

Observations to be made **hourly** during resuscitation and any other phase of critical illness

Is the patient in pain?

Pulse

Respiration

Temperature

Blood pressure (if sites of wounds and/or dressings permit)

Conscious level (use Glasgow Coma Scale)

Fluid balance
  Input – intravenous, oral, nasogastric
  Output – urine, vomit, nasogastric, stool (esp. diarrhoea)

(Food intake – calculate and record daily)

Table 12.5 Signs of adequate resuscitation

Urine volume	> 1 ml/kg/h
Temperature	Skin warm Core/skin temperature difference few degrees
Pulse	Not more than 25% above normal
Respiration	Not more than 25% above normal
Blood pressure	Normal NB: Low BP means significant hypovolaemia (or pain)
Conscious level	Normal Easily roused if asleep

ing blood. The signs of adequate resuscitation are summarised in Table 12.5.

Urine output is an important guide to fluid therapy, firstly because adequate perfusion of the kidneys means that other vital tissues are being adequately perfused, and secondly because renal failure must be prevented. A useful rule is that 1 ml urine per kilogram body weight per hour is satisfactory.

Insufficient urine nearly always means insufficient fluid, and will respond to an increased drip rate. If the hourly urine output falls below the desired rate, increase the drip rate by the same volume as the shortfall in hourly urine. **Never** give diuretics as the first treatment of a low urine output.

If the patient is up to date with the planned fluid regimen but is still only producing a few ml of urine per hour (*oliguria*), give a *bolus* of one hour's fluid and then continue the infusion at a rate increased by the same amount as described above, provided the patient is not showing any signs of fluid overload. Note that no urine at all is most likely to be due to a blocked catheter. If the patient has clinical signs of fluid overload, insert a central venous catheter and treat as below.

If the patient still does not produce urine, insert a central venous line (see practical procedure, p. 379) and measure **central venous pressure.** If CVP is low, give fluid rapidly until it is only just normal (at the lower end of the normal range). If the urine output does not then increase, treat as described on p. 92. **Acute renal failure** is a serious complication of burn shock and its management is described on pp. 91–96.

Monitoring nutrition

The patient should be weighed regularly and accurately, at least once a week, until the wound is fully healed. Note that the patient will gain weight during the first 2 days because extra fluid is being given and leaking into the tissues, so the baseline weight should be measured as soon as possible after admission, as soon as analgesia has been given and a drip started.

KEY POINT
Weight loss should never be allowed to exceed 10% of admission weight, and should preferably be less than this.

The main problems with feeding, particularly via the nasogastric route, are diarrhoea and vomiting. These should be managed by temporarily decreasing the amount and concentration of feeds, or spreading daily feeds over a longer period. Try to avoid stopping feeding. If these measures fail, diarrhoea can sometimes be controlled by giving codeine phosphate orally or via the feeding tube.

Blood urea and electrolytes should be checked twice a week if the patient is progressing satisfactorily, and daily or more often if the patient is critically ill. Blood glucose should be measured at least daily during feeding using stick tests, and abnormal results confirmed by the laboratory.

If more carbohydrate is given than the patient can metabolise, blood glucose will rise. This should respond to a moderate decrease in the amount of carbohydrate in the diet. Occasionally burns or other major injuries can precipitate diabetes in susceptible patients, which may require treatment with insulin.

Total parenteral nutrition, if available, is occasionally required if ileus continues for more than 2 or 3 days after the resuscitation phase, or is present for more than a few days at any other stage.

Infection – diagnosis and treatment

Infection is the most likely reason for the patient to become critically ill during the recovery phase. After the burn wound itself, the respiratory tract is the commonest site of infection. Any other tissue in the body may also become infected. The investigation, diagnosis and treatment of respiratory and other infections are no different for burns patients than for others, but infections of the burn wound itself have a number of difficulties with respect to diagnosis and treatment.

The general signs of infection

These are changes in one or more of the regular observations, such as a change in temperature, pulse rate, respiratory rate, or conscious level. Children particularly may get gastrointestinal problems such as not eating, diarrhoea, and vomiting without apparent direct relation to the site of infection.

Rapid and large changes are the most significant, but any change should be treated with suspicion. Temperature is a useful example. Very commonly it is elevated during the first few days after a burn, and gradually decreases to normal. As long as the patient is otherwise well this temperature is not of concern, but a departure from the pattern, such as a rapid large rise (or fall) in temperature, or other evidence of infection, is an indication for action.

There may be signs of infection in the lungs or elsewhere, which must be investigated and treated, but always **suspect the burn wound**. Bacteria are nearly always found on the surface of burn wounds. They cause illness when they invade the living tissue beneath the burn wound. This invasion may be accompanied by death of the living tissue and conversion of the wound to a deeper one (for example from partial to full thickness), a sign which is pathognomonic of invasive burn infection, but invasive infection can occur in the presence of a clean, healthy-looking wound. The appearance of conversion to a full-thickness wound is that of enlarging single or multiple patches of dark-red, brown or black.

Diagnosis of the site and nature of infection

This is by clinical examination and laboratory investigations. Include a chest X-ray and microbiological culture of specimens of blood (which should also be examined for malarial parasites), urine (especially if the patient is or has been catheterised), and any other possible source or site of infection such as intravenous catheter tips. Other investigations, such as lumbar puncture, are performed if indicated clinically.

One difficulty with respect to infected burn wounds is that the results of surface culture are not a totally reliable guide to the nature of the infection and hence to antibiotic treatment. One reason is that different organisms may be present on different parts of the wound, and culture results depend on where samples are taken from and how many are taken. Secondly, the organisms invading the wound and causing infection may be different from those obtained by surface culture. Blood culture, if positive, is reliable.

The general treatment of burn infection

This consists of intravenous fluids and intravenous antibiotics, and blood transfusion may be beneficial, especially if haemoglobin is below normal, and if fresh blood is used. Appropriate antibiotics to use before a bacteriological diagnosis has been obtained should cover staphylococci, streptococci, and Gram negatives such as *E. coli* and *Pseudomonas*. A suitable combination would therefore be gentamicin and cloxacillin, but any bacteria which have already been cultured from the wound should also be covered.

It is often found that burns seem to render patients liable to attacks of malaria. It is always reasonable to try as hard as possible to diagnose malaria in any burns patient who becomes ill and to give antimalarial treatment if indicated.

The therapeutic difficulty with infected burn wounds is that they may cover a large area and represent a very large mass of infected tissue, within which bacteria cannot be reached by parenterally administered drugs. This problem can be approached by one or a combination of methods of local treatment:

1. Topical antibacterial agents can also be applied; most however will not penetrate the eschar and reach the organisms. Mafenide (Sulfamylon), if available, will penetrate and is a useful treatment.
2. The infected wound can be excised at operation. This procedure may be limited by bleeding requiring blood transfusion, when blood is in short supply. The wound should be excised, including underlying fat down to the level of the deep fascia, using a scalpel. If the wound is on a limb, use a tourniquet. If no blood is available, there is one type of wound which can still be usefully treated: sometimes there is a hard eschar with pus underneath it – this will be easy and the whole eschar can be excised with little bleeding. The wet necrotic slough underneath cannot be excised without bleeding, but simply removing the hard eschar may have a beneficial effect similar to draining an abscess.
3. Antibiotics, diluted and infiltrated under the eschar in the area believed to be infected, can limit extension of the infection. Potentially toxic substances such as gentamicin should not be used.

Conclusions

Burns are an important cause of surgical pathology and mortality in the tropics and the main indications for admission to a critical care area are for management of fluid therapy and respiratory injuries in the immediate post-injury period, and later for the treatment of life-threatening complications, which are nearly all infections.

At all stages there is a need for prevention. Firstly the prevention of the injury itself, programmes for which do not at present exist in most countries. Secondly for prevention of infection, and thirdly for prevention of deformity and disability by physiotherapy, splintage, and skin grafting in good time.

While a substantial number of patients die from very large burns, either from burns shock or from rapidly supervening and overwhelming infection, a large number, particularly paediatric patients, die from the infective complications of much smaller and often partial thickness wounds. A reliable means of preventing this in the tropics remains to be found.

> **KEY POINT**
>
> The most likely ways of decreasing the mortality of burns are prevention of infection and careful attention to nutrition. Complete records should be kept and analysed to establish whether these measures work in your institution.

Further reading

Website for McComb Foundation which supports burns projects in SE Asia http://www.mccomb.org.au

Websites for burn associations often with useful and free links. News of meetings and of EMSB courses.
www.anzba.org.au
www.bba.co.uk
www.journalofburns.com

General articles

ARORA S, ANTIA NH. Treatment of burns in a district hospital. *Burns* 1977;4,49–51; and *SDMH Journal* 1982;6:89–95.
ARTZ CP, MONCREIF JA, PRUITT BA. *Burns: A team approach*. Philadelphia: Saunders, 1979.
MCGREGOR JC, GEORGANTOPOULU A. Retrospective analysis of the Bangour Burn Unit. *J R Coll Surg Edinb* 1992;37:381–4.
MUGUTI GI et al. A review of burns treated over a one year period at Mpilo Central Hospital, Zimbabwe. *J R Coll Surg Edinb* 1994;39:214–7.
OLABANJI JK, OGINNI FO, BANKOLE JO, OLASINDE AA. A Ten-Year Review of Burn Cases Seen in a Nigerian Teaching Hospital. *J Burns Surg Wound Care* 2003;1 www.journalofburns.com
RAMZY PI, BARRET JP, HERNDON DN. Thermal injury. *Crit Care Clin* 1999;333–52.
SOWEMIMO GO. Burn care in Africa: reducing the misery index: the 1993 Everett Idris Evans Memorial Lecture. *J Burn Care Rehabil* 1993;589–94.

Inhalational burns

LANGFORD RM, ARMSTRONG RF. Algorithm for managing injury from smoke inhalation. *BMJ* 1989;299:902–5.
LUND T, GOODWIN CW, MCMANUS WF et al. Upper airway sequelae in burn patients requiring endotracheal intubation or tracheostomy. *Ann Surg* 1985;201:374–82.
PAPINI RP, WOOD FM. Current concepts in the management of burns with inhalational injury. *Care Crit Ill* 1999;20:61–6.
PAUL S, BUENO R. The burned trachea. *Chest Surg Clin N Am* 2003;13:343–8.
RABINOWITZ PM, SIEGEL MD. Acute inhalational injury. *Clin Chest Med* 2002;23: 707–15.

Early management and resuscitation

FRAME JD, KELLY DA, CLARKE J. Early and late management of burns. *Surgery* (The Medicine Group) 1992;109–19 (two articles).
GRAVES TA, CIOFFI WG, MCMANUS WF et al. Fluid resuscitation of infants and children with massive thermal injury. *J Trauma* 1988;28:1656–9.
KRAMER GC et al. Oral and Enteral Resuscitation of Burn Shock: the historical record and implications for mass casualty care. www.journalofburns.com Volume 1.
STONE CA, PAPE SA. Evolution of the Emergency Management of Severe Burns (EMSB) course in the UK. *Burns* 1999; 25:262–4.
YOWLER CJ, FRATIANNE RB. Current status of burn resuscitation. *Clin Plast Surg* 2000; 27:1–10.

Metabolic issues

ALEXANDER JW, MACMILLAN BG et al. Beneficial effects of aggressive protein feeding in severely burned children. *Ann Surg* 1980;192:505–17.

DEMLING RH, SEIGNE P. Metabolic management of patients with severe burns. *World J Surg* 2000;24:673–80.

GALLAGHER G, RAE CP, KINSELLA J. Treatment of pain in severe burns. *Am J Clin Dermatol* 2000;1:329–35.

HALEBIAN P, ROBINSON N, BARIE P et al. Whole body oxygen utilization during carbon monoxide poisoning and isocapneic nitrogen hypoxia. *J Trauma* 1986;26:110–7.

Infection

EDWARDS-JONES V, GREENWOOD JE. What's new in burn microbiology? James Laing Memorial Prize Essay 2000. *Burns* 2003;29:15–24.

PRUITT BA. The diagnosis and treatment of infection in a burn patient. *Burns* 1984;11:79–91.

Symposium on Infection Control in Burns. *J Hosp Infect* 6(SupplB) 1985.

The burn wound

DING YL, HAN CM. Recent advances in burn wound management in China. *Acta Chir Plast* 1989;31(2):84–91.

WALLACE AB. The exposure treatment of burns. *Lancet* 1951;1:501.

Burned hands

GIBRAN NS, HEMIBACH DM. Current status of burn wound physiology. *Clin Plast Surg* 2000;27:11–22.

LUCE EA. The acute and subacute management of the burned hand. *Clin Plast Surg* 2000;27:49–63.

MAHLER D, HIRSHOWITZ B. Tangential excision and grafting for burns of the hand. *Br J Plast Surg* 1975;28:189–92.

TILLEY W, MCMAHON S, SHUKALAK B. Rehabilitation of the burned upper extremity. *Hand Clin* 2000;16:303–18.

Unusual burns

KOUMBOURLIS AC. Electrical injuries. *Crit Care Med* 2002;30:S424–30.

MOZING DW, SMITH AA, MCMANUS WF et al. Chemical burns. *J Trauma* 1988;28:642–7.

GHISLAIN PD, ROUJEAU JC. Treatment of severe drug reactions: Stevens–Johnson syndrome, toxic epidermal necrolysis and hypersensitivity syndrome. *Dermatol Online J* 2002;8:5.

STRATTA RJ, SAFFLE JR, KRAVITZ M et al. Management of tar and asphalt injuries. *Am J Surg* 1983;146:766–9.

AMY BW, MCMANUS WF, GOODWIN CW, PRUITT BA. Lightning injury with survival in five patients. *JAMA* 1985;253:243–5.

13
Perioperative care

This chapter describes the preoperative preparation for surgery and anaesthesia, recovery of the patient who has just been operated on and the principles of postoperative care. Incorrect perioperative care may cause critical illness, transforming a straightforward safe situation into a life-threatening one. About 40% of critically ill patients require surgical treatment, so that good understanding of perioperative care is essential.

Preoperative care

Anaesthesia and surgery stress patients, particularly those suffering from cardiovascular, respiratory, renal or metabolic disease. Anaesthesia causes changes in cardiac output, blood pressure and respiratory depression. Major surgery may be accompanied by bleeding or significant fluid loss. Careful preoperative preparation of the patient gives him the best chance of successful surgery.

The time available to prepare a patient will vary from a few minutes, in an emergency such as a ruptured ectopic, to several days for an elective case. In all cases a history and examination should be carried out, appropriate investigations ordered (Table 13.1), and blood cross-matched if necessary. Unexpected problems detected preoperatively may delay surgery to allow investigation and treatment. Occasionally elective cases are cancelled by the anaesthetist in theatre. In Lusaka this is most commonly due to uncontrolled hypertension, anaemia or lack of cross-matched blood. When a patient is cancelled at this stage everyone's time is wasted, particularly the patient's.

Neurological problems
Depressed conscious level

Determine the conscious level using the Glasgow Coma Scale. Establish the cause, e.g. head injury, and correct any reversible factors. Postoperatively the conscious level may be depressed by anaesthesia and the patient may be unable to maintain his own airway.

Epilepsy

Treatment should be continued over the operative period. Certain anaesthetic drugs, e.g. methohexitone, enflurane, should be avoided.

Head injury

Raised intracranial pressure (see p. 178) should be treated with mannitol (200 ml 20% over 15 min or 0.25–0.5 g/kg in a child) during transfer to theatre for burr holes. Hypercarbia or hypoxia raise intracranial pressure and must be avoided. Postoperative ventilation may be indicated. Around 30% of head injuries have other major injuries, which can complicate anaesthesia.

Table 13.1 Preoperative checklist

History	
Current illness	Relevant details; if an emergency, last oral intake
Previous illness	Any serious illnesses, particularly previous operations, anaemia, asthma or other respiratory disease, cardiac, rheumatic fever, bleeding tendencies, hypertension, diabetes, renal, jaundice, epilepsy
General condition	Exercise tolerance, dyspnoea, angina, peripheral oedema, palpitations, fainting episodes, orthopnoea, productive cough, wheezing, dyspepsia with reflux, urinary symptoms, current pregnancy, smoking, alcohol intake
Drug history	Previous anaesthetic problems, drug allergies, current drug therapy
Examination	
General	Teeth, mouth opening, neck mobility, anaemia, jaundice, cyanosis, clubbing, nutrition, hydration, pyrexia
Specific	Conscious level, pulse, BP, heart sounds, respiration, abdomen
Laboratory	
Haemoglobin	Major cases, clinically anaemic patients, where peroperative blood transfusion likely
Coagulation	History of abnormal bleeding. Jaundiced patients – prothrombin time
Electrophoresis	Anaemic children, suspected sicklers
Sickledex	Suspected sicklers
U & E	Patients on diuretics, hypertensives, renal disease, peritonitis, bowel obstruction, severe vomiting or diarrhoea
LFTs	History of liver abnormality
ECG	Heart disease, arrhythmias, cardiac failure, hypertension
Chest X-ray	Heart failure, significant respiratory illness
Respiratory tests, e.g. peak flow	Asthmatics, chronic chest problems
Blood gases	Severe respiratory disease

Cardiovascular problems

Patients most at risk are those with cardiac failure, ischaemic heart disease, valvular heart disease and those with arrhythmias (especially ventricular).

Cardiac failure

This should be controlled following the guidelines on p. 52. Patients who have ischaemic heart disease should be medically treated to control angina. Always try to postpone patients for 6 months after an infarct (this reduces the chances of perioperative reinfarction). Arrhythmias should be diagnosed if possible on an ECG. Control atrial fibrillation by digitalisation until the apex beat is below 100/min. Check serum postassium in patients on digoxin and diuretics to ensure there is no hypokalaemia.

Reducing postoperative risk of myocardial infarction

To reduce the risk of postoperative myocardial infarction in patients who have cardiac disease it is important to reduce myocardial oxygen consumption. This is achieved by reducing heart work, though not at the expense of inducing cardiac failure. The aim is to minimise pain, shivering, reduce the heart rate (preoperative and perioperative beta-blockers such as propranolol) and afterload. Hypotension and hypoxaemia should be avoided and in certain circumstances inotropes should be used to improve myocardial contractility. The decision making is facilitated by use of cardiovascular system technology to monitor blood, central venous and pulmonary capillary wedge pressures.

Hypertension

Untreated, this may result in exaggerated swings in blood pressure during the perioperative period and so should be well controlled for a few days before operation. Aim to reduce the blood pressures to 160/100 mmHg. Uncontrolled blood pressure may cause cerebral haemorrhage, cardiac ischaemia or cardiac failure. Episodes of low pressure may cause an impaired cerebral or cardiac blood flow. Antihypertensive drugs should be given in the morning of operation and continued postoperatively. Avoid hypotension (e.g. shock) by maintaining circulating volume.

Uncontrolled hypertensives requiring emergency surgery: pain and anxiety should be relieved (opiate ± diazepam) and severe hypertension controlled with a parenteral drug such as hydralazine. A beta-blocker may be indicated if there is associated tachycardia provided that there is no history of asthma or cardiac failure. (*Note:* A systolic blood pressure of 100 mmHg may represent shock in a hypertensive patient.)

Murmurs

These are due to turbulent blood flow. In pregnancy or severe anaemia a systolic flow murmur may be heard owing to a high cardiac output. Providing that the cardiovascular system is otherwise normal, and the patient has a reasonable exercise tolerance, anaesthesia and surgery are likely to be safe. Diastolic murmurs or abnormal systolic murmurs (loud or accompanied by a thrill, or alteration in the heart sounds) are signs of underlying heart disease and should be fully assessed before elective surgery. Monitor the patient carefully during surgery. Patients at risk of endocarditis should be given suitable antibiotic prophylaxis.

Hypovolaemic shock

Restore blood volume before theatre and monitor urine output with a catheter during and after surgery (see p. 26).

> **KEYPOINT**
>
> Patients with shock, hypertension or cardiac disease should be catheterised during major surgery.

Anticoagulant therapy

Warfarin should be discontinued 5 days before surgery to allow the prothrombin time to return to around one and a half times normal. Heparin (s.c.) can be given to patients at high risk of embolisation (e.g. prosthetic valves). If there is liver disease or jaundice give i.v. vitamin K 10 mg and check prothrombin time before surgery. In an emergency 1 or 2 units of fresh frozen plasma will replace the deficient clotting factors. Heparin may be reversed with protamine given slowly i.v. (1 mg for every 100 units of heparin given in the last 4 h). The half-life of heparin is 4–6 h so that there is little risk of bleeding if surgery can be delayed for 6 h after discontinuing heparin.

Thromboembolism

Patients at risk of deep-vein thrombosis and pulmonary embolism include those with a history of venous thrombosis, obesity, major or pelvic surgery, prolonged inactivity, use of oral contraceptives, pregnancy, old age, cardiorespiratory disease, sepsis and cancer. There are a number of different methods designed to reduce the incidence of what may be a fatal complication:

1. Anti-thromboembolism elastic stockings (graded compression by the stockings up the calf).
2. Subcutaneous heparin 5000 units subcutaneously started with the premedication (or earlier if the patient is

bedridden) and continued postoperatively 8 or 12 hourly hourly until the patient is ambulant. Recently, 20–40 mg of low-molecular-weight heparin once daily has been introduced as an alternative. The combination of subcutaneous heparin and anti-thromboembolism graded compression stockings seems particularly effective.
3. Dextran 70 500 ml perioperatively and 500 ml daily until ambulant.

The management of deep-vein thrombosis is described on p. 262.

Anaemia

Anaesthesia is more of a risk if the haemoglobin (Hb) is below 8 g/dl because of reduced oxygen-carrying capacity. Reductions in cardiac output will reduce tissue oxygenation, and excessive fluids are prone to cause cardiac failure because the heart is already stressed. In patients with ischaemic heart disease a Hb of 10 g/dl is safer.

Patients who are chronically anaemic (Hb 6–8 g/dl) cope well with minor surgery, as they develop compensatory mechanisms such as better oxygen delivery to the tissues due to haemoglobin releasing oxygen more readily at tissue level (oxygen dissociation curve shifts to the right) and an increased cardiac output. Patients with acute haemorrage take a few days to compensate fully and are therefore at greater risk from anaesthesia. Where possible postpone surgery until the Hb is above 8 g/dl. If preoperative transfusion is required, do this at least 24 h in advance (consider covering with furosemide). Avoid surgery in patients with Hb less than 8 g/dl unless life-saving. Local anaesthesia is generally safe; where general anaesthesia is used give oxygen postoperatively and avoid fluid overload.

Sickle cell disease

Avoid cold, dehydration, tourniquets and hypoxia which can trigger haemolysis and precipitate a crisis (p. 38). In major surgery consider transfusion to raise the Hb to greater than 8 g/dl resulting in a Hb A 50% of the total Hb.

Further reading

DANZER BI, BIRNBACH DJ, THYS DM. Anesthesia for the parturient with sickle cell disease. *J Clin Anesth* 1996;8:598–602.

DIX HM. New advances in the treatment of sickle cell disease: focus on perioperative significance. *AANA J* 2001;69:281–6.

VICHINSKY EP, NEUMAYR LD, HABERKERN C, *et al*. The perioperative complication rate of orthopedic surgery in sickle cell disease: report of the National Sickle Cell Surgery Study Group. *Am J Hematol* 1999;62:129–38.

Respiratory disease

Assess exercise tolerance, cough, sputum production, wheeze and cyanosis; investigate as shown in Table 13.1. In the immediate postoperative period the patient may breathe inadequately (especially after thoracotomy and laparotomy) due to pain, muscle spasm, drug depression and deranged lung physiology. During surgery, secretions will gather in the bronchial tree. Increase the frequency of suction and physiotherapy postoperatively to clear these secretions. If the patient has recently been in respiratory failure, or is at significant risk of failure, postoperative ventilatory support may be indicated. In those patients receiving oxygen therapy it should be continued during transfer to and from theatre. Local anaesthesia or spinals have little effect on respiratory function and may be preferred if the patient can lie flat.

Asthma

This should be controlled before surgery. In all asthmatics give two puffs of a salbutamol inhaler either with the premedication or immediately before induction in the anaesthetic room. Continue the patient's normal medication perioperatively. Patients on oral steroids benefit from 100 mg of hydrocortisone i.v. at induction. This should be continued until the patient is able to take his oral medication again. Treat bronchospasm in symptomatic asthmatics undergoing emergency surgery before induction but do not give intravenous aminophylline if the patient is already taking it orally. Ketamine, halothane and ether are bronchodilators and safe in asthma.

EXAMPLE
A 45-year-old lady was ventilated for 10 days following a flail segment caused in a road traffic accident. Two days after being weaned from the ventilator she went to theatre to have a fractured femur internally fixed. The anaesthetist gave a spontaneous breathing anaesthetic without major problems and left her in the recovery room breathing room air. Shortly after she become cyanosed and had a cardiac arrest.

LESSON Patients who have poor respiratory function require careful anaesthesia and recovery. Good oxygenation at all times must be maintained; this lady arrested in recovery from hypoxia.

Jaundice

This predisposes to postoperative renal failure (hepatorenal syndrome). Renal failure is more common in dehydrated patients, so that intravenous fluids should be administered 12 h before theatre to prevent dehydration. The use of mannitol to promote a diuresis during and after surgery is thought to be beneficial. All patients should be catheterised and mannitol (150–200 ml of 20%) can be given if urine output falls below 0.5–1 ml/kg/h. A CVP line will help guide fluid replacement if the patient becomes oliguric.

Patients with jaundice are also more likely to bleed due to deficient clotting factors. Always give vitamin K (10 mg daily) for at least 3 days before elective surgery and check the clotting time or prothrombin index in all jaundiced patients.

Renal failure

Patients may be anaemic, hypertensive, acidotic or hyperkalaemic. Anaemia is well tolerated and most can safely be operated on providing their Hb is above 6 g/dl, and blood loss is replaced with blood. Patients on dialysis should be in fluid balance before operation, and hyperkalaemia corrected to 5.5 mmol/l or below (see p. 85 for the emergency management of hyperkalaemia). Since salt and water excretion is impaired, do not administer excessive i.v. fluids. Patients who pass low volumes of poor-quality, dilute urine may suffer further renal damage when dehydrated. Maintain patients' normal fluid intake and replace surgical losses with appropriate fluids. Maintaining fluid balance is difficult; consider monitoring central venous pressure. Also monitor serum K^+ and urea. Certain drugs such as gentamicin are potentially toxic to the kidney and their dosage needs to be reduced.

Diabetes

See pp. 107–110.

Emergency surgery

This has a higher mortality than elective surgery. The time available for preparation is limited; concentrate on diagnosis, investigation and resuscitation, which may be life-saving. Aim for a normal circulating blood volume, and normal urea and electrolytes. If there is difficulty in assessing the blood volume or the cardiac function in a hypotensive patient, then a central venous pressure (CVP) line should be inserted (see practical procedure, p. 382). Any patient who is shocked should be catheterised to measure urine output hourly. Occasionally patients may have to be anaesthetised before they have been fully resuscitated. For example, a patient with a ruptured spleen may need an urgent laparotomy to stop the bleeding and it may not be possible to restore his blood pressure to normal before surgery. In contrast, there is no excuse for a patient with bowel obstruction going to theatre with a low BP.

Respiratory distress should be managed as described on pp. 6–9. Emergency cases often have a paralytic ileus or full stomach which makes the induction of general anaesthesia dangerous because of the risk of regurgitation and aspiration. Patients at risk should have a nasogastric tube passed and the stomach contents aspirated and be left on free drainage. Stop tube feeds at least 6 h preoperatively. Patients who have had intestinal obstruction for several days may be severely dehydrated and hypokalaemic. If the K^+ is <3.0 mmol/l, an attempt should be made to correct this before operation. Anaesthesia in patients with K^+ <2.5 mmol/l is risky, and should only be done in an emergency.

KEYPOINT
A nasogastric tube in the stomach does not guarantee the stomach is empty.

Traumatised patients need careful handling of fractured limbs and it is wise to have plenty of people to help with the lifting. If there is any danger of there being a fractured cervical spine, then stabilise the neck (pp. 202–5). A senior person should supervise the lifting personally. Patients with fractured ribs should have an intercostal drain inserted (see p. 205) to prevent a tension pneumothorax developing under anaesthesia.

Postoperative recovery from anaesthesia

During an operation the patient is closely observed by the anaesthetist and following surgery the patient should be transferred to a specially equipped recovery area (Figure 13.1). The immediate recovery from anaesthesia should be supervised by a trained nurse until the patient is ready to return to the ward. Table 13.2 shows the checks that should be made in recovery and some of the problems that can arise.

KEYPOINT
Check recovery equipment daily.

The nurse should check what sort of anaesthesia and surgery the patient has had and whether the anaesthetist has any special instructions. The patient should be nursed on his side or three-quarters prone unless there are contraindications to this position, e.g. a fractured cervical spine. The aim is to prevent aspiration of secretions or vomit, and to maintain the airway by causing the tongue to fall forwards rather than backwards. An oropharyngeal (Guedel) airway may also help. Until the patient is awake, observe for obstruction (listen) and adequacy of breathing (colour of tongue, chest movements, auscultation). Measure the pulse and BP regularly. If the patient vomits or is at risk of aspiration (for example after ENT surgery), tilt the trolley head down. Most airways can be protected and maintained by these simple methods, though occasionally the anaesthetist may need to reintubate someone whose breathing is inadequate. When there is inadequate breathing, give oxygen and intermittent positive pressure ventilation with an Ambu bag until definitive treatment is decided.

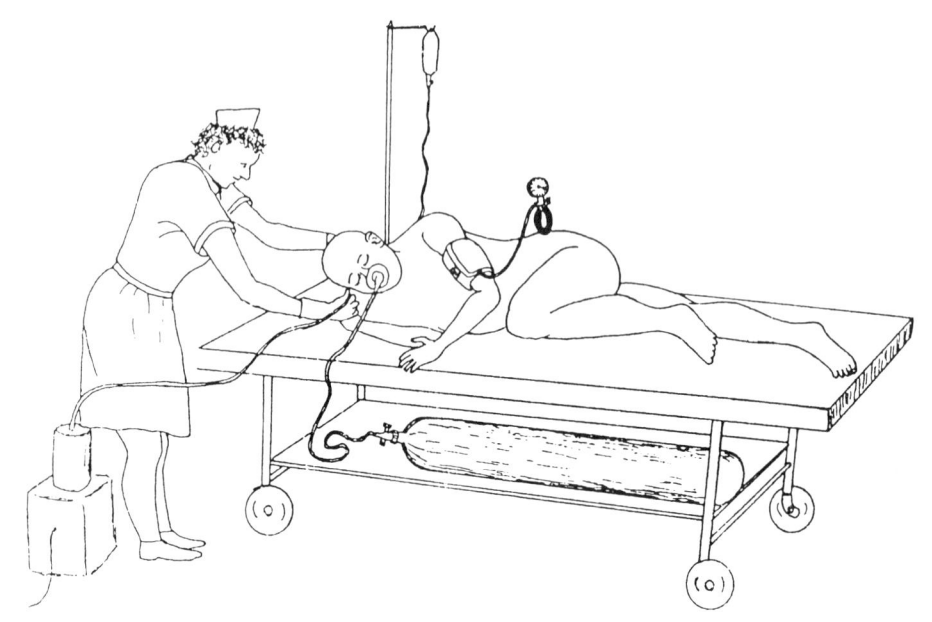

Figure 13.1 Supervision of the postoperative patient during recovery from anaesthesia. Note that the trolley should have sides to prevent the patient falling off.

Laryngospasm is where spasm of the vocal cords prevents breathing. The patient struggles for breath, often making a crowing noise on inspiration. He will quickly become cyanosed. The airway should be rapidly cleared by suction, oxygen administered and the airway supported (if possible without the use of a Guedel airway, which occasionally may stimulate laryngospasm). Most cases settle spontaneously with simple care, but you should send for the anaesthetist as some of these patients require reintubation.

Most patients are *extubated* by the anaesthetist in the operating theatre but patients who are not ready to support their own airway will come to recovery with a laryngeal mask or endotracheal tube in place. Determine what the anaesthetist wishes you to do. Usually the mask or tube can be removed once the patient is awake and has good airway reflexes. If you have been instructed to remove them, keep the patient on his side breathing extra oxygen until he has adequate airway reflexes, then suction the pharynx and remove the tube. If you are not sure what to do with an endotracheal tube, ask for advice because some patients who have had operations on the head and neck may require the tube to be left in position for some hours postoperatively. In such cases explain what is happening to the patient when he wakes up since he will be unable to speak and may be anxious. Do not allow patients to extubate themselves; restrain if necessary.

KEYPOINT
An unconscious patient must never be left unsupervised.

In recovery all patients who have had a general anaesthetic should be given oxygen until they are fully awake. Those who have had major surgery should be given oxygen over the next 2–3 days, as should

Table 13.2 Recovery checklist

Check	Problem	Common causes
1. Position	Airway obstruction	Obstruction, laryngospasm
	Nerve trauma from pressure	
2. Breathing	Noisy	Obstruction, laryngospasm
	Inadequate	Anaesthetic drugs e.g. opiates, muscle relaxants, kinked endotracheal tube, surgical pack in mouth
3. Pulse	Weak	See BP low
	Bradycardia	Hypoxia, anaesthetic drugs, e.g. neostigmine, head injury
	Tachycardia	Hypotension, pain, anaesthetic drugs, e.g. atropine, fever
	Irregular	Arrhythmias – respiratory failure, heart disease, anaesthesia drugs, e.g. halothane
4. BP	Low	Hypovolaemia, cardiac failure, anaesthesia overdose, respiratory failure
	High	Hypertensive disease, pain, respiratory failure, full bladder
5. Conscious level	Prolonged unconsciousness	Anaesthetic overdose, respiratory failure, hypoxia peroperatively, medical problem, e.g. CVA, metabolic, hypoglycaemia (children)
	Restless	Hypoxia, pain, cold, full bladder, muscle relaxant still acting, halothane shivers, painful positioning, ketamine
6. Notes	Instructions	Drugs, fluids, post-op ward care, oxygen

anyone with anaemia or chronic cardio-respiratory disease. Give 4 litres a minute via a face mask or 3 litres a minute via nasal spectacles.

The patient should return to the ward only when the following criteria are satisfied:
1. He is conscious and able to control his airway.
2. He is breathing well with a good colour.
3. Blood pressure and pulse are stable.
4. Muscle power has recovered – test for this by checking that the patient can lift his head off the pillow and hold it off for at least 5 sec.
5. The drip is running and fluids are up to date.
6. The surgeon's post-operative orders are clear and understood.
7. The drugs which were ordered have been given.
8. Pain is adequately controlled.

KEYPOINT
Never send a patient back to the ward until he is fully recovered.

EXAMPLE

A healthy 25-year-old primagravida had an emergency Caesarean section for fetal distress, under general anaesthesia. At the end of the operation she was turned on her side and extubated. In recovery the patient was allowed to slide onto her back and when she vomited shortly afterwards she aspirated. The suction machine would not work and the patient died.

Postoperative recovery from surgery

Patients recovering from major surgery account for 30–40% of patients needing critical care. The aims of postoperative care are:

Table 13.3 Common postoperative surgical problems

First 48 hours	After 48 hours
Hypotension	Bronchopneumonia
Fluid balance	Wound infection
Oliguria	Recurrent sepsis
Atelectasis	Deep-vein thrombosis
	Prolonged paralytic ileus
	Pressure sores

1. support of the circulation and maintainance of major organ function, particularly the lungs, heart and kidney;
2. monitoring for complications;
3. maintaining fluid and electrolyte balance;
4. providing adequate analgesia; and
5. treatment of specific problems.

The common problems in the postoperative period (Table 13.3) can often be prevented by adequate preoperative and immediate postoperative care.

Support of failing systems

The management of respiratory, cardiac and renal failure is discussed in Chapters 1, 3 and 5. Major organ failure in relation to hypovolaemic shock is discussed in Chapter 2.

Monitoring for complications

Monitoring of the postoperative patient includes regular recording of the pulse, blood pressure, respiratory rate, pattern of breathing, colour of the tongue, conscious level, temperature and urine output. These should be recorded every 15 min for the first 2 h, followed by every 30 min for 2 h. Once the patient has been stable for 4 h, hourly monitoring should be sufficient. If the patient is unstable or has major problems then more frequent monitoring may be necessary.

Various investigations may be indicated such as urea and electrolytes, blood glucose, haematocrit and chest X-ray. The choice of investigations will be determined by the original problem or associated medical diseases. For example diabetics undergoing surgery should have the blood glucose and urea and electrolytes checked within an hour or two of the operation. The patient with respiratory impairment would have blood gas analysis or oxygen saturation monitoring if available. The role of investigations for different systems is discussed in the relevant chapters.

Fluid and electrolyte balance

All patients undergoing major surgery must have fluid balance charts on which all fluid input and output is accurately entered. In a patient with normal renal function, urine output should be at least 0.5 ml/kg/h. In the postoperative period failure to pass adequate amounts of urine usually means dehydration and hypovolaemia.

Fluid input must include both maintenance requirements (Table 4.1) and extra fluids to account for losses from nasogastric tubes, drains and fistulae. In calculating the total output 500–1000 ml of insensible loss should be allowed in the adult (12 ml/kg in a child). If the patient is febrile the insensible loss is increased about 12% per 1°C.

Tables 4.1 and 4.2 show the maintenance and electrolyte requirements. As a general rule in the adult give 1 litre of normal saline or Ringer's lactate for every 2 litres 5% dextrose. In babies and neonates it is best to use quarter-strength Darrow's (alternate half-strength Darrow's with 5% dextrose). Table 4.4 shows the electrolyte content of different intravenous fluids.

Gastric and intestinal secretions are rich in sodium and potassium. If gastrointestinal losses are high give extra sodium and potassium. When a patient has over 500 ml of nasogastric aspirate give 2 litres of normal saline or Ringer's lactate for every litre of 5% dextrose and add 3 g potassium chloride to each litre (1 g KCl = 13.5 mmol). The constitutents of various gastrointestinal secretions are shown in Table 4.3.

Oliguria should be managed according to the flow chart in Chapter 5 (p. 92).

Drains

An accurate description of where drains have been placed should be recorded in the operation notes. Those responsible for postoperative care should know which drain is which and record the output from each drain separately. If possible a drainage bag should be used to collect the effluent from a corrugated drain. This enables the output to be recorded and minimises discomfort to the patient from damp dressings and bed linen. Tube drains may be of suction or non-suction type. The output may be collected directly into a bag using appropriate connections in a non-suction drain. With suction drains it is important to check that the suction bottle has been attached correctly so that suction is being effectively applied.

Analgesia

The postoperative patient who is breathing spontaneously is in need of analgesia rather than sedation. This may be provided either by intermittent doses of opiate or by continuous infusion. Intermittent bolus injection may produce periods of oversedation followed by poor analgesia, but is the most widely used and safest option for the general wards. Constant infusion may result in accumulation of the analgesic drug. Pethidine infusions of 0.1–0.4 mg/kg/h often produce good pain relief without respiratory depression provided that the infusion is meticulously controlled and the patient closely observed. Alternative methods include epidural analgesia (epidural bupivacaine + diamorphine or fentamyl or intercostal nerve block (total dose bupivicaine should not exceed 2 mg/kg every 4 h) if the skill to do these has been acquired. Epidural opiates may cause respiratory depression up to 12 h after injection so patients need to be nursed on ICU to monitor the respiratory rate in case of inadequate breathing.

Critically ill patients have increased sensitivity to opiates. Morphine is metabolized by the liver, and its metabolites, which are also active, accumulate in renal failure.

In addition to analgesia, the postoperative patient receiving artificial ventilation may require sedation with diazepam or propofol to make ventilation tolerable without distress. Midazolam is similar to diazepam but with more potent amnesic properties and a short half-life of 2 h so that if it is available it is preferred. The use of sedation and muscle relaxants in ventilated patients is discussed on p. 338.

Treatment of specific problems

When examining a patient after surgery follow the checklist shown in Table 13.4. This will enable you to detect the most important postoperative problems.

The most common important postoperative problems are discussed as follows:
- hypotension;
- the postoperative chest;

Table 13.4 Postoperative checklist

Conscious level	Oral hygiene
Pain	Thirst
Respirations	Gastrointestinal recovery
Rate	Abdominal distension
Depth	Bowel sounds
Pattern	Flatus and stool
Colour of tongue	Urine output
Chest auscultation	Fluid balance
Pulse	Drains
Blood pressure	Legs
Temperature	Wound
Drug therapy	Pressure areas

- the postoperative abdomen and return of gastrointestinal motility;
- wound care;
- pyrexia;
- deep-vein thrombosis.

Hypotension

Examine the patient to determine the cause and take appropriate action according to Table 13.5. Work through the causes listed in Table 13.5 from top to bottom. After excluding hypoxia (which may be rapidly fatal) you will find that inadequate fluid or blood replacement in theatre is the commonest cause. Septicaemia is the next most likely, particularly when there has been a septic focus at surgery (e.g. peritonitis) or instrumentation of the urinary tract.

In hypothermia associated with surgery in critically ill patients, warming the patient will be associated with a reduction in peripheral vasoconstriction. This may result in a further fall in blood pressure and will require volume replacement.

The postoperative chest

Atelectasis means collapse of areas of the lung which then become unavailable for gas exchange. Atelectasis is most common in the first 24–48 h after an operation and may be complicated by pneumonia if not treated aggressively.

The main reasons for atelectasis are:
1. underventilation of the lungs due to pain and abdominal distension;
2. retention of airway secretions during and after anaesthesia.

Prevention of atelectasis in patients breathing spontaneously requires good postoperative analgesia and early chest physiotherapy; the latter includes deep-breathing exercises and coughing. Chest physiotherapy should assist the patient rather than exhausting him (p. 349). Early mobilisation of the patient will also help to minimise atelectasis.

Table 13.5 Causes and management of postoperative low blood pressure

Possible causes	Look for	Action required
1. Hypoxia	Obstructed airway Noisy breathing Cyanosis Inadequate breathing Dyspnoea	Clear airway Correct position Oxygen by mask Ventilatory support Consider diagnosis of aspiration/myocardial infarction/pulmonary embolus
2. Inadequate fluids	Cold peripheries Weak thready pulse Operative blood loss not replaced Negative fluid balance	Blood replacement Increase intravenous fluids
3. Bleeding (a) Continued oozing from raw surfaces (b) Reactionary haemorrhage (c) Slipped ligature	Pale tongue and conjuctivae Weak thready pulse Bleeding from wound or drains	Moderate loss 500–1000 ml, replace blood Continuing or massive bleeding – take patient back to theatre once BP restored
(d) Clotting defect or DIC, massive transfusion	Bleeding from wound or drains	Coagulation defect – give fresh blood Fresh plasma or cryoprecipitate
4. Septicaemia	Often warm peripheries, bounding pulse Weak, thready pulse Septic focus at operation Instrumentation of the urinary tract	Support circulation with i.v. fluids Oxygen therapy Appropriate i.v. antibiotics

Table 13.5 Causes and management of postoperative low blood pressure (*continued*)

Possible causes	Look for	Action required
5. Cardiogenic		
(a) Myocardial infarction	History of cardiovascular disease Chest pain	ECG for diagnosis Treat failure
(b) Cardiac failure	Breathless, raised JVP Basal creps	Furosemide 80 mg Restrict fluids
(c) Pulmonary embolus	Chest pain, cyanosis, raised JVP	Oxygen, chest X-ray, ECG, heparinise
6. Hypothermia (p. 114)	Subnormal temperature Especially in baby	Warm
7. Anaphylaxis (p. 30)		
(a) Blood transfusion reaction (p. 33)	Pyrexia Petechial rash Correct blood given?	Stop blood Manage as described on p. 33
(b) Drug allergy	Recent administration of antibiotics? Allergic history?	Cancel prescription on chart Support circulation if severe

Atelectasis is suspected when there is reduced air-entry in the lung bases, and dullness to percussion and is confirmed by signs of lung collapse on X-ray. If an entire lung collapses owing to a mucous plug in the main bronchus the affected side of the chest will have restricted movement.

The treatment is oxygenation, aggressive physiotherapy with percussion, deep breathing and coughing. If this is not successful in clearing a large area of collapsed lung, bronchoscopy and suction of a mucous plug under direct vision should clear the airway and allow ventilation of the affected area.

Antibiotic therapy with penicillin, co-trimoxazole or ampicillin should be given if the patient has fever, signs of pulmonary infection or underlying lung disease.

Failure to treat atelectasis properly may result in pneumonia, which prolongs postoperative stay and may be fatal in the elderly.

Pneumonia is treated by chest physiotherapy and an appropriate antibiotic (e.g. penicillin).

The postoperative abdomen and return of gastrointestinal motility

Gastrointestinal motility returns to normal within the first 2–3 days after a laparotomy. The recovery may be prolonged if there is hypokalemia, peritonitis or a retroperitoneal haematoma. Small intestinal motility normally resumes after a few hours, gastric motility after 24 h and colonic motility after 48 h.

Bowel sounds resume, then the patient passes flatus and finally stool. Any distension should resolve and the abdomen is soft when the flanks are palpated. (Do not palpate the abdomen near the wound as this is painful.) Often the patient experiences colicky pains as areas of small bowel contract against segments which are still paralysed. Once the patient passes flatus these colicky pains subside. The first bowel actions may be loose especially when there has been peritonitis or intestinal obstruction. Diarrhoea usually resolves within 2–3 days of the first bowel action and is a normal occurrence at this stage of recovery. Later on diarrhoea may be associated with a pelvic or other intra-abdominal abscess or prolonged antibiotic therapy.

Nasogastric tubes help to decompress the stomach but have the disadvantage of being uncomfortable and making it hard for the patient to cough. The normal aspirate from a nasogastric tube is about 300 ml/24 h, although daily gastric secretions usually amount to 1.5 litres. They are normally removed between 24 h and 48 h after surgery once the aspirate is less than 400 ml/24 h. If it is greater than this for more than 48 h then the most likely cause is prolonged paralytic ileus.

Paralytic ileus occurs to some extent after nearly all abdominal operations. When it is prolonged there is often no obvious reason but the known precipitating causes should be considered:
1. recurrent intra-abdominal sepsis;
2. a leaking anastomosis;
3. retroperitoneal haematoma;
4. hypokalaemia or uraemia;
5. sympathomimetic, anticholinergic or opiate drugs.

The treatment is expectant unless an underlying cause is suspected. Postoperative intestinal obstruction must be ruled out. Consider a diagnosis of intestinal obstruction if ileus persists beyond 5 days, or the aspirate becomes faeculent, dirty or foul-smelling. Postoperative intestinal obstruction requires urgent reoperation.

Wound care

Wounds expected to heal without infection are closed primarily with sutures. It makes little difference whether the patient has interrupted or continuous sutures.

In wounds where infection is anticipated the skin is left open to allow drainage and cleaning. After 5 days or so open wounds granulate and closure is achieved either by secondary suturing or by waiting for healing by secondary intention. To close a wound when surgery has been performed in the presence of sepsis invites the development of wound abscess, which may delay recovery, cause septicaemia and confuse the clinical picture.

The purpose of a dressing is to protect the environment from the patient, not vice versa. Wounds that are not bleeding or oozing pus do not require dressings. Unless the surgeon specifies to the contrary it is better for the wound to be exposed after the first day. The wound should be inspected daily. Wound infection does not normally occur before the fourth or fifth day. The signs of wound infection are redness, tenderness, oedema and low-grade fever. Pus may be seen around the sutures or leaking between the edges of the wound. The treatment of a wound infection is removal of the skin sutures in the area of infection to allow free drainage of the pus. Antibiotics are not required. The fever will subside when the wound is drained by suture removal.

Wounds left open should be cleaned three times daily with Eusol, normal saline or other suitable solution. Gradually, over 2–3 weeks, the subcutaneous tissue granulates, any discharge subsides and the wound becomes clean and bright red. Thin patients do not normally need secondary suturing since by the time the wound is clean it is almost healed. In fat patients secondary suturing may shorten the postoperative stay in hospital by about a week or so.

Pyrexia

A slight fever is common in the first 24 h after anaesthesia and surgery. If it settles no action is necessary.

The causes of persisting or high fever include the following:

1. Atelectasis and bronchopneumonia – usually develop in the first few days after surgery.
2. Bacteraemia and septicaemia: diagnose by blood culture, suspect if instrumentation of urinary tract has been performed or if there are indwelling central venous lines or catheters. Remove catheters and CVP lines if they are suspected of being the cause. Septicaemia is discussed on p. 133.
3. Wound infection (after third day).
4. Recurrent sepsis.
5. Malaria.
6. Urinary tract infection, particularly where there is an indwelling catheter.
7. Deep vein thrombosis (pyrexia low grade).
8. Unsuspected pressure sores.

The treatment of pyrexia depends on the underlying cause and is discussed in the appropriate sections throughout the book.

Deep vein thrombosis

Thrombosis may occur in the veins of the calf, thigh or pelvis. Surgery, infection, obesity, major surgery, prolonged bed rest, oral contraceptives, pregnancy, cancer, old age and Caucasian race are predisposing factors. The true incidence of postoperative deep vein thrombosis in Africans is not known. The clot can dislodge from the veins and pass to the lungs where it causes pulmonary embolism, which is sometimes fatal.

The classical signs of deep-vein thrombosis are a warm, swollen, painful limb and low-grade fever. A clinical diagnosis is inaccurate but can be confirmed by venography and ultrasound when they are available. If there is swelling and tenderness extending to the thigh and groin then there is likely to be femoral and iliac vein thrombosis, which may cause a massive or fatal pulmonary embolus.

The affected limb should be elevated until the swelling subsides and if femoral or iliac venous thrombosis has developed the patient should be fully anticoagulated (pp. 446 and 455).

Treatment for calf vein thrombosis may be by elevation alone or combined with heparin 5000 units 8 hourly subcutaneously rather than full intravenous heparinisation.

Ileofemoral thrombosis requires full heparinisation and anticoagulation can be maintained as an outpatient for 1–3 months using warfarin.

Pulmonary embolism

The management of pulmonary embolism is discussed on p. 69. Patients who suffer from acute chest pain after surgery should be suspected of having either a myocardial infarction or a pulmonary embolism. A chest X-ray, ECG and careful examination of the legs for venous thrombosis will help differentiate the two conditions.

14

Critical illness in obstetrics and gynaecology

Pre-eclampsia and eclampsia

Definitions

Pre-eclampsia is a syndrome peculiar to pregnancy that may be initiated by a maternal immunological reaction to the feto-placental unit, resulting in defective development of the placenta. It can occur whenever there is living placental tissue even in the absence of a fetus, as in the post-partum period or in the rare condition of hydatidiform mole. It may also be superimposed on an underlying tendency to maternal hypertension. The hypertension may have been present before conception or may develop only in later life. There may be underlying renal disease.

The syndrome is defined by its clinical features of hypertension and proteinuria. Pregnancy-induced hypertension (PIH) is the term used to describe the development of hypertension alone. There may also be oedema, but this is only likely to be significant if of rapid onset, generalised and associated with excessive weight gain (Table 14.1).

Eclampsia is defined as convulsions associated with pre-eclampsia in the pregnant or post-partum patient (within 14 days of delivery). Of these fits 70% occur before, 10% during and 20% after delivery. Imminent eclampsia is severe pre-eclampsia (proteinuria++ and a blood pressure of 160/100 or more) plus symptoms.

Table 14.1 Classification of hypertensive disease during pregnancy

1. Pregnancy-induced hypertension (after 24 weeks' gestation)
   (a) Pre-eclampsia
      BP rises – systolic >30 mmHg over pregnancy
      – diastolic >15 mmHg over pregnancy
      BP >140/90 with proteinuria
      +/– oedema or excess weight gain
   (b) Eclampsia – pre-eclampsia + convulsions
   (c) Pregnancy-induced hypertension without proteinuria

2. Chronic hypertension +/– superimposed pre-eclampsia
   Diastolic >90 mmHg before 20th week of pregnancy

3. Chronic renal disease with associated hypertension and proteinuria.

Pre-eclampsia may first be recognised late in the second trimester and convulsions (eclampsia) may occur with little warning before, during or after labour. In other patients the course is more chronic and the fetus growth retarded. In pre-eclampsia early delivery may be beneficial to the fetus, but the timing of delivery will also depend on the facilities available for neonatal intensive care. Once eclampsia has developed or is imminent then rapid delivery is in the best interests of both the mother and the fetus.

Severe pre-eclampsia, eclampsia and their complications are associated with increased maternal and fetal mortality. There is a reduced circulating plasma volume due to a contracted vascular space and interstitial oedema due to a low serum albumin and leaky capillaries. Despite the low circulating volume the central venous pressure is usually normal and the patient is prone to develop pulmonary oedema.

Clinical recognition

Hypertension is frequently the first sign to be detected, and is sometimes associated with excessive weight gain, though clinical evidence of oedema may be absent. Proteinuria usually appears last and signifies vascular and renal disease. Proteinuria may have been present for several weeks or may develop over a few hours but it is rarely absent in eclampsia. The presence of pre-existing hypertension or renal disease, may complicate the clinical picture.

In severe pre-eclampsia symptoms such as headache, blurred vision, epigastric pain and vomiting are indications of impending eclampsia. Other warning signs include a rapid rise in blood pressure, oliguria, localised or generalised twitching, restlessness and brisk tendon reflexes. Many patients fit before admission to the hospital. In the tropics pre-eclampsia may quickly progress to severe pre-eclampsia or eclampsia. Since the blood pressure may be variable it should be measured repeatedly and patients may fit with a single BP reading as low as 120/90 mmHg. Fits may occur with increasing frequency and may result in hypoxic brain damage and/or respiratory failure. The more serious the maternal condition the worse the prognosis for the fetus.

Fits, occurring in late pregnancy, labour or the immediate post-partum period (usually less than 48 h but sometimes as long as 14 days post delivery), associated with proteinuria with or without hypertension, should be managed as eclampsia until proved otherwise. Differential diagnoses include acute hypertension due to ergometrine, cerebrovascular accident, cerebral malaria, meningitis, hypoglycaemia, epilepsy or electrolyte imbalance.

Relevant investigations

Laboratory tests do not usually help with the diagnosis of pre-eclampsia. However, investigations may help to detect complications early, for example intra-uterine growth retardation may be shown on ultrasound. Urea, electrolytes and creatinine levels are indicated when there is oliguria or renal disease is suspected. Blood film for malaria parasites, lumbar puncture and blood glucose may help to exclude other causes of convulsions or coma. A chest radiograph is indicated for pulmonary complications.

Management

Transfer

The patient with severe pre-eclampsia should be managed in a specially equipped area of the hospital or the labour ward with facilities for immediate resuscitation and airway management including intubation. Trained midwives and doctors familiar with this condition must be in constant attendance, under the supervision of a senior doctor or obstetrician. The patient should be nursed in a room with adequate lighting to allow observation. If severe pre-eclampsia or eclampsia develops in a peripheral centre the patient must be urgently transferred to hospital, after receiving sedation. The patient should be accompanied by a trained midwife with an eclampsia tray containing: oropharyngeal airway, mucus extractor, oxygen mask, swabs, syringes and needles, and drugs including

Table 14.2 Aims of management in pre-eclampsia and eclampsia

Preservation of a clear airway
Control of convulsions.
Deliver fetus and placenta.
Control blood pressure.
Treat complications:
  Oliguria, renal failure;
  Cerebral oedema or CVA;
  Pulmonary oedema or aspiration pneumonia;
  Disseminated intravascular coagulation (DIC).

diazepam. It is recommended that ambulances with oxygen cylinders should be available to bring such patients to referral centres. The priorities in management are listed in Table 14.2.

Intensive care

The only cure is delivery of the fetus and placenta. All other forms of treatment aim to protect the mother from complications.

Maintenance of a clear airway using posture, oropharyngeal airways or an endotracheal tube and control of fits take priority. Close monitoring of the conscious level (Glasgow Coma Scale), blood pressure and pulse rate should be done every 15 min. Where possible the ECG should be monitored. Cardiac failure can occur very suddenly and should be actively looked for and promptly treated. The bladder must be catheterised and an accurate input–output chart kept. Proteinuria and haematuria should be recorded, and blood sent to the laboratory for estimation of urea and electrolytes, and haemoglobin. Cross-matching of blood is done in patients who may require operative delivery. Although the development of DIC is rare it may be detected by measuring the platelet count and coagulation times. In patients who are deeply unconscious it is wise to pass a nasogastric tube to reduce the risk of aspiration. Magnesium trisilicate 15 ml given 2 hourly either orally or down the nasogastric tube will increase gastric pH and minimise the consequences of aspiration should it occur. Sodium citrate or H_2 antagonists are alternative therapies.

The main complications of severe pre-eclampsia for the mother are cerebrovascular accident, cardiac failure, pulmonary oedema, renal failure and convulsions (Table 14.2).

Control of convulsions

The patient with convulsions needs delivery and the longer the fit–delivery interval the worse the prognosis. Unless labour is advanced and particularly where sophisticated fetal (e.g. cardiotocograph) and maternal monitoring is not possible the best option is a Caesarean section under general anaesthesia.

KEYPOINT
Prevent hypoxia during convulsions.

The options for controlling the convulsions are magnesium sulphate, diazepam and clomethiazole (Heminevrin). The simplest, cheapest and most effective method which is safe for the fetus is the magnesium sulphate regimen shown in Table 14.3. Magnesium sulphate can be easily prepared by all pharmacies. The intramuscular injections are best given with a large bore needle (16–18 gauge) and local anaesthetic makes the injection less painful.

Diazepam is given in an initial dose of 10–20 mg intravenously to control or prevent the onset of fits. A state of drowsiness can be maintained by an infusion of 80 mg diazepam in 1000 ml 5% dextrose. The mother should not be deeply sedated because of the risk of airway obstruction and aspiration of vomitus. A drip rate of 20–30 d.p.m. should be titrated against the patient's response. The dose of diazepam should not exceed 30 mg if the patient is

Table 14.3 Magnesium sulphate regimen

1. Give 4 g of magnesium sulphate as a 20% solution intravenously at a rate of 1 g/min.
2. Follow this immediately with a deep intramuscular injection of 5 g of 50% magnesium sulphate solution into each buttock (total 10 g). If convulsions persist after another 15 min, give up to 2 g more intravenously as a 20% solution (4 g in a large patient).
3. Every 4 h give an injection of 5 g of 50% magnesium sulphate in alternate buttocks.
4. Check before each injection:
   (a) The patellar reflex is present.
   (b) Respiration is not depressed.
   (c) Urine output over the previous 4 h was 100 ml.
   If any of the above conditions are not met withold the injection. If respiratory depression occurs give 1 g of calcium gluconate slowly intravenously (10 ml of 10% solution).
5. Discontinue magnesium sulphate 24 h after delivery.

Magnesium sulphate is easily prepared by most pharmacies.
Local anaesthetic should be added to i.m. injections as the injection is best made with wider (16–18) gauge needles.

going to be delivered within 15 h of admission because of the risks of hypothermia, hypotonus and hypoglycaemia to the neonate. Clomethiazole has less sedative effect. Clomethiazole is not stable in hot climates and comes in powder form. We have little experience of its efficacy, as it is expensive and not widely available. If the convulsions do not quickly respond to the above measures then the mother should be anaesthetised with thiopentone, paralysed with a muscle relaxant, intubated and ventilated, since anaesthesia itself will control convulsions. To prevent convulsions following delivery phenytoin (oral, nasogastric or intravenous p. 453) may be useful if magnesium sulphate has not been used or in rare cases was not effective.

Further reading

GREENE MF. Magnesium sulfate for preeclampsia. *N Engl J Med* 2003;348:275–6.
ELTZSCHIG HK, LIEBERMAN ES, CAMANN WR. Regional anaesthesia and analgesia for labor and delivery. *N Engl J Med* 2003;348:319–32.
Magpie Collaborative Group. Do women with pre-eclampsia, and their babies, benefit from magnesium sulphate? The Magpie trial: a randomised placebo-controlled trial. *Lancet* 2002;359:1877–90.

Delivery

The cure of the disease lies in the delivery of the fetus and placenta. Delivery should be by Caesarean section unless labour is progressing satisfactory. When delivering the patient with severe pre-eclampsia vaginally, close monitoring of the fetus (e.g. by cardiotocograph) is mandatory. Vaginal delivery may be assisted by epidural analgesia, which minimises the stress of labour, facilitates blood pressure control and optimises placental perfusion. Epidurals are contraindicated in the presence of a coagulation defect, thrombocytopenia or haemorrhage. Attempts at vaginal delivery should be abandoned if convulsions, blood pressure and oliguria cannot be controlled. Other reasons for abandoning vaginal delivery are if active labour is not occurring within 4 h of rupture of the membranes, or if there is a failure of labour to progress as plotted in the partogram, or fetal distress. Persistent hypertension means that the second stage of labour should be shortened by the use of an episiotomy, vacuum extraction or forceps delivery. In cases of eclampsia, delivery of the fetus should never be delayed. The fit–delivery interval influences the maternal and perinatal mortality significantly and if the fit–delivery interval exceeds 4 h, there is a marked increase in both fetal and maternal mortality. Syntometrine (engometrine + oxytocin) or ergometrine must not be used in third-stage management, except in the case of severe post-partum haemorrhage, because ergometrine causes vasoconstriction, which raises the blood pressure. When indicated oxytocin may be given by i.v. infusion.

Anaesthesia

The patient should always be positioned in the lateral tilt position to avoid pressure from the uterus on the vena cava, which reduces venous return and causes hypotension. Endotracheal intubation may raise the blood pressure, which may occasionally cause cerebral haemorrhage, cardiac ischaemia or cardiac failure. These risks are minimised if the blood pressure is controlled before anaesthesia as outlined below. However, delivery should not be delayed by attempts to control the blood pressure. Intubation may be difficult because of laryngeal oedema and a selection of endotracheal tubes and introducers should be available. Pre-induction alfentanil, labetalol or magnesium have been shown to reduce the hypertensive reponse to intubation. Aaesthetic drugs may depress the myocardium and cause vasodilation, which results in hypotension. Patients who have had magnesium sulphate therapy are more sensitive to muscle relaxants. Blood loss during Caesarean section should be replaced accurately, if necessary with the aid of CVP monitoring. Urinary output must be closely monitored. Ketamine, Syntometrine and ergometrine all raise the blood pressure and should, in general, be avoided. During the recovery phase the patient must be carefully observed and should only be extubated when she can maintain her own airway and respiration is adequate.

Epidural anaesthesia is used in some units for operative deliveries in obstetric practice, and provided hypotension is avoided and there are no contraindications (detailed above), is usually safe in pre-eclampsia when administered by an experienced anaesthetist. It is less suitable for eclamptics because of the risk of fitting on the operating table. Spinal anaesthesia is also commonly used, although rapid-onset hypotension should be anticipated and treated.

Control of blood pressure

The drug of choice is hydralazine, a peripheral vasodilator which lowers blood pressure while maintaining placental perfusion. Add 40 mg of hydralazine to 500 ml of normal saline and start the infusion at 10 d.p.m. increasing to a maximum of 30 d.p.m. The drug should be titrated against the blood pressure with the aim of achieving a diastolic pressure of between 90 and 100 mmHg and a systolic below 160 mmHg. If the blood pressure falls markedly it may further reduce blood flow to an already underperfused placenta. During the infusion the blood pressure should be monitored every 15 min until the desired level is achieved. Small bolus doses of hydralazine (5–10 mg i.v.) may be used in an emergency and this may be safer where supervision of an infusion is poor.

In the absence of hydralazine, diazoxide may be effective but is less predictable and should be given as 30 mg intravenous boluses every 5 min with continuous or repeated blood pressure monitoring. Do not give 150 mg or 300 mg as a single i.v. dose. Do not exceed 300 mg in one hour. The drop in blood pressure may be severe and fatal. In our experience hydralazine has provided good control of blood pressure and it should be regarded as an essential drug. Tachycardia may develop in association with hydralazine or diazoxide. If this is severe it may be controlled by intravenous labetalol, which also has a useful antihypertensive action. Methyldopa is an effective antihypertensive drug (oral or i.v. – see p. 450) but requires several hours to take effect. Adding methyldopa to the initial dose of hydralazine allows antihypertensive control to be taken over by methyldopa after a few hours.

Severe hypotension complicating treatment is due to reduced circulating volume aggravated by peripheral vasodilatation. The treatment is to position the patient head down and resuscitate with intravenous fluids.

Complications

The natural history of oliguria and interstitial oedema in pre-eclampsia is resolution commencing with a diuresis within 24 h of delivery.

Oliguria

This may be due to hypovolaemia and dehydration due to the constricted circulation and/or renovascular damage from the hypertension and pre-eclampsia process. Any attempt to give rapid volume replacement is unwise, especially before delivery. Oliguria is an indication for delivery of the fetus. Insertion of a CVP line allows blood and fluid losses during delivery to be accurately replaced. Delivery also acts as a fluid challenge in that retraction of the uterus increases the venous return to the heart. This is likely to be less than in a normal pregnancy but none the less the underlying insterstitial oedema makes excessive volume replacement unwise before delivery.

When oliguria persists or develops in the post-partum period CVP monitoring is also indicated. If the CVP is normal or low and there are no signs of fluid overload (basal crepitations in the lungs) then a fluid challenge of either 500 ml of normal saline or 250 ml of dextran 70 is safe. Only once the circulating volume is restored should a diuretic challenge (furosemide 80 mg) be given. If diuretics are given before hypovolaemia is corrected then any urine produced represents further loss of intravascular fluid, and severe hypotension may result occasionally. The blood pressure should also be controlled since it is difficult to achieve a good urine output when there is persistent severe hypertension. When the patient does not respond to fluids or diuretics then an infusion of 2.5–5 µg/kg/min of dopamine is indicated. If this fails to produce urine and the urea continues to rise then the patient will need peritoneal or haemodialysis. The management of oliguria and renal failure are discussed more fully in Chapter 5 (see flow chart Figure 5.2). Most patients with oliguria respond to fluids. The urea and electrolytes should be measured daily.

Pulmonary oedema

This has a high mortality in the pre-eclamptic patient. Furosemide 80 mg should be given and repeated as necessary provided the kidneys are capable of excreting urine. The patient should be sat up, started on oxygen and have her fluids restricted (p. 54). Ventilatory support may be necessary. If there is renal failure dialysis should be commenced. Removal of 500 ml of blood may also help if fluid overload or cardiac failure is present. Cardiac disease in pregnancy is discussed on p. 71).

Renal failure

Renal function is compromised by both renovascular damage (as evidenced by proteinuria) due to the pre-eclamptic process and reduced renal perfusion due to hypovolaemia. Renal damage is minimised by blood pressure control and delivery. Fluid therapy aims to maintain perfusion of the kidney in an attempt to avoid acute tubular necrosis. Hourly urine output, proteinuria and specific gravity should be monitored in addition to the blood urea. If acute renal failure develops the patient can be treated conservatively awaiting resolution. Signs of fluid overload, a rapidly rising urea or hyperkalaemia mean that peritoneal or haemodialysis is necessary. Peritoneal dialysis can be commenced even within 48–72 h of Caesarean section.

Coma

The causes of coma in pre-eclampsia and eclampsia are cerebral oedema, cerebral haemorrhage or hypoxic damage during a fit. A rapid fall in blood pressure in response to antihypertensive therapy or blood loss may reduce cerebral perfusion and cause a cerebrovascular accident. There is no specific management, but all general measures in the care of the comatose patient should be given. Exclude other causes of coma. The general management of the comatose patient is described on p. 175. Await recovery since this may be complete despite a low coma scale on admission.

Post-delivery

During the 48 h following delivery intensive observations must be continued, as the mother is still at risk from convulsions and renal failure. The blood pressure must be controlled if the diastolic is above 120 mmHg, or if less severe hypertension does not settle within 12 h of delivery. If hypertension does not settle by 6 weeks post-partum the patient will require long-term anti-hypertensive therapy.

Breast feeding

If mother and baby are able, breastfeeding should be encouraged even if this means rearranging the usual division of care between the neonatal and intensive care units.

Counselling

The patient should be advised that the problems encountered in the management of severe hypertensive disease in pregnancy may be prevented by good ante-natal care. Primiparous patients will probably not have a recurrence of pre-eclampsia in their next pregnancy. Multiparous patients may be advised to undergo tubal ligation.

Obstetrical haemorrhage

Obstetrical haemorrhage means bleeding associated with pregnancy and includes abortion, ectopic pregnancy, choriocarcinoma, ante- and post-partum haemorrhage, and coagulation failure due to causes such as amniotic fluid embolism and septic shock.

Antepartum haemorrhage is bleeding from the placental site occurring after 28 weeks of gestation. The common causes of severe haemorrhage are placenta praevia and placental abruption.

Postpartum haemorrhage is bleeding from the genital tract after delivery of the fetus.

The effects of haemorrhage are more severe when superimposed on pre-existing anaemia or if there is associated malaria, sickle cell or cardiac disease. Cardiac disease may make blood transfusion precarious. Haemorrhage may also be associated with septic shock in cases of septic abortion, prolonged obstructed labour and ruptured uterus. Clotting defects may complicate haemorrhage in placental abruption, septic shock, longstanding intra-uterine death, amniotic fluid embolism eclampsia and massive blood transfusion.

Treatment aims to stop the bleeding by dealing with the underlying cause and transfusion of fresh whole blood or fresh frozen plasma, either of which will help replace clotting factors, as well as blood volume. In the case of placental abruption the clotting mechanism rapidly recovers once the fetus and placenta have been delivered.

General anaesthesia in the presence of severe anaemia must be induced with great

Abortion

When incomplete, the cervical os will usually be open and removal of the products of conception from the cervical canal with ovum forceps may help control shock before formal evacuation in theatre. This may be carried out under pethidine analgesia. Evacuation should not be delayed by resuscitation and blood transfusion if active bleeding continues. Septic abortion should be managed as described in the section on pelvic sepsis (p. 276).

Ectopic pregnancy

These patients usually present after 6 weeks amenorrhoea, although the history may be atypical due to irregular vaginal bleeding or denial of pregnancy. Lower abdominal pain usually precedes slight vaginal bleeding. The cervix is acutely tender on gentle palpation and the os closed unless a decidual cast has been passed. The uterus may be ill defined owing to surrounding blood clot and a separate adnexal mass is seldom distinguished. The beta human chorionic gonadatrophin (HCG) will normally be over 1000 iu in an ectopic pregnancy. The diagnosis should be confirmed by ultrasound or laparoscopy if available. Laparoscopy is the most accurate diagnostic procedure but is not always available. Ultrasound (abdominal or vaginal) may confirm the diagnosis and demonstrate fluid in the pelvis but a negative scan does not exclude ectopic pregnancy unless it shows an intra-uterine pregnancy – a twin ectopic is very rare.

A culdocentesis is another possible procedure to confirm the presence of a haemoperitoneum (Figure 14.1).

care, and oxygen should be administered postoperatively. Mechanical or manual ventilation should be maintained until all danger of hypoventilation has passed.

This will require a syringe with a long needle, a vaginal speculum and a movable light source. After careful insertion of the needle at the apex of the posterior vaginal fornix it should be withdrawn slowly under vision with negative pressure. A false positive result may occur due to puncture of a vessel on the posterior surface of the uterus, especially if retroverted or if the adnexae are adherent in this area. A small amount of blood is often aspirated into the syringe as the needle is withdrawn through the wall of the posterior fornix. A false negative result can occur if the blood is loculated by adhesions. Pus or strawcoloured fluid almost excludes ruptured ectopic pregnancy but it is possible for the needle to collect fluid from an ovarian cyst and miss the loculated blood.

In cases of suspected ectopic pregnancy with shock, laparotomy should not be delayed by diagnostic procedures. The priority is to clamp the bleeding vessel. Resuscitation should be carried out en route to theatre and if the condition is not improving, surgery to clamp the bleeding vessel should proceed as part of the resuscitation process. Autotransfusion can be used if the bleeding is fresh (<6 h).

Further reading

PISARSKA MD, CARSON A, BUSTER JE. Ectopic pregnancy. *Lancet* 1998;351:115–20.

Chorioncarcinoma

This is a malignancy of placental tissue which usually follows a hydatidiform mole by some weeks or months but may follow a normal pregnancy, abortion or ectopic pregnancy. The bleeding may be vaginal, or intraperitoneal or from distant metastases such as in the lungs. Diagnosis is by

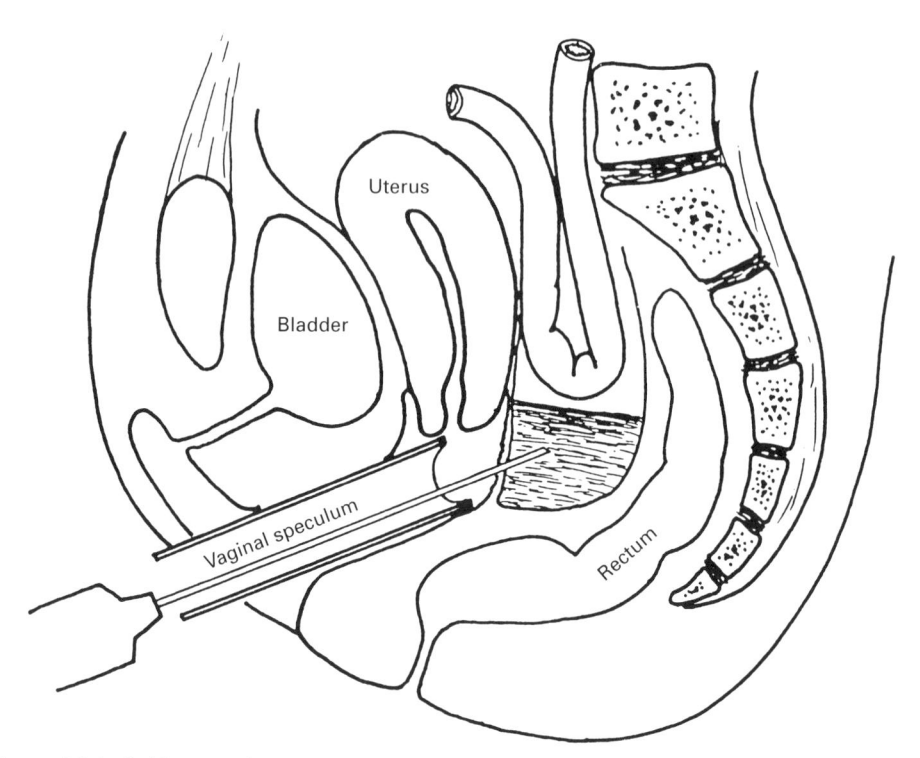

Figure 14.1 Culdocentesis.

a positive pregnancy test in serial dilutions of urine to give a titre of HCG. A chest X-ray should be taken to look for pulmonary metastases. Surgery may be extremely hazardous and chemotherapy too slow to control haemorrhage. Hysterectomy may be the only method of controlling uterine bleeding. Haemorrhage from vaginal lesions may be controlled by careful undersewing. The need for a repeat evacuation in a patient with a history of abortion should alert one to the possibility of a chorioncarcinoma and the products should be sent for histology.

Ante-partum haemorrhage (APH)
(Figure 14.2)

In severe cases the cause will be either placenta praevia or placental abruption. The definition of severe and the decision whether to treat the condition conservatively for the sake of a pre-term fetus or to avoid a Caesarean section for a dead fetus will depend on the availability of blood for transfusion. Placenta praevia may be suspected when the APH is painless and the presenting part high and possibly not cephalic. If quickly available, an ultrasound scan can confirm the diagnosis. Vaginal examination on the ward must be avoided and examination under anaesthesia (EUA) undertaken with a 'double set up' prepared for immediate Caesarean section.

In the case of abruption revealed blood loss is less than actual blood loss and the patient may be severely shocked despite little external haemorrhage. Patients with pre-eclampsia are prone to abruption and a normal blood pressure reading may in fact represent hypotension. Pain usually starts

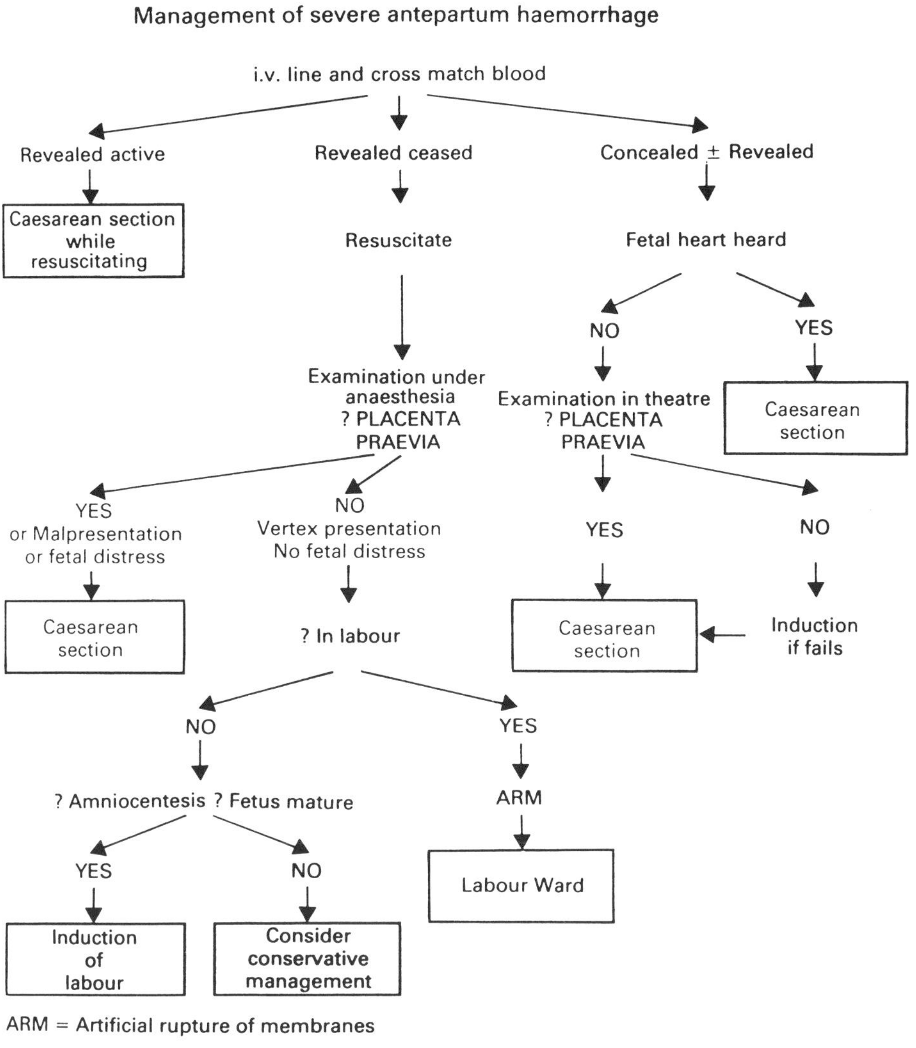

Management of severe antepartum haemorrhage

Figure 14.2 Management of severe ante-partum haemorrhage.

suddenly and is continuous; the uterus feels hard and does not relax, even although labour may have been precipitated. The fetus is likely to be dead.

In some cases it may be difficult to differentiate between placenta praevia and abruption because both bleeding and pain are present. If the patient is in labour and the head is entering the pelvis a major degree of placenta praevia is unlikely. If there is a small possibility of placenta praevia the patient should be examined in theatre but anaesthesia is not necessary unless the likelihood of this is high.

Adequate blood replacement may require CVP monitoring and should accompany induction of labour or precede Caesarean section. Any clotting defect recovers soon after delivery but it is important to keep the uterus contracted and empty by manual compression and oxytocics (ergometrine 0.5 mg i.v. stat or

Syntometrine one ampoule i.m. followed by oxytocin 10 units in one litre of intravenous fluid) until it has recovered or post-partum haemorrhage will be added to the ante-partum. Renal failure may occur and the urine output must be monitored. Induction of labour should be abandoned in favour of Caesarean section in the absence of normal progress or if there is evidence of oligura or continued bleeding.

Vasa praevia is a rare cause of APH. It is due to bleeding from fetal vessels lying in the membranes and overlying the cervical os. A small bleed of fetal blood is associated with fetal distress and a high perinatal mortality. If recognised in time the fetus should be delivered by immediate Caesarean section and then transfused.

Post-partum haemorrhage (PPH)
(Figure 14.3)

This is especially dangerous if it follows APH (both placenta praevia and abruption predispose to it) or pre-existing anaemia. The bleeding may be from lacerations of perineum, vagina, cervix or body of the uterus. Uterine bleeding may be from an atonic uterus or a rupture. The uterine rupture may result in blood loss through the vagina or into the peritoneal cavity or the broad ligament. A broad-ligament haematoma may be recognised by a pelvic swelling displacing the uterus laterally. A cervical tear may extend into a uterine laceration and therefore repair of the cervix must be seen to reach the apex of the laceration or else laparotomy should be

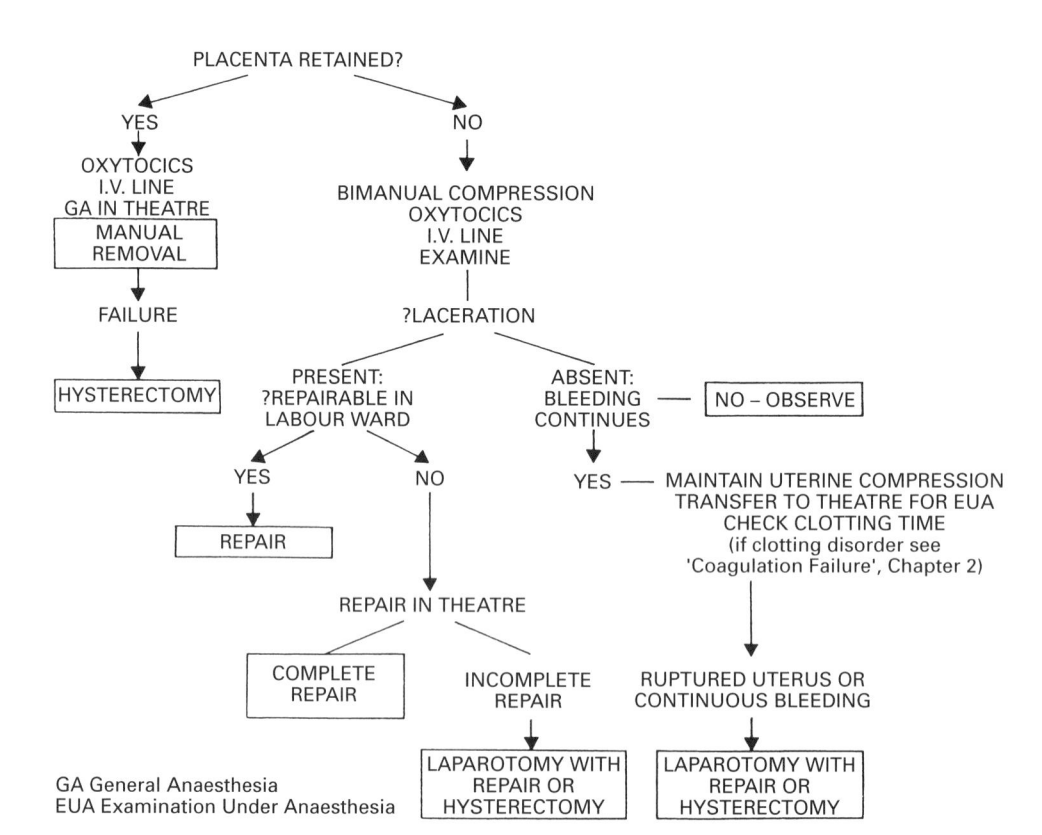

GA General Anaesthesia
EUA Examination Under Anaesthesia

Figure 14.3 Management of severe post-partum haemorrhage.

undertaken. In obese patients the extent of intraperitoneal blood loss may not be appreciated until the patient is in shock.

The first priority is control of haemorrhage. If the placenta has been expelled completely, bimanual compression will reduce uterine blood loss whether due to atony or to uterine rupture. If the uterus is allowed to fill up with blood, the area of the placental site is stretched and the 'living ligatures' rendered less effective, thus setting up a vicious circle of bleeding and further distension. Second, one or more large intravenous (i.v.) cannulae should be inserted and blood volume replacement started. Third, blood is cross-matched (a sample should be taken when setting up the drip and certainly before the administration of any dextran). At the same time oxytocics are given. Ergometrine or Syntometrine may be repeated once intramuscularly or intravenously when there is an intravenous infusion running. Oxytocin up to 40 units/l is given continuously for 2 h, slowly reducing the rate of infusion. After examination any surgery required is carried out according to the flow chart (Figure 14.3).

If the placenta is retained and not easily removed in labour ward at the time of delivery then its removal will require a general anaesthetic in theatre. Oxytocics are used to limit blood loss while this is being arranged. Ergometrine will tend to close the cervix for 20–30 min. Morbid adherence may be due to placenta accreta and may require hysterectomy.

Secondary PPH (24 h to 6 weeks postpartum) is most likely to be associated with sepsis and/or retained products of conception. EUA will be required with removal of any products by gentle digital and blunt curretage avoiding perforation of the soft uterus. If bleeding is not controlled or if there is any suggestion of scar dehiscence following Caesarean section laparotomy and possibly hysterectomy may be required.

Secondary haemorrhage after hysterectomy may require ligation of the anterior divisions of one or both internal iliac arteries.

Amniotic fluid embolism

This is a rare cause of disseminated intravascular coagulation, which may then result in haemorrhage. It is associated with shock, dyspnoea, cyanosis and a clotting defect and has a high mortality. It may be due to intact membranes in advanced labour, especially if there is polyhydramnios. Treatment is that of shock, coagulation failure and hypoxia.

Post-partum collapse

Haemorrhage may be hidden as described under post-partum haemorrhage. This includes haemorrhage into paravaginal or vulval tissues, which may be detected on vaginal examination or EUA and will require evacuation and haemostasis.

Uterine inversion causes shock, whether partial with dimpling of the fundus or complete with the fundus presenting at the introitus having passed through the cervix. If recognised at the time of occurrence it may be replaced immediately. Later, resuscitation, general anaesthesia and digital manipulation or hydrostatic pressure will be necessary to replace it. Inversion of the uterus must be distinguished from prolapse of a submucosal pedunculated fibroid.

Amniotic fluid embolism may present post-partum, having occurred just before delivery. Anaesthetic complications include total spinal block, hypoventilation following general anaesthesia and Mendelson's syndrome following inhaled vomit. Treatment of the latter follows the guidelines given on p. 13. Medical causes include cardiac disease with failure following delivery, malaria and pulmonary oedema, possibly due to overtransfusion of a chronically anaemic patient. The differential diagnosis of the unconscious patient post-partum is given in the section on eclampsia.

Obstetrical and gynaecological sepsis
(Figure 14.4)

Introduction

Pelvic sepsis of obstetrical and gynaecological origin includes septic abortion, often with perforation of the uterus, puerperal sepsis, and neglected salpingitis in the non-gravid uterus associated with abscess formation and peritonitis. The signs indicating the anatomical location and severity of the condition are both local and systemic. Pelvic sepsis refers to infection above the pelvic diaphragm and while it is likely to be associated with vaginal discharge the latter may also be due to vaginitis or cervicitis in the absence of pelvic sepsis. Peritonitis may be localised in the pelvis or generalised.

Apart from history and clinical examination, help in making the diagnosis may be obtained from examination under anaesthesia (EUA) and culdocentesis (see p. 272). While laparoscopy is useful in the diagnosis of stages 1 (uncomplicated salpingitis) and 2 (adnexal swelling), and especially in differentiating ectopic pregnancy, it is not likely to be helpful and may be dangerous in more advanced disease. Ultrasound scanning will show whether there is a fetus in the uterus, whether the membranes are intact and whether the fetus is alive. EUA should be undertaken only after obtaining consent from the patient for any operative procedures that may be indicated.

When the gravid or recently gravid uterus is the source of serious sepsis it will have to be removed. The non-gravid uterus associated with pelvic peritonitis arising in the fallopian tubes may usually be conserved.

In all these conditions septic or endotoxic shock may be a complication (see p. 27). Antibiotic therapy will usually need to be broad spectrum and parenteral. Anaerobic organisms are especially likely to be implicated in infections of the gravid uterus. Rarely, gas gangrene and tetanus may complicate infections of the gravid uterus and appropriate prophylaxis with active or passive immunisation may be wise in post-abortal and puerperal patients. Specimens should be taken for culture and sensitivity examination including blood culture. Start antibiotic therapy before results are available; crystalline penicillin, gentamicin and metronidazole is usually an effective combination but a cheaper one that is also useful is crystalline penicillin and chloramphenicol. The latter may be given orally in the absence of vomiting.

Further complications include the formation of subphrenic and multiple peritoneal abscesses. These conditions are usually treated by a general surgeon.

Septic abortion

Septic abortion may present with a threatened or incomplete abortion, i.e. the cervix may be closed or open. Sepsis complicating spontaneous incomplete abortion is seldom severe unless there has been gross delay in evacuating the products of conception. Sepsis resulting from criminal interference with the gravid uterus may be severe in the presence of a closed cervix or may fail to respond to antibiotic cover and evacuation in the presence of an open cervix.

There may be perforation of the uterus into the peritoneal cavity with signs of peritonitis. If the patient requires evacuation culdocentesis can be performed at the same time, which may reveal blood or pus in the pouch of Douglas. Perforation may also occur into the broad ligament, in

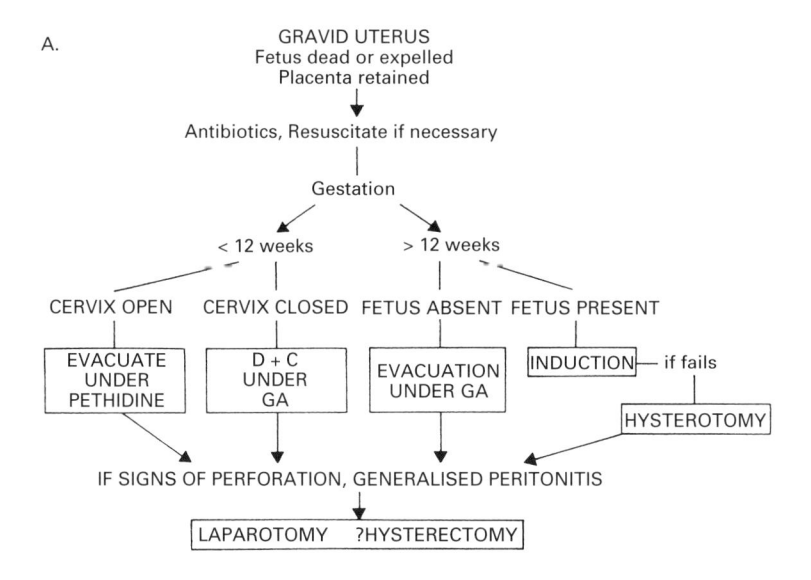

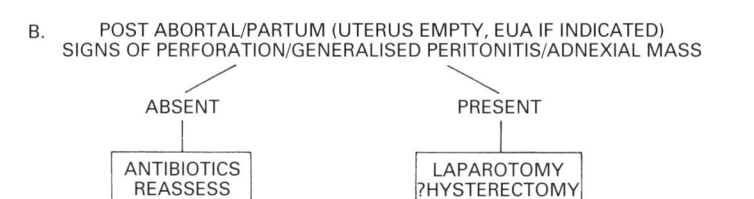

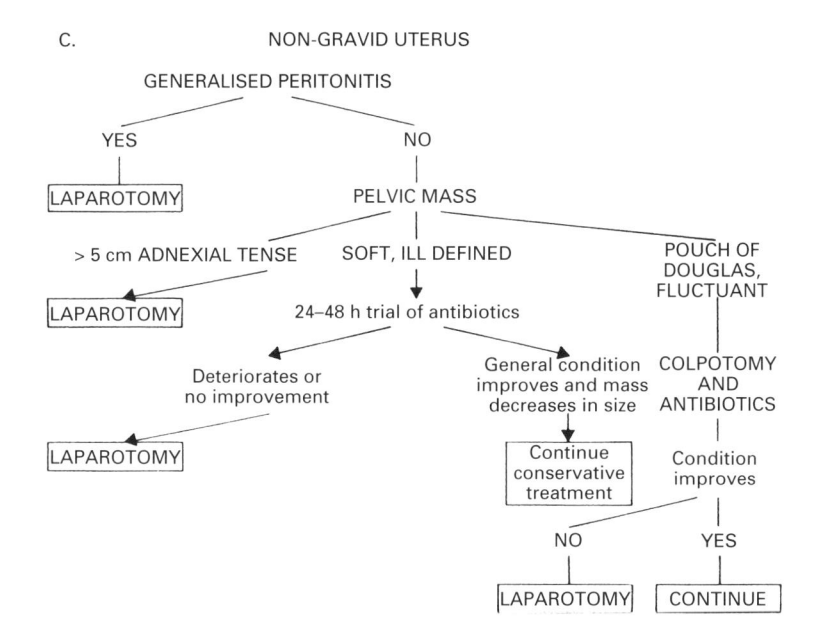

Critical illness in obstetrics and gynaecology 277

Figure 14.4 Flow chart of management of pelvic sepsis.

which case inflammatory thickening or abscess formation may be felt in the parametrium between the fingers lateral to the cervix on pelvi-rectal examination. In cases of doubt laparotomy must be performed. Broad ligament induration may be the only evidence of a small uterine perforation (even at laparotomy), but hysterectomy is essential and often bilateral salpingo-oophorectomy.

Before evacuation and/or laparotomy, resuscitation and antibiotic cover may be required but the surgery should not be unduly delayed.

Puerperal sepsis

Puerperal sepsis following vaginal delivery should, if possible, be treated with antibiotics that will not harm the breast-fed baby. However, no antibiotic should be witheld if the mother's condition demands it. Penicillins, gentamicin, cephalosporins and metronidazole are suitable. (If chloramphenicol has to be used breastfeeding should be continued despite the slight risks to the baby.)

A pyosalpinx may be difficult to detect alongside the involuting uterus and in case of doubt laparotomy is indicated.

A gangrenous uterus may follow Caesarean section complicated by sepsis from a prolonged or obstructed labour and in the presence of a classical or 'T' incision in the uterus. If the patient's condition (pulse rate, respiration rate, abdominal tenderness and distension) is deteriorating and vaginal examination reveals foul black lochia or dehiscence of a lower-segment uterine scar, laparotomy is indicated. The patient and surgeon should be prepared for hysterectomy.

Adnexal abscesses of the non-gravid uterus

Salpingitis is usually a bilateral disease, but in the case of recurrent infections one tube may become much more swollen than the other, giving the impression on vaginal examination of unilateral disease. Abscess formation may be within the tube (pyosalpinx) or outside the tube sealed off by bowel and omentum (tubo-ovarian abscess).

Non-gravid patients with salpingitis associated with adnexal swellings and pelvic peritonitis are usually managed with parenteral antibiotics for 24–48 h. The patient's condition must be carefully monitored and laparotomy performed if she deteriorates, if the swelling increases in size or has not been reduced in size by the end of this time, or if there is any doubt about the diagnosis. A considerable amount of tubal swelling may be due to oedema, which can subside. By waiting, surgery is sometimes avoided, and if an operation is required later it may be less extensive. Rupture of a pyosalpinx results in an acutely ill patient with septic shock and has a high mortality. Whenever this diagnosis is suspected laparotomy should be performed following urgent resuscitation.

Occasionally a fluctuant swelling in the pouch of Douglas dissecting down the rectovaginal septum will be found, indicating an abscess that may be drained by colpotomy. However, the abscess formation is likely to be multilocular (except in postoperative infection following hysterectomy), and subsequent abdominal surgery may be required if signs of sepsis persist after colpotomy and antibiotic therapy.

Antibiotics

Severe infection of obstetric and gynaecological origin is usually due to a mixed infection of Gram-negative bacilli and anaerobes. Thus gentamicin (or kanamycin) with penicillin and metronidazole is the first choice (an alternative regime is penicillin and chloramphenicol). Gonoccal infection may have been the primary infection in up to 50% of cases of tubo-ovarian sepsis and when it is found appropriate treatment should be given, according to local sensitivity patterns. *Chlamydia trachematis* may be present and after control of the acute sepsis a course of tetracycline is wise.

Further reading

DE MUYLDER X. Pelvic inflammatory disease in Zimbabwe. *Trop Doct* 1988;18:44–8.

Management of the newborn baby

The normal healthy newborn

The majority of newborn babies do not require any resuscitation. Fetal lungs contain a significant volume of lung fluid (about 40 ml/kg). Compression of the baby's chest during passage through the birth canal results in some of this fluid being expelled from the lungs via the mouth and nose. It is therefore normal for the baby to have some fluid draining from the mouth and nose during delivery and vigorous suction is not necessary. Excess fluid can simply be wiped away with gauze. A number of tactile and other sensory and biochemical stimuli result in the baby's first breath. This draws air into the lungs and increases flow of blood from the placenta. Reduction in pulmonary artery pressure results in increased pulmonary blood flow and independent respiration is established. Over-enthusiastic efforts using suction to resuscitate babies who do not need it may well be detrimental, resulting in damage to the fragile nasopharyngeal mucosa and possibly inducing reflex bradycardia. Suction is really only needed in the situation of perinatal asphyxia and where there is heavy meconium staining of the liquor (see below). Following delivery the baby should be dried and covered to avoid heat loss and placed on the mother's abdomen while the cord is being clamped and cut. The baby should then be given to the mother to cuddle. Following uncomplicated deliveries there is no urgency to cut the cord. Once in the mother's arms the baby should be allowed to suckle. This stimulates the release of oxytocin, which helps to reduce blood loss, assists mother–baby bonding and encourages the establishment of breast-feeding.

The baby in trouble – neonatal resuscitation

AIMS OF RESUSCITATION
1. Assist neonatal breathing to oxygenate the blood. 2. Maintain body temperature. 3. Assist the circulation to oxygenate the tissues.

Perinatal asphyxia

If the baby's brain becomes hypoxic during labour or delivery, it may not respond to the stimuli which normally induce the onset of spontaneous respiration and other cardiopulmonary adjustments. The baby is asphyxiated and resuscitation for such babies is a matter of urgency. Every health facility delivering babies must be prepared for neonatal resuscitation and should have a warm place near the delivery beds with a resuscitation trolley containing the equipment listed in Table 14.4.

The Apgar score (Table 14.5) is widely used to determine the baby's degree of hypoxia at birth and the response to resuscitation. While a single 1-minute Apgar score is not predictive, the change in Apgar over 5–10 min is a useful but not infallible indicator of outcome. In practice the 1-minute Apgar score is assigned

Table 14.4 Equipment for resuscitation of neonates

1. Warm towels to dry baby
2. Suction catheters with side ports 5 and 10 Fr and source of controlled suction
3. Neonatal resuscitation bag with pressure relief safety valve (e.g. Penlon, Laerdal or Ambu bag) and face masks of differing size
4. Overhead heater (ideal) or well wrapped hot water bottle at body temperature and resuscitation tray with a 30° tilt
5. Neonatal laryngoscpe with straight blade, batteries and bulbs
6. Endotracheal tubes sizes 3.5, 3, and 2.5 mm internal diameter with connectors to fit ventilation bag
7. Drugs: naloxone, dextrose, sodium bicarbonate, adrenaline (and water for injection for dilution)
Vitamin K, antibiotic eye ointment
8. Syringes, needles, umbilical catheters, cord clamps, scalpel blades, sterile swabs
9. Oxygen source (though this is not essential – and room air may be better!)
10. Guedel's airways of appropriate size (not essential, but handy to have available)

retrospectively after the initiation of resuscitation in a baby who does not breathe spontaneously after delivery.

The procedures for neonatal resuscitation are essentially the same as for resuscitation in older children and adults. However the **A (airways)** and the **B (breathing)** are by far the most important aspects. If the A and B are correctly managed the vast majority of asphyxiated babies will take care of the C (cardiac/circulation) themselves. Drugs (D) are only considered if the baby is still not improving after Airways and Breathing have been correctly attended to.

Procedure of resuscitation

(Resuscitation is easier with two pairs of hands than one – get assistance if available.)

- **Keep the baby warm** at all times. Dry the baby with a warm towel or cloth.
- **Place the baby head down on a gently sloping resuscitation table.**
- **Clear the airways** (nose, nasopharynx and pharynx) of mucus, meconium, blood or fluid using a soft suction catheter (a negative pressure of 50 cmH$_2$O is usually adequate). This is best done under direct vision using a laryngoscope as a light source.

Table 14.5 Apgar score

	0	1	2
Appearance (Colour)	Pale or centrally and peripherally cyanosed	Centrally pink peripherally cyanosed	Pink centrally and peripherally
Pulse (Heart rate)	0	<100/min	100/min or >
Grimace (Response to stimulation)	Nil	Grimace	Cry or cough
Activity (Muscle tone)	Completely floppy	Reduced/No active movement	Normal activity
Respiration	Absent	Gasping/Irregular	Regular/Crying

- **Get air or oxygen into the baby.** Air may be as good as oxygen for neonatal resuscitation. The absence of an oxygen supply is therefore not an impediment to good neonatal resuscitation.

  Bag and mask is the best method of resuscitation for all but the most severely asphyxiated babies. Every health facility should have a working neonatal resuscitation bag and masks of varying sizes. Round masks with a pneumatic cuff are best. The mask should fit snuggly round the baby's nose and mouth. The baby's chin should be lifted gently, and the neck straightened into the neutral position, but care should be taken not to hyperextend the neck (this closes rather than opens the airway). The bag is squeezed at a rate of about 30/min, and chest expansion with each inspiration should be visible. An appropriately sized Guedel's airway may be used but is not essential.

  Intubation should be reserved for the most severely asphyxiated babies – those who are pale or blue with no respiration and a pulse rate below 60/min (Apgar 2 or less) – and for those in whom bag and mask ventilation is not producing the desired result. Neonatal intubation (use a size 3.5 endotracheal tube for big babies, a size 3 for small babies and a size 2.5 for the very small babies) is a specific skill. It is much better to provide good effective bag and mask ventilation than to waste time failing in attempts to intubate.

  Mouth to face (nose and mouth) resuscitation can be used in the absence of bag and mask or intubation equipment
- In the vast majority of cases the heart rate will increase with adequate ventilation. **If there is still severe bradycardia** (pulse rate below 60/min) **after adequate ventilation is achieved, cardiac massage** using two fingers to depress the mid sternum at a rate of 100/min **may be tried** (three compressions to one breath). If this is unsuccessful **adrenaline 0.1 ml/kg of 1 in 10 000** (dilute 0.5 ml 1 in 1000 adrenaline with 4.5 ml normal saline or water for injection) may be given intravenously, or down an endotracheal tube.
- If spontaneous respiration does not occur within 5 min of commencing adequate ventilation and achieving oxygenation (as determined by a pulse rate of >100/min), or if there is persistent bradycardia the **administration of drugs** (naloxone, sodium bicarbonate, dextrose) **should be considered.**

  If mother has had pethidine or other opiate analgesia within 8 h of delivery **naloxone 10 μg/kg** can be given i.v. or i.m.

  The possibility of continuing acidosis should be considered in babies who have been severely asphyxiated and **sodium bicarbonate (1 ml/kg of 8.4% or 2 ml/kg of 4.2%)** given i.v.

  The possibility of hypoglycaemia should always be considered and if possible blood sugar checked with a Dextrostix test. In proven (blood sugar of <2 mmol/l) or suspected hypoglycaemia **10% Dextrose 3–5 ml/kg or 50% dextrose 1 ml/kg** should be given i.v.

  If peripheral venous access is not achieved relatively quickly, an umbilical venous catheter should be inserted (a size 5 or 8 Fr feeding tube can be used if necessary). The cord is cut 2–3 cm above the umbilicus. Bleeding can be controlled by compressing the cord. The catheter should be inserted to a distance of two-thirds of the distance between the umbilicus and the shoulder. It may be necessary to clamp the umbilical arteries, and a purse-string suture should be applied. If the catheter is to be left in for any length of time. The drugs given i.v. (by either route) should always be flushed through with normal saline.

> **PRACTICE POINT**
>
> 1. Air is probably as good as oxygen for neonatal resuscitation.
> 2. Every health worker attending deliveries should be familiar with the use of the neonatal bag and mask, and every health centre should have a working bag and mask.
> 3. It is much better to use a bag and mask well than to waste time trying unsuccessfully to perform neonatal intubation.

Prevention of meconium aspiration

Once thick, viscid meconium has been aspirated into the lungs, there is little that can be done other than supportive treatment. It is thus important that meconium aspiration be prevented if at all possible.

During labour

Where there is heavy staining of the amniotic fluid with thick, viscid meconium, meconium washout should be performed. This is done by inserting a 22 Fr catheter through the cervix and irrigating with **warm** normal saline, allowing the saline and meconium stained fluid to drain out. The first 500 ml is run in quickly and a further 500 ml over an hour. This not only washes out the meconium but also supplements the amniotic fluid volume, minimising umbilical compression by fetal parts.

At delivery

The baby's upper airways should be sucked out as thoroughly as is possible as soon as the head is delivered and before the delivery of the body. It is helpful to have an assistant for this. Delivery can then be completed, the cord clamped and cut, and the baby carried immediately in a dry warm towel or cloth to the resuscitation area.

If the baby is delivered before suction can be performed suction before the baby takes a deep breath may prevent aspiration. The chest should be gently compressed to discourage breathing while suction is being performed. This is the only intervention that takes priority over drying and wrapping the baby.

On the resuscitation tray any remaining meconium should be sucked out under direct vision. If the resuscitator is skilled in neonatal intubation, and if meconium is visible below the vocal cords an endotracheal tube should be passed and the trachea sucked out, either through a suction catheter passed through the endotracheal tube, or by applying suction to the tube itself during slow extubation.

Post-delivery care of asphxiated babies

Babies with mild degrees of asphyxia usually do well, and can generally be looked after by their mothers with regular observation by nursing staff.

Babies with severe asphyxia have high mortality and high morbidity. There may be a deceptive period of several hours when the baby seems reasonably well, but this if often followed by the development of major neurological dysfunction as raised intracranial pressure develops. Convulsions, apnoea, and metabolic disorders including hypoglycaemia (the most common), hypocalcaemia and hyponatraemia are frequent.

Treatment is primarily supportive – maintaining temperature, oxygenation, and blood sugar levels. Phenobarbital is usually given to prevent fits and paraldehyde or diazepam to control them (be aware that the combination of phenobarbital and diazepam may produce respiratory depression). Phenytoin may be used if preventative treatment with phenobarbital is inadequate. Steroids and mannitol are often given but of no proven benefit. Fluid administration is reduced to two-thirds maintenance (40 ml/kg) or less.

Survivors of severe neonatal asphyxia are often severely and permanently neurologically damaged.

Every effort should be made to prevent perinatal asphyxia by detecting high-risk pregnancies, making sure that the affected mothers are referred to facilities offering the highest available level of obstetric and neonatal care and paying due attention to the basic obstetric rules of labour and delivery. Fetal heart rate monitoring may detect signs of early fetal distress, allowing for early intervention. A fetal stethoscope, if used correctly, is almost as efficient as a cardiotocogram.

> **PRACTICE POINT**
>
> The outcome for severely asphyxiated babies is very poor. Efforts must be directed at prevention of neonatal asphyxia.

Further reading

Advanced Life Support Group. Resuscitation at birth. In: *Advanced Paediatric Life Support. The Practical Approach*. 3rd edition. London: BMJ Books, 2001:59–67.

SLATTERY MM, MORRISON JJ. Preterm delivery. *Lancet* 2002;360:1489–97.

15
Nutritional support in the critically ill

Definitions

Normal nutrition supplies the body's requirements in terms of energy, protein, vitamins and trace elements. The protein must contain sufficient essential amino acids and the energy source must include both carbohydrate and fat, including essential fatty acids. Malnutrition implies undernutrition or obesity.

In critical illness the major problems are lack of nutrition and accelerated catabolism. Patients whose critical illness accompanies or complicates underlying malnutrition, particularly children, carry a much worse prognosis. They are more susceptible to infection, they have reduced immunological function and poorer wound healing. Grossly obese patients are also more prone to complications of a critical illness such as pneumonia and thromboembolism.

The energy contained in the fat deposits (approximately 141 000 kcal in a 70 kg man) is largely unavailable during critical illness and the small store of glucose in the blood and glycogen in the liver are quickly utilised, which leads to a breakdown of protein from muscle for energy supplies. The loss of protein or lean body mass results in impaired immunity and healing and weight loss. These effects develop rapidly unless nutritional intake can be maintained and arise sooner in patients who were already malnourished when they became ill.

The metabolic demands are far less in starvation than in critical illness. This is because the starving patient can adapt and utilise fat stores to provide energy and so reduce the catabolism of protein. A starving but otherwise healthy adult survives 4–8 weeks, whereas a critically ill patient receiving no nutritional intake from the onset of illness may live only 10–21 days.

Recognition of malnutrition

It is fairly easy to recognise the severely wasted individual with marked weight loss due to muscle and fat atrophy. However visual assessment is usually inaccurate unless the malnutrition is extreme. By the time the patient is obviously malnourished it may be too late to save him.

Unfortunately there is no single test which can be interpreted as meaning a patient is malnourished. As a result, different tests have been developed which in combination provide a profile of nutritional status. These tests are listed in Table 15.1.

Many people do not know their normal weight. Some tropical countries have developed standard weight-for-height or weight-for-age charts for children but there is little data for adults. Triceps skinfold thickness and arm-muscle circumference also lack standardised charts in many developing countries.

Nutritional support in the critically ill

Table 15.1 Measurements of nutritional status

Physical
  Weight for height or age[1]
  % weight loss, % ideal weight for height or age
  Arm muscle circumference[1,2]
  Triceps skin-fold thickness
  Hand-grip dynamometry

Biochemical
  Albumin[1]
  Prealbumin
  Transferin or total iron binding capacity (TIBC)
  Creatinine (creatinine–height index)

Immunological
  Total lymphocyte count[1]
  Hypersensitivity to common antigens by skin tests

[1] Denotes simplest and most reliable tests in each group.
[2] Arm muscle circumference (cm) = Arm circumference (cm) − (0.314 × Triceps skin-fold thickness) (mm)

In hospitals where laboratory services are poor, nutritional assessment is probably best determined by measuring height, weight, arm muscle circumference and skin-fold thickness. You need only skin calipers, bathroom scales and a tape measure. Children can be weighed by the nurse weighing first herself alone and then herself holding the baby. If skin calipers are not available arm circumference, measured at the midpoint of the upper arm between the olecranon and the acromion, will approximate well to arm muscle circumference in individuals who do not carry a lot of subcutaneous fat (Figure 15.1). In critically ill patients daily weight change is a more accurate measure of fluid balance than of nutritional status.

If laboratory facilities for measuring the total lymphocyte count and serum albumin are available then nutritional status is fairly accurately assessed by arm muscle circumference, serum albumin and total lymphocyte counts.

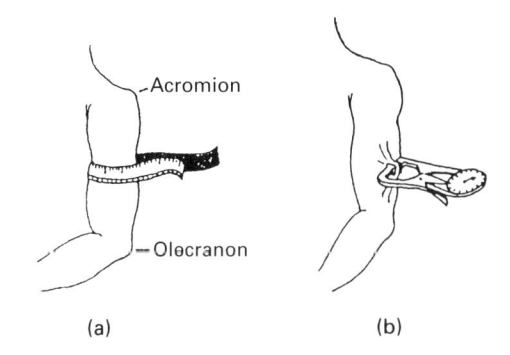

Figure 15.1 Nutritional status: assessment of (a) arm circumference and (b) skin fold thickness measured at a point midway between between the acromion and olecranon.

Moderate nutritional failure may be defined as weight loss of over 10%, total lymphocyte count less than $1500/mm^3$ and albumin less than 30 g/l. The arm muscle circumference will be below 21 cm in the adult male and 18 cm in the adult female.

Severe malnutrition may be defined as weight loss over 30% normal, total lymphocyte count less than $1000/mm^3$ and albumin less than 22 g/l. Arm muscle circumference will be below 18 cm in the male and 16 cm in the female.

Once fat stores are being utilised for energy the urine will contain ketones. Protein and nitrogen balance can be easily calculated according to the formula:

$$\textit{Intake} \quad \frac{\text{protein (g)}}{6.25} = \text{nitrogen (g)}$$

$$\textit{Output} \quad 24\,h\ \text{urine urea (mmol)} \times 0.035 + 2 = g\ \text{nitrogen}/24\,h$$

When nitrogen balance is negative it means there is a net breakdown of protein for energy requirements. A negative nitrogen balance is inevitable in the first few days of a critical illness. The 2 g in the formula represents skin and faecal loss of nitrogen. Urine urea is not a difficult test to perform but it must be done on a 24 h sample since there is a wide variation in urea excretion throughout the day.

Nutritional support

Ideally, nutritional failure should not be allowed to develop in the critically ill patient. The key to successful nutritional support is to supply the predicted nutritional requirements in a utilisable form as soon as possible and for as long as is necessary.

Energy requirements

Exact energy expenditure can be measured only as a research technique. Therefore energy requirements must be estimated according to diagnosis, weight of the patient and age.

Energy requirements are based on resting metabolic expenditure and energy expenditure due to activity. Although a labourer may need up to 4000 kcal per day a sedentary person may only use 2000 kcal. Studies on surgical patients suggest that the resting metabolic expenditure is 1000–1200 kcal per day, depending on the disease process, the magnitude of the operation, and the age and weight of the patient. If the patient is septic then the energy expenditure is increased by 200–300 kcal and if recovering from an operation another 200 kcal. Thus most surgical patients require fewer than 2000 kcal per day, probably fewer than 1500 kcal if the patient weighs less than 50 kg and is not septic. The only category of critically ill patient who is markedly different is the patient with burns. These patients have a vastly increased energy expenditure and about 500 kcal should be added for each 10% area of burn.

KEYPOINT
Burned patients have increased nutritional requirements.

A critically ill patient cannot handle extra calories. During a critical illness it is not possible to improve a patient's nutritional status but only to maintain it and prevent loss of lean body mass. Excessive calories will provide metabolic stress producing hyperglycaemia, fatty liver with cholestasis and sometimes hyperosmolar coma.

A good rule of thumb is to provide 25 kcal/kg in older children and adults. Add 5 kcal/kg if the patient has had major surgery and another 5 kcal/kg if the patient is septic. This should be enough in the non-burned, critically ill patient to maintain lean body mass. Add 1 kcal/kg/1% area of burn (see p. 241).

In protein–calorie malnutrition in children give 150 kcal/kg/day (p. 290).

Protein and nitrogen requirements

The average adult needs about 70 g protein per day. This can be provided by soya bean, sour milk and eggs if the gastrointestinal tract is functioning, as these foodstuffs contain all the essential amino acids. If intravenous nutrition is to be given then amino acid solutions are used. Since amino acids contain nitrogen it is usual to talk about nitrogen requirements. There is 1 g of nitrogen in 6.25 g of protein, so the average adult needs 11–12 g nitrogen. One aim of nutritional support is to keep the patient in positive nitrogen balance. Provide slightly more (1–2 g extra) nitrogen than is being lost. Nitrogen is normally lost in the urine (mainly as urea), in the faeces, and from the skin by cell loss. Excess losses occur from intestinal secretions where there is a fistula or from open wounds such as burns. Nitrogen loss can be calculated from the formula on the page 285. In practice, if 12–14 g of nitrogen (70–90 g protein) are given daily this will preserve the lean body mass.

In protein–calorie malnutrition in children give 4 g/kg/day of protein.

Vitamins and trace elements

These must be provided in long-term nutritional support. See under specific regimens (Table 15.3). Folic acid (5 mg twice weekly) is indicated in patients with increased red cell turnover, e.g. severe haemolysis.

Who needs nutritional support?

Any patient who is unlikely to resume a normal oral diet within 5 days is likely to need nutritional support. This will include patients with coma, tetanus, bulbar palsy, prolonged endotracheal intubation, and those with gastrointestinal failure due to small-bowel fistula, short-bowel syndrome, abdominal tuberculosis, complicated pancreatitis and intra-abdominal sepsis.

KEYPOINT
If the gastrointestinal tract is functioning always use enteral nutrition.

Enteral nutrition

Enteral nutrition is given by mouth, by nasogastric tube or by 'ostomy feed. If fine-bore nasogastric tubes are used then commercial feeds will have to be given. These are relatively expensive, are not widely available in developing countries and confer little benefit over locally made liquidised food given through a normal, plastic, wide-bore nasogastric tube. The wide-bore tubes are more irritant and uncomfortable but we have found them to be satisfactory and have not yet seen complications such as oesophageal ulcers or strictures, even in patients fed for some weeks.

KEYPOINT
Ensure the nasogastric tube is in the stomach before commencing feeds.

The method of inserting a nasogastric tube is described on p. 374. Feeding should be gradually increased in both concentration and volume. Table 15.2 shows how we increase the feed, reaching 2 litres of full strength after 4 days. It is often possible to reach full-strength feeds and full volumes within 2–3 days. The feed should provide the nutritional requirements already described. One should be guided by the response of the gastrointestinal tract to feeding. High aspirates, vomiting, abdominal distension or diarrhoea are signs that feeding must be either reduced or stopped.

It is possible to give enteral nutrition continuously using a drip (often with an infusion controller), or by bolus injections down the tube. In our unit we use the latter method as it is more economical in nursing time and also more physiological. There is probably little to choose between the methods.

The main complications of enteral nutrition are diarrhoea and fluid and electrolyte imbalance. If severe diarrhoea occurs then stop the feed for 1–2 days and recommence once it has settled. The diarrhoea can often be controlled using oral rehydration salt for 24–48 h. If milk is used in the enteral feed try stopping the milk as some patients are lactose-intolerant. Another complication is the development of gastric or intestinal ileus, resulting in increased nasogastric aspirations. If this occurs correct any electrolyte imbalance, maintain the patient on intravenous fluids and wait until aspirations subside before attempting to reintroduce the feeds.

Aspiration pneumonia may occur owing either to a misplaced nasogastric tube

Table 15.2 Build-up of nasogastric feeding

Day 1	1	litre quarter-strength
2	1.5	litres half-strength
3	2	litres three-quarters-strength
4	2	litres full-strength

(Figure 15.2) or to regurgitation up the oesophagus. If the patient is conscious sit him upright for feeds. Otherwise lay him on his side if the airway is not protected by an endotracheal tube.

Other complications are due to the constituents of the feed. There may be excessive glucose causing hyperglycaemia. Complications due to the feed are much less likely to occur in enteral than parenteral nutrition. The introduction of infection is rare. Changes in liver function tests may develop in patients on long-term feeding but these reverse once the patient is eating normally.

Parenteral nutrition

Patients who require a nutritional support and whose gastrointestinal tract is not functioning need parenteral nutrition. Parenteral nutrition costs $US50–100 per day (which is about the same as an expensive antibiotic, e.g. cefotaxime, or anticancer cytotoxic therapy). Its use may be appropriate in carefully selected patients with a good prognosis in some institutions in developing countries.

A typical regimen for parenteral nutrition in critically ill patients is shown in Table 15.3. Parenteral nutrition is normally given through a central venous line because of the high osmolarity of the solutions given, which rapidly thrombose peripheral veins. It is however possible to change veins daily and give adequate nutritional support via peripheral veins, but the method is troublesome. A central vein with a subcutaneous tunnel to minimise the risk of infection is the simplest and most convenient method (see p. 384). Mixing compatible solutions in a 3-litre bag allows for much simpler administration of the nutrients and reduced risk of infection. They can also be given using multiple bottles and Y connections with giving sets but the amino acids and calories should be given simultaneously to avoid the amino acids being metabolised to supply energy needs rather than being incorporated in protein synthesis.

The complications of parenteral nutrition are shown in Table 15.4 (see also p. 391). Daily use of Intralipid is associated with fewer metabolic complications so that 25–50% of the calorie requirements are given in the form of fat. Intralipid is a more expensive energy

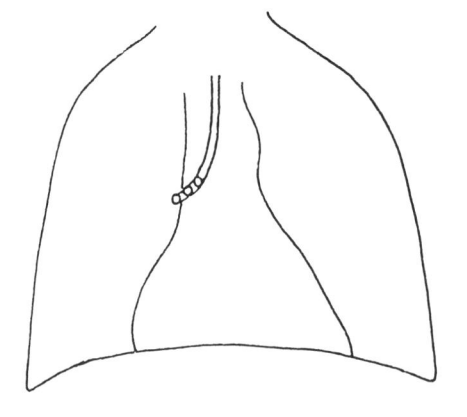

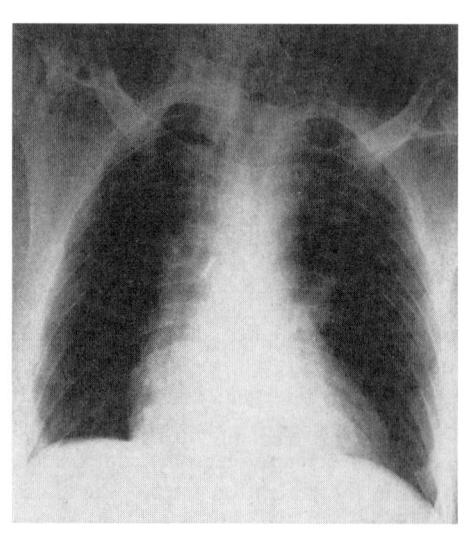

Figure 15.2 The importance of checking the position of a nasogastric tube: note the tip of the nasogastric tube is in the right main bronchus. This tube was NOT checked before feeding was commenced and the patient developed a pneumonia as a result.

Table 15.3 Parenteral feeding regimen

Synthamin 14	1000 ml	14 g nitrogen as amino acids
Dextrose 20%	1500 ml	1200 kcal energy[2]
Intralipid 10%	500 ml	500 kcal energy[2]
Addamel	3 vials per week	Trace elements
Soluvit	3 vials per week	Water-soluble vitamins
Vitalipid	3 vials per week	Fat-soluble vitamins
Electrolyte requirements		(total per day)[1]
Sodium		120 mmol
Potassium		70 mmol
Calcium		10 mmol
Phosphate		30 mmol

1 Calculate electrolytes in the above solutions and add extra as required to reach total amount. More electrolytes will be needed if there are increased losses as in intestinal fistula. Refer to Table 4.3 for electrolyte content of various intestinal secretions.

2 If Intralipid 10% once or twice a week is to be given then make up daily energy needs using dextrose on days when Intralipid is not being given. With dextrose as the only energy source it is likely that 40–80 units per day of insulin should be given in the 3 litre bag. Titrate dose of insulin against the blood glucose.

Table 15.4 Some complications of parenteral nutrition

Complication	Avoidance	Action
Related to central venous line		
On insertion		
Pneumothorax	Correct technique	Chest drain
Vascular damage	Correct technique	Remove, reinsert
Air embolism	Head-down tilt	Thoracotomy, aspirate ventricle
Presence of line		
Thrombosis	Place in large central vein	Remove line
	Heparin	
Infection	Subcutaneous tunnel	Remove line
	Meticulous care of catheter site	
	Ensure sterility of solutions	
	Change giving sets daily	
Catheter migration	Secure properly	Remove, reinsert
Catheter blocked	Supervision of flow	Remove if not detected immediately
Related to nutrients		
Hyperglycaemia	Insulin	Increase
	Use Intralipid daily	Insulin
Hyperosmolar syndrome	Reduce osmolarity	
	Rehydrate	
Fatty liver	Use Intralipid daily	
Venous thrombosis	Reduce osmolarity of solutions	

source than dextrose. To supply essential fatty acids it need only be given once or twice a week and if unavailable the patient can be anointed with sunflower oil which enables essential fatty acids to be absorbed through the skin.

Stopping nutritional support

Patients receiving nutritional support are expected to recover. It can be discontinued once an adequate oral diet is being taken. In the case of parenteral nutrition the

Table 15.5 Feeding regimen for protein–calorie malnutrition in children

Protein–calorie mix	
Skimmed milk powder	124 g
Sugar	130 g
Oil	80 ml
Add water to make	1000 ml
Lactose-free mix	
Casilan	45 g
Sugar	60 g
Oil	150 ml
Add water to make	1000 ml

Both feeds are given at a rate of 100 ml/kg/day. Feed every 3 h, omitting the 0300 h feed and give 14 ml/kg/feed. This regime provides 150 kcal/kg/day and 4 g protein/kg/day.

support can be tailed off over 1 or 2 days as the patient's oral intake increases. If at any time the prognosis changes and becomes hopeless then nutritional support should be stopped.

The child with critical malnutrition

Severely malnourished children usually die of infection – often gastroenteritis – compounded by dehydration, electrolyte imbalance or severe anaemia. Therefore a critically-ill malnourished child is managed so as to detect and treat infection (including malaria), electrolyte abnormality (especially potassium) and severe anaemia. This is additional to enteral nutritional support in children who cannot take sufficient nutrient by mouth. If nasogastric tube feeding is required the feeding regime in Table 15.5 has proved satisfactory. Oil should be omitted if diarrhoea is severe. If the child recovers from the acute illness nutritional rehabilitation and education of the family is necessary to prevent recurrence.

Further reading

ALLISON SP. Nutritional problems in intensive care. *Hospital Update* 1984 Dec;1001–12.

BLACKBURN GL, *et al.* Nutritional and metabolic assessment of the hospitalized patient. *JPEN J Parenter Enteral Nutr* 1977;1:11–22.

GRIFFITHS RD. Specialized nutrition support in critically ill patients. *Curr Opin Crit Care* 2003;9:249–59.

MACFIE J. Energy requirements of surgical patients requiring intravenous nutrition. *Ann R Coll Surg Engl* 1984;66:39–42.

MARIK PE, ZALOGA GP. Early enteral nutrition in acutely ill patients: a systematic review. *Crit Care Med* 2001;29:2264–70.

PRESS M, HARTOP PJ, PROWEY C. Correction of essential fatty acid deficiency in man by the cutaneous application of sunflower seed oil. *Lancet* 1974;i:597–8.

RYAN JA, PAGE CP. Intrajejunal feeding: development and current status. *JPEN J Parenter Enteral Nutr* 1984;8:187–98.

WERNERMAN J. Glutamine and acute illness. *Curr Opin Crit Care* 2003;9:279–85.

16
Nursing critically ill patients

Problems of nursing critical illness

Without good nursing care many seriously ill patients will die regardless of the medical treatment; both patients and doctors rely heavily on the nurses in critical illness. Patients are usually bedridden and dependent for virtually all bodily needs. In addition most will need emotional support and reassurance. Nurses should always talk to their patients, even if unconsious, explaining what they are doing, however ordinary it may seem to them. Always assume that every patient can hear and so may be comforted by conversation, but may also be distressed by discussion about the prognosis at the bedside. The doctors rely on the nurses for accurate monitoring of the patient's progress, for prompt and effective action if there is sudden deterioration and for reliable administration of treatment.

In this chapter the importance of established routines of nursing care is emphasised and less well-known procedures and important routines in seriously ill patients are described.

Standard nursing care

Positioning the patient

The position of seriously ill patients can significantly influence the outcome.

Prevention of venous thrombosis

Try and prevent patients lying with their legs crossed as this may predispose to impaired venous return and deep calf vein thrombosis. Frequent leg and foot movements should be encouraged as a further measure against venous thrombosis.

The unconscious patient

The first priorities are to safeguard the airway and also the cervical spine in cases where cervical spine injury has not been ruled out. When spinal injury is not a concern the correct position for a patient in coma is three-quarter prone as shown in Figure 16.1. In this position the tongue cannot fall back and block the airway, oral secretions or vomit cannot be inhaled and the neck is not twisted into an unnatural position. The other positions shown (Figure 16.1) are not safe unless the patient is intubated. If the patient is lying on his back the tongue will occlude the airway and oral secretions or vomit may be inhaled leading to pneumonia and either way the patient will die. Twisting the head to one side does not safeguard the airway and may obstruct venous drainage from the head, leading to a rise in intracranial pressure. The comatose patient is usually nursed with the head of the bed elevated 15°.

The hypotensive patient

Unless he is also dyspnoeic the hypotensive patient should be nursed with the end

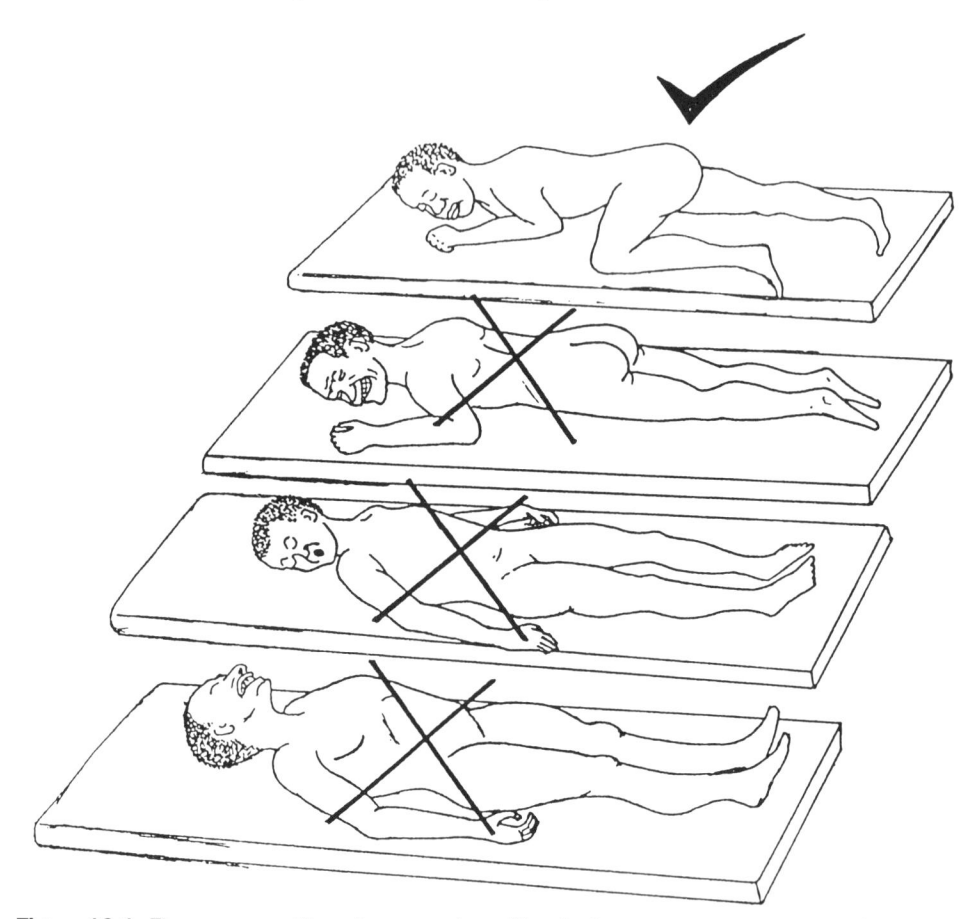

Figure 16.1 The coma position: the correct position is three-quarters prone, as shown.

of the bed elevated to aid the return of blood to the heart. If hypotension is associated with severe dyspnoea the patient will need to be propped up despite the low blood pressure unless ventilatory support can be given.

The breathless patient

Patients with severe dyspnoea cannot lie flat as pressure from the diaphragm further hinders breathing. The patient should be made comfortable sitting up with pillows and if possible a backrest. If in addition to dyspnoea the patient is comatose or hypotensive then ventilatory support is desirable as the patient is safer if nursed flat.

The patient with an unstable neck or spine

To reduce the risk of damage to the spinal cord by movement or poor positioning the patient is usually treated by traction (Figure 11.7), which stabilises the spine. Before traction is applied great care is needed when positioning or moving the patient. With fractures of the neck a senior nurse or doctor must be given the sole responsibility of holding the head and maintaining it in neutral alignment (p. 203) when moving the patient. In bed the patient should be kept flat and the position of the head and neck maintained with sandbags or use a Stiffneck collar if available (Figure 11.5).

Nursing of patients with injuries of thoracic or lumbar vertebrae is more difficult because there is no simple way these bones can be immobilised. The patient must be nursed flat and when moved every effort should be made to keep the spine straight. The impact at the time of injury sufficient to damage the vertebrae is so great that gentle movement of the patient is unlikely to cause additional damage to the spinal cord. The ideal way of nursing these patients is on a Stryker frame, but this is unlikely to be available. A simple alternative is to place wedges under the mattress to lift the patient's weight off the side being wedged.

The postoperative patient

Patients who have not recovered consciousness should be positioned in the same way as other comatose patients (Figure 16.1) Once the airway is safe and the blood pressure stable the position will depend on the operation performed. Following abdominal surgery the patient should be encouraged to sit up and breathe deeply to prevent chest infections.

Mouth cleaning

Patients who cannot take oral fluids and those with an orotracheal tube are prone to develop dirty mouths which predispose to infection. Mouth cleaning (with saline or sodium bicarbonate) should be carried out at least 4 hourly and more often if necessary. Keep lips moistened to prevent cracking.

Eye care

Unconscious patients who are unable to blink or to protect the eyes are at special risk of corneal damage and of eye infections. The eyes should be kept closed using Lacri-Lube and Glad wrap or OpSite. An alternative is paraffin gauze laid over the upper lid and brought down onto the cheek; the same effect can be obtained using Micropore or Sellotape but strapping should not be used because it will damage the skin. Four hourly ocular lubricants (e.g. artificial tears, carmellose sodium, hypromellose, Lacri-Lube) help prevent drying of the cornea and 4 hourly irrigation with normal saline helps to prevent infection. If there is conjunctivitis (manifest by a red eye with sticky secretions) then an antibiotic ointment (e.g. chloramphenicol or tetracycline) should be instilled after cleaning.

Pressure area care

Prolonged pressure on the skin overlying boney prominences impedes the skin circulation, leading to ischaemia and necrosis. The main pressure points are over the sacrum, the hips, the heels, the spine, the shoulders, the elbows and the back of the head (Figure 16.2a). Pressure sores can

(a)

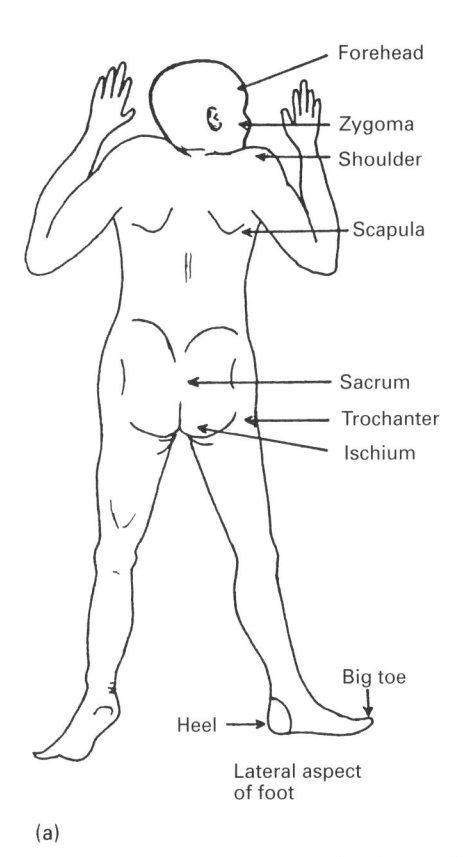

Figure 16.2 (a) Pressure areas to be observed and protected.

be graded (Figure 16.2b). They are usually the result of neglecting pressure areas and indicate inadequate nursing. They jeopardise the patient's chances of recovery, cause considerable pain and prolong the time in hospital. When extensive, pressure sores may need complicated reconstructive surgery.

> **KEYPOINT**
>
> You cannot turn a comatose patient on your own.

Pressure points can be protected by placing sheepskins under the bottom sheet and by using protective rings (water-filled surgical gloves are a substitute). Pressure area care must be given at least 2 hourly.

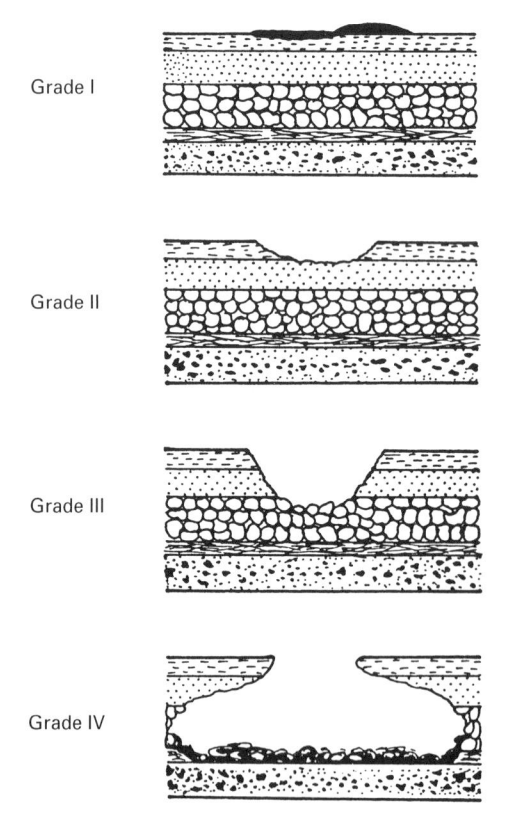

Figure 16.2 (b) Grades of pressure sores.

Table 16.1 Measures which prevent pressure sores

2 hourly turning.
2 hourly inspection of pressure areas.
Lifting not dragging the patient.
Keeping the skin dry and clean.
Changing the sheets when they are wet.
Avoiding adherent strapping.
Use of sheepskin or a ripple mattress.
Water-filled gloves to protect the heels.

Avoid dragging; lift the patient as the friction of dragging the patient across sheets damages the skin (Table 16.1).

Further reading

BADER DL. (ed.) *Pressure Sores – A Practical Problem*. Basingstoke: Macmillan, 1990.
DESFORGES JF. Pressure ulcers among the elderly. *N Engl J. Med* 1989;320:850–3.

Nutrition

Providing there are no contraindications, oral or nasogastric feeding should be commenced within 2 or 3 days to prevent acute nutritional or calorie deficiency. Patients who cannot take by mouth require nasogastric (enteral) or intravenous (parenteral) feeding. Feeding may also be given via a gastrostomy or jejunostomy tube when indicated. Details of nutritional requirements and of enteral and parenteral feeding are described in the chapter on nutrition (p. 286). Only general aspects of nutrition as they relate to nursing are discussed in this section.

In patients taking by mouth the main problem encountered will be unwillingness to eat. The nurse must try and overcome this by patient persuasion, which takes time and effort. Some patients can be encouraged if the relatives bring in food the patient wants from home. Those with normally functioning intestines who cannot take by mouth (e.g. comatose patients) are fed through a nasogastric tube. The feed supplied for 24 h should contain all nutritional and fluid requirements and is usually given as 6–8 feeds in the day. Before each feed always check the position of the nasogastric tube (p. 374) and aspirate the nasogastric tube. If more than 100 ml is aspirated omit the feed. After each feed a small amount of water should be given to clean the nasogastric tube.

Parenteral feeding is considered only when oral and enteral feeding are not possible and is discussed more fully on p. 288. Parenteral feeding requires a central venous line and special care is needed to prevent its accidental removal or the introduction of infection.

Fluid balance

In patients taking by mouth fluid intake must be recorded and must be adequate. Those who are unable to take fluids orally will require nasogastric or intravenous fluids and the duty of the nurse is to ensure the prescribed amount of fluid is given and recorded.

In calculating fluid requirements the current fluid balance must be considered, which includes the patient's hydration and any positive or negative balance of the previous day. The formula for calculating daily fluid requirements is:

$$\frac{intake}{24\,h} = \text{measured output in previous 24 h,}$$

plus estimated insensible loss in 24 previous hours,

plus or minus previous day's balance.

The practice of recording a cumulative balance is seldom useful and may cause confusion. In a patient who is well hydrated the aim is to replace the previous day's fluid losses (i.e. urine, vomit, nasogastric aspirate, diarrhoea and drains), plus insensible loss which is usually 500 to 1000 ml. Insensible losses are increased by excessive sweating, oropharyngeal suction of secretions, hypersalivation, warm weather, fever and endotracheal intubation without humidification. In patients in negative or positive balance from the previous day the fluid needs are increased or reduced respectively. Concentrated urine and, in the absence of renal failure, a urine output of less than 50 ml/h in an adult suggests inadequate fluid intake.

Bowels

Constipation or diarrhoea may complicate the progress of a serious illness. Bowel movements should be recorded and the presence of diarrhoea reported. In a patient taking food orally or being fed by nasogastric tube, bowel movements should occur approximately every 2 or 3 days. If they fail to do so then rectal examination should be performed and if the rectum is empty a suppository given. Bowel movements are normally infrequent in patients not taking by mouth and in postoperative patients following laparotomy. Laxatives and suppositories should not be given without discussing it with the doctor. Faecal impaction causes abdominal distension and the rectum contains hard faeces; it should be treated with an enema. But if this fails manual removal is required.

Special nursing procedures

These are described in detail because of their importance in the care of critically ill patients.

Care of intravenous lines

Infection is the commonest problem of intravenous cannulae and may be localised

(thrombophlebitis) or may progress to septicaemia. Careful technique during insertion and when caring for intravenous lines will reduce the risk of infection. Special attention should be given to the following aspects:
1. Use aseptic technique during insertion.
2. Only use sterile cannulae.
3. Leave the site of insertion and surrounding skin exposed or cover with a loose dry dressing which must be changed daily.
4. Inspect the infusion site regularly and if the patient complains of pain at the site or along the limb.
5. Use aseptic technique when changing the infusion or the giving set.
   Clean the site of insertion twice daily with dilute Savlon or another antiseptic and report if it appears infected.
6. Resite the cannula:
   (a) whenever there are local signs of inflammation;
   (b) if possible routinely every 48 h;
   (c) whenever flow is unsatisfactory and not improved by flushing.

In addition care must be taken to infuse the correct fluid at the correct rate. Errors commonly arise from the following:
1. *Unclear medical instructions.* If medical instructions cannot be understood ask the doctor to clarify his order.
2. *The wrong blood or fluid.* If blood is being transfused check the patient's name and group against the blood pack and check the pack number against the laboratory's report of the cross match. It is wise for two people to check blood.
3. *Drug errors.* Two people should check any additives to the infusion against the drug orders. Additives must be inserted with a sterile needle and syringe (see also i.v. administration of drugs, pp. 302, 435).
4. *Infusion at the wrong rate.* Infusions given too slowly or too fast are dangerous and the rate of infusion needs frequent checking. It may be difficult to adjust the rate for very slow infusions (commonly needed in children). In such circumstances try and use a paediatric giving set and burette or an infusion controller (e.g. a Dialaflo or Accudrop). Electronic pumps and flow meters are rarely needed. They are expensive and frequently go out of order, becoming useless unless there is an after-sales service.

The rate of infusion depends on the size of the drop (and therefore the number of drops per ml). In adult infusion sets 1.0 ml is contained in 15 drops whereas in most paediatric sets (including burettes) 1.0 ml is contained in 60 microdrops. To calculate the number of drops to be given per minute for a given number of ml per hour use the following formula:

$$\text{drops per min} = \frac{\text{drops/ml} \times \text{ml/h}}{60}$$

EXAMPLE

You are instructed to give 1000 ml over 24 h.

This means you must give 1000 ml divided by 24 every hour which equals 41.6 ml – say 40 ml/h. If you are using an adult giving set the calculation is:

$$\frac{15 \times 40}{60} = 10 \text{ drops/min}$$

This infusion rate would be unlikely in an adult but quite probable in a child. If you are using a paediatric giving set the calculation is:

$$\frac{60 \times 40}{60} = 40 \text{ microdrops/min}$$

Thus when using a paediatric giving set delivering 60 microdrops per millilitre the number of drops per minute equals the number of millilitres per hour.

Central venous lines are long catheters inserted into major veins such as the subclavian, the jugular or the femoral. They are difficult to insert and care must be taken to avoid their accidental removal by a restless patient or when turning the patient. The catheter site should be cleaned and dressed twice daily and the giving set changed daily whenever possible. If a central line is in position, central venous pressure (CVP) monitoring may be requested. The technique for measuring CVP is described on p. 388. Always ensure the drip is running again after measuring the CVP. Failure to recommence the infusion may result in the line becoming blocked. Whenever a central venous line is removed the tip should not be contaminated but should be cut off using sterile scissors and placed in a sterile container to be sent for culture.

Care of urethral catheters

The main problem associated with urethral catheters is infection. The catheter should be inserted with aseptic technique and the urethral meatus and external part of the catheter should be cleaned at least twice daily with an antiseptic which will not burn the urethra (avoid iodine or spirit; use dilute Savlon, chlorhexidine gluconate or even normal saline).

Urine may be drained continuously or intermittently. Intermittent drainage is recommended for patients with retention of urine due to injuries of the spine, as this helps to maintain bladder tone and later development of reflex bladder emptying. When drainage is intermittent the bladder should be emptied at least every 4 h. A closed system should be used for continuous drainage and the collecting bag should always remain below the patient. Distension of the collecting bag should be avoided. A patient who is catheterised and appears not to be passing urine may have a blocked, misplaced or dislodged catheter.

PRACTICE POINT
If the patient is not passing urine check the catheter is not blocked or misplaced.

Care of a nasogastric tube

A nasogastric tube may be required for gastric aspiration or for feeding and drug therapy. The *position* of the tube must be checked as soon as it is passed. The easiest way to confirm it is in the stomach is to fill a 10-ml syringe with air and blow this down the tube while listening with a stethescope over the epigastrium for the noise of the air entering the stomach. No whoosh of air means the tube is not in the stomach; remove it and start again. Never put fluid down a nasogastric tube until the position in the stomach is certain. Another way of checking the position of a nasogastric tube is to test the aspirate for acid. Nasogastric tubes with radio-opaque ends can be seen on X-ray.

Having positioned the tube correctly, record the length of tube outside the nose for future reference and secure it firmly. Care should be taken to avoid pressure from the tube causing damage to the nostril. The nose and mouth need extra cleaning when a nasogastric tube is in place. The presence of a nasogastric tube may make it difficult for the patient to cough, and chest physiotherapy is advisable. If the nasogastric tube is intended to keep the stomach empty continuous drainage is more satisfactory than intermittent aspiration.

Care of the endotracheal tube

Insertion of an endotracheal tube is described on p. 331. The normal upper airway functions of protection against infection, humidification of inspired air and expectoration of sputum by coughing are lost when an endotracheal (or tracheostomy) tube is in place. Nursing care must

replace these functions as far as possible and this requires the following:
1. frequent chest physiotherapy (p. 349);
2. aseptic suction of the airways (p. 352);
3. humidifying inspired air or gases (p. 347).

In addition, endotracheal tubes need to be firmly secured to prevent their dislodgement.

The position of an endotracheal tube should be checked repeatedly by the following means:
1. Checking the length of tube outside the patient's mouth or nose against the measurement made on insertion. Portex tubes and most red rubber tubes have centimetre markings from the tip. If not use a measuring tape (Figure 16.3) and always put a label above the patient's bed with the intubation details.
2. Examination of chest movements and breath sounds at regular intervals. If the tube dislodges out of the trachea chest movement and air entry will be greatly diminished on both sides. If the tube slips down it may enter the right main bronchus, preventing ventilation through the left main bronchus and chest movement and breath sounds of the left chest will be diminished or absent (Figure P2, p. 333). Problems with endotracheal tubes are discussed more fully on p. 333.

Cuffed endotracheal and tracheostomy tubes may cause pressure damage to the larynx. The risk is greater if the cuff is over-inflated and is less of a problem with Portex tubes. If rubber tubes are used deflation of the cuff at 2-hourly intervals is recommended. Before deflating the cuff oral secretions should be sucked out to prevent them being inhaled. In patients who are being ventilated through a cuffed tube ventilation should be increased when the cuff is released to compensate for the leak around the tube. In children (<11 years), non-cuffed tubes are usually used but if a cuffed tube has been inserted the cuff should not be inflated.

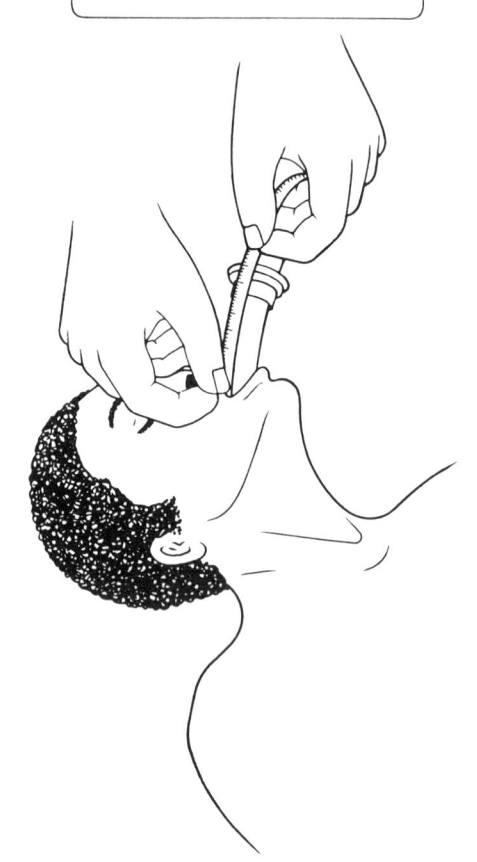

Figure 16.3 Measuring the position of an endotracheal tube. Measure the distance from the patient's upper teeth (or nose in the case of a nasal tube) to the endotracheal tube connector with a tape measure. Always check with the label above the bed that the tube remains in the same position.

Chest physiotherapy

The importance of chest physiotherapy in all seriously ill patients cannot be over emphasised. It prevents patients dying from accumulated secretions; it reduces the risks of pneumonia; it helps prevent collapse of parts of the lung; it is essential for patients with endotracheal or tracheostomy tubes in place and it is part of the treatment of virtually all acute chest problems.

Few hospitals in developing countries have enough physiotherapists for any patient to receive more than daily treatment from them. Seriously ill patients require chest physiotherapy every 4 h and it has become part of the nursing care of these patients. Ideally nurses should receive instruction in the techniques from a physiotherapist. The techniques are breathing exercises, postural drainage, chest vibration, encouragement of coughing, assisted coughing and suction of the airways and are described in detail in the section on practical procedures (p. 349).

Monitoring progress

The 'what' and 'why' of monitoring

Monitoring is the regular measurement and recording of certain physiological parameters, chosen because they are judged to be the best indicators of significant change in condition for that patient. Progress or deterioration results in altered observations, which may indicate the need to adjust treatment. For monitoring to be effective:
1. the observations carried out must be appropriate to the problem;
2. the frequency of observation must be sufficient to detect change in time for remedial action;
3. observations must be measured and recorded accurately;
4. the significance of changing observations must be known;
5. the action to be taken in the event of change or deterioration must be known;
6. that action must be taken.

It follows that inappropriate, infrequent, inaccurate or inadequately recorded observations are either misleading or useless. Also, monitoring is time wasted if nursing or medical staff fail to take appropriate action. However excessive observations (either too many or too frequent) are time-consuming for busy nurses, disturbing to the patient and more likely to be inaccurate.

Clinical observations (e.g. temperature, pulse rate, respiration rate, blood pressure, fluid intake and output recording, general or local skin or mucous membrane colour, peripheral pulses, mental state and Glasgow Coma Scale) requiring nothing more sophisticated than a thermometer, a watch with a second hand, a sphygmomanometer, a measuring jug, and a torch give sufficient information in most cases. The temptation to invest in more sophisticated monitoring equipment should be resisted unless the equipment can be adequately maintained, will aid management in a significant number of patients and is understood by the staff.

Which observations to monitor?

The temperature, pulse rate, respiration rate, conscious level, blood pressure and intake and output charting are relevant to all seriously ill patients. The diagnosis dictates additional observations required. Examples include the Glasgow Coma Scale (see below) for unconscious patients, blood sugars for diabetic ketoacidosis, the presence of cyanosis in respiratory distress, foot colour and pulses in a newly plastered leg and the number of ventricular ectopics in a patient with myocardial infarction.

How frequently to monitor?

The severity of illness, the probability of rapid change, the diagnosis and sometimes the treatment influence the optimum frequency of observation. The observations required may not all need to be done with the same frequency. In general, the more seriously ill the patient is the more frequent the observations will need to be and in rapidly changing situations (e.g. active bleeding) quarter-hourly measurements may be necessary. As a patient's condition stabilises the frequency can be reduced.

Recording the observations

Easily read charts with recordings shown graphically are preferred. More than one chart may be needed and special charts for specific problems are useful. Examples of charts used at the University Teaching Hospital, Lusaka, Zambia, are shown in Chapter 17. It is economical to use both sides of the paper, though preferably not for observations on the same day. Observation charts should be kept with the hospital record after the patient is discharged as they are often helpful when later reviewing management of patients.

Special monitoring

The Glasgow Coma Scale

This is a method of monitoring conscious level by recording eye opening, response to verbal commands and response to pain in a standardised way. It is indicated in all unconscious patients and is fully described in the chapter on coma (p. 166).

ECG monitoring

Continuous recording of cardiac rate and rhythm requires a special monitor and is generally not necessary except in patients with recent myocardial infarction or those at risk from serious arrhythmias (e.g. tetanus, chloroquine poisoning). Recognition and management of arrhythmias are described on pp. 56–65. The cost of ECG monitoring can be reduced by attaching the skin electrodes to a used infusion bag which is opened out (Figure 16.4). This way one set of electrodes can be used for up to ten patients but there is a risk of cross-infection and the method is not recommended unless electrodes are in very short supply and the benefits of cardiac monitoring outweigh the risks of cross infection.

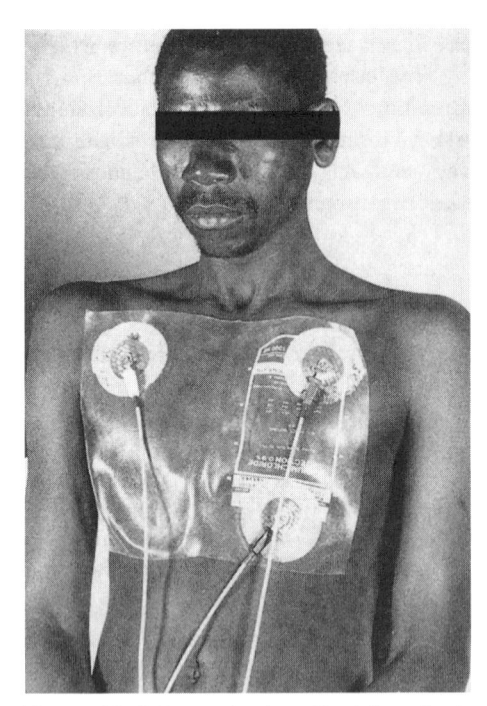

Figure 16.4 Improvised method for attaching ECG electrodes. A used plastic infusion bag is slit open and holes are made for the electrodes. The electrodes are secured with tape and then the plastic bag is attached to the patient's chest or back. As this system cannot be sterilised it is a potential source of cross-infection.

Central venous pressure monitoring

A cannula placed in a major vein allows the venous pressure to be measured. Examination of the major veins in the neck gives the same information but is considerably less accurate. If the neck veins are abnormally full the central venous pressure (CVP) is raised whereas if they are 'empty' when the patient is lying flat the CVP is an accurate reflection of the venous return to the right side of the heart and gives a good indication of the blood volume in relation to the capacity of the vascular bed. In patients with a low blood pressure the CVP helps to define the cause as it is low in hypovolaemia and raised in cardiogenic shock. CVP monitoring may be helpful in preventing fluid overload. Measuring the CVP is simple and requires only a central venous catheter and a ruler. It is fully described on pp. 388–392.

Administration of drugs

In seriously ill patients there is no room for error in drug administration. The use of intravenous drugs and dangerous drugs increases the risk of mistakes being fatal.

General precautions

1. Before giving any drug check for a history of drug reactions and any contraindications.
2. Drugs must be given in the correct dose by the correct route at correct time intervals and these details should be checked against the doctor's prescription.
3. Clearly record the dose and time of administration for each drug. This reduces the risk of a drug being omitted or given twice when nurses change shifts.
4. When giving drugs by injection use only sterile equipment and carefully disinfect the site of injection with a suitable antiseptic. This is especially important if you are injecting into an intravenous drip.
5. During intramuscular injection try and make the patient relax; use only those sites shown in Figure 16.5. Check that the needle is not in a blood vessel by aspirating before intramuscular injection.

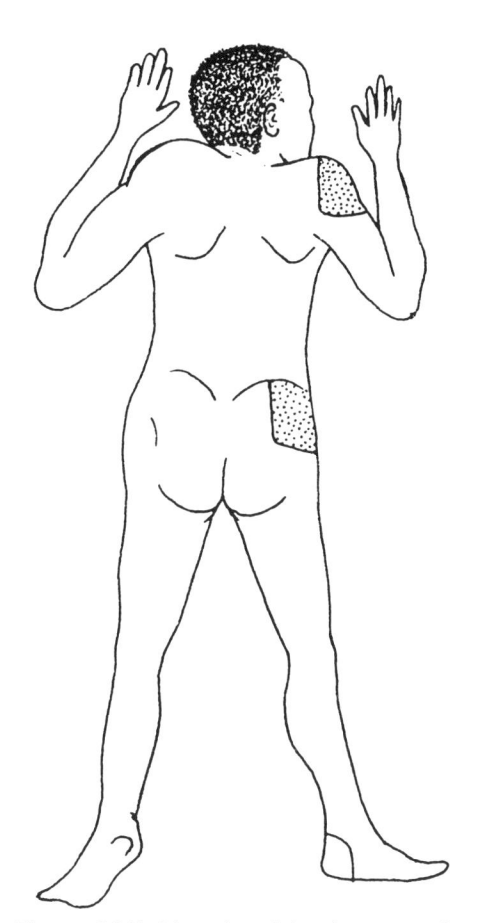

Figure 16.5 Sites for giving intramuscular injections.

Safe administration of intravenous drugs

Drugs are given intravenously to ensure a rapid onset of action, to accurately titrate dose against response, or the drug may be too irritant to give intramuscularly. Nurses caring for seriously ill patients are often asked to accept responsibility for administering and controlling intravenous drug therapy.

Intravenous drugs reach the circulation (and therefore the heart and brain) quicker and in higher concentrations than drugs given by other routes. Intravenous drugs must be injected slowly and the patient watched for any side effects or signs of an allergic reaction. When using sedatives or analgesics inject until the desired effect is obtained and then stop. Regular intravenous drugs are best given via an intravenous infusion. The risks are minimised by following these guidelines:

1. Exclude previous reactions to the drug in use.
2. Always follow the manufacturer's instructions exactly.
3. Give bolus injections over 1 to 2 min (unless the instructions actually state otherwise); aminophylline for example is given over 10 min.
4. Observe the patient's condition carefully throughout the injection.

To the above should be added the following guidelines in the administration of drugs by intravenous infusion:

1. The infusion pack containing the drug should not be the same one being used for routine hydration. (It can be given through the same cannula by using a Y-connection or inserting a needle into the rubber tubing at the end of the giving set, providing neither infusion fluid interacts with the drug.)
2. The amount of drug added to the infusion fluid should be clearly indicated in the infusion bottle or pack.
3. Add drugs only to infusion fluids mentioned in the manufacturer's instructions.
4. Frequently used drug infusions should have a standardised concentration (e.g. dopamine, p. 445).
5. Use sterile technique to add the drug to the infusion.
6. Make up a new infusion every 24 h.
7. Discard the whole solution if it becomes opaque after adding the drug.
8. If you are the prescriber make sure you have given clear instructions regarding:
   (a) the amount of drug and type and volume of infusion fluid to which it is to be added;
   (b) the rate of flow in drops per minute;
   (c) the type and frequency of observation required to monitor the infusion;
   (d) indications for changing the rate of the infusion;
   (e) the direction and degree of rate change.

EXAMPLE

Which of the following instructions would you prefer to receive?

Rx Quinine 10 mg/kg/8 hourly as a 1.8% solution in 5% dextrose water by i.v. infusion.

OR

Rx Add 1.8 g quinine to 1.0 litre of 5% dextrose water and infuse 20 drops per hour for 4 hours at 8-hour intervals.

Investigations

Investigations usually require samples to be taken from the patient and may be carried out in the laboratory or by the bedside. They are used for diagnosis and in assessing progress. Nurses assist by collecting samples and by doing some bedside tests. The nurses also usually receive the results of investigations before the doctor and should be able to recognise important abnormalities so that they know when to inform the doctor urgently.

Collecting the sample

Results of laboratory investigations may be misleading if samples are collected in the wrong way or placed in the wrong containers or if there is delay before they get to the laboratory. The nursing staff may be requested to collect blood samples and nurses should be taught the technique of venepuncture.

When collecting blood samples make sure blood is put in the right container(s) for the tests required. Material collected for culture must not be contaminated during collection and should be placed in sterile containers. There are special bottles for blood cultures. Samples for culture should reach the laboratory as soon as possible. If there is an unavoidable delay then blood cultures should be kept at room temperature (unless they can be out in a laboratory incubator) and other samples should be placed in the fridge.

Prevention of infection

Critically ill patients may have become ill because of infection and are at special risk of secondary infection. This section is primarily concerned with prevention of the spread of infection from patient to patient, nurse to patient and patient to nurse. The medical aspects of management of serious infections are discussed in Chapter 8.

The nature of infection

Infection is the result of invasion of the body by harmful organisms – commonly bacterial but sometimes viral, fungal or protozoal. Infection usually leads to illness through tissue destruction or the production of toxins.

Sources and spread of infection

Organisms responsible for infection may be introduced to the patient from outside (*exogenous*) or may be due to organisms arising from within the patient (*endogenous*).

Exogenous infections enter the body through the skin, the lungs and the intestinal tract or may be transferred into the body by blood transfusion, insect bites, sexual intercourse and invasive medical procedures. Exogenous infection may come from another patient, contaminated stock solutions or equipment, a member of staff or a dirty environment. Thus infection may spread from patient to equipment to another patient, or a patient to nurse's hands to another patient, or from a nurse through air to patient. In the context of the critically ill patient infection is most commonly spread by staff from hands, stock solutions or equipment. Spread through the air, through food or water and by insect bite is uncommon.

PRACTICE POINT
Unwashed hands spread infection from patient to patient.

Endogenous infection is due to commensals, which are micro-organisms which normally live in harmony on or in us. Common commensals include strains of *Escherichia coli* in the bowel, *Clostridium welchi* and *Staphylococcus aureus* on skin and *Streptococcus viridans* in the mouth. In a healthy person these organisms in these sites are harmless and may even be beneficial (e.g. normal intestinal organisms prevent harmful bacteria becoming established in the gut, and their destruction by antibiotics predisposes to serious gut infections). However in patients already seriously ill with other problems commensals may spread from their normal sites and become pathogens.

Factors determining the development of infection

The development of infection following exposure to a micro-organism depends on the route of infection, the infecting dose, the nature of the organism and on the body's defence mechanisms including the immune system.

The organism, dose and route of infection

Some organisms cause greater problems than others by the nature of the illness they cause and the ease with which they can be treated. For any given organism the greater the number of organisms that enter the patient the more severe will be the illness. Although aseptic technique may not guarantee sterility it will greatly reduce the number of organisms contaminating the area. Introduction of organisms directly into the bloodstream bypasses the local defence mechanisms and generally results in a more severe illness.

The body's defences

There are local and general defences against infection. The skin is one of the more important local defences and few organisms can enter through intact skin. Following skin trauma or burns, organisms can easily invade the underlying tissue and local or generalised infection follows. If the blood supply is poor infection is more likely to become established and tissue ischaemia predisposes to infection with organisms such as those of gas gangrene and tetanus, which prefer hypoxic conditions (anaerobes). Other local defences include saliva, gastric acid, mucosal epithelium and other mucosal secretions.

General defence depends initially on white cells and macrophages and later on antibodies and tissue immune responses. White cells and antibodies are carried to the site of infection by the bloodstream; ischaemic tissue is at high risk of infection. Conditions which impair the production of white cells (e.g. leukaemia, cancer therapy or irradiation) or of antibodies (e.g. steroid therapy and infection with the human immune deficiency virus) impair the immune response. Other conditions associated with impaired immunity are malnutrition, alcoholism, acute infections such as malaria, chronic infections such as tuberculosis, and any serious chronic debilitating illness.

Special problems of infection in the seriously ill

Infections create major problems in the care of critically ill patients because the illness may be due to a particularly virulent organism, immunity may be comprised or the primary condition may cause depressed immunity. In addition, critically ill patients have greater exposure to micro-organisms because of frequent invasive procedures (e.g. catheters, i.v. cannulae, surgical drains), i.v. fluids and blood, antibiotic resistance and loss of commensals due to antibiotic therapy, sharing of specialised equipment among patients and frequent nursing, which allows greater opportunity for spread of infection by nurses. This includes infection arising in a nurse (e.g. a hand infection with *Staphylococcus aureus*) as well as transmission from patient to patient through hands or contaminated equipment.

If a special unit is run for critically ill patients, hospital organisms may develop resistance to numerous antibiotics and patients nursed in this environment are at serious risk of overwhelming untreatable infections. A register in which site, organisms and antibiotic sensitivity for each infection are entered allows early recognition and corrective action if there is a rising incidence of cross-infection and the emergence of multi-resistant organisms. A change in antibiotic prescribing practice will usually reverse the emergence of such organisms.

Staff caring for seriously ill patients must take great care not to spread infection. Many precautions which prevent cross-infection between patients also reduce the risk of staff acquiring infections. Skin or mucous membrane contamination by blood, other tissue fluids or excreta are the major sources of infection for staff.

Preventing spread of infection

Preventing infection requires knowledge, care and time. A shortage of staff may make some of the suggestions given below impossible but the price of secondary infection is high.

To prevent cross-infection take the following steps:
1. Have separate basic equipment for each patient and always sterilise equipment between patients. This applies to thermometers, sphygmomanometer cuffs, suction catheters, etc., as well as more complicated equipment such as ventilator tubing.
2. Use disposable equipment (e.g. syringes, needles, catheters, intravenous cannulae, endotracheal tubes).
3. Wash hands properly before each patient using at least soap and if available a disinfectant solution. If running water is not available, wipe both hands with a disinfectant solution containing alcohol.
4. Ordinary towels are a serious risk and wherever possible use paper towels.
5. Use careful aseptic technique for all invasive procedures.
6. Keep wounds and sites of insertion of intravenous lines clean.
7. Disinfect contaminated linen.
8. Maintain a clean environment, washing down table tops, working surfaces, sinks, basins and the sluice with disinfectant and wash ward curtains frequently.

Barrier nursing

Patients are usually barrier-nursed to prevent them transmitting infection. This might be appropriate for a patient with a staphylococcal infection that is resistant to all antibiotics. Occasionally barrier nursing is implemented to protect the patient from infection (reversed barrier nursing), which might be appropriate for example in a patient with severe neutropenia.

Properly done, barrier nursing is time-consuming, with repeated washing and donning and removing gowns, gloves, masks and shoe covers. Unless properly done, barrier nursing does not prevent the spread of infection and may actually reduce patient care if staff are busy. Therefore barrier nursing should only be ordered when considered essential and there must be adequate staff and equipment.

Protecting staff from infection

Hepatitis B and C

This is a special risk to all health workers exposed to blood or other tissue fluids in developing countries where hepatitis B carrier rates are high. However, indigenous staff of these countries often have natural immunity and the main risk is to staff from countries where hepatitis B infection is uncommon. As hepatitis B can be fatal and it is not always possible to avoid contact with body fluids, the safest policy is to vaccinate non-immune staff. The absence of antibodies to hepatitis B antigen in the blood indicates the absence of immunity. These tests are usually available only in major centres. In the event of a needle-stick injury from a patient known or suspected to have hepatitis B infection, a non-immune staff member can be protected by administration of anti-HBV globulin and vaccination.

Staff deserve to know their risks and be protected. The risk of transmission of hepatitis B or C from infected staff to patients is small but real.

Human immune deficiency virus (HIV) (pp. 164–165)

This is spread the same way as hepatitis B, but the risk of infection has been found to be very much lower because the virus is more fragile and a larger 'dose' is needed. At present good practice minimises the risk of transmission, but post-exposure prophylaxis should be considered following significant exposures.

Other infections

These are seldom a risk to staff, providing they practise safe nursing techniques which are taught in basic training. Occasionally a particular infection will cause concern (e.g. pneumonic plague) and senior medical staff should then arrange chemoprophylaxis or vaccination for the staff.

Good habits reduce your risk of getting infections from patients. They include the following:

1. Avoid needle-stick injuries; do not resheath a used needle (Figure 16.6) but dispose of it into a 'sharps box'. If a needle-stick injury does occur then the area should be cleaned with antiseptic and a doctor informed.
2. Wear gloves whenever exposed to blood, excreta or body fluids. Gowns and waterproof aprons offer further protection in heavily contaminated areas, but must be removed and placed in disinfectant immediately after use. Masks offer very little protection against organisms coughed out by patients and are not recommended.

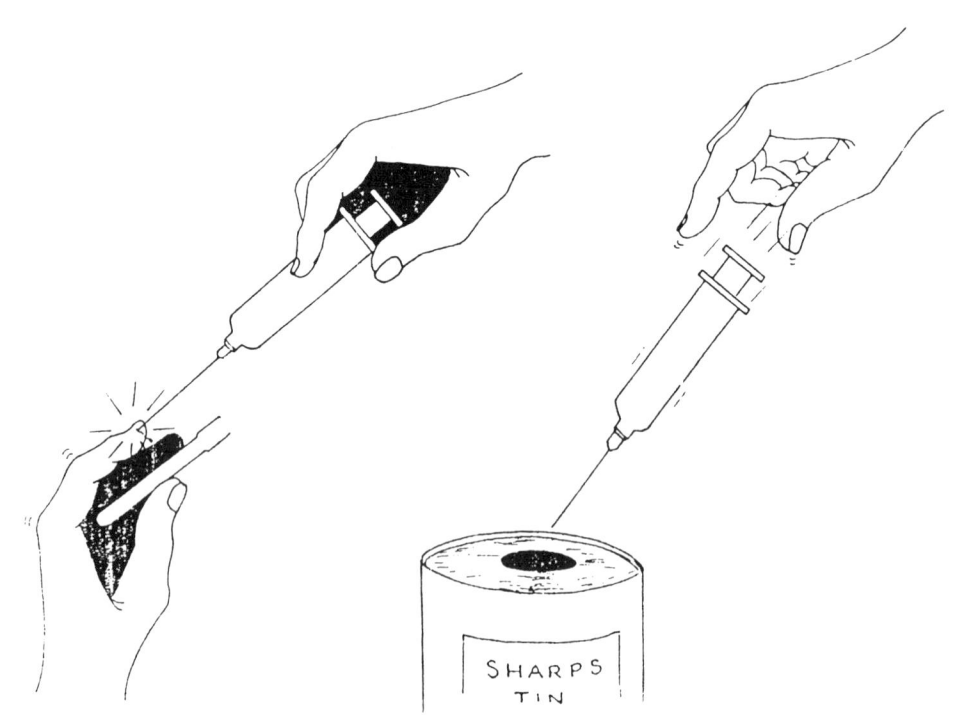

Figure 16.6 Prevention of needle stick injuries. Prevent injuries by using a sharps tin. Do not resheath needles.

3. If blood or other body fluids from a patient splash into the eyes, irrigate immediately with tap water or normal saline. Some hospitals provide protective eye gear to prevent this.
4. Any area contaminated by a spillage of blood or other body fluids should be cleaned promptly with sodium hypochlorite (bleach) or other antiseptic.

Sterilisation

All items of patient care equipment can be divided into three groups.
1. Instruments inserted into the patient for procedures such as LP, cut down, CVP catheter and for operation must be **sterilised**, which means that all living organisms, including spores, in contact with the article are killed.
2. Items which come into contact with mucous membranes but do not normally enter sterile tissues, such as endotracheal tubes should preferably be **sterile**, but sterility is not absolutely essential and **high-level disinfection** is adequate. High-level disinfection kills bacteria, spores, fungi and non-lipid viruses. Disinfection is defined as freeing an article from some or all of its burden of live pathogenic micro-organisms.
3. Items which do not come into contact with mucous membranes e.g. Ambu bags, walls, floor, sheets, furniture, stethoscopes, etc., should be **cleaned** with detergent in water.

Autoclaving

This is the best method of sterilising instruments. Some items are unable to withstand the heat (121°C at 15 lbf/in^2 (approx. 103 kPa) for 15 min) and should be soaked in 2% glutaraldehyde for 6–10 h after precleaning with detergent and water. Then rinse in sterile water and store in a sterile container. Gluteraldehyde (Cidex) has been replaced in some countries by disinfection with hydrogen peroxide or paracetic acid, particularly for the cleaning of endoscopes. Hydrogen peroxide is an alternative for delicate equipment such as cameras, telescopes and micro instruments. Autoclaving can be achieved by using a domestic pressure cooker. Autoclave pressures need to be increased at altitude. There will be an appropriate adjustment in use in your hospital.

Boiling

Boiling at 100°C for 5–10 min will kill all non-sporing organisms and many sporing organisms and can be used if other methods are not available. Steaming at 100°C for 90 min is also effective. However, boiling does not produce 100°C except at sea level. In Kampala, Uganda (c. 1500 m), water boils at 94°C, while in Addis Abbaba, Ethiopia (c. 2000 m), it boils at 92°C. Boiling is not safe above sea level if absolute sterility is required.

High-level disinfection

This can be achieved using 2% glutaraldehyde or boiling in water for 20 min.
Disinfection of items which do not come into contact with mucous membranes can be carried out in a room at an intermediate level using 1% hypochlorite (bleach). This is suitable for toilets, bedpans, urinals and cleaning body fluid spills in the ICU.

Fumigation

There is no need to fumigate rooms following cases of gas gangrene, tetanus, AIDS or TB. The only indication for fumigation is anthrax.

Hand washing

Hand washing should be with soap and water or with Hibiscrub (chlorhexidine

0.5% in aqueous solution). Skin preparation should be with 0.5% chlorhexidine in 70% alcohol or washed with 3% hexachlorophene detergent and painted with 1% iodine.

Cleaning

This involves the use of detergent not disinfectant.

Linen should be placed in waterproof bags or containers and removed from the ward for washing and disinfection, which should include at least 10 min at 65°C.

Cardiorespiratory arrest

When cardiac arrest occurs there is acute cessation of blood flow to the tissues. If the circulation is not re-established within 3 min the brain becomes severely hypoxic and irreversibly damaged. If immediate resuscitation is carried out, around 20% of patients may recover. The prognosis depends on the cause, the speed of initial resuscitation, the underlying disease and the general condition of the patient. The management of cardiac arrest is described in the section on practical procedures (p. 396).

Can cardiorespiratory arrest be prevented?

Many cardiorespiratory arrests are preventable and resuscitation is often unsuccessful. Proper monitoring (p. 299) will often allow cardiorespiratory arrest to be anticipated. Relieving airway obstruction, mechanical ventilation for respiratory failure, rapid correction of hypovolaemia and control of serious cardiac arrhythmias are all methods of preventing cardiorespiratory arrest. It is good practice to explore the cause of each arrest with a view to preventing the same mistake being made in other patients.

Who to resuscitate

Cardiopulmonary resuscitation (CPR) should always be attempted in patients in whom recovery is expected and in those in whom the prognosis is uncertain. CPR should generally not be attempted in patients with diseases with a poor prognosis for quality of life or survival. It is helpful to the nursing staff if doctors can indicate, in advance and with an explanation, those patients for whom attempts at resuscitation are inappropriate.

How to recognise cardiorespiratory arrest

Cardiorespiratory arrest is present when there is no pulse palpable in major arteries (femoral and carotid) and the patient is unconscious. Cessation of respiration, fixed dilated pupils and cyanosis are usually present. An unconscious patient with gasping respiration, marked bradycardia or an impalpable brachial pulse has to all practical purposes 'arrested'. When in doubt treat the patient as if he has arrested.

The resuscitation trolley

The speed of response to and therefore the outcome of cardiorespiratory arrest depends in part on the quick availability of equipment and drugs. The equipment and drugs should always be intact and in working order. Therefore the set should be replaced immediately after use and should be checked by a senior member of staff at frequent intervals – with every shift handover or at least daily.

The patient's family

Communicating

Communication is *two-way*. We need to *listen* to the relatives (which we are bad at)

as well as *talk* (which we think we are good at). Our objectives in communicating with the family are:
1. to fill in gaps in the patient's history;
2. to elicit the family's fears and worries;
3. to inform them of the patient's problem, management and prognosis;
4. to answer their queries;
5. to involve them in decision making.

With good communication the burden of anxiety for the family is less; they may be able to assist in management, e.g. by sitting with a restless patient or helping with feeds; they may bring in special foods; they are able to donate blood and sometimes they can arrange for supplies of needed drugs and equipment. In this way they are reassured by being able to participate in the patient's care and are of real help to staff.

Who is responsible

Responsibility for communicating with the family of ill patients is shared between the nursing and medical staff. It is important for each to understand and implement their respective duties and to avoid giving conflicting information. It is also important to pass information received from the family to other medical and nursing staff.

Whom to talk to

Early in the illness the next of kin or a senior member of the family should be identified and the names of people entitled to receive information obtained from him/her. Information should not be released to others without express permission. In the case of a large family it is wise to identify a single senior family member as the representative of the family who will act as the communication link between hospital staff and the whole family. This prevents unecessarily frequent enquiries and reduces the risk of the family receiving apparently conflicting reports.

What to tell them

In most countries it is not acceptable for medical staff to withold information about patients since the immediate family need to understand the nature of the problem and the likelihood of recovery. The family should be informed (and sometimes consulted) about management and they should receive progress reports. In conscious patients the family may be consulted on how much the patient is told about his illness.

How to tell them

Worldwide the health professions are known for their inability to communicate with people. Many unjustified adverse comments about hospitals stem from our inability to explain things. Good communication will gain the confidence of the family and reduce their distress, as well as improving the public's image of the hospital.

Discussion is usually with a lay person who may be distressed as well as nervous. A few minutes spent in general conversation allowing both sides to 'feel their way' is time well spent. The problem should be explained at a level that can be clearly understood by the person receiving the information. This may be difficult to do in a single session, particularly if the person is finding it difficult to concentrate or the problem is particularly complicated. Two or three short sessions may be preferable to one intense, exhausting and distressing session.

Who tells them

Staff should have clear guidelines as to who may give information to family members. The initial interview should be with a doctor. It may be advisable to have another staff member present as a witness that the correct information was given. Progress reports may be given by identified nursing or medical staff. Adverse developments are best communicated by a doctor or senior nurse. Other staff should refer enquiries to the right person.

Spiritual care

Visits from the hospital chaplain or a minister of the same religion as the patient should be encouraged and they should be considered as part of the care team.

Visiting

Visiting regulations should be as relaxed as possible without detriment to the patient or other patients. Often visiting should be limited to close family, who should however be given reasonably free access in controlled numbers. Staff should be prepared to inconvenience themselves for the sake of the family and the patient.

Futher reading

McIvor D, Thompson FJ. The self-perceived needs of family members with a relative in the intensive care unit (ICU). *Intensive Care Nursing* 1988;4:139–45.

Reporting to the next shift

Continuity of care is of particular importance in seriously ill patients and requires a considerable exchange of information between nursing shifts. This is usually achieved through the verbal and written nursing report. A written report is necessary, but it is difficult to find the correct balance between an over-detailed report which 'loses' essential information and a shorter report that omits essential information. At a minimum the written report should include the eight points shown in Table 16.2.

Table 16.2 Contents of the written report for each individual patient on changing nursing shift

1. Any major change in the patient's condition.
2. Specific changes in management.
3. The time drugs and other treatments are next due.
4. The latest communication with relatives.
5. Unexpected events such as press or police enquiries.
6. Any difficulties with drugs, supplies or equipment.
7. Communications with doctors and the laboratory.
8. Urgent outstanding matters such as blood being cross-matched or awaiting a time to go to theatre.

The verbal report is best given at the bedside, which allows the staff of both shifts to double check. At the bedside the nurses can discuss changes in observations and in management and demonstrate important points about the patient (but with care, since even unconscious patients can hear). These details do not need to be duplicated in the written report. A suggested check list for the nurse coming on duty is given in Table 16.3.

Housekeeping

Good housekeeping – an essential for tranquility in every home – is also essential to the survival of seriously ill patients. It requires organisation by senior staff and cooperation from all staff.

It includes:

1. maintaining sufficient supplies of frequently used materials, including drugs;
2. anticipating unavailability of fresh supplies over weekends and public holidays;
3. arranging regular servicing of all equipment;

Table 16.3 Contents of the verbal report at bedside handover

For new patients (away from the bedside): 1. The diagnosis. 2. The systems which have failed. 3. The management plan. 4. The information given to the family. And for all patients (at the bedside): 1. Greet the patient. 2. Note conscious level and mood. 3. Respiration 　Are colour and breathing all right? 　Is the patient on oxygen? 　If on a ventilator: 　　Is the tube in the correct position? 　　Is the chest movement symmetrical? 　　Are the breath sounds equal? 　　What are the ventilator settings? 4. Circulation 　Is the skin warm or cold? 　Are recent pulse and BP recordings all right?	5. Position 　Is it correct? 　When were the pressure areas last inspected? 6. Fluid balance 　Is the i.v.i. running? 　What rate should it be running at? 　Is the i.v.i. site all right? 　Are the medical instructions clear? 　Is the fluid input recorded up to date? 　When was the urine bag last changed? 　Was the amount drained entered? 　Is the overall fluid balance all right? 　Is the adding up of the fluid chart correct? 7. Nutrition 　Are there any special requirements? 8. Drugs 　When are they next due? 9. Progress 　Is the patient stable, deteriorating or improving?

4. having telephone numbers for the key people concerned with supplies and maintenance to contact them 'out of hours';
5. maintaining general cleanliness and order;
6. maintaining good relationships with all those on whom you depend.

17

Organisation and management

Definitions

Intensive care means doing the best for critically ill patients with the resources available.

Critical illness can be defined as an acute disease process which may result in death if not treated promptly. The patient's condition requires aggressive treatment and frequent monitoring, so that any changes which might alter therapy can be detected early and acted upon. Sometimes a less severe acute illness may require intensive care because of an underlying chronic disease. Patients should be regarded as potentially salvageable before being admitted to an intensive care area or unit, or at least there should be sufficient doubt about their prognosis to warrant making every effort.

An *intensive care unit (ICU)* is the place where critically ill patients are grouped together for observation and treatment. It may be a separate ward or, in smaller hospitals, an area of a ward. The aim is to provide the best care possible in that hospital by:
1. providing a high ratio of nurses to patients,
2. concentrating limited resources and skills in one area of the hospital,
3. reserving expensive drugs and therapies for patients being treated by doctors and nurses who are able to choose who are most likely to benefit, and to ensure that such therapies are properly administered so as to obtain maximum effectiveness.

Benefits of an ICU

Appropriate treatment protocols can be established which should result not only in better management of patients but also in more efficient use of resources, thereby reducing the total cost of care of the critically ill by the hospital. The reputation of the hospital and morale among the staff should improve, while difficult and often dangerous transfer of very ill patients can be minimised. When good intensive care results in a reduction of the number of medical evacuations from a country, scarce foreign exchange is also conserved.

The potential disadvantage of setting up an ICU is that costs are greatly increased if the level of technology is inappropriate and if the wrong patients are admitted (Figure 17.1). The ability of nurses in the general wards to look after serious cases may be undermined and ward doctors may resent the loss of clinical control over their patients.

These disadvantages can be minimised by ensuring that the allocation of resources to intensive care is appropriate to the needs of the whole hospital. Ward nurses can be given experience in the ICU and their overall confidence is likely to increase if they are able to do their job properly because they have been relieved of the extra demands of a very sick patient, who they cannot care for effectively without neglecting their other ward duties. There is little doubt that critically ill patients do

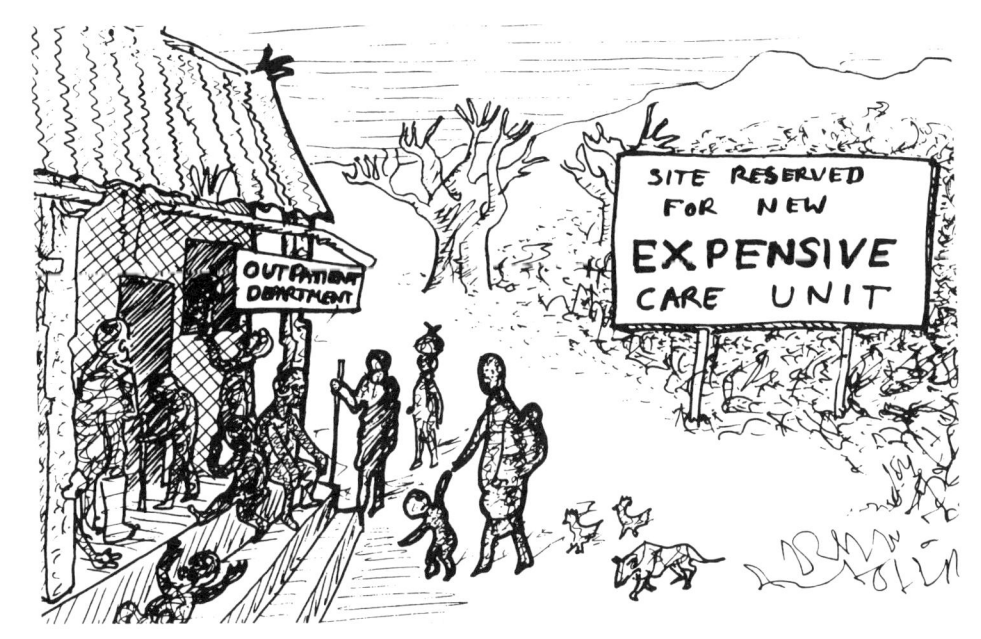

Figure 17.1 Intensive or expensive care?

better in special units, so that the loss of clinical responsibility should be seen as an opportunity for sharing expertise for the benefit of the patient. Admitting doctors or firms should always maintain some involvement in the management of their patient, which helps to make both ICU and ward doctors more knowledgeable.

> **KEYPOINT**
>
> Appropriate intensive care means valuable resources are used effectively.

Planning and costs

In large hospitals 1–2% of hospital beds should be assigned for the critically ill. Thus a 1000-bed hospital would have ten beds, a 400-bed provincial hospital four beds. In smaller hospitals slightly more beds would be required, so that a 150-bed district hospital might allocate three beds. However, the bed allocation does depend on whether severely malnourished children or severe burns will be treated in the ICU, and if so for how long. The percentage of intensive care beds will also rise in hospitals serving an older population, doing a lot of major elective general surgery and pursuing a policy of day surgery, short stay or early discharge (up to 3–4%).

The standard of care appropriate for critically ill patients in the tropics can be considered on three different levels. It is important to note that for level 1 and 2 care equipment forms a small percentage of the total cost of care (Figure 17.2).

Level 1 care

This provides basic monitoring of the pulse, blood pressure, respiration, temperature, conscious level and urine output. The patient can be regularly turned, infusions can be supervised, nasogastric feeding given, and intubated patients suctioned. Mechanical ventilation and cardiac monitoring are not available at this level. The equipment needed is simple and

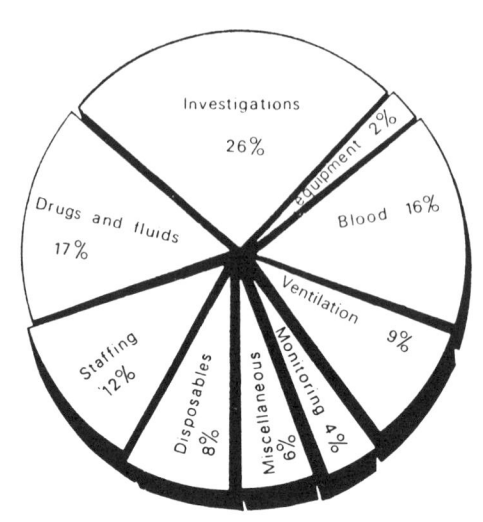

Figure 17.2 Piegraph showing the proportional breakdown of costs in intensive care in Zambia during the period 1986–7.

Investigations 26%
Equipment 2%
Blood 16%
Drugs and fluids 17%
Ventilation 9%
Staffing 12%
Disposables 8%
Miscellaneous 6%
Monitoring 4%

averaged out over a few years is likely to cost only a few dollars per day. Even without an ICU this amount is likely to be spent on a critically ill patient treated in a general ward since the major part of the cost is due to infusions and drugs.

Level 2 care

This aims to provide mechanical ventilation and cardiac monitoring facilities over and above the basic care of level 1. The overall cost of care is about $US100 per patient per day.

The cost of care in our ICU (5 level-1 and 5 level-2 beds) in Zambia in 1987 is shown in Figure 17.2. The cost per patient per day was $US76, which was similar to cost of a night in one of the international hotels. Equipment contributed little to cost and even mechanical ventilation using the Oxford Mk. II ventilator at $US35 per patient per day was cheaper than some antibiotics or cytotoxic drugs. Cardiac monitoring cost $US9 per patient per day. The most expensive treatment given was a unit of blood, which cost $US40 per unit.

Every hospital would need to make an assessment of its own costs and clearly almost two decades later these costs quoted in our study will have changed.

Level 3 care

In many developing countries this is unlikely to be affordable or appropriate, except in teaching institutions and central referral hospitals. The daily cost of this level of care is in excess of $US500–1000 in developed countries and includes facilities for total parenteral nutrition, haemodialysis, cardiac pacing, Swan–Ganz catheters and CT scanning.

A more complete list of equipment and drugs needed for level 1 and 2 care is provided at the end of the chapter (Tables 17.1 and 17.2).

Design and location

The critical care area should be centrally located in the hospital and spacious. Space is needed, both around the bed and behind the head of the bed, to perform procedures, to resuscitate the patient in an emergency and to keep equipment at the bedside. The unit should be well lit, preferably with an overhead strip light for each bed. If possible the unit should be close to the emergency area, labour ward and theatre, as the transfer of critically ill patients can be precarious. There must be plenty of storage space for equipment, disposables, and drug stocks. Simple sideroom investigations such as a malaria film should be available in larger ICUs. Nurses should not have to leave the ICU to drink tea. Larger ICUs will benefit from a staff refreshment room and a reception area for relatives.

Each bed area should be well fitted with electrical sockets (Figure 17.9). About 6 to 8 sockets are needed for level-2 beds. If the hospital has piped oxygen and central suc-

Table 17.1 Essential drugs at different levels of intensive care

Level 1 drugs:

atropine	insulin	penicillin (oral/i.v.)
adrenaline (epinephrine)	heparin	chloramphenicol (oral/i.v.)
calcium gluconate	digoxin	gentamicin (i.v.)
lidocaine (i.v.)	morphine	metronidazole (oral/p.r.)
50% dextrose	pethidine	ampicillin (oral/i.v.)
10% mannitol	propranolol	cefotaxime (i.v.)
suxamethonium	furosemide	ketoconazole (i.v.)
tubocurarine	phenobarbital	quinine
pancuronium	phenytoin	chloroquine
naloxone	dexamethasone	chloramphenicol (eye)
hydrocortisone	hydralazine	oxytocin
aminophylline	diazoxide	protamine sulphate
potassium chloride	vitamin K	cloxacillin (oral/i.v.)
lidocaine spray	1% lidocaine	warfarin (oral)
magnesium trisilicate	magnesium sulphate	salbutamol
diazepam	chlorpromazine	sodium bicarbonate
isoprenaline	lactulose	desferrioxamine
anti-tetanus serum	snake anti-venom	acetylcystine
activated charcoal	methionine	
Resonium A (polystyrene sulphonate resin)	pralidoxime	

Level 2 ICUs in central hospitals should also have:
Cardiac: verapamil and amiodarone, labetalol.
Shock: dopamine, dobutamine, noradrenaline (norepinephrine)
Gastrointestinal: cimetidine, vasopressin.
Antibiotics: metronidazole (i.v.), cefotaxime or some other third/fourth generation cephalosporins/penicillins.

Level 3:
A much wider range of drugs is likely to be available, including:
nitroprusside;
parenteral nutrition;
atenolol, practolol, acebutalol.

tion this should be available on every bed. Backup oxygen cylinders and electrical suckers should be available, as central units may fail. The bed itself should be mobile and capable of height adjustment, tilting head-up and head-down and have an adjustable backrest to allow patients to sit up. The head of the bed must be completely removable (or sawn off) to allow easy access to the airway for intubation and internal jugular vein cannulation. The mattress should have a watertight cover to prevent contamination.

Each bed area should have its own stethoscope, sphygmomanometer, Ambu bag, suction apparatus and a basin or sink for hand washing. The space for one bed should be three bed areas of a Nightingale ward. Curtains help maintain a sense of privacy and reduce the feeling of dehumanisation, but may spread dust and contribute to airborne infection. Screens should not be placed where they will interfere with practical procedures such as insertion of central venous lines. The cost of this basic equipment for the bed area is

Table 17.2 Treatment, monitoring and investigations required at the three levels of intensive care

Treatment	Monitoring	Investigations
Level 1		
Airway suction	Temperature	Blood film
Oxygen	Pulse, BP	CSF examination
Ambu bag	Fluid balance	Blood glucose
Bed without head	Conscious level	Haematocrit/FBC
Enteral nutrition	Chest – auscultation	Plain 'X-rays
Peritoneal dialysis	Pupils, fundoscopy	Urea and electrolytes
		ECG
Level 2		
Ventilation	Cardiac monitor	Microbiological culture
Infusion controller	Pulse oximetry	Angiography
Defibrillation	Central venous pressure	Coagulation tests
		Endoscopy
		Liver function tests
		Calcium, magnesium
Level 3		
Haemodialysis	Intra-arterial BP	Blood gases
Haemofiltration	Swan–Ganz catheter	Cardiac output
Parenteral nutrition	Intracranial pressure	CT scanning
Cardiac pacing	Capnometer	Isotope scanning
		All biochemical tests

very small (around $US1 per patient per day). For many hospitals, creating the space may be the greatest problem in setting up a critical care area.

There should be pictures or posters on the wall, and a clock which the patient can see when supine or sitting. The monotony of looking at a blank wall destroys patient morale and adds to the stress of being critically ill. Soft music is also beneficial.

Organisation of care

Nursing

An essential principle of critical care is a high nurse-to-patient ratio. Level-1 beds should have one nurse for every two patients, while level-2 beds should have one nurse for every patient. This ratio must be maintained at all times throughout the 24 h of the day. Critically ill patients are as much in need of intensive care during the night as during the day. Five posts are needed to have one nurse for 24 h if there are three shifts. This allows for leave, illness and other absences. If the unit is quiet, intensive care nurses can be encouraged to nurse in the general wards where they will have the opportunity to impart their skills to others.

EXAMPLE

A 400-bed hospital which might have four level-1 ICU beds would need to allocate ten nurses to ensure a 1:2 ratio throughout the 24-h period.

A 1000-bed hospital which might have five level-1 and five level-2 beds would need seven or eight nurses at all times. Thus 35–40 posts would need to be created. A ten-bedded intensive care unit should have a senior nurse on every shift and so the number of sisters' posts allocated for the unit should be three to five. This provides opportunities for promotion, which helps to keep experienced nurses in the unit.

The authors ran a ten-bedded ICU (five level-1 and five level-2 beds) in a 1500-bedded teaching hospital admitting 95 000 patients per annum. Elsewhere there were three special observation beds in obstetrics, three high-care beds in paediatrics and a separate neonatal unit. In 1987 the ICU admitted 750 patients with an average bed-occupancy of six patients per day. Although the nurse allocation allowed four nurses at night, shortages of staff reduced this to three. During the two day shifts there were four trained nurses, student nurses and an ICU-trained sister. When the unit was busy at night either with three or four ventilated patients and/or eight or nine admissions more mistakes were made because three nurses were too few. Visiting hour at 6.30 a.m. and handover at 7.30 a.m. were particularly dangerous times.

Documented reports on patients' condition are required by matrons and also by the next shift of nurses. It is important that nurses do not spend so much time writing such reports that the patients are neglected. The forms we developed in order to save nurses' time and improve the quality of information are shown in Figures 17.3 and 17.4.

The inequalities of life ensure that ICUs treat a disproportionate number of VIPs. A senior nurse who has the support of the hospital administration should be put in charge of the unit. Firm handling of relatives and attendants is often required. VIPs should not be admitted to ICU unless they are critically ill.

Approximately one-third of patients admitted will die. Death involves compassionate handling of relatives, which is part of the critical care team's responsibility. Senior staff may need to give advice and support to junior members of the team when there are disappointing or unexpected deaths and when mistakes (which are inevitable) have been made.

Clinical

One person must have overall responsibility for running an ICU. The admitting doctor or medical units should remain involved in the patients' care at the same time.

Our ICU in Lusaka had a consultant in charge whose full-time responsibility was to run a surgical unit. He, together with other senior doctors, ensured that all patients are seen first thing in the morning and as often as necessary throughout the day. The admitting firms were encouraged to join the morning ICU round to discuss their patients. At night, the on-call medical and surgical teams provided emergency cover to the unit. There were no resident ICU staff, although postgraduates were occasionally posted for 1–3 months as part of their training.

This system worked fairly well during the day. Standards of clinical care fell at night because the nursing staff had no senior ICU doctors to consult. The junior medical staff called to the unit from the on-call teams frequently mismanaged the patient. Whenever possible the level of medical cover to ICU should be maintained throughout the 24-h period. In Lusaka this was not possible owing to shortages of doctors.

Charts and protocols

Good care cannot be provided without simple and clear observation charts. Many ICUs use a single large chart to record all nursing observations, results of investigations, doctors' orders and drugs prescribed. Such charts greatly assist nursing management but should not become a substitute for detailed clinical notes in the patient's file. In Lusaka we used a chart based on the Glasgow Coma Scale (Figure 17.5), a fluid balance chart and a drug chart. We had a special respiratory observation chart

Date:	Name:	Age:	Sex:
Diagnosis	Date of admission		
Shift	Morning	Afternoon	Night
Failed system			
Progress			
Observations T P R BP Urine output Fluids in			
Nursing care Next due at: Observations Mouth care Pressure areas Cuff release Chest physio NG feed			
Drugs next due:			
Special comments Weaning for transfer to Ward, not for resuscitation relatives informed, drugs not available, etc. tests done			

Key   Failed systems

A = Airway (i.e. intubated)
R = Respiratory (i.e. ventilated)
BP = Blood pressure (i.e. syst<80)
C = Coma
H = Heart failure
R = Renal failure (i.e. on dialysis)
L = Liver/jaundice
O = Nil

Condition

S = Satisfactory
P = Poor
C = Critical

Figure 17.3 Nursing shift report chart: one for each patient.

Daily matron's report from ICU						NB New page/day			
Date									
Name	Total no. of patients:					Admissions:	Discharge:	Deaths:	
	Age	Sex	Diagnosis	Condition	Progress		Failed systems	Comments	

Conditon   Progress
S = Satisfactory   S = Stable
P = Poor   I = Improving
C = Critical   D = Deteriorating

Failed systems

A = Airway (i.e. intubated)   C = Coma   L = Liver/jaundice
R = Respiratory (i.e. ventilated)   H = Heart failure   O = Nil
BP = Blood pressure (i.e. systolic<80)   R = renal failure (i.e. on dialysis)

Figure 17.4 Matron's report containing essential information on all patients in the unit.

for patients being weaned from the ventilator (Figure 17.6).

Management protocols for common conditions should be devised. The protocols should be easily accessible or even put up on the wall of the unit. This should maintain a consistent standard and educate those using the protocols. The effectiveness of each protocol should be reviewed from time to time by careful audit or prospective study.

Paraclinical departments

Every department of the hospital will be able to contribute to effective clinical care in the ICU (Figure 17.7).

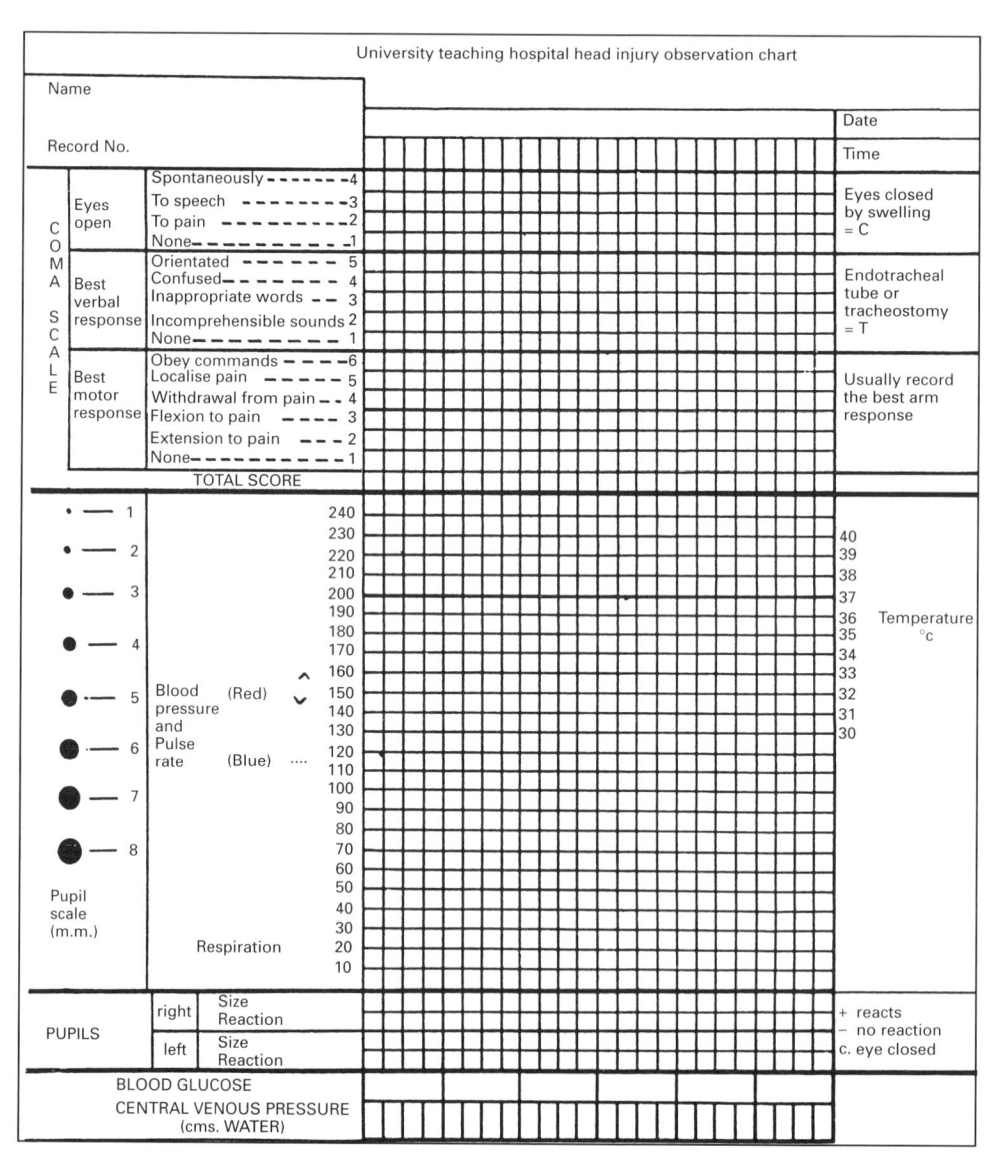

Figure 17.5 The Glasgow Coma Scale chart combined with recording of pulse, BP, pupil size, blood glucose and central venous pressure.

Time	Oxygen flow/ conc.	Resp. rate	Colour tongue	Air entry R L	Sedation	E.T. tube measure	Tidal vol.	Sweat +/−	Signature

Figure 17.6 Respiratory observation chart.

The results of investigations must be available rapidly. X-rays requested should be taken at the bedside and films sent to the unit as soon as possible. Laboratory and radiography staff should give priority to ICU patients. Good communications and liaison between ICU and the laboratory or X-ray department should ensure that a workable system can be established.

The physiotherapist has a significant contribution to make to the care of the critically ill. In large hospitals there should be a 24-h service, but unfortunately in the tropics much of the physiotherapy will have to be administered by nurses. Whenever possible physiotherapists should be allocated specifically to ICU.

The dieticians and catering department should ensure the right food is available for nasogastric feeding (p. 286). Some foodstuffs may need to be liquidised.

The ICU must also keep good stocks of all lifesaving drugs. This involves co-operation with the hospital pharmacy. The system of ordering drugs only on a patient's chart is unacceptable for critically ill patients, who cannot wait until pharmacy opens.

All equipment should be checked daily. Emergency and resuscitation equipment should be checked at the start of each shift. Checklists should be used to ensure this is done thoroughly. If a laryngoscope bulb is blown or a large blade lost in a drawer a patient may die. The hospital workshop should be involved in the ICU, coming each day to solve problems. Whenever possible one nurse should be made responsible for equipment and all members of the team should be instructed on how to use and look after equipment. In Lusaka one of the senior doctors also met with the workshop team on a regular basis to discuss major problems with faults and spares.

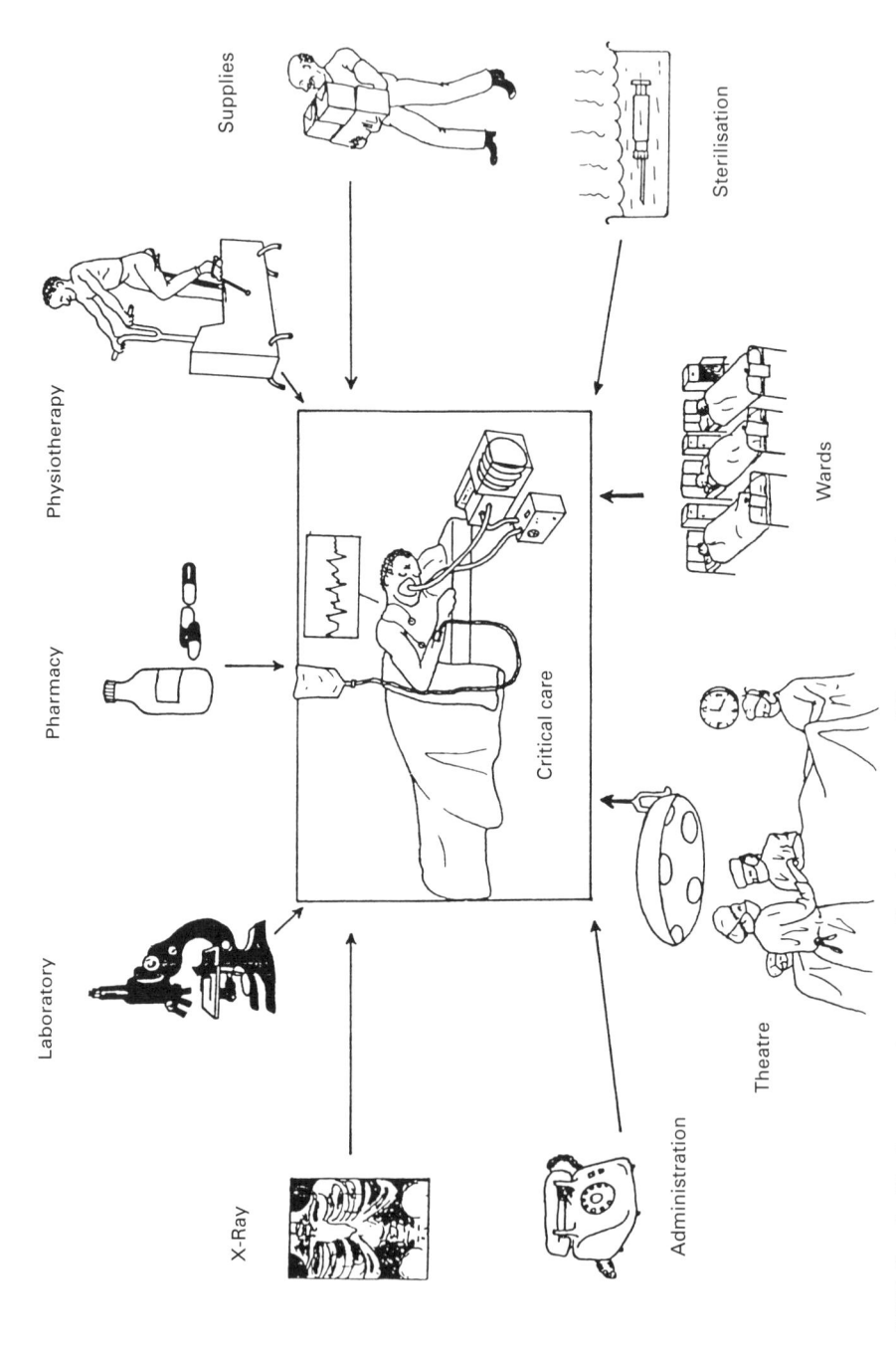

Figure 17.7 Good critical care requires cooperation between many different hospital departments.

Patient selection

An ICU is not a casualty department which conducts primary assessment and treatment of accident and emergency cases. Although trauma is responsible for a significant proportion of admissions to an ICU in developing countries (25% in Zambia), the responsibility for resuscitation, initial assessment and emergency treatment, at least in a large hospital, belongs to the emergency staff and on-call doctors.

ICU is not a terminal care unit. Dying patients with incurable disease should not be nursed there. This would be unfair both to the terminally ill and the critically ill.

An admission and discharge policy should be established. The aims of such a policy are to reserve intensive care for those who are critically ill but with some chance of survival. Once the patient can be properly managed in the general wards the patient should be discharged. A ward should either keep one vacant bed for each patient it has in the ICU or it should have some means of creating a bed as soon as a patient is discharged from ICU.

KEYPOINT
A patient should not be kept in ICU because the ward is full.

If patients remain in ICU because the ward is full then the unit becomes crowded and those with critical illness receive substandard care.

During the period of development in our ICU the yearly admissions rose from 450 to more than 900 over 4 years. This increase was contained by keeping an average bed-occupancy rate of six patients per day throughout. We allowed an open admission policy, believing it to be safer for the patients if a doctor could admit all those he considered to have a reversible critical illness. The ICU team concentrated on prompt diagnosis and treatment and insisted on discharge once the decision to discharge had been made regardless of the availability of beds in the general wards. The decision to discharge the patient was the responsibility of the ICU team. Sometimes the admitting firm was available to discuss this, but it was usually not practical to wait for their appearance before discharging the patient. We followed up all our patients on the ward so as to ensure that our criteria for discharge were realistic.

Measuring effectiveness

Since an inappropriate ICU may consume valuable resources it is important to have some means of measuring effectiveness.

The outcome of a critically ill patient is affected by the diagnosis, the severity of the illness, the standard of monitoring and the treatment available.

Some form of audit should be kept whereby each patient admitted to the unit should have the name, age, sex, date of admission, date of discharge or death, treatment, ICU outcome and eventual ward outcome recorded. Although the information can be recorded by a ward clerk, the accuracy of the information must be checked by the nursing and medical staff. Without such information there can be no evidence of the effectiveness of care, nor can the size of some problems be appreciated.

A medical summary of the diagnosis, problems and treatment of each case should be made by a senior nurse or senior doctor. Post-mortems (hard to obtain in the tropics) on unexplained deaths will result in improved standards of care.

The concern to give appropriate intensive care has resulted in the development of systems to classify the severity of illness. Although certain diagnoses may have a higher mortality than others, the severity of illness also affects outcome.

One example of this is head injury. In our ICU in a study of 214 head injuries there was a 50% mortality. This means very little when stated like this. When graded the severity of head injury according to the admission Glasgow Coma Scale (see Chapter 10) we found that patients with GCS 3–5 had a 91% mortality, 6–8 had 21% and 9 or more had 20%. Most of the deaths in the patients who had a GCS of 9 or more died of other injuries. Thus it is important not only to diagnose a head injury but also to grade the severity and to know if there are associated injuries which might affect outcome. When two places grade head injuries according to the Glasgow Coma Scale they can then compare their results of treatment and make recommendations for improvement.

There are different ways of classifying the severity of critically ill patients with different diagnoses. Some Western ICUs have a system called APACHE II which stands for Acute Physiology And Chronic Health Evaluation. This attempts to classify the severity of illness for all patients admitted to ICU. It is often not possible to use APACHE II in the tropics because it relies on laboratory tests which may not be available, such as blood gases and serum creatinine. Throughout this book we have referred to some ways of classifying the severity of illness. Examples are the Glasgow Coma Scale for head injuries and percentage area of burn in burns. In Lusaka we also developed a method of scoring the severity of illness using only clinical variables – a *clinical sickness score*. Scores are allocated for pulse rate, systolic blood pressure, respiratory rate, urine output, temperature and the Glasgow Coma Scale. The method of scoring is shown in Figure 17.8.

Wastage of resources

The expense of medical care is increased by wrong and inappropriate use of resources. The wrong equipment may be used, or it may be used to treat the wrong patients. If the patient is not at risk of developing the complications for which he is being monitored then the monitoring is unnecessary. Sometimes monitoring (e.g. central venous line) carries its own risks to the patient (infection). If scarce resources are wasted on a patient with no chance of survival then the cost of intensive care is increased without benefit and there may be less resources with which to treat other salvageable patients. Wrong use of an expensive machine by someone unfamiliar with its workings may result in it being damaged. Resources are also wasted when therapeutic intervention is delayed. It is a great deal cheaper and more effective to treat sepsis early than to wait for complications and septic shock to develop. Late drainage of acute osteomyelitis will result in bone death and chronic osteomyelitis, requiring months or years of dressings and prolonged hospital stay. Failure to resuscitate a patient adequately before theatre may result in cardiac arrest on induction of anaesthesia. In the developing world a key part in the management of acute illness is the prevention of life-threatening complications and thus the need for intensive care. If prompt treatment can prevent chronic morbidity then both the patient and those paying for health care will benefit.

Teaching and training

Where medical students, postgraduates, nurses and clinical officers are trained an effective ICU will improve standards of teaching. Trainers should keep in mind the ultimate work environment with regard to the level of care affordable and what equipment is available.

Teaching and training activities should include audit, research, autopsy, review, mortality meetings, case conferences, books

Organisation and management 325

Day	0	1	2	3	4	5	6	7
Date								
Pulse								
Systolic B.P.								
Respiratory rate								
Urine output								
Pyrexia								
15 – G.C.S.								
TOTAL								

SCORING TECHNIQUES

SCORES	4	3	2	1	0	1	2	3	4
Pulse	>180	140–179	110–139	—	70–109	—	55–69	40–54	<40
Systolic BP	>200	170–199	150–169	140–149	100–139	80–99	60–79		<60
Respiratory Rate	>50	35–49		25–34	12–24	10–11	6–9		IPPV
Urine Output	anuria		<50/h		50–200/h		>200/h		
Temperature °C	≥40	39		38	36–37	33–35	31–32	30	29

Glasgow Coma Scale: Subtract from 15 (*in postoperative patients score after waking from anaesthesia)

Mark T for endotracheal tube
Mark C for eyes closed by oedema etc.
Mark S for sedation

Figure 17.8 Clinical sickness score.

and journals, teaching juniors, workshops and conferences.

Specific requirements

These will be described under the following categories:
- bedside equipment;
- unit equipment;
- standard software (catheters, disposables, etc.);
- standard drugs;
- standard investigations.

Level 3 care is beyond the scope of this book, so that the lists which follow deal only with levels 1 and 2.

As far as possible, equipment should be standardised throughout a country, so that the ordering of spare parts can be simplified, with the hope of improving availability and knowledge of what is needed by those responsible for purchasing and supplies. The purpose of these lists is to act as a guide. Local circumstances and pathology will influence the choice of what is required in a particular hospital.

Technicians should be trained to repair the ICU equipment and the equipment chosen should be relatively simple to maintain.

Equipment should be checked on every nursing shift and made part of nursing reports on handover and to the matron's office. Standardisation of equipment will allow nursing familiarity with the available equipment and this would enable equipment to be used safely.

Bedside equipment (Figure 17.9)

Level-1 beds

Each bed should have the following standard equipment:

1. Bed with a movable head to allow access which can be tilted both head-up and head-down. The bed should have wheels for safe transfer of patients.
2. Waterproof mattress.
3. 2–4 electrical sockets per bed.
4. Suction machine.
5. Oxygen cylinder.
6. Oxygen flowmeter.
7. Wall-mounted sphygmomanometer.
8. Stethoscope.
9. Ambu bag.
10. Face mask for ambu bag.
11. Oxygen mask or nasal prongs.
12. Drip stand.
13. Thermometer and tube with disinfectant.
14. Suction tray (contents – see below).
15. Hand washing bowl with disinfectant and towel.
16. Bin.
17. Sharps tin.

Two oxygen cylinders should be available for each bed unless there is piped oxygen from a central tank. (If there is a central tank one backup cylinder should be available for each bed.)

The suction should be electrical or an efficient foot sucker. Even if there is a central suction unit providing vacuum from a socket on the wall there should still be one backup sucker for each bed.

Level-2 beds

1. 6 electrical sockets per bed.
2. Mechanical ventilator (e.g. East Radcliffe, Manley, Bird or Oxford).
3. Humidifier (kettle) if not standard with ventilator.
4. Ventilator alarm if not standard with ventilator.
5. Cardiac monitor and electrodes.
6. Infusion controller (pump or means of gravity flow control).

Unit equipment

All ICUs should have the following standard unit equipment:

1. ECG machine
2. 2 torches, bulbs and batteries.
3. Ames glucometer and Dextrostix sticks.
4. Ophthalmoscope, auroscope.
5. Battery charger and rechargeable batteries to fit all equipment.
6. Intubation trolley (see below).
7. Intercostal drains, bottles (2) and necessary connections and clamps.
8. Tracheostomy tray and full range of tracheostomy tubes (21–42 Fr guage, majority should be 33–42 Fr guage).
9. Burr hole tray (this should be immediately available if not kept in the ICU).
10. Chest aspiration set.
11. Cutdown set.
12. Lumbar puncture set.
13. Food liquidiser for tube feeding.
14. Steam tent.
15. Refrigerator.
16. Kettle.
17. Defibrillator (level 2).
18. Access to rigid bronchoscope and foreign body grasping forceps.
19. Access to a mobile operating light (level 2)

Suction tray (see p. 352)

1. 2 suction catheters, one for the mouth and one for the endotracheal *or* tracheostomy tube.

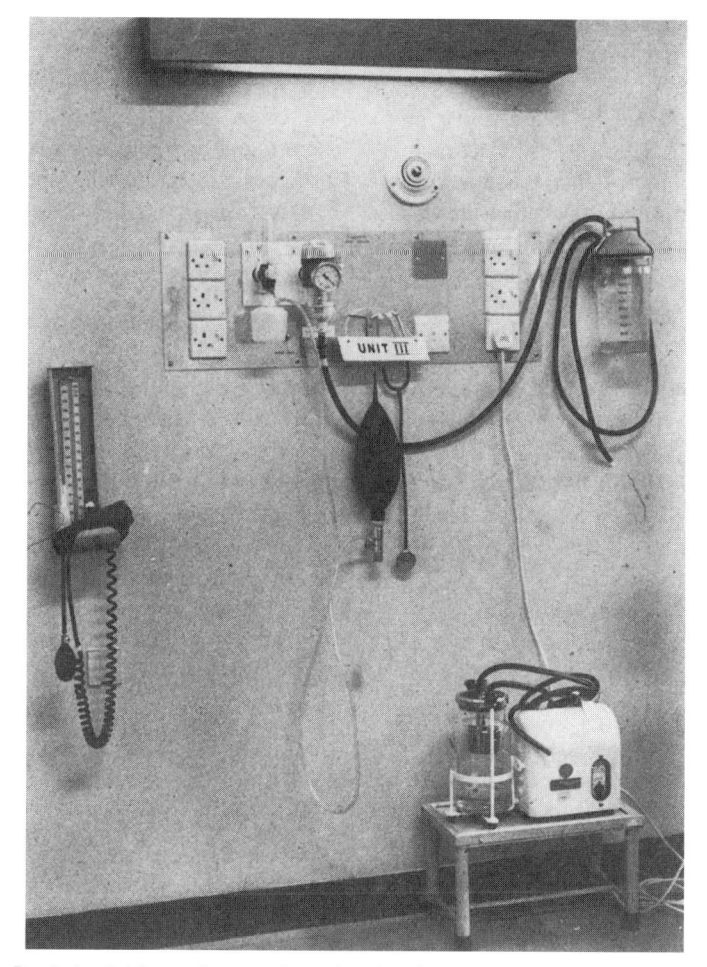

Figure 17.9 Basic bedside equipment for a level-1–2 bed.

2. 2 receivers with disinfectant, one for each catheter.
3. 1 bowl of sterile water.
4. Gauze swabs.
5. Sterile forceps for using no-touch technique with suction catheters.
6. Guedel (or oropharyngeal) airway.

Intubation trolley (see p. 331)

1. 2 laryngoscopes with working bulbs and batteries. Spares should be available.
2. Full range of adult and paediatric laryngoscope blades.
3. Yankauer metal sucker.
4. Introducer for ETT.
5. Endotracheal tubes, sizes 3–9 in half-sizes.
6. Connectors for ETT already fitted.
7. 10-ml syringe (non-sterile) to blow up balloon of ETT.
8. Catheter mount
9. Guedel airways – range of sizes.
10. Magill's forceps.
11. Mouth guard, adult and paediatric size.
12. Ambu bag.
13. Ambu valve connected to bag.
14. Ambu face mask (range of sizes to fit all patients).
15. Oxygen cylinder.
16. Oxygen masks.

17. Variable diameter oxygen tubing.
18. Scissors.
19. Bandage and tape to secure ETT.

Standard software

1. Central venous catheter (Cavafix).
2. Endotracheal tubes with high-volume, low-pressure cuffs (Portex, definitely not red rubber tubes).
3. Disposable condenser humidifiers (e.g. Humidivent – Portex).
4. Disposable condenser humidifiers for tracheostomy (e.g. Trachivent – Portex).
5. Nasogastric tubes.
6. Urinary catheters (Foley).
7. Paediatric buretrols.
8. Infusion gravity flowmeters.
9. Suction catheters (2 per patient per shift; 6 per day).
10. Tracheostomy tubes (cuffed and uncuffed 21–42 Fr gauge).
11. Lumbar puncture needles.
12. Syringes and needles of all sizes.
13. Steinman or Denham pins plus hand-drill for skeletal traction.
14. Colostomy and drainage bags.
15. ECG electrodes (where cardiac monitors available – level 2).
16. Ventilator tubing autoclavable (level 2).
17. Ventilator tubing lightweight (level 2).
18. Disposable nebulisers.

Standard drugs

Both oral and parenteral preparations should be available when drugs can be given by either route. All drugs should be available in the ICU in large hospitals or immediately available from the pharmacy in small hospitals. A refrigerator should be available in ICU for storage of heat-labile drugs.

Standard investigations

1. Urea and electrolytes.
2. Haemoglobin, white count and haematocrit.
3. Blood glucose.
4. Urine microscopy and urinalysis.
5. Blood slide for malaria parasites and trypanosomes.
6. Lumbar puncture, CSF microscopy, biochemistry.
7. X-rays.
8. Liver function tests, serum calcium, magnesium, phosphate, amylase (level 2).
9. Coagulation tests (level 2).
10. Angiography (level 2, central hospital).
11. Microbiology, culture and sensitivity for blood, sputum and urine.
12. Stool microscopy.

All units should have a glucometer (around $US120), Dextrostix sticks.

In larger hospitals a microscope, white-cell counting chamber, haematocrit scale, capillary tubes and sealing wax, centrifuge, microscope slides and stains in a side-room next to the ICU will enable rapid diagnosis and early institution of correct treatment.

Further reading

ENGLEHARDT HT, RIE MA. Intensive care units, scarce resources and conflicting principles of justice. *JAMA* 1986;255:1159–64.

JENNETT B. Inappropriate use of intensive care. *BMJ* 1984;289:1709–11.

KNAUS WA. Rationing, justice and the American physisician. *JAMA* 1986;255:1176–88.

KNAUS WA, DRAPER EA, Wagner DP, ZIMMERMAN JE. Apache II: a severity of disease classification system. *Crit Care Med* 1985;13:818–29.

SCHMULIAN C. *Organization of critical care Surgery*. Medicine Group Surgery, 1998:73–7.

WATTERS DAK, WILSON IH, SINCLAIR JR, and NGANDU N. A clinical sickness score for the critically ill in Central Africa. *Intensive Care Med* 1989;15:467–70.

Practical procedures
Endotracheal intubation

In conscious patients this can be performed by giving the patient a short anaesthetic and a short-acting muscle relaxant such as suxamethonium (see p. 454) or by using local anaesthesia to the airway and larynx (see p. 427). If the patient is unconscious and has no gag reflex, intubation can be performed without any anaesthetic. In unconscious patients with a gag reflex, either general or local anaesthesia may be used. Ideally intubation should be performed by someone with experience. Hypoxic and severely ill patients do not tolerate intubation well. If you have no staff with anaesthetic experience, intubation under local anaesthesia is the safest option.

The use of muscle relaxants by staff without anaesthetic experience can be very dangerous. Do not use them unless you are certain you will be able to ventilate, and never use them in patients with upper airway obstruction or upper airway abnormalities.

Types of endotracheal tube

For intubation in excess of 24 h a plastic endotracheal tube is required because the older red rubber, re-usable anaesthetic endotracheal tubes cause swelling in the airway. If red rubber tubes are left in the larynx for longer than 24 h laryngeal and tracheal inflammation and oedema will result. Plastic (PVC) tubes (e.g. Portex) with an inscription 'IT Z 79' are ideal. This means it is implant-tested and is unlikely to provoke an inflammatory reaction in the airway. Plastic endotracheal tubes come in two varieties, tubes with a low-volume, high-pressure cuff and tubes with a high-volume, low-pressure cuff which should be used on ICU. High-pressure cuffs can be modified if the cuff is stretched by overfilling it with hot water and then emptying it before use. If this is done carefully the cuff will not rupture and will behave just like a high-volume, low-pressure cuff. Plastic high volume, low pressure tubes have been used for several weeks in the same patient but tracheostomy is more common as endotracheal tubes are often more difficult to manage than tracheostomy tubes and are associated with complications (Table P2). Other disadvantages are that patients require more sedation, and weaning patients off ventilation is easier if a tracheostomy has been performed. Once ventilation has been commenced, the decision whether to perform a tracheostomy will depend upon the answers to the following questions:

1. Are plastic tubes available?
2. How long is ventilation likely to be required?
3. Can an endotracheal tube be managed safely?
4. Can tracheostomy be performed safely?

Table P1 Average sizes of endotracheal tube, tracheostomy tube and suction catheter sizes

Age	Size (mm internal diameter)	Tracheal tube Length (oral) (cm)	Tracheal tube Length (nasal) (cm)	Tracheostomy tube (mm internal diameter)	Tracheostomy tube Fr[1]	Suction catheter Fr[1]
Neonates						
1 kg	2.5	7.5	9.0			4
2 kg	3.0	9.0	10.5			6
3 kg	3.0	9.5	11.0	3.0		6
Months						
0–3	3.5	11.0	14.0	3.5	14	8
3–6	4.0	12.0	15.0	4.0	16	8
6–12	4.5	12.5	15.5	4.5	18	8
Years						
2	5.0	13.0	16.0	5.0	20	10
3	5.0	13.5	16.5	5.0	20	10
4	5.5	14.0	17.0	5.0	20	10
5	5.5	14.5	17.5	5.0	20	10
6	6.0	15.0	18.0	6.0	24	10
7	6.0	15.5	18.5	6.0	24	10
8	6.5	16.0	19.0	6.0	24	10
9	6.5	16.5	19.5	6.0	24	10
10	7.0	17.0	20.0	7.0	28	10
11	7.0	17.5	20.5	7.0	28	10
12	7.5	18.0	21.0	7.5	30	10
13	7.5	18.5	21.5	7.5	30	10
14	8.0	21.0	24.0	8.0	33	12
Adult female	7.5 or 8.0	21.0	24.0	8.0	33	12
Adult male	8.5 or 9.0	22.0	25.0	9.0	36	14

1 French gauge.

Size of endotracheal tubes

Table P1 gives the tube sizes, lengths and suction catheter sizes for all ages. Tracheostomy tube sizes are also listed. An easy guide to the size of the trachea is the width of the thumb.

Endotracheal intubation in children less than 10 years

Never use a cuffed tube, as this can cause severe airway oedema at the level of the cricoid cartilage, which is the narrowest part of a child's airway. Always ensure that there is a leak round the tube after intubation. This will ensure that the tube will not cause pressure on the tracheal mucosa which will impair blood flow and result in pressure necrosis and stricture. In children the width of the little finger is a good guide to the tube size or the following formula can be used:

Endotracheal tube size = Age/4 + 4

Nasotracheal intubation

This type of intubation is better tolerated than orotracheal intubation and is useful in long-term ventilation. It should not be used in patients with severe facial injuries, frontal or basal skull fractures.

Procedure

The procedure of intubation can only be learned by practising under careful supervision. Ask your anaesthetist to show you. The important points are described below. The description assumes that you are using a curved (Macintosh) blade; if you are using a straight (Magill) blade, position it as described under paediatric intubation.

Preparation

Check the contents of your intubation tray regularly (see p. 327) and use cricoid pressure during intubation if the patient is at risk of regurgitation (see. p. 424). A period of pre-oxygenation is useful to help prevent any hypoxia during intubation.

KEY POINT
Check you have everything you may need before starting, including the estimated size of endotracheal tube and one smaller.

Method (Figure P1)

1. Position the head correctly by placing it on a pillow which raises it off the bed, resulting in cervical spine flexion and extension at the atlanto-axial joint. In this position (sometimes referred to as the sniffing position) the larynx is in the best position for intubation in an adult patient (Figure P1a).
2. Insert the laryngoscope (holding it in your left hand) into the right side of the mouth until you are level with the uvula. Move the blade into the midline, pushing the tongue over to the left with the left side of the blade and identify the epiglottis by gently inserting the blade further into the mouth, at the same time lifting the laryngoscope in the direction shown, which will expose the epiglottis. Do not lever the laryngoscope on the front teeth (Figure P1b).
3. Place the tip of the laryngoscope in front of, and at the base of, the epiglottis (Figure P1c). Lift the laryngoscope as described and you will see the larynx appearing (Figure P1d). Sometimes pressure by an assistant on the front of the thyroid cartilage will expose the cords more easily.
4. Intubate the patient with your right hand, passing the correct size of tube gently through the cords and around 5 cm into the trachea. Inflate the cuff with just enough air to seal the trachea when the lungs are inflated with an Ambu bag.

KEY POINT
Do not allow the patient to become hypoxic during intubation.

5. *Difficulties* These often result because the laryngoscope has gone too far into the pharynx and has passed the epiglottis. Bring it back until the larynx and epiglottis appear. If this is ineffective get an assistant to press firmly on the thyroid cartilage.
   (a) Secretions obstruct the view. Suck these out and intubate. If the patient vomits or regurgitates before you secure the airway immediately place him on his left side, head-down, to prevent aspiration. Suction the pharynx clear.
   (b) The endotracheal tube bends and will not go through the cords. Use a smaller tube or stiffen the tube with a suitable introducer. In some cases only part of the larynx may be seen; these patients are best intubated using a flexible introducer, which is placed between the cords and then the endotracheal tube is pushed over it into the larynx.

(c) Failed intubation. The priority is to maintain oxygenation and protect the airway. If you have paralysed the patient ventilate him via a face mask until spontaneous respiration is re-established. If he is at risk of regurgitation, position him on his left side, head-down.

(d) Paediatrics. Babies and small children (<2 years) have relatively large heads and the larynx is positioned higher in the neck. They are best intubated without a pillow using a straight-bladed paediatric laryngoscope. Perform the procedure as before, but this time find the epiglottis and pick it up to expose the cords when using a straight blade. Insert the tube until a reasonable length of tube (2–3 cm) is in the trachea. Do not use a cuffed tube below the age of 10 years.

After intubation

Check that air entry is present in both lungs by listening in the axillae. Secure the tube by tying or taping it firmly in place.

Nursing care

The nursing care of patients with endotracheal tubes is discussed on p. 297 and aims to avoid the complications listed below. Every hour the chest movement on breathing, air entry and respiratory rate should be monitored. The position of the tube as measured from the lips to the connector should be recorded (Figure 16.4). The cuff pressure should be checked 4 hourly and should not exceed 30 cmH$_2$O (normal 15–25 cmH$_2$O).

An endotracheal tube bypasses the normal means of humidification in the nasopharynx and protection against infection, stops the patient from coughing and

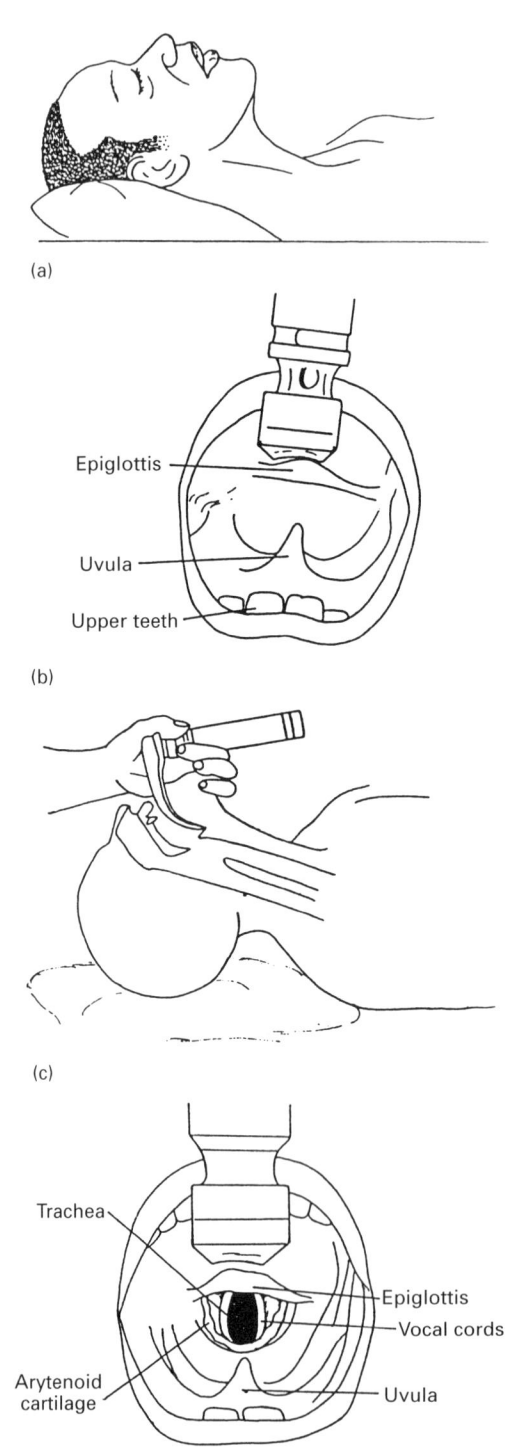

Figure P1 Intubation.

clearing airway secretions. Artificial humidification (p. 347) is essential and bagging and suction must be performed with a meticulous aseptic technique to keep the airway clear of secretions.

Complications of endotracheal intubation
(Table P2)

If an endotracheal tube is pushed too far it will pass into the right main bronchus (Figure P2). This results in collapse of the left lung with mediastinal shift to the left. Always ensure both lungs are being ventilated after intubation by listening to both sides of the chest in the axilla.

The endotracheal tube may become blocked, dislodged or kinked. All of these conditions may prove fatal. Cuff deflation due to a torn cuff results in a leak and may cause underventilation. Regular measurement of the position of the tube using a mark is important (Figure 16.4 – some tubes have marks on them; otherwise, a mark can be made with an indelible pen when the tube is inserted). Humidification and regular suction will reduce the incidence of blocked tubes. If it is difficult to pass the suction catheter through the endo-

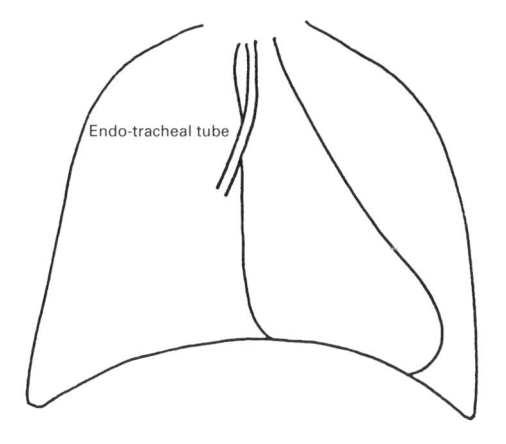

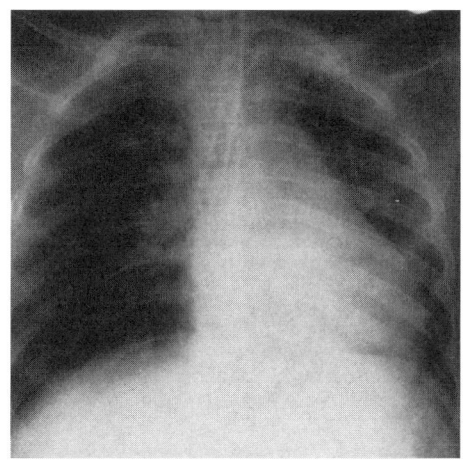

Figure P2 Chest X-ray showing an endotracheal tube that has been pushed in too far and is lodged in the right main bronchus. The tip should be in the mid-tracheal position.

Table P2 Complications of endotracheal intubation

Complication	Result
Failed intubation	Hypoxia
Trauma to the larynx	Haemorrhage and oedema
Tube dislodging into the oesophagus	Hypoxia
Tube dislodging into right main bronchus	Collapsed left lung and hypoxia
Kinked tube	Hypoxia
Tube blocked by secretions	Hypoxia
Cuff leak	Aspiration and under ventilation
Overinflated cuff	Tracheal ulceration and stenosis
	Obstruction of the tube by herniation over the end
Sputum retention	Pneumonia
Introduction of infection	Pneumonia

tracheal tube this indicates either kinking or blockage. When this occurs change the tube.

The endotracheal tube may cause airway oedema and ulceration which subsequently heals with fibrosis. Either the vocal cords or the trachea may be affected.

Following extubation *laryngeal oedema* may be recognised by difficulty in breathing, noisy breathing, stridor or retention of secretions. Treat with dexamethasone 4 mg 8 hourly. Confirm diagnosis by laryngoscopy. If reintubation is necessary then consider tracheostomy to remove source of irritation.

Tracheal stenosis presents with symptoms and signs similar to laryngeal oedema. The site of stenosis is usually where the endotracheal or tracheostomy tube cuff was situated. Secure the airway by tracheostomy if necessary and confirm the diagnosis by bronchoscopy. Treatment is by repeated dilatation. If this fails, tracheal resection or reconstruction will be necessary.

KEY POINT

Use the correct size of tube and do not overinflate the cuff. Never insert a tube that is a tight fit.

Patients who self-extubate may damage their vocal cords. They may self-extubate because they are left intubated too long or are not properly restrained or sedated.

Since endotracheal intubation bypasses the normal protective mechanisms of the airway it provides a potential route of infection. Pneumonia, often due to multi-resistant Gram-negative organisms, is one of the more serious complications of intubation and ventilation. Patient circuits must be properly sterilised (see p. 307) and the correct technique for suction used (p. 352).

Extubation

Before extubating a patient the following criteria must be satisfied:
1. There has been adequate spontaneous breathing following a successful period of weaning and there is no doubt about the patient's ability to breathe adequately.
2. Sedation or muscle relaxants should not have been given within the previous 4 h.
3. The patient should be capable of protecting and clearing his airway by coughing and preventing his tongue from obstructing the upper airway. Thus there should be a good cough and gag reflex.
4. Secretions should not be excessive and an ETT should no longer be considered necessary for suction.
5. There should be no anticipated airway problems – in patients where an airway problem is anticipated or in patients with excessive airway secretions, tracheostomy should be considered rather than extubation.

Unless supervision is adequate as a general rule **do not**:
1. extubate at night;
2. extubate when no one is available to reintubate.

Ensure the following are immediately available:
1. equipment for reintubation;
2. suction;
3. anaesthetic drugs and suxamethonium;
4. an oxygen mask and oxygen.

The patient must have an intravenous line *in situ* and should have an empty stomach. In conscious patients extubation should be performed with the patient on his side or sitting up, while an unconscious patient should be extubated on his side. Bag and suck the patient for the last time, explain what you are going to do and suck out all the secretions from the mouth and pharynx. Deflate the cuff of the endotracheal tube and withdraw it carefully but swiftly at the end of the patient's inspiration. Give the patient oxygen to breathe by face mask and do not leave him.

Observe the patient carefully, monitoring pulse, respiratory rate, respiratory pattern, colour and consciousness level. Listen for wheeze or stridor. Stridor is a serious sign which may be caused by laryngeal oedema, ulceration or partial blockage of the airway by slough or thick secretions. Reintubation may be necessary.

> **KEY POINT**
>
> Do not leave the patient after extubation. Stay and observe.

Postoperative patients

Most postoperative patients recover quickly and some will extubate themselves if not promptly extubated once they are awake. The anaesthetist will usually give advice on when to extubate a postoperative patient.

Ventilation

Many of the terms used in this section are explained in the A to Z of Ventilation (p. 422).

Once the decision to ventilate a patient has been made the patient's trachea should be intubated.

Setting up the ventilator

Before connecting the endotracheal tube to the breathing circuit of the ventilator check the following:
1. Catheter mount connections.
2. Breathing circuit and humidifier.
3. Power supply.
4. Oxygen supply.
5. The ventilator:
    (a) turn on;
    (b) set tidal volume;
    (c) set frequency;
    (d) set oxygen concentration or flow.

Check for leaks by pressure testing the circuit. This is done by occluding the patient end of the ventilator circuit. If this does not generate 60 cmH$_2$O pressure when occluded (or the preset pressure limits) or if there is an audible leak then find and seal the leak before connecting the patient.

Connect the patient to the ventilator by connecting the catheter mount to the endotracheal tube connector. Ensure there are no leaks at this point and check that the chest is moving. Listen to the chest and record the time, ventilator settings and initial observations.

Decide on the oxygen concentration desired and add oxygen to the ventilator by using the table shown in Table P3. Many ventilators allow you to dial the oxygen concentration directly. The percentage of oxygen you use will vary from 100% in severe lung disease with grossly inadequate oxygen diffusion to 30% if the patient is being ventilated for airway problems without an oxygen diffusion defect. Avoid hypoxia and try to avoid ventilating patients with concentrations of oxygen over 60% for periods over 24 h as this can cause oxygen toxicity (p. 347). Give PEEP if required.

Management of a ventilated patient

A nurse should be beside the patient at all times. She should watch for sweating, restlessness, 'fighting' the ventilator and movement of the chest wall. The pulse, blood pressure, colour of the tongue, ventilator settings and position of endotracheal tube must be monitored hourly or more often if there is a problem. The general care for an unconscious patient also applies, including turning, mouth care and pressure area care. The nurse should always speak to the patient, to explain and reassure even if the patient is heavily sedated or unconscious. Continuous pulse oximetry is ideal.

Table P3 Inspired oxygen concentration during ventilation. If the minute volume is calculated and the flow of added oxygen is known, the resulting oxygen concentration is shown in the table

Added oxygen (l/min)

		1	2	3	4	5	6	7	8	9	10	11	12	13	14	15
	3	47	74	100												
	4	41	60	80	100											
	5	37	53	68	84	100										
Ventilator	6	34	47	60	74	87	100									
minute	7	32	44	55	66	77	89	100								
volume	8	31	41	51	60	70	80	90	100							
(l/min)	9	30	39	47	56	65	74	82	91	100						
	10	29	37	45	53	60	68	76	84	92	100					
	11	28	35	42	50	57	64	71	78	86	93	100				
	12	28	35	41	47	54	60	67	74	80	87	93	100			
	13	27	34	39	45	51	57	64	70	76	82	88	94	100		
	14	27	33	38	44	49	55	60	66	72	77	83	89	94	100	
	15	26	32	37	42	47	53	58	63	68	74	79	84	89	95	100

> **KEY POINT**
>
> A nurse should be beside a ventilated patient at all times.

Equipment

An Ambu bag or Mapleson C circuit and a sterile tray containing a suction catheter, gloves and forceps for endotracheal suction should be at the bedside.

An intubation trolley (p. 327) and emergency drugs including muscle relaxants, sedatives and anaesthetic drugs should be immediately available.

Suction

The technique is described on p. 352. Hypoxia during suction, accidental ventilator disconnection, ventilator leaks or ventilator failure are potentially lethal. Constant bedside vigilance is the only way to minimise ventilator accidents. Tracheal secretions should be sucked out as often as required. Pre-oxygenate the patient with 100% oxygen if possible. When sucking hold your breath in expiration for the duration of the procedure so as to avoid hypoxia. Even the length of time a healthy nurse can hold her breath in expiration may be too long for some patients. Bagging and sucking is a form of chest physiotherapy and should be performed 4 hourly or more often if required. Two people are needed to bag and suck safely and efficiently, one to bag and the other to suck.

> **KEY POINT**
>
> Breathe out and hold your breath when you are suctioning a patient to make yourself aware of the duration of apnoea.

Monitoring

The signs of hypoxia and hypercarbia are listed in Table 1.1. If any of these are present you must act immediately and try to determine the cause. Careful observation of colour, sweating, pulse rate (constant pulse oximetry is preferable if you have a monitor), blood pressure, movement of the chest and conscious level are all essential. Review the FiO_2 every few hours, as this may need to be increased if there are signs of hypoxia. The minute volume should be increased if CO_2 retention is suspected (e.g. patient breathing against the ventilator).

KEY POINT

Unexpected bradycardia in a ventilated patient equals hypoxia.

Observations

The following observations should be performed and charted at least hourly:
1. pulse rate and oxygen saturation;
2. blood pressure;
3. colour of tongue (if no pulse oximeter available);
4. consciousness level;
5. ventilator rate;
6. air entry left and right;
7. tidal volume;
8. inspired oxygen concentration;
9. peak inspiratory pressure;
10. endotracheal tube position;
11. cuff pressure (4 hourly).

Investigations

Blood gas analysis and oximetry are discussed on p. 355 and are of considerable help in the management of these patients. However, these measurements are often unavailable and ventilatory support can be performed safely and effectively without them provided careful clinical monitoring is performed. An initial chest X-ray is advisable, and this should be repeated when indicated.

Sedation

Patients vary in their responses to intubation and ventilation. Those who are exhausted, unconscious or very unwell often do not require sedation. However, many other patients do require intravenous sedation and an intravenous infusion is preferable to bolus doses providing the infusion can be properly supervised. Unsedated patients who cough and breathe against the ventilator are at risk of under-ventilation or self-extubation. The requirements for sedation are increased if the patient is intubated (rather than if he has a tracheostomy); some conditions require a lot of sedation, e.g. tetanus. Agents commonly used include morphine, pethidine, fentanyl, alfentanil, midazolam, propofol and diazepam. Propofol is expensive but wears off predictably. Pethidine may accumulate as norpethidine, which is toxic and limits its suitability. Alfentanil is expensive but does not accumulate in renal failure.

Dosages may need to be increased considerably and if an infusion is being given start with the p.r.n. dose as a bolus and then maintain sedation by infusion. Often the best regimen is a combination of an opiate and midazolam.

Opiates not only sedate the patient but also help settle him on the ventilator owing to their depression of respiratory drive and cough reflex. When given intravenously these drugs have a rapid onset of action. They should all be given slowly and the blood pressure should be monitored. If the opiate drugs are given by infusion, the length of time the patient takes to wake will depend on the duration of the infusion, but it will be rarely longer than 6 h. The commonest problem is hypotension and bolus doses of these drugs should be given with great care in shocked patients. Morphine releases histamine and should be avoided in asthmatics.

Muscle relaxants

These act at the neuromuscular junction producing skeletal muscle paralysis. They paralyse the muscles of respiration and have no effect on the central nervous sys-

tem, so that the patient will not be asleep or sedated in any way.
Indications:
1. To facilitate intubation of the trachea.
2. In conjunction with sedation in some ventilated patients.

Their use in artificial ventilation has advantages and disadvantages:

Advantages:
- Tracheal intubation is easier.
- The patient will not fight the ventilator.
- Ventilation is efficient.
- The patient cannot extubate himself.

Disadvantages:
- Must be used with caution if intubation is to be performed by someone who is inexperienced.
- Ventilator disconnection will be fatal if not recognised.
- Communication with the patient is impaired.
- Inadequate sedation is difficult to recognise.
- Fits and spasms are masked and may therefore go untreated.

PRACTICE POINTS
1. Do not use a muscle relaxant to intubate a patient unless you are sure you can ventilate and intubate.
2. Never assume the patient is unconscious because they cannot move.
3. Give adequate sedation using clinical signs as a guide to efficacy (pulse, blood pressure, pupil signs and sweating).
4. The patient should be closely supervised to avoid ventilator disconnection.
5. During suction the patient may become hypoxic. Always hold your breath in expiration when suctioning a patient.

Suxamethonium is a depolarising muscle relaxant, is short-acting (4 min) and is used to produce a brief period of paralysis for intubation. It should never be used to maintain muscle relaxation in ventilated patients.

Non-depolarising muscle relaxants such as pancuronium have a longer duration of action and are used to maintain paralysis, when required, on the ventilator. In renal failure atracurium is the muscle relaxant of choice. Never use gallamine in renal failure. Tubocurarine should be used with caution in patients with shock.

In general, we try not to use muscle relaxants, preferring instead to use adequate amounts of opiate and midazolam sedation. However, in a few patients who prove difficult to ventilate (i.e. those with poor lung compliance or who do not settle after adequate sedation and effective ventilation), we occasionally use relaxants to facilitate ventilation. Sedation is always given at the same time to prevent the patient waking up while paralysed.

Physiotherapy, endotracheal intubation, tracheostomy, and ventilation all inhibit the patient's ability to cough. This will lead to retention of secretions and alveolar collapse which predispose to pneumonia. Regular bagging and suction and chest physiotherapy are essential, as often as required to keep the chest clear (pp. 349–351).

Problems in ventilated patients

The solution lies in careful examination of first the patient and then the equipment.

The chest is not moving

Causes
1. Endotracheal tube (ETT) is in wrong position.
2. ETT is kinked or blocked.
3. ETT cuff is deflated.

4. Ventilator problem – circuit leak, disconnected from patient, stopped working, power failure.

Action

Immediately disconnect the patient from the ventilator, connect an Ambu bag with oxygen to the endotracheal tube and ventilate by hand. If the chest starts to move this means there has been a problem with the ventilator. Maintain ventilation by hand until the problem is identified and rectified. The chest compliance can be easily appreciated when bagging the patient. Auscultate both sides of the chest.

If the chest still does not move and ventilation feels easy then listen for a leak. If the problem is not a deflated cuff then it is likely that the endotracheal tube is displaced. If ventilation feels difficult then a kinked or displaced tube may be the cause. The kink may be obvious or it may be impossible to pass a suction catheter down the tube. Remove the ETT, ventilate by face mask and reintubate. If there is a high inflation pressure and only one side of the patient's chest is moving properly consider the possibility of a tension pneumothorax (p. 341) or intubation of the right main bronchus.

KEY POINT
Whatever the problem disconnect the patient from the ventilator and ventilate using an Ambu bag.

The patient breathes against or fights the ventilator

Do not sedate a patient who is fighting the ventilator until you have ensured that:
1. the ETT is in the trachea;
2. the ETT is not touching the carina;
3. the ETT is not blocked;
4. the patient does not need to be suctioned;
5. the patient is not cyanosed or hypotensive or retaining CO_2;
6. there is bilateral air entry in the chest;
7. the bladder is not distended and there is no other cause for the patient to be in pain, such as a fracture;
8. the patient is actually fighting and not fitting.

The underlying principles of management are: hyperventilate the patient by hand. Check the ventilator pressure and look for leaks in the ventilator circuit, for a deflated ETT cuff or dislodged tube. Listen to the chest: is there bilateral air entry? Is the patient sweating or cyanosed? Check blood gases and/or oxygen saturation if available.

If other causes of restlessness are excluded then sedate the patient as described previously. When putting the patient back on the ventilator consider increasing the rate and/or tidal volume if it is thought that the problem was CO_2 retention.

Hypotension, tachycardia, bradycardia

These may be due to underventilation and hypoxia. Check that the chest is moving with the ventilator. If it is not then disconnect the ventilator and ventilate by hand with an Ambu bag. Treat and consider causes as above. If bradycardia develops during suction, immediately reconnect the patient to the ventilator and give 100% oxygen. Other causes of bradycardia include brain stem damage, heart block or drugs such as beta-blockers or digoxin.

The deteriorating patient

In patients whose observations detriorate (bradycardia, tachycardia, consciousness level, hypotension or sweating), check for chest wall movement, air entry, adequate ventilator pressures and function. Often the deteriorating patient will fight against the ventilator. Check the blood gases and/or oxygen saturation if these are available.

Rising ventilator pressures

The normal ventilator pressures should be between 15 and 30 cmH$_2$O. The causes of rising pressures are the following:
1. blocked or kinked ETT;
2. stiff lungs due to pulmonary oedema or ARDS (stiff, low, compliant lungs can be recognised by increased resistance to ventilating the patient by hand);
3. tension pneumothorax;
4. bronchospasm;
5. fighting the ventilator (see above);
6. incorrect ventilator settings.

Treat according to cause. The higher the pressures needed to ventilate the patient, the greater the possibility of a pneumothorax or pressure damage to the lungs. Check a chest X-ray.

Low ventilator pressures

The chest wall may not be moving adequately with the ventilator. The possible causes are leak, disconnection, tube dislodgement, cuff deflation or incorrect ventilator settings.

Ventilate the patient by hand until you have rectified the problem.

Pneumothorax

This may be due to rupture of a lung bulla or ventilation with too high an inflation pressure. Because air is being forced into the lungs by the ventilator, a pneumothorax in a ventilated patient will always be under tension. If it is not recognised and relieved then hypotension and cardiac arrest will develop. The signs of pneumothorax are as follows:
1. reduced air entry on the affected side;
2. hyper-resonant percussion note on the affected side;
3. tracheal deviation away from the affected side;
4. decreased chest movement on the affected side;
5. an appearance of overinflation of the chest on the affected side;
6. increased ventilator pressures;
7. hypotension, tachycardia;
8. raised JVP and CVP;
9. bradycardia (end-stage).

An urgent chest X-ray should be taken to confirm the diagnosis (Figure 1.4) and an intercostal drain inserted (p. 365). If the patient is deteriorating rapidly then the affected side can be decompressed by inserting a wide-bore cannula into the pleural cavity in the anterior axillary line (6th intercostal space). Patients with fractured ribs are at risk of developing a tension pneumothorax on the ventilator and should have a prophylactic chest drain inserted.

Self-extubation

Patients usually extubate themselves by pulling out the tube or dislodging it when they turn the head from side to side.

The causes are: inadequate sedation; inadequate nursing supervision (sometimes due to too many patients and not enough nurses); failure to secure the endotracheal tube properly; deflation of the cuff or failure to record the distance of the end of the endotracheal tube from the teeth at regular intervals.

Self-extubation can damage the larynx and may be fatal if the patient cannot maintain his airway.

Self-extubation should be prevented rather than treated. Once it happens a decision needs to be made as to whether the patient can maintain his own airway or whether he should be reintubated.

How long should a patient be ventilated?

Ventilate until the cause of respiratory failure is better and the patient can breathe spontaneously via the endotracheal tube on 30% oxygen or less, maintaining oxygenation without tiring. Shocked patients or those with septicaemia should not be weaned until their general condition is improving and any other major problems are corrected. If the patient has gross pathology in the chest such as pneumonia wait until this is clearing before you attempt weaning. Do not try to wean patients before pleural effusions or empyemas are drained.

Are the pressures required to ventilate the patient high? If so he is not ready for weaning. You can assess the compliance of the chest for yourself by ventilating the patient with an Ambu bag. If the lungs feel stiff the patient is not ready for weaning.

Patients who have been given muscle relaxants will not breathe spontaneously until the muscle relaxants have worn off (which may take up to 4–6 h or longer if there is renal failure). Heavy sedation may also suppress breathing.

To determine whether a patient will breathe spontaneously, connect the patient to a breathing circuit or attach an Ambu bag and give 10% more oxygen. Ventilate by hand at a slow rate of 5–6/min. Watch for spontaneous movement of the chest. Explain to the patient that you want him to breathe. It may take 60 seconds or more for the patient to start breathing, particularly if the ventilator has been set at a fast rate of 15–18 breaths/min. This may have reduced the carbon dioxide tension in the blood and thus the CO_2 drive to breathing. Keep a finger on the pulse and watch the oxygen saturation while waiting for him to breathe.

Once the patient is breathing you must decide if the tidal volumes are adequate. Feel the amount of air being expired by placing your hand near the ETT. A Wright's respirometer (see A to Z of Ventilation, p. 434) can be used to measure tidal volume (normal tidal volume is 7–10 ml/kg). Ausculate the chest and assess air entry.

Respiratory rate and pattern are just as important as tidal volume. Initially the patient may breathe at 40–50 breaths/min. If this does not quickly settle to a rate below 30 the patient is not yet ready to be weaned. Watch the pattern of breathing. If the chest fails to expand reasonably he is probably not ready for weaning. Signs of hypoxia such as tachycardia, restlessness, sweating and hypotension are evidence that the patient is not ready for weaning.

How do I wean a patient off the ventilator?

The underlying condition should be better and the patient must be able to breathe well spontaneously for at least 15 min without developing tachycardia, cyanosis, hypotension or distress.

Sometimes weaning may take days and at other times the patient can be extubated immediately he comes off the ventilator. In general, the longer someone has been ventilated, the longer is the weaning process. Oxygen therapy and humidification should continue through a weaning circuit (p. 426). Continuous positive airways pressure (CPAP) may still be necessary. During the period of weaning the nurse should carefully observe the patient, monitoring pulse rate, blood pressure, respiratory rate, respiratory pattern and oxygen saturation. The nurse should note too whether the patient gets restless or starts to sweat – these are both signs of respiratory distress and hypoxia. Some patients require heavy sedation to re-establish the ventilation after a period of spontaneous breathing. Unfortunately the effects of the sedation may persist into the next period of weaning. When prolonged weaning is anticipated and sedation is a problem, tracheostomy will help because less sedation will be required.

Classical weaning: allow the patient to breathe spontaneously for 10 min in the hour and increase the time period gradually.

Other types of gradual weaning: ventilators that have different modes make weaning simpler. From controlled ventilation, change the mode to 'pressure support'. This means the patient's own effort to breathe will be assisted by the ventilator and the amount of assistance from the ventilator gradually reduced. SIMV (synchronised intermittent mandatory ventilation), which provides a specified number of breaths per minute (see p. 427) may also be used. If positive airways pressure is still needed after weaning CPAP mode can be used. When available, pulse oximetry should be monitored during weaning. It is possible to recognise clinically that the patient is not suitable for weaning before severe blood gas abnormalities develop.

Blood gas analysis

Blood gases and oximetry should not become a substitute for clinical examination and monitoring of the patient. The decision to wean and extubate can usually be made on clinical grounds and although blood gas analysis may help it is not essential. Patients who have a PaO_2 of less than 8 kPa on 40% oxygen or more are unlikely to wean successfully. Patients who have a raised CO_2 after a period of spontaneous breathing when weaning should not be extubated.

Lung protection strategies during ventilation

It is known that positive pressure ventilation may result in ventilator-induced lung injury. This may be caused by pressure-induced overdistension of alveoli, and damaging shear forces during repeated opening and closing of alveoli. Protective strategies being explored include:

- Avoiding unnecessarily high inspired oxygen concentrations by monitoring against oxygen saturations.
- Limiting inspiratory pressures (<35 cmH$_2$O) by using pressure control ventilation and smaller tidal volumes around 400–500 ml.
- 'Permissive' hypercapnia – allowing the $PaCO_2$ to rise to reduce ventilator pressures. Acidosis occurs, but is rarely a problem if the pH remains >7.25.
- Positive end expiratory pressure (PEEP) can prevent cyclical collapse and opening of alveoli. Levels of 10–12 cmH$_2$O are commonly used.
- Inverse ratio ventilation (IRV) allows the duration of inspiration to be extended and the duration of expiration shortened. Arterial oxygenation improves by recruiting lung alveoli and reducing shunt but also through increasing mean airway pressure.
- Prone position is known to improve oxygenation rapidly in patients with ARDS due to improved regional ventilation. It has not yet been shown to improve survival.

Non-invasive ventilation

This is a technique that ventilates the patient via a nasal or full-face mask. It is most commonly used in chronic respiratory failure patients such as those with an exacerbation of COAD.

Ethical problems and ventilation

Artificial ventilation can save the lives of critically ill patients. It can also prolong the suffering of patients who have an incurable illness. It is preferable to identify the patients who are incurable before ventilating them and avoid ventilation. This is often a very difficult decision and as a result incurable patients are sometimes ventilated. In these circumstances, once the decision has been made that the underlying cause is untreatable, a decision to withdraw ventilation should be made. Depending on local practices, full explanations should be given to the family and often the patient. Ventilation is easier to reduce and withdraw when the patient is well sedated.

Further reading

BROWER RG, FRESSLER HE. Mechanical ventilation in acute lung injury and acute respiratory distress syndrome. *Clin Chest Med* 2000;21:491–510.

The Acute Respiratory Distress Syndrome Network. Ventilation with lower tidal volumes as compared with traditional tidal volumes for acute lung injury and the acute respiratory distress syndrome. *N Engl J Med* 2000;342:1301–8.

Oxygen therapy

Anyone who is hypoxic requires oxygen therapy. Several techniques are available to administer oxygen including masks, nasal spectacles or nasopharyngeal catheters.

Masks

Fixed-performance masks

Sometimes called venturi masks, these deliver an accurate, fixed concentration of oxygen at a high flow-rate. This type of mask has instructions on it to tell you how much oxygen to add and what percentage will result. Models are available to deliver 24%, 28%, 35%, 40% or 60% oxygen. A common example of this mask is the Ventimask. Such masks are particularly useful for when you need to provide an exact percentage of oxygen (see controlled oxygen therapy, p. 347).

Variable-performance masks

These include all other masks and provide a flow of oxygen which the patient breathes along with air drawn in from around the outside of the mask. When breathing in there is a peak inspiratory flow rate of about 30 l/min. This means that the oxygen concentration administered by this type of mask will vary according to the flow of oxygen and the characteristics of the mask. The same factors affect nasal spectacles and cannulae.

Nasal spectacles

These deliver oxygen at the nostrils and depend on the oxygen being carried down through the nose during inspiration. They are inefficient if the patient is breathing through the mouth.

Naso-pharyngeal cannula

This is a piece of soft tubing which is inserted into the nasopharynx, often with some local anaesthetic gel to make it comfortable. The cannula should be inserted into the nose until the tip can just be seen appearing below the soft palate and then taped at the nose. Using this technique oxygen is delivered into the airway and it is a convenient method of administration if no masks are available. Some patients dislike the drying of the mucosa that this technique produces. This is also a suitable method of giving oxygen to patients who have oropharyngeal airways in place if the cannula is inserted into the airway. Because of the high pressures in oxygen delivery systems the cannula must never be able to enter the oesophagus, as this might lead to gastric distension or even damage to the oesophagus. The safest way to use these cannulae is with a T-piece arrangement (Figure P3), which allows any excess pressure which would be caused by misplacement of the cannula to be blown off. In normal use the trap should not bubble and the end of the T-piece should be just far enough under

Table P4 Methods of oxygen delivery compared

Method	Oxygen flow[1] (l/min)	Approximate concentration delivered
Venturi masks	4–8	24–60%[1]
Plastic masks	4–12	30–60%
Nasal spectacles or catheter	2–6	30–50%

[1] Depends on the model and the manufacturer's recommendations. Lower flows are needed in children, particularly for nasopharyngeal cannulae.

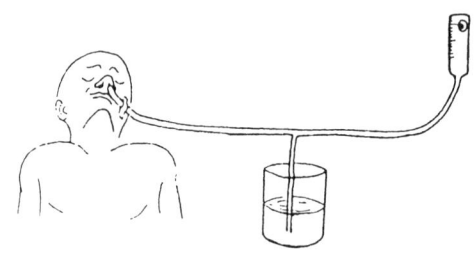

Figure P3 T-piece arrangement for nasopharyngeal oxygen using a nasogastric tube. The underwater T-limb prevents excess oxygen pressures being delivered to the patient. The tip should be far enough under water to prevent it bubbling when the nasal catheter is in the correct position. This is usually around 10 cm below the surface, but depends on the size of the tubing and the flow of oxygen employed. If bubbles appear during use it is likely that the catheter has become misplaced or kinked, and its position should be checked. If the catheter is correctly sited then put the T-limb further under water until the bubbling stops.

water to prevent bubbling but not exceed 30–40 cm (usually 10 cm is adequate).

The approximate concentrations delivered by these methods are indicated in Table P4.

When using masks, spectacles and cannulae the patient always draws in atmospheric air with the oxygen to some extent. This means that it is impossible to give more than 50–60% oxygen from a standard delivery system. The only way to give a patient 100% oxygen (e.g. for preoxygenation) is with a specialised circuit such as a Mapleson C circuit, or using an Ambu bag with an oxygen reservoir (see A to Z of Ventilation, p. 427).

Administration of oxygen

Oxygen should be ordered specifying the mask and the flow of oxygen to be used. The patient must be supervised to ensure that the prescribed oxygen is being received as intended (Figure P4).

A guide to the percentages achieved by simple plastic face masks is shown in Table P5.

In mild hypoxia (PaO_2 >9.3 kPa), start with nasal spectacles or cannula (2–3 l/min oxygen) or a simple plastic mask (4 l/min) is acceptable. In moderate hypoxia (PaO_2 6.7–9.3 kPa) use a simple mask (6–12 l/min) or a 50–60% Ventimask. Monitor response to oxygenation by patient colour, general condition, blood gases or oximetry and adjust your therapy accordingly. If despite high-flow oxygen

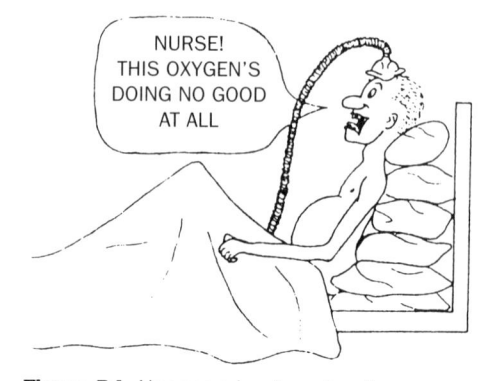

Figure P4 Unsupervised oxygen therapy.

Table P5 Plastic face mask oxygen delivery rates

Oxygen flow (l/min)	Approximate oxygen
4	35%
6	45%
8	50%
10	55%
12	60%

therapy the patient deteriorates it is likely that artificial ventilation will be required.

Controlled oxygen therapy

Patients who have had a long history of severe chronic obstructive airways disease (COAD) and present in respiratory failure require special care with their oxygen therapy. Some of these patients chronically retain CO_2 and rely on a lower than normal PaO_2 to stimulate respiration. The effect of breathing a high concentration of oxygen in these patients is to temporarily improve their PaO_2 but paradoxically reduce their respiratory drive, causing more CO_2 retention and worsening their respiratory failure. When dealing with these patients you should use the most accurate oxygen masks you have. Start controlled oxygen therapy at a concentration of 24% using a fixed-performance venturi mask and increase the oxygen to 28% after an hour if there is no respiratory deterioration (this is best determined by blood gas analysis; a rising $PaCO_2$ indicates that the respiratory drive is failing). The principle behind controlled oxygen therapy is to provide improved oxygenation without compromising respiratory drive.

Oxygen toxicity

An uncommon complication of oxygen therapy, this is caused by prolonged administration of excessive oxygen. It is a serious problem in premature neonates causing retrolental fibroplasia and excess oxygen therapy should always be avoided in premature babies. Toxicity is less common in older patients.

The priority with any oxygen therapy is to keep the patient well oxygenated. This should be achieved without using excessive oxygen and if blood gas analysis or an oximeter are available they can usefully guide oxygen therapy. During oxygen therapy the concentration of oxygen should be reduced regularly and the effect assessed by pulse oximetry.

In patients who are ventilated, the addition of positive end expiratory pressure (PEEP) whenever more than 50% oxygen is required will often assist in oxygenation, and this is preferable to increasing the inspired oxygen concentration. If hypoxia is still present despite PEEP values of 10 cmH_2O and O_2 concentration of 60%, then you must increase the O_2 concentration up to a point where hypoxia is overcome, accepting that O_2 toxicity is a theoretial problem.

Humidification

Medical oxygen is dry and may cause an uncomfortable drying of the mucous membranes, especially when used with nasal spectacles or cannulae. Certain oxygen equipment manufacturers produce water humidifiers which fit on the bottom of the oxygen flow meters to overcome this problem. These are probably beneficial, especially with nasal cannulae or catheters, though they are not vital. Some patients dislike the resulting water droplets falling on their face. A common problem with these humidifiers is that they may leak oxygen. If this occurs then disconnect the humidifier and make sure the patient gets all the oxygen. Never use a humidifier in the oxygen delivery line when you are feeding oxygen into a ventilator or nebuliser, as these devices humidify the oxygen by a different means. A simple bubble humidifier can be made by bubbling oxygen through water before it reaches the patient.

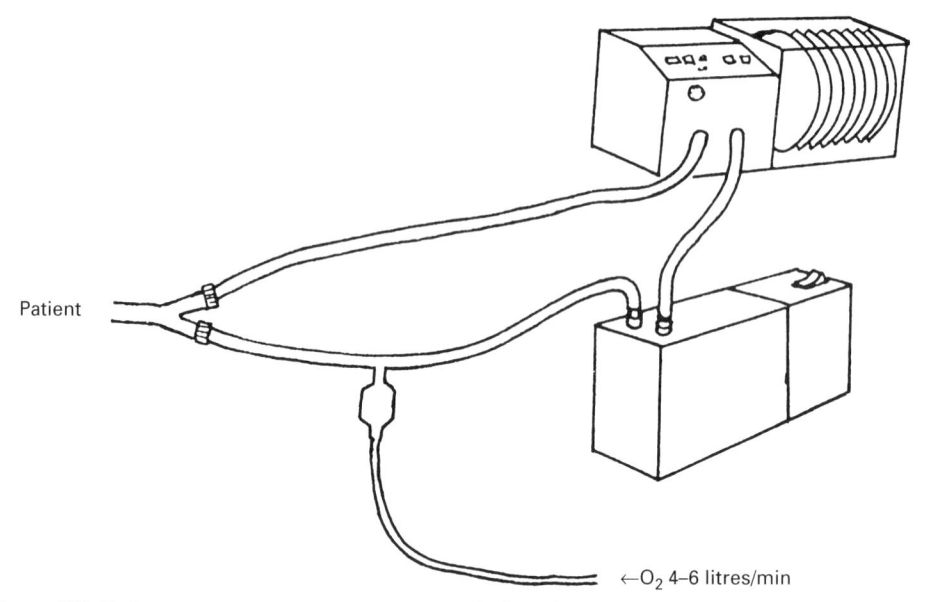

Figure P5 T-piece arrangement to connect a nebuliser into the inspiratory tube.

Nebulisers

These devices produce very small droplets of liquid drugs when a flow of oxygen is passed through them. The patient breathes the oxygen and the drug passes to the bronchi where it either acts directly or is absorbed. The most common drugs used in this way are the bronchodilator drugs such as salbutamol, terbutaline and ipratropium. When you are using a nebuliser decide the correct dose of drug you wish to use, dilute it to 4 ml with the recommended diluent and place it in the chamber. (You need around 4 ml to make the nebuliser work efficiently). Connect the oxygen source at 6–8 l/min and arrange the patient so that they are sitting with the nebuliser in a vertical position. You will see a fine mist of liquid coming out of the nebuliser, which the patient breathes.

If you wish to use a nebuliser with a patient on a ventilator, check if there is a special facility on the ventilator for doing so (e.g. Puritan Bennett and Siemens ventilators may have a nebuliser in the inspiratory tube). With other ventilators you must put the nebuliser in a T-piece arrangement in the inspiratory tube (Figure P5). This arrangement means that you are adding oxygen to the ventilator tubing which increases the tidal volume by the amount of oxygen which goes through the nebuliser during inspiration. If the ventilator is delivering 20 breaths/min with a normal inspiratory: expiratory time ratio (1:2) then each inspiration will take 1 second. If 6 litres a minute of oxygen are being delivered to the nebuliser then 100 ml extra oxygen will be delivered to the patient with each breath. This will not matter in an average adult but may require changes to the ventilator setting in children.

An alternative is to hand ventilate the patient while the nebuliser is being used in a T-piece arrangement in your manual circuit. This is particularly useful for children.

Nasopharyngeal oxygen in children

Giving oxygen by nasophanyngeal catheter in children is described on page 369.

Chest physiotherapy

Indications

The primary purpose of chest physiotherapy is to remove airway secretions and to prevent and treat chest infections. In critically ill patients it is also used to prevent accumulation of secretions which may lead to infection and which may precipitate or aggravate respiratory failure. It is particularly indicated in patients with inadequate ventilation and in intubated patients and those with a tracheostomy.

Specific conditions requiring physiotherapy include:
- unconsciousness;
- following abdominal or chest surgery or trauma;
- inadequate coughing due to muscle weakness or lung disease;
- primary lung disease with sputum retention;
- the presence of a nasogastric tube.

In these conditions chest physiotherapy prevents accumulation of secretions, reduces the risks of pneumonia and helps prevent pulmonary collapse. Chest physiotherapy may precipitate bronchospasm and may aggravate hypoxia and in very ill people it may cause exhaustion. Particular care is needed in critically ill patients.

Breathing exercises

Breathing exercises encourage full expansion of all parts of the lung and help to prevent pneumonia and lung collapse (atelectasis). Deep breathing should be encouraged frequently and in different positions. The use of an incentive spirometer may be helpful (Figure P7). If there is sputum these exercises can be combined with assisted coughing (see below).

Postural drainage

Sputum in the lower airways does not stimulate coughing. Postural drainage is designed to allow gravity to assist in draining secretions. It is indicated in all patients who have or may get sputum retention.

Technique

1. The procedure is explained to the patient.
2. The patient is placed in the correct position to drain the affected lobe(s).
3. Chest vibration (see below) should be done for 1–2 min at about 5 min intervals.
4. When the patient coughs the cough should be assisted (see below) and if this is ineffective the airways should be sucked out as often as necessary.
5. Drainage should continue for between 5 and 20 min depending on the volume of secretions.
6. In intubated patients the final stage of the treatment is airway suction (see below).

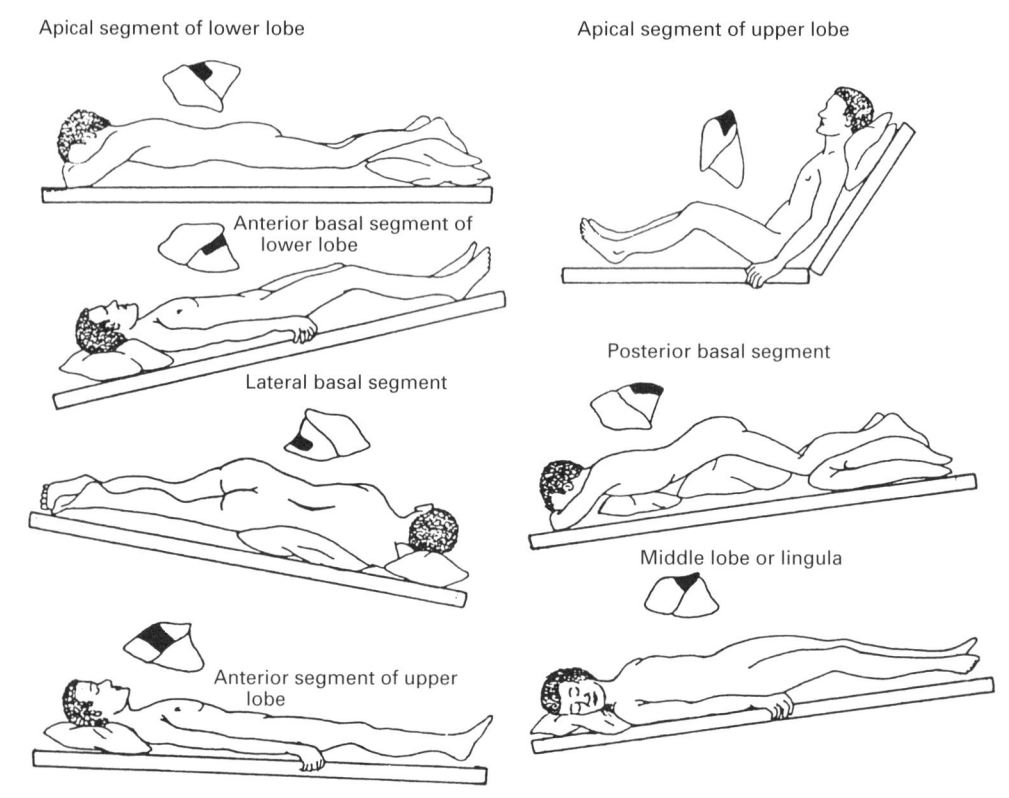

Figure P6 Chest physiotherapy for particular lobes of the lung.

7. The treatment is then repeated with the patient lying on the opposite side.

Chest vibration

Thick sputum may adhere to the bronchial walls and chest vibration is carried out during postural drainage to 'shake' secretions into the bronchi.

Techniques

1. Explain what you are doing to the patient.
2. Cup both hands.
3. Slap the lower chest fast with alternate hands.

Never vibrate the chest with the hands flat; this causes pain.

Assisted coughing

Weak patients and patients with chest diseases lose the power to expel sputum by coughing. Assisted coughing is designed to increase the force of expiration during a cough.

Technique

1. Grip the lower part of the chest between both hands.
2. During the expiratory phase of coughing squeeze the chest firmly.

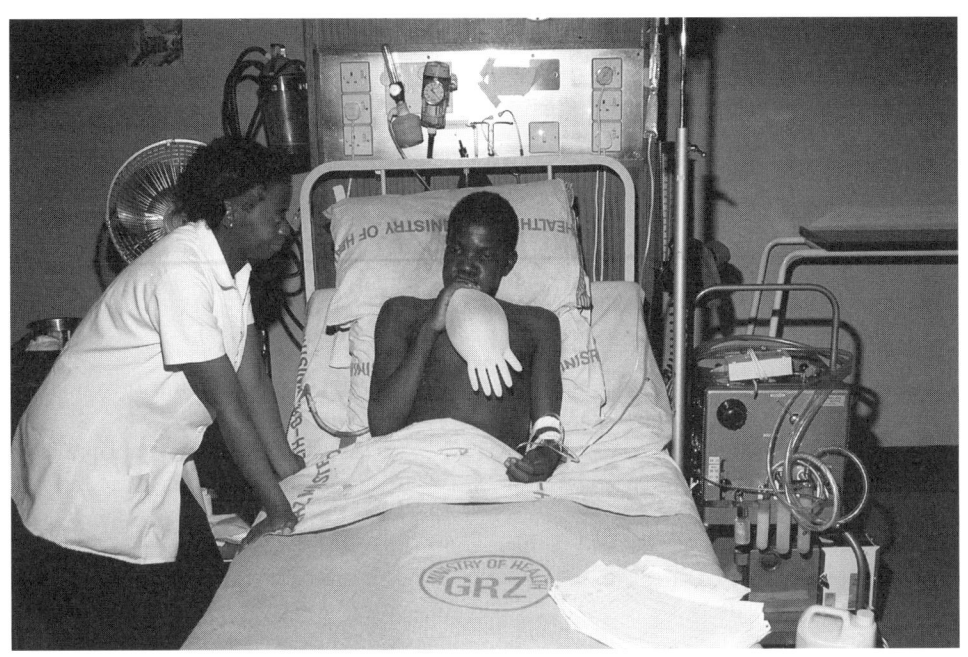

Figure P7 Chest physiotherapy and incentive spirometry: The effort of blowing up a surgical glove is an inexpensive way of making the patient work to expand and clear his lungs. This reduces atelectasis and subsequent infection of collapsed alveoli providing more open alveoli for gas exchange. Once the patient understands what is required they can continue with their own chest physiotherapy during the rest of their critical period. A 1970s East Radcliffe ventilator is shown on the right of the picture.

In patients who are on a ventilator, assisted coughing requires manual control of breathing using a bag and 100% oxygen.

Further reading

SELSBY DS. Chest physiotherapy. *BMJ* 1989; 298:541–2.

Airway suction

When the cough is ineffective because the patient is intubated or too weak, suction is used to remove sputum from the main airways. It cannot be performed unless the patient is intubated or has a tracheostomy. The airway should be sterile and a no-touch technique is used to prevent infection being introduced.

Technique (Figures P8–P11)

In patients breathing spontaneously

1. Use a no-touch technique.
2. Check the sucker is working.
3. Attach a correctly sized sterile catheter to the sucker (p. 422).
4. Turn the sucker on.
5. Explain what you are doing to the patient. Preoxygenate.
6. Disconnect the patient from the humidifier (or ventilator).
7. Block the suction by squeezing the suction catheter near its attachment to the sucker using forceps in your left hand.
8. Using forceps in your right hand, insert the catheter into the endotraceal tube and gently push it down as far as it will go.
9. Release the catheter from the forceps in your left hand to allow suction – slowly withdraw the catheter with a twisting movement. Reconnect patient.
10. Clear the catheter by sucking up a small amount of sterile water.
11. Repeat the process until secretions are cleared.
12. Suck out the mouth **after** completion of airway suction.
13. Turn the sucker off.
14. Place the catheter in the 'used' bowl.

When suction catheters are in short supply catheters can be re-used providing the tracheal catheter is always kept separate from that used for oral suction and they

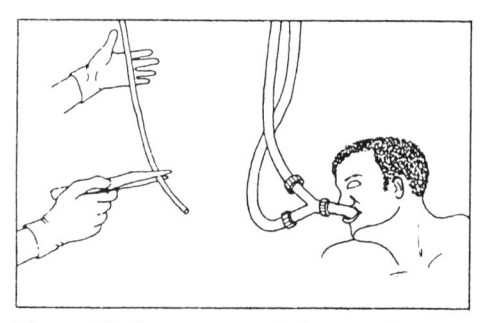

Figure P8 Preoxygenate **before** suction.

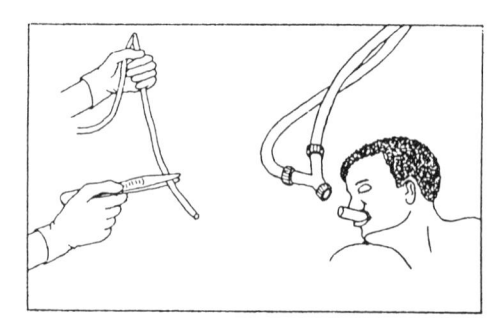

Figure P9 Disconnect the ventilator circuit, occlude the suction catheter, and using sterile forceps or disposable gloves, insert the suction catheter down the endotracheal tube.

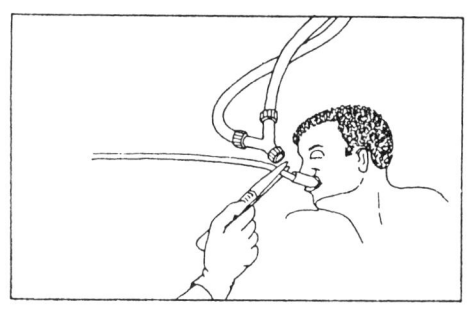

Figure P10 Suction the patient while slowly withdrawing and rotating the catheter.

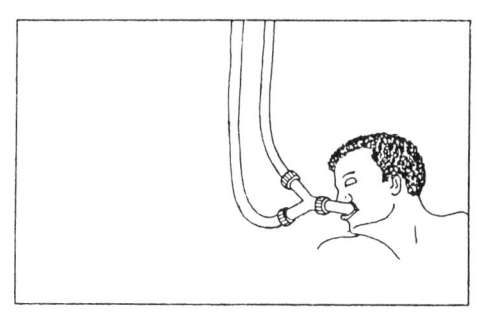

Figure P11 Reconnect the patient to the ventilator.

are soaked in separate bowls and covered with disinfectant between use. Before use rinse the catheters in sterile water.

PRACTICE POINT
Suction of the trachea after oral suction without changing the catheter causes respiratory infection.

In patients on a ventilator

Patients needing ventilatory support do not breathe sufficiently on their own and may develop serious hypoxia during airway suction. To prevent this, two nurses are needed; maximum oxygenation is given before suction and the time without ventilation should not exceed the time a person can hold their breath in expiration without discomfort. In children the safe time without ventilation is even shorter. Additional steps to make suction safe for these patients are:

1. Ventilate the patient with 100% oxygen using a bag for 10 'breaths' immediately before commencing suction (p. 422).
2. Never take longer than 15 seconds (or as long as you can hold your breath) to insert and withdraw the suction catheter and recommence ventilating the patient with 100% oxygen.
3. Check the colour of the tongue for hypoxia during the procedure.
4. Give the patient a further 10 'breaths' of 100% oxygen before repeating suction.
5. On completion reconnect the patient to the ventilator, adjust the concentration of oxygen to its previous level and check the endotracheal tube position (p. 298).

PRACTICE POINT
Hold your breath in expiration when suctioning a patient who is not breathing spontaneously. A patient cannot do without ventilation for longer than you can hold your breath. Ventilated patients become hypoxic quickly.

Problems with airway suction

1. The catheter will not pass down the endotracheal tube.
   (a) Check the catheter is not too large for the size of tube (p. 423).
   (b) Check the position of the tube.
   (c) Try moistening a dry catheter with a small amount of saline.
   If this is unsuccessful it is likely that the tube is kinked or blocked and will need replacing urgently.
2. Secretions are very thick and difficult to suck out: try injecting 2–3 ml of sterile saline down the endotracheal tube and sucking the patient out again.

Thick secretions are normally due to inadequate humidification and if left untreated may eventually block the tube.
3. When the patient is sucked out he develops cyanosis and bradycardia. This is due to lack of adequate preoxygenation, carrying out suction for too long or using too large a suction catheter.

Airway suction can be dangerous in asthmatics and head-injured patients. In asthmatic patients on the ventilator, airway suction can provoke severe bronchospasm and should not be performed until bronchodilation therapy has commenced. Patients with severe head injury can respond to airway suction with large increases in intracranial pressure. This effect can be blunted by ensuring that head-injured patients receive a dose of i.v. opiate before airway suction to ensure they are adequately sedated for the procedure.

Blood gas analysis

Blood gases are measured using a special analyser and give information about oxygenation, carbon dioxide excretion and the acid–base balance of the body, which reflects its metabolic condition. Blood gases are useful in guiding treatment of critically ill patients but are expensive and dependent on advanced technology, and for these reasons they are not available in many hospitals in developing countries.

Taking the sample

The radial, brachial and femoral arteries are suitable for sampling. Note the time of sampling, the patient's temperature, oxygen flow rate and ventilator settings if relevant.

1. Clean the skin over the intended site with a suitable antiseptic solution and ask an assistant to be ready to help hold the limb.
2. Add about 0.2 ml of heparin (strength 1:1000) to a 2 ml or 5 ml syringe and work the plunger up and down a few times to coat the inside of the syringe with heparin. Finally attach a fresh needle (25 gauge for the arm; 23 or 21 gauge for the femoral) and expel all heparin and air from the syringe. (The amount of heparin left at the tip of the syringe will anticoagulate the sample.)
3. Palpate the artery gently with the fingers of your left hand and introduce the needle using a no-touch technique into the artery with your other hand, maintaining a slight negative pressure on the plunger all the time. When sampling from the arm keep the syringe at an angle of 45° to the skin; in the groin the needle should be almost at 90°. When taking samples from the arm it is a good idea to infiltrate the subcutaneous tissues with a small volume of 1% lidocaine before starting.
4. As soon as you see blood enter the syringe, stop advancing the syringe, aspirate 2 ml of blood, then take the needle out. If you do not obtain blood draw the syringe back slowly in case you have gone right through the artery. Place a cotton wool ball on the puncture site and ask your assistant to press firmly on it for a minimum of 5 min to prevent haematoma formation which may be a particular problem after arterial puncture because of the high pressures in arteries.
5. Remove the needle from the syringe and expel any air bubbles which have entered the blood during sampling. Cap the syringe with an airtight cap and carry out analysis. If there will be a delay of 10 min or more before analysis, or you have to send the sample to a laboratory, put the syringe into a plastic bag with a few pieces of crushed ice.
6. Check the site of your puncture for swelling or bleeding.

Table P6 Normal arterial blood gas values

PaO_2	11–13 kPa (83–98 mmHg)
$PaCO_2$	4.8–6.0 kPa (36–45 mmHg)
pH	7.36–7.44
Haemoglobin O_2 saturation	≥95%
Bicarbonate	22–26 mmol/l
Base excess	– 3 to + 3

To convert kPa to mmHg multiply by 7.5.

Blood gas results

Most blood gas analysers give values for the following parameters (normal values are given in Table P6).

PaO_2

This is the partial pressure of oxygen in arterial blood. Atmospheric pressure is made up of the different gases which form air, and the pressure varies with altitude. At sea level normal atmospheric pressure is said to be 1 atmosphere. Different units are used for measuring pressure, so that 1 atmosphere of pressure can be expressed as 14.7 pounds per square inch (lbf/in^2), 100 kilopascals (kPa) or 760 millimetres of mercury (mmHg). At sea level 21% of air is oxygen, so the partial pressure of oxygen in the air is 21% of 1 atmosphere, i.e. 21 kPa or 159 mmHg. When a liquid is exposed to a gas the amount which dissolves in the liquid is determined by the pressure of the gas. The higher the pressure of the gas, the more will dissolve. We can measure the pressure of dissolved oxygen in the blood and this tells us how well the lungs are transferring the oxygen from the atmosphere to the blood. At normal altitudes the pressure should be 11–13 kPa (83–98 mmHg) when breathing air. Elderly patients have lower arterial oxygen tensions than young people. Any values below 11 kPa indicate hypoxia.

$PaCO_2$

The partial pressure of carbon dioxide in arterial blood. Normal value is 4.8–6.0 kPa (36–45 mmHg). Values above 7.3 kPa usually represent respiratory accumulation of CO_2 due to inadequate ventilation. A $PaCO_2$ of below 4.8 kPa represents hyperventilation.

Oxygen saturation

This is the percentage of the total haemoglobin combined with oxygen. This is usually 95% or more in normal people and values below 90% reflect serious hypoxia (see p. 429).

pH

This is a measure of the number of free hydrogen ions in a solution. Excess hydrogen ions means acidosis, lack of hydrogen ions means alkalosis. The normal pH of the blood is in the range of 7.36–7.44. Abnormalities of pH may be due to respiratory or metabolic problems. A pH below 7.2 represents severe acidosis.

Standard bicarbonate

This indicates the arterial level of sodium bicarbonate, which is an alkaline buffer the body uses to keep itself in the correct pH range. The body varies the level of bicarbonate to compensate for disturbances in the acid–base balance. The normal level is 22–26 mmol/litre.

Base excess

This indicates the activity of all of the metabolic bases that act as buffers to minimise changes in blood pH. These bases comprise bicarbonate, phosphate and protein. If the figure for base excess is positive it means there are excess circulating bases (alkalis), while if it is negative there is a reduced amount of circulating bases.

Interpretation of blood gas results

The results of blood gas analysis should always be considered in relation to the clinical presentation of the patient. The extra information gained will confirm or in some cases refute your diagnosis but will always guide your therapy. They are of particular value in monitoring the progress of patients with respiratory disease and in metabolic problems such as diabetic ketoacidosis. A guide to their interpretation follows.

Respiratory failure

Blood gases of PaO_2 less than 8 kPa (60 mmHg) or $PaCO_2$ greater than 7.3 kPa (55 mmHg) indicate respiratory failure. In patients who become acutely hypoxic the $PaCO_2$ may be low owing to increased ventilation stimulated by the hypoxia from inadequate gas exchange across the alveolar capillary membrane (e.g. due to pneumonia or pulmonary oedema). In some texts this is called type 1 respiratory failure. In other patients with inadequate breathing or an obstructed airway the PaO_2 is reduced and the $PaCO_2$ is raised. This is sometimes called type 2 respiratory failure or ventilatory failure. Many patients who initially present with type 1 failure develop type 2 as they become exhausted. Less commonly, $PaCO_2$ is raised with a normal PaO_2; this may occur for example in a chronic bronchitic who receives too much oxygen for his respiratory drive (see controlled oxygen therapy) or in postoperative cases on oxygen who have respiratory depression due to opiates.

Acid–base balance

Acids are formed in the body during metabolism, the most important being carbonic acid (H_2CO_3), lactic acid and ketone bodies. The body's enzyme systems function best with a normal pH and the body has several mechanisms to maintain pH within the normal range of 7.36–7.44: (1) the buffering action of circulating alkalis or bases such as bicarbonate, phosphate and protein, (2) CO_2 excretion in the lungs (thus regulating the amount of carbonic acid: less CO_2 = less carbonic acid = fewer hydrogen ions), and (3) excretion of hydrogen ions and bicarbonate via the kidney.

The amount of circulating bases or buffers is limited, as is the body's ability to generate them in response to imbalance. Thus large changes in blood hydrogen ion concentration must also be compensated for by the lungs and the kidneys. Excretion of acid by the kidneys is much slower than by the lungs. The ability to maintain acid–base balance via the lungs or the kidneys is dependent on normal function of these organs. Thus acidosis not only accompanies respiratory and renal failure but the ability to compensate for acid–base imbalance is limited by their integrity.

Acidosis may be due to respiratory or metabolic causes. The compensatory mechanisms may be completely effective in maintaining normal pH or may only be partially effective. Thus the blood gases may show a mixture of abnormalities.

Respiratory acidosis

This is caused by an accumulation of CO_2, as occurs in respiratory failure. The body

Table P7 Respiratory acidosis

	Uncompensated	Compensated
pH	Low	Normal
$PaCO_2$	High	High
Base excess	Normal range	Positive
Bicarbonate	Normal range	High

Table P8 Metabolic acidosis

	Uncompensated	Compensated
pH	Low	Normal
$PaCO_2$	Normal range	Low
Base excess	Negative	Negative
Bicarbonate	Low	Low

Table P9 Respiratory alkalosis

	Uncompensated	Compensated
pH	High	Normal
$PaCO_2$	Low	Low
Base excess	Normal range	Negative
Bicarbonate	Normal range	Low

Table P10 Metabolic alkalosis

	Uncompensated	Compensated
pH	High	Normal
$PaCO_2$	Normal	High
Base excess	Positive	Positive
Bicarbonate	High	High

responds to this by buffering the acids and by making and conserving alkaline substances called bases (metabolic compensation) by which it attempts to return the pH to normal (see Table P7).

Metabolic acidosis

This occurs when the body retains abnormal amounts of acidic products of metabolism, as in renal failure or diabetic ketoacidosis. The body responds to this by hyperventilation to remove more CO_2, which will bring the pH back towards normal. See Tables P7 and P8.

When we examine the blood gases of a patient with acidosis we will see either an uncompensated or a compensated acidosis. The PaO_2 and the oxygen saturation will vary depending on the cause of the problem.

Alkalosis

This may be respiratory or metabolic in origin. In *respiratory alkalosis* there is hyperventilation (which may be a response to hypoxia or due to excessive ventilation), causing an increased excretion of CO_2 which makes the patient alkalotic. *Metabolic alkalosis* can occur for two reasons; either the patient loses excess acid (e.g. prolonged loss of hydrochloric acid from the stomach through a nasogastric tube) or gains alkali as in an overdose of sodium bicarbonate at cardiac arrest. As in acidosis compensation will take place by either the metabolic or the respiratory route. The blood gases will be as shown in Tables P9 and P10.

Metabolic and respiratory derangements may be complex, for example a patient may develop two abnormalities, e.g. a diabetic with ketoacidosis who aspirates and develops respiratory failure. He would show a mixed picture of hypoxia and metabolic acidosis and the $PaCO_2$ would depend on the severity of the respiratory problem.

Note that full compensation may not occur in some patients and blood gas interpretations may occasionally be difficult.

What is the difference between the oxygen saturation obtained at blood gas analysis and the value given by a pulse oximeter?

The value given by the oximeter is measured directly and the blood gas value is calculated from a standard Hb oxygen dissociation curve and PaO_2 value. Therefore the oximeter is more accurate!

Tracheostomy

A tracheostomy is an opening in the trachea to provide access to the airway below the larynx.

Indications

1. Obstruction of the upper airway due to trauma, tumour, bilateral paralysis of the vocal cords, foreign bodies, inflammation or oedema, facial or airway burns, snake bite, dental or oropharyngeal infection or trauma and haematoma to the upper airway, or head and neck tumour.
2. Airway toilet in patients with prolonged retention of bronchial secretions due to bronchopneumonia, chest trauma, chronic pulmonary disease and paralysis of intercostal muscles such as Guillain–Barré syndrome.
3. In ventilated patients, tracheostomy:
   (a) makes nursing of the ventilated patient easier;
   (b) should be performed after 24–48 h if plastic endotracheal tubes are unavailable;
   (c) can help in weaning patients from a ventilator.
4. Laryngectomy for carcinoma of the larynx.
5. Patients at risk of aspiration of gastric contents with bulbar palsy.

Cricothyrotomy (Figure 11.1)

For immediate, emergency access to the airway due to obstruction above the larynx. Use a wide-bore intravenous cannula inserted into the larynx via the cricothyroid membrane (Figure P12) in the midline. See Figure 11.1 on p. 197.

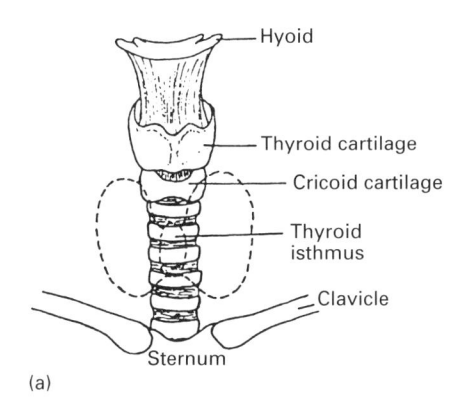

Figure P12 (a) View of the larynx and trachea from the front.

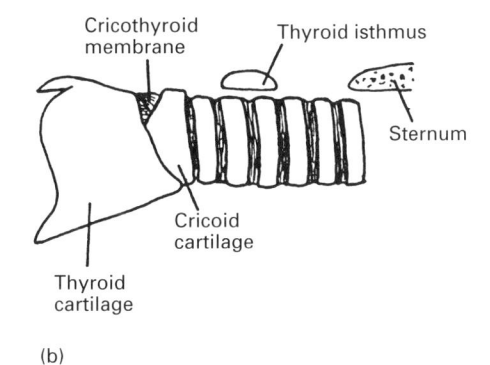

Figure P12 (b) Lateral view of the anatomy of the larynx.

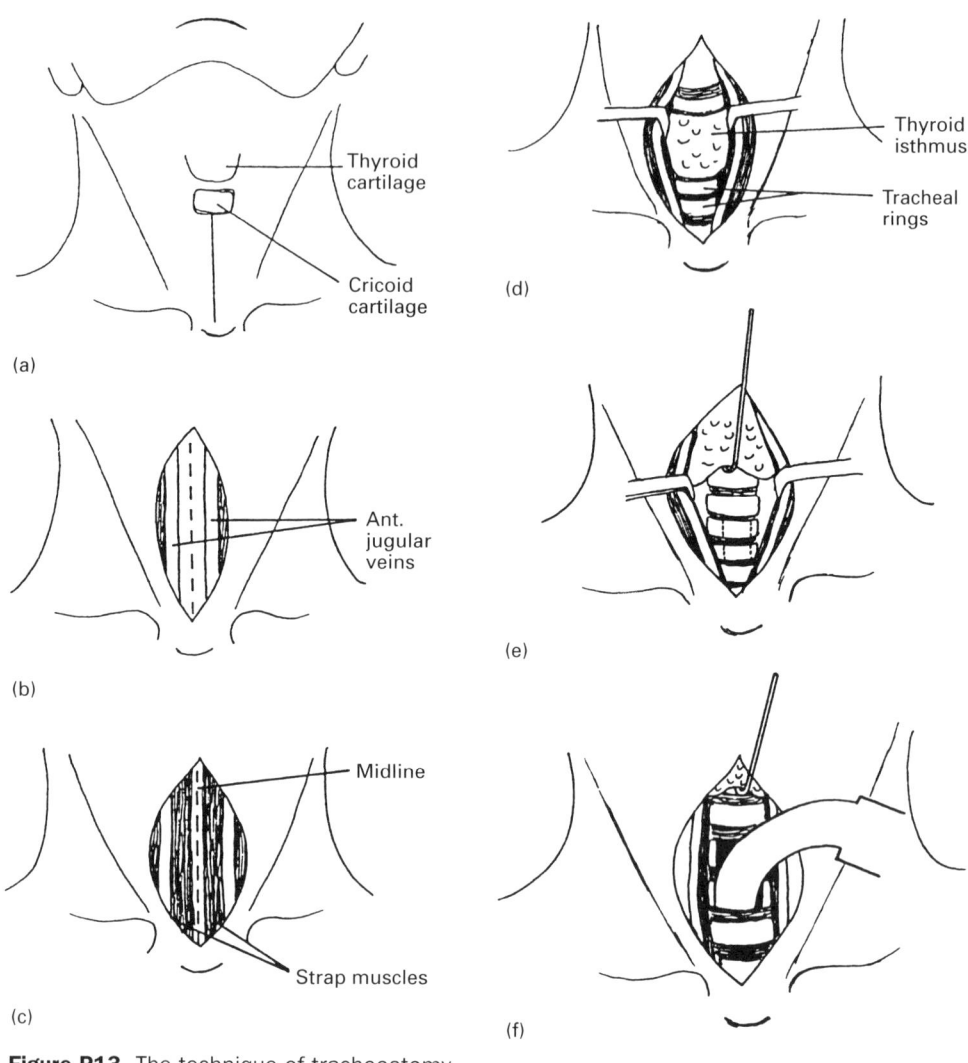

Figure P13 The technique of tracheostomy.

Tracheostomy (Figure P13)

Equipment

1. Good light.
2. Tracheostomy tubes: sizes 30–39 Fr in an adult, size of little finger in a child (p. 330), and tape to secure tube.
3. Suction.
4. Scalpel.
5. Artery and dissecting forceps, and retractors.
6. An assistant.

Ensure you have good light and a sterile tracheostomy set if there is time. An assistant makes the procedure easier. Feel the trachea below the cricoid cartilage.

Anaesthesia

Local or general anaesthesia can be used. Local anaesthesia is advised for anyone with airway obstruction in whom intubation could be a problem. It is advisable in an intubated patient to have someone, preferably an anaesthetist, looking after the endotracheal tube and general condition of the patient. In a deeply comatose patient anaesthesia is unnecessary and if the patient's airway is completely obstructed, but cannot be sorted by intubation or a mask and airway, anaesthesia causes delay.

Check that all connectors and tubing are available to attach the patient to a ventilator, anaesthetic circuit or Ambu bag before you start.

Procedure

1. The anatomy of the larynx and trachea is shown in Figure P12.
2. Make a midline incision, 4–5 cm long from the cricoid cartilage to the sternal notch (Figure P13a).
3. In an emergency divide all midline structures including the thyroid isthmus, ignore the bleeding and open the trachea between the 3rd and 4th rings. Insert a tracheostomy tube, suck out the airway and then stop the bleeding.
4. If there is time, identify the layers as you deepen the midline incision:
   (a) Skin, subcutaneous fat, and platysma muscle.
   (b) Investing layer of cervical fascia; the anterior jugular veins lie on either side of the midline (Figure P13b).
   (c) The strap muscles sternohyoid and behind it sternothyroid; these are separated from their twin on the other side rather than divided (Figure P13c). If you cannot identify the midline between the strap muscles feel the underlying trachea and continue your incision through the muscles towards the trachea.
5. The thyroid isthmus is exposed by the assistant retracting the strap muscles on either side (Figure P13d); the isthmus can be retracted superiorly with a blunt hook pulling it up towards the cricoid cartilage or divided between artery forceps; the blunt hooked retractor can then be inserted immediately below the cricoid to pull the trachea superiorly.
6. The rings of the trachea with the pretracheal fascia overlying them (Figure P13e); if you cannot feel tracheal rings which are firm, cartilaginous structures you are not in the midline and you may be about to open the carotid artery!
7. Cut a section out of the anterior trachea with a fine blade between the 2nd and 3rd or 3rd and 4th rings (Figure P13f). The diameter of the hole will be almost as big as the anterior surface of the trachea if a size 39 Fr tube is being inserted in an adult. Do not worry if you perforate the cuff of an endotracheal tube already in the trachea. In children incise the trachea but try to avoid excising a large portion of the anterior trachea. Never include the 1st tracheal ring in your tracheostomy since this may cause tracheal stenosis later.
8. If the patient is intubated withdraw the endotracheal tube to a point just above the tracheotomy and insert the tracheostomy tube by curving the tube downwards through the hole and into the lower trachea.
9. Suction the trachea and connect the anaesthetic circuit or Ambu bag as appropriate.
10. Inflate the cuff in adults; children will have a non-cuffed tube.
11. Ventilate and continue resuscitation as necessary.
12. Ligate any bleeding vessels.
13. Strap securely using the tapes that pass through the slots in the wing of the tube.
14. If necessary close the skin with one or two 3/0 sutures above and below the tracheostomy tube. Dress the wound around the tube. Change the dressing 2–3 times daily or more often if required.

Changing the tube

The tube should not be changed for the first 7 days. The first time the tube is changed have a tracheostomy set, tracheal dilators and equipment for orotracheal intubation and resuscitation with O_2 and suction available in case you fail to insert the new tube. The tube can be changed when needed by an experienced nurse thereafter.
1. Wear gloves and treat as for a sterile procedure.
2. Always have smaller-sized tracheostomy tubes available in case you cannot reinsert one of the same size.
3. Tell the patient what you are going to do; sedate if necessary.
4. Cut the tapes.
5. Suction the patient.
6. Remove the tracheostomy tube with your left hand and immediately reinsert the new one with your right, curving it in and down the trachea.
7. You may need to suck to see the hole if the patient coughs up thick or blood-stained secretions.

Final removal

Before removal check that the patient can breathe around the tube by occluding it with a cork or your thumb. Alternatively, a speaking tube can be inserted. If the patient becomes distressed do not remove the tube.

Once made, a tracheostomy should be maintained for at least 5–7 days. Before final removal smaller tubes can be inserted on alternate days and then the tube simply removed and the hole covered with a swab.

Care of a tracheostomy tube

A cuffed plastic tube may be inserted initially in adults, but it is important that the pressure in the cuff does not impair the microcirculation in the tracheal mucosa. After a few days, if the patient is not on a ventilator and not at risk of aspiration, the cuffed tube can often be replaced by a non-cuffed tube which may be made of plastic or silver. While a cuffed tube is in place the cuff must be deflated at regular intervals (2–3 minutes every hour) or use a high-volume, low-pressure cuff (p. 329) and check the cuff pressure at regular intervals.

Tracheostomy bypasses the normal humidification of inspired gases that occurs in the nasopharynx. A condenser humidifier such as a Trachivent or Humidivent (Portex) should be applied if possible (Figure V6, p. 426). Alternatively, moisten a swab and place it over the tracheostomy (see humidification, p. 425).

The patient will require regular suction and chest physiotherapy (pp. 349–351).

Any skin sutures can be removed after 7 days.

Complications

These are similar to those of endotracheal intubation and are discussed under intubation (p. 333). Infection is a real risk of tracheostomy in critically ill patients, especially in the presence of respiratory infection, and infection at the tracheostomy site should be vigorously treated and the site kept clean and dry.

Minitracheostomy

This is really a cricothyrotomy.

Indication

Airway toilet in a patient breathing spontaneously or emergency access to the airway owing to life-threatening laryngeal obstruction (as in cricothyrotomy, p. 197).

Procedure

Under local anaesthetic a size 4 PVC endotracheal tube is inserted through the cricothyroid membrane. The part of the tube outside the patient is then split to allow the tube to be strapped around the neck.

The access provided to the airway enables suction and chest physiotherapy to avoid endotracheal intubation or formal tracheostomy. The patient is able to speak with the minitracheostomy in place, but cannot breathe entirely through it.

Removal

Explain what you are going to do, suction the patient and pull out the tube.

Percutaneous tracheostomy

Percutaneous tracheostomy is performed on intubated patients in the ICU using a percutaneous technique. Various kits are available, the most common one being the Ciaglia model made by Cook. The technique is best learned from someone who has experience in the technique and detailed instructions are supplied with all kits.

1. After positioning the patient with the head extended and a rolled towel between the shoulders, perform laryngoscopy and withdraw the endotracheal tube until the cuff can be just seen appearing through the vocal cords. Place an extra 10 ml of air in the cuff, and arrange for an assistant to hold it in place. Some leakage of ventilator gas will occur, check the tube is stable and ventilation is still adequate.
2. Locate the cricoid cartilage and the sternal notch. Infiltrate lidocaine 1% and adrenaline 1 : 200 000 subcutaneously into the tissues at the level of the estimated 3rd tracheal ring. Make a 2-cm horizontal incision, and dissect bluntly using a pair of forceps in the midline until a finger can palpate the tracheal rings.
3. Insert the needle into the trachea between rings 2/3 or 3/4 and check that you can aspirate air (Figure P14a). Slide

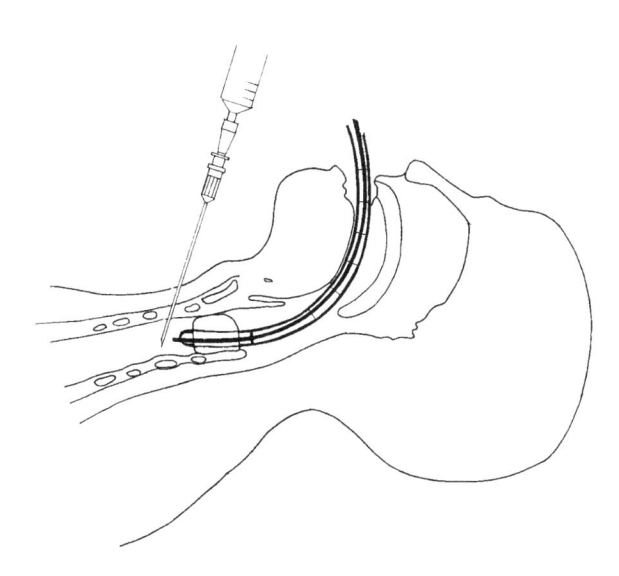

Figure P14a The needle is inserted into the trachea between rings 2/3 or 3/4 after checking that you can aspirate air.

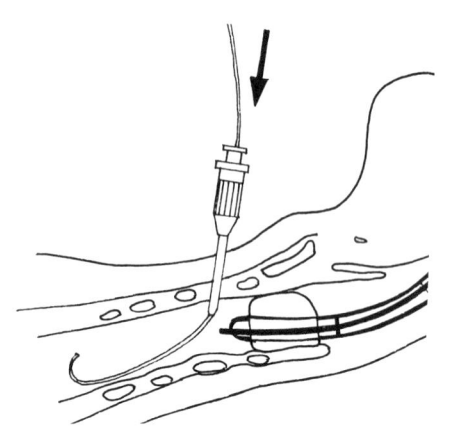

Figure P14b The cannula is slid over the needle and then the wire is inserted into the trachea.

the cannula over the needle and then insert the wire into the trachea (Figure P14b). A flexible bronchoscope is useful, but not essential, at this stage to confirm the correct midline placement of the wire.

4. Dilate the track with the dilators (Figure P14c) and then insert an appropriately sized tracheostomy tube over one of the dilators (Figure P14d). A twisting motion will help it pass into the trachea. Fix the tracheostomy tube in the normal fashion. See Figure 14c and d.
5. Bleeding is usually minimal with careful blunt dissection and can be controlled with pressure or a surgical tie.
6. If any difficulties are encountered the endotracheal tube should be re-inserted into the tracheal after removing and re-inflating the cuff. Ask for surgical help.

An alternative kit made by Portex dilates the track using a pair of specially designed re-usable tracheal dilating forceps.

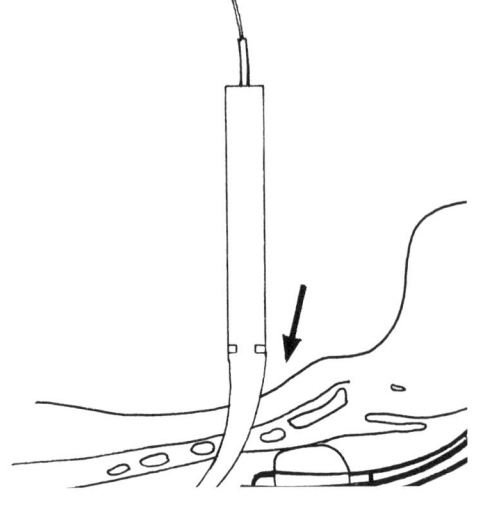

Figure P14c Dilating the track prior to insertion of the tracheostomy tube.

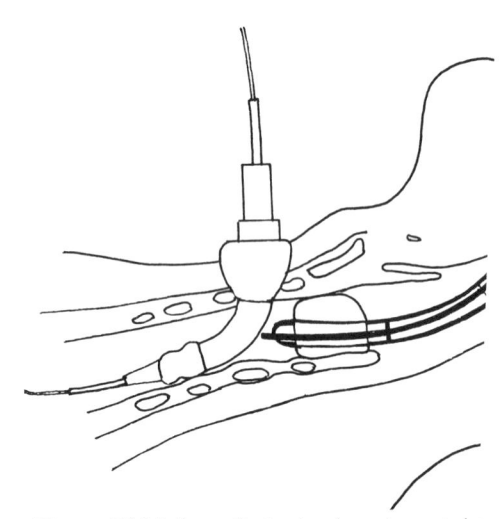

Figure P14d Inserting a tracheostomy tube over a dilator.

Further reading

ROGERS S, PUYANA JC. Bedside percutaneous tracheostomy in the critically ill patient. *Int Anesthesiol Clin* 2000;38:95–110.

Insertion of an intercostal drain

Indications

Intercostal drains are normally inserted to drain air, blood, pus or fluid from the pleural cavity. Sometimes they are inserted prophylactically in patients with fractured ribs who require general anaesthesia or mechanical ventilation.

In an emergency when a patient is suspected of having a tension pneumothorax and is shocked and cyanosed, a wide-bore intravenous cannula can be inserted directly into the pleural cavity to relieve tension as a temporary measure. This cannula should be left in until a proper intercostal drain is inserted.

Equipment

Intercostal drain, an introducer and a trocar and cannula, a scalpel, artery forceps and needle holder, local anaesthetic, connectors, clear tubing, a bottle and sterile water.

Fill the bottle so that the inlet tube lies beneath the water level (Figure P15). Make sure everything connects before you start.

Types of drain

1. Argyll or Portex drains are supplied with a trocar introducer, which is used to penetrate the chest.
2. Malecot drains are inserted using a trocar and cannula and the wings of the malecot prevent accidental removal. A catheter introducer with a blunt tip is used to insert the malecot drain through the cannula.
3. In an emergency and where the correct tubes are not available any suitable sterile tube may be used (e.g. a Foley catheter).

The danger with trocars is that they may puncture the lung or heart. If should not

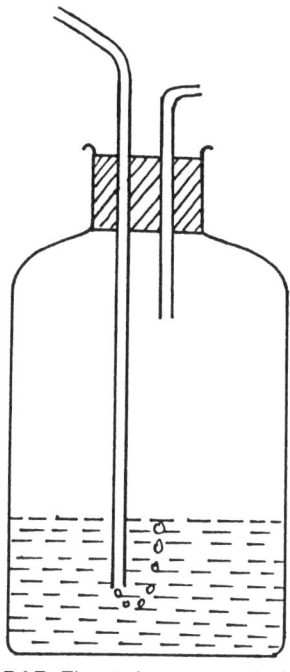

Figure P15 The tube connected to the patient must be below the water level. There must be a second tube to allow air to escape.

be necessary to use a trocar. If a trocar is used it should be understood that it may go too far and an introducing trocar can often be removed to feed the drain into pleural space after cutting down to the pleura.

Technique

The sternal manubrium is adjacent to the second rib. Count the ribs from this point and insert an intercostal drain in the **5th intercostal space in the anterior or mid-axillary line**. Rarely an anterior intercostal drain will be inserted for pneumothorax in the 2nd or 3rd intercostal space in the mid-clavicular line, but this site should not be used in traumatised patients, as it does not drain blood.

Clean and drape the patient.

Infiltrate local anaesthetic subcutaneously and down to the upper border of the rib below the intercostal space chosen.

Make a 2–3 cm incision (Figure P16) and deepen this to the upper border of the lower rib. Palpate the intercostal space and deepen the incision with blunt dissection through the intercostal muscles until you feel the pleura. Dissect, using forceps carefully, a little at a time, palpating for the pleura after each little cut.

> **PRACTICE POINT**
>
> The key to safe insertion is making a deep incision and opening the pleura, with blunt dissection wide enough to admit your drain. Keep the incision closer to the lower rib than the upper (Figure P16).

When down to the pleura, open it with the finger or forceps and insert the drain (Figure P17). A soft drain can be inserted using the forceps as an introducer or guide. Grasp the tube between the jaws of the

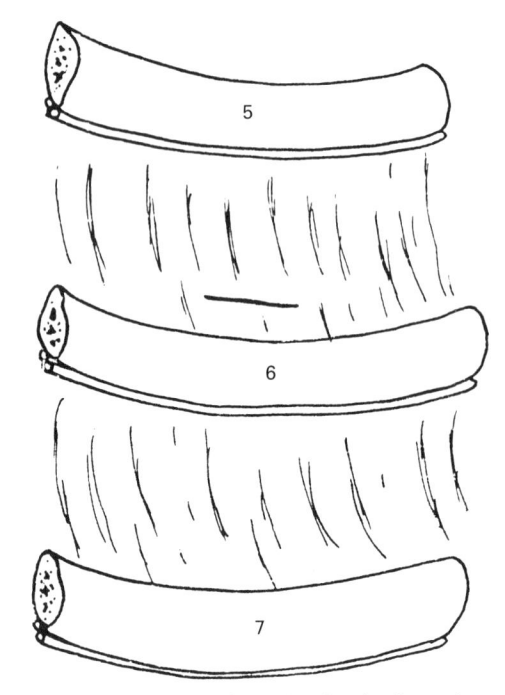

Figure P16 Site of incision for the insertion of an intercostal drain.

forceps. The drain should be passed posteriorly and to the base of the chest so it will drain with a minimal risk of dislodgment. Once the drain has passed into the pleural cavity remove the introducer or forceps and clamp the drain with artery forceps. Connect the drain to the tubing and the underwater-seal bottle. Secure the drain with a suture, and perform a purse string. Ensure that all the holes in the drain have entered the chest.

As soon as the drain is connected and the artery clamp is removed there should be air bubbling through the water. Air will continue to bubble out until all the air from the pleural cavity has been removed. Thereafter, only if the patient coughs might some air bubble out. If the drain was inserted for blood, pus or fluid then there may be no bubbling initially but rather drainage of whatever fluid was in the pleural cavity.

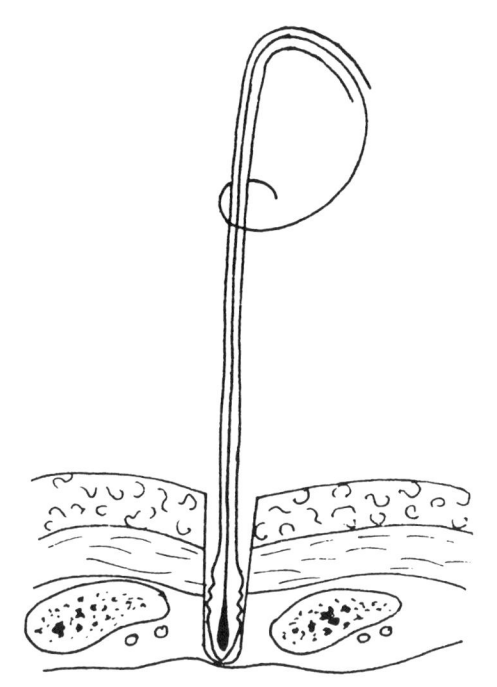

Figure P17 Insertion of the drain.

Take a chest X-ray at this point, if available, to check the position of your drain.

Care of an intercostal drain

Make sure that all the connections are secure and that the tubing is not kinked. There should be an artery forceps beside the bed or clamped to the bedsheet. The chest drain bottle should rest on the floor below the level of the patient and the intercostal drain should be clamped whenever the patient is being moved (Figure P18).

Once the visceral pleura lies against the chest wall the drain will record swings in intrapleural pressure but will not bubble. The fluid in the drain tube will rise on inspiration and fall on expiration. This is known as the drain 'swinging'. The swinging will stop after a few days because the area around the drain becomes sealed off from the rest of the pleural cavity. A drain that is not swinging can be removed with

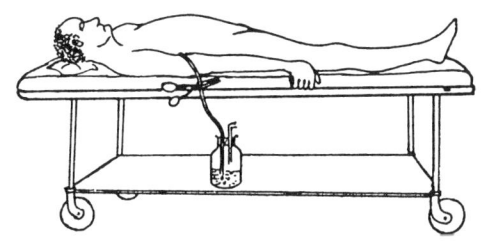

Figure P18 Correct positioning of the underwater drain.

only a small risk of pneumothorax. Swinging drains require the wound to be sealed (usually by suture) on removal and dressed firmly to block communication between the atmosphere and the pleural cavity. When a drain is no longer draining or swinging it is blocked or misplaced or unnecessary.

When reviewing a patient with a chest drain, examine the chest and ask yourself the following questions:
1. Is the drain bubbling or swinging? If not, is it blocked, misplaced or sealed off? How much drainage has there been from the drain?
2. Is there a large artery forceps beside the bed in case of accidental disconnection?
3. Is the drainage tubing lying in the right position? Check for kinking and for the patient lying on the tubing.
4. Is a chest X-ray necessary?

Antibiotics are not given routinely but only if indicated for other reasons.

Problems

Blockage

Patients with empyema are particularly prone to blockage. This is recognised by the fact that the drain does not swing, despite the lung not being fully expanded, nor is the pleural cavity clear.

Clamp the drain and disconnect it from the tube connecting with the bottle. Using an aseptic technique, flush the tube down to the bottle. Some drains become blocked because soft rubber tubing is used which kinks easily. If soft rubber tubing is autoclaved it becomes sticky and the inner surfaces of the tube may adhere and obstruct the lumen. Some drains are blocked by blood clot or pus. If the blockage is in the chest drain itself, try milking the clot out by squeezing along the drain or flush the drain gently with sterile saline.

If you cannot unblock the drain, remove it and take a chest X-ray. Do not try to readjust the position of a drain in the chest. Rather remove it and insert another.

Chest drains may become dislodged and lie in the chest wall. Check the drain and the suture where it enters the chest when the drain is not working. A chest X-ray may show the misplaced drain.

A blocked chest drain can be dangerous, particularly in ventilated patients in whom there was pneumothorax. A blocked drain might lead to tension pneumothorax.

Persistent bubbling

Persistent bubbling means that there is still a leak from the lung into the pleural space. As the leak gets smaller there will only be air bubbling on forced breathing or coughing. Persistent bubbling without re-expansion of the lung suggests a bronchopleural fistula. This should seal within a week of the original injury and then the lung should expand. Low-pressure suction is occasionally applied to the underwater seal bottle in order to encourage full re-expansion of the lung if collapse persists for more than a few days.

Removal

To remove a chest drain have sutures and a sterile dressing ready. Infiltrate local anaesthetic if you need to suture the wound. Sometimes a purse string suture was inserted originally to allow the drain site to be sealed by suturing on removal. Suturing is not usually necessary. Ask the patient to breathe out and pull the drain out firmly and quickly during expiration. Strap a sterile dressing on the wound.

Giving oxygen by nasopharyngeal catheter

A thin flexible tube is passed through the nose until its tip lies in the patient's throat just beyond the soft palate (Figure P19a). The catheter is passed for a distance equal to that from the side of the nostril to the front of the ear (Figure P19b). Note that the catheter should be pushed straight backwards (towards the back of the head), not upwards towards the top of the patient's head. The tip of the catheter should be visible just below the uvula when the mouth of the child is open. The nasopharyngeal catheter is known in some places as an oropharyngeal catheter, because its tip lies in the patient's oropharynx.

The advantages of this method are that the lowest flow rate of oxygen is required to achieve a given concentration in the airways, the concentration is not reduced if the patient's nostrils are blocked, the catheter can easily be secured in place so that it is unlikely to be dislodged, and there is no danger of hypercarbia (carbon dioxide accumulation) if the oxygen is turned off or the tubing disconnects. With a nasopharyngeal catheter, an oxygen flow of 1 l/min delivers between 45% and 60% of oxygen to a 5 kg child. When oxygen is supplied from a cylinder with a flowmeter, the use of a nasopharyngeal catheter can

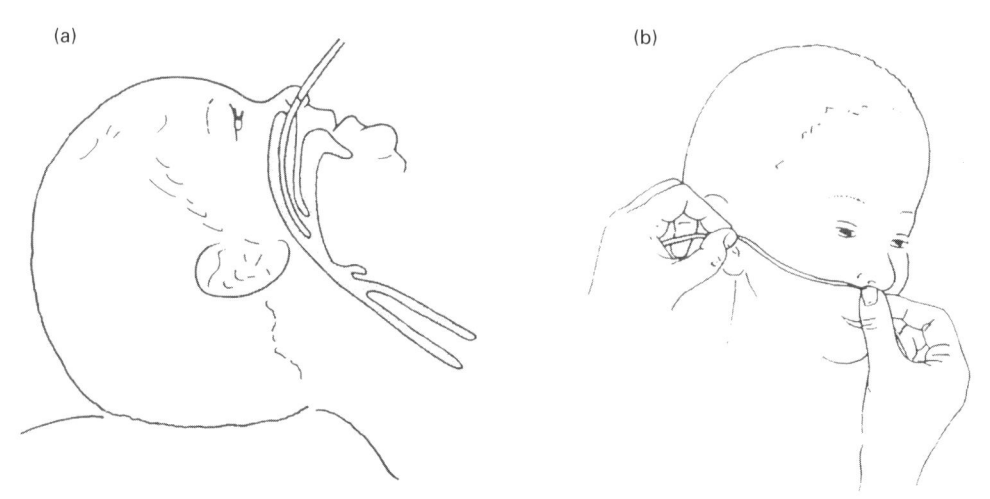

Figure P19a Pass the tube through the nose until its tip lies in the child's throat, just beyond the soft palate.
Figure P19b The catheter is passed for a distance equal to that from the side of the nostril to the front of the ear.

result in considerable savings over other methods of administration.

However, the gas should be humidified (to avoid drying of the pharyngeal mucosa and reduce the likelihood of inspissated secretions which can block the catheter and cause airway obstruction), the catheter must not be pushed in too far (because gastric distension may result), the flow rate must not be greater than 1 l/min in an infant or 2 l/min in a child (because of the risk of gastric distension), and the catheter must be taken out and cleaned at least twice a day (so that mucus does not block the holes of the catheter). A low-flow flowmeter (giving approximately 0–3 l/min) is required because standard flowmeters (approximately 0–16 l/min) cannot be adjusted accurately to deliver 1–2 l/min. Some children will cough and gag, or even vomit, when a nasopharyngeal catheter is first put in. Some will keep on coughing and gagging, and the catheter should then be withdrawn slightly. Occasionally, a nasopharyngeal catheter will cause obstruction of the airways or even apnoea; continuous and skilled nursing care is needed to prevent or treat these rare but potentially fatal complications. If a nasogastric tube and a nasopharyngeal catheter are used at the same time, they should be placed in the same nostril.

Further reading

KLEIN M, REYNOLDS LG. Nasopharyngeal oxygen in children. *Lancet* 1989;i:493–4.

SHANN F. Nasopharyngeal oxygen in children. *Lancet* 1989;i:1077–8.

SHANN F, GATCHALIAN S, HUTCHINSON R. Nasopharyngeal oxygen in children. *Lancet* 1988;ii:1238–40.

Peritoneal dialysis and lavage

Equipment

1. Peritoneal catheter and introducer.
2. Connecting tubing.
3. Isotonic dialysate fluid × 36 1-litre bags. Y-configuration giving set tubing.
4. Measuring jug.
5. Scalpel and suture material.
6. Iodine or chlorhexidine solution for skin cleansing.
   1% lidocaine local anaesthetic.

Indications

Patients in renal failure with a good prognosis (young, with an acute insult and one system disease) who present clinically with:
1. anuria or oliguria; with
2. decreasing conscious level; and/or
3. evidence of pulmonary oedema; and/or
4. uraemic frost; or
5. pericardial friction rub.

Biochemically those patients with:
1. dangerous resistant hyperkalaemia (greater than 7 mmol/l).
2. a serum urea rising faster than 8 mmol/l in 24 h; or
3. a urea greater than 40 mmol/l;

Contraindications

1. Abdominal sepsis.
2. Abdominal surgery less than 3 days previously.
3. A relative contraindication is a patient with a poor prognosis.

Special considerations

1. Strict asepsis.
2. Constant nurse attendance to monitor fluid balance.
3. The bladder should be emptied with a catheter before insertion of the peritoneal dialysis catheter.
4. If there has been a previous laparotomy then a 5-cm incision should be made and the catheter inserted under direct vision.
5. If there is a previous midline scar use the iliac fossa.
6. If there is evidence of a pelvic fracture then insert the catheter 3 cm above the umbilicus.

Technique of insertion

1. Scrub and put on sterile gloves.
2. Shave and clean the skin below the umbilicus and then infiltrate with 1% lidocaine.
3. Make a 2 cm midline incision 2 cm below the umbilicus.
4. Keep cutting down through the abdominal wall until you reach the peritoneum but do not cut through the peritoneum.

5. Separate the subcutaneous tissues with a pair of artery forceps and then insert the catheter on the introducer.
6. You will feel a definitive 'give' as you perforate the peritoneum.
7. Advance the catheter off the introducer in the direction of the left iliac fossa.
8. Withdraw the introducer and push the connecting tubing onto the end of the catheter.
9. Tie a purse string suture around the wound and catheter and then infuse 2 litres of dialysate over 30 min and drain off immediately.
10. Thereafter infuse 2 litres over 30 min, allow to dwell for 60 min, then drain out over 30 min.
11. Should there be problems with fluid overload or pulmonary oedema then add 50 ml of 50% dextrose to each litre of the dialysate fluid to make a hypertonic solution that will enable more fluid to be removed.

Figure P20 shows the different sites which can be used to insert a peritoneal catheter.

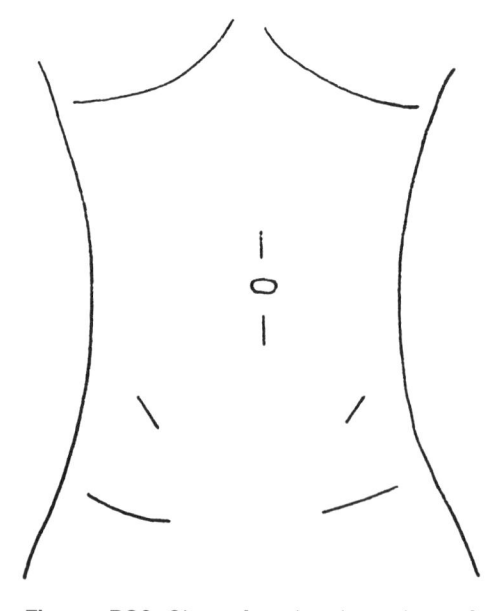

Figure P20 Sites for the insertion of catheter for peritoneal dialysis.

Monitoring

Chart fluid in, dwell time and fluid out. Calculate any positive or negative balances and summate these every five cycles. Regularly check the neck veins and lung bases for evidence of fluid overload and also check for signs of hypovolaemia; a central venous line may be useful when fluid status is difficult to assess. Monitor urine output with a catheter, at least initially. Check the urea and electrolytes daily. The majority of patients will respond to initial therapy with 36 cycles. If the urea remains high and/or the urine output is less than 0.5 ml/kg/h then a further 36 cycles are indicated. If, after this, the urine output *still* remains less than 0.5 ml/kg/h then the doctor will have to decide objectively whether the patient is likely to benefit from further therapy. Factors that should guide this decision include the presence of other disease processes, the age and clinical state of the patient, the potential reversibility of the original insult and available resources.

Problems

Fluid will not flow in/out of the catheter

Try flushing the catheter with saline or dilute heparin solution. Routine use of heparin (and antibiotics) is of no benefit. Try withdrawing the catheter slightly in order to free the tip, which may be plugged with omentum or lying against viscera. Check that the inflowing dialysate fluid is high enough on the drip stand to have a good flow. Check that the outflow is below the level of the patient and sit the patient at 45° or more, if conscious.

Fluid oozes around the site of insertion

Tie a purse string suture around the catheter and skin at the insertion site. If this does not work then stop the dialysate flow for 2 h before recommencing.

Infection of the peritoneum

This will be shown by milky fluid on draining and/or intermittent blockage to flow. Withdraw the catheter and, if it is essential, insert a new one in another site. Try adding gentamicin 80 mg to the next six cycles to help clear the infection. It may be that there is sepsis throughout the peritoneum, in which case there is no alternative but to abandon peritoneal dialysis.

Electrolyte imbalance

This may be corrected by the use of appropriate i.v. solutions.

Peritoneal lavage

1. Infuse 1 litre of normal saline into the peritoneal cavity.
2. Massage the fluid around and then place the empty saline bag on the floor still connected to the peritoneal cavity.
3. Fluid will flow out of the peritoneal cavity owing to the syphon action aided by the vacuum in the collapsed saline bag.
4. If you are able to read newsprint through the peritoneal effluent after the first few hundred ml have drained then there is an insignificant amount of blood in the peritoneal cavity. To do this place the drip tubing over a page of newsprint.
5. For a more accurate result use a cell counting chamber. More than 50 000 red blood cells per cubic mm is significant. More than 25 white cells per cubic mm is suggestive of an inflammatory stimulus in the peritoneal cavity. If more than 6 h have elapsed since the injury then the white cells will always be raised if there is a ruptured viscus.
6. Perform a laparotomy if there is a positive result for red cells (newsprint obscured), white cells or bile in the lavage fluid.
7. Once the saline has been drained from the peritoneal cavity, pull out the catheter and dress the wound.

Peritoneal dialysis in children

1. Before inserting the trocar and dialysis catheter it is a good idea to instil 25 ml/kg of warmed dialysis fluid into the peritoneal cavity over 15 min via a Dwellcath.
2. In small children it may be necessary to cut off a part of the perforated catheter tip.
3. Use 50 ml/kg of warmed dialysis fluid for each cycle.
4. Infuse the fluid over 10 min, leave to equilibrate for 30 min and drain out over 20 min – each cycle thus taking 60 min.

Removal of the catheter

Explain the procedure to the patient. Sedation is not required. Cut the sutures holding the catheter and pull the catheter out briskly. Dress the wound with an ordinary sterile dressing. Any discharge from the wound usually settles within a few days and further suturing of the wound is not required.

Insertion of a nasogastric tube

Indications

1. Aspiration of gastric contents and decompression of the upper gastrointestinal tract in patients with gastric stasis, paralytic ileus or intestinal obstruction. In upper gastrointestinal bleeding a nasogastric tube helps to remove blood from the stomach.
2. To protect an anastomosis in the oesophagus, stomach or duodenum.
3. Enteral nutrition.

Contraindications

1. Fracture to base of skull.
2. Maxillary fractures.
3. Epistaxis (use other nostril).
4. Nasopharyngeal tumours.
5. Coagulopathy.

Special considerations

Patients who require gastric lavage for poisoning should have this performed with a wide-bore gastric lavage tube passed through the mouth and not a nasogastric tube, which is too narrow to lavage the stomach effectively. Only perform gastric lavage with a nasogastric tube if no gastric tube is available.

Method of insertion

Conscious patient

Before inserting the tube, estimate the length required by holding the tube alongside the patient.

Insert with the patient sitting or lying on his left-hand side. The head and neck should be flexed. Explain the procedure. Use plenty of lubricant and spray the nose and pharynx with 1% lidocaine. The nostrils are horizontal, so pass the tube horizontally through the nose until the tip reaches the nasopharynx. Once the tube reaches the pharynx ask the patient to swallow.

Unconscious patient

Either use the left lateral position or the tube can be passed under direct vision with a laryngoscope and Magill's forceps.

General points

If the tube keeps coiling up in the mouth try a different position or technique. It is often discomfort that makes the patient struggle and seem unco-operative. Try to keep the patient relaxed; use local anaesthetic. Sometimes swallowing water with the tube helps.

Correct positioning of a nasogastric tube is essential. On insertion of the tube the patient should not cough unduly which might suggest it has been misplaced in the trachea. Gastric juice should be aspirated from the stomach. Air should be injected down the tube with a 10 ml syringe. When you listen over the stomach with a stethoscope a 'whoosh' of air will be heard clearly on injection, confirming the position of the tube. If there is doubt about the position take a chest radiograph if the tube tip has radio-opaque bearings (Figure 15.2). Having checked the position of the tube, its length should be recorded at the nose and it should then be well secured. If the position changes feeding should be stopped until the correct position has been reconfirmed. Nurses should be capable of determining the position of a nasogastric tube without the help of a doctor.

The chest X-ray in Figure 15.2 shows an incorrectly placed nasogastric tube in the right main bronchus. Feeding down this tube resulted in severe pneumonia. It is normally wise to check the position radiologically before starting feeding.

Aspirating the tube

A nasogastric tube should normally be allowed to drain freely. The collecting bag should be below the level of the stomach to encourage emptying of gastric contents by syphon.

Since a nasogastric tube rarely empties the stomach completely, free drainage can be combined with hourly aspiration. The practice of spigoting a nasogastric tube to block it and only aspirate at intervals is unnecessary.

It is not necessary to change modern plastic tubes providing they remain patent and do not become dislodged.

Complications

1. Oesophageal ulceration – this was more common when red rubber nasogastric tubes are used and, in our experience, is very rare.
2. Impairment of coughing – it is uncomfortable to cough with a nasogastric tube in place. It predisposes to bronchopneumonia.
3. Misplacement may result in fluid entering the lung as described above.
4. Otitis media due to the irritant effect of the tube at the opening of the Eustachian tube.

Puncture suprapubic cystotomy

Indications

Failed urethral catheterisation, due to either an impassable outlet obstruction or urethral injury in association with fracture of the pelvis.

In hospitals where commercially prepared pre-packed suprapubic cystotomy kits (e.g. Cystofix) are not available the usual practice is to perform an open formal suprapubic cystotomy. This is a relatively elaborate procedure performed in the operating theatre and the puncture suprapubic cystotomy as described below is an alternative, highly effective, inexpensive and safe bedside procedure for all cases of failed urethral catheterisation in which the bladder is distended and there is no suprapubic scar. An open suprapubic cystotomy is always safe, but there are often delays in getting a patient who is suffering in acute retention into theatre to perform the procedure.

Where ward ultrasound is immediately available bladder distension can be confirmed on ultrasound if the distended bladder is not obviously palpable. The author (B. Elem) has successfully used the puncture technique described below for many years in the tropics.

Contraindication

Previous suprapubic surgery.

Precaution

The bladder should be palpably distended or you should be able to fill the bladder with saline to make it palpably distended.

Equipment (Figure P21a)

1. A trocar and cannula used for aspiration of a hydrocoele.
2. 1 m of a used intravenous drip tubing sterilised in Cidex (glutaraldehyde) with an identifying mark of black silk tied around the tube at 15 cm from one end. The lowermost 10 cm of the tube distal to the mark is split on one side.
3. A 5-ml syringe with a needle.
4. A small surgical blade or a sterilised razor blade.
5. A No. 1 cutting silk suture.
6. 1 or 2% lidocaine.

Technique

1. Clean the suprapubic area with antiseptic solution.
2. Infiltrate the proposed puncture site with local anaesthetic, two fingers' breadth above the symphysis pubis, strictly in the midline, down to the bladder. The presence of a dilated bladder is confirmed by aspiration of a few ml of urine with the same syringe.

Practical procedures 377

(a)

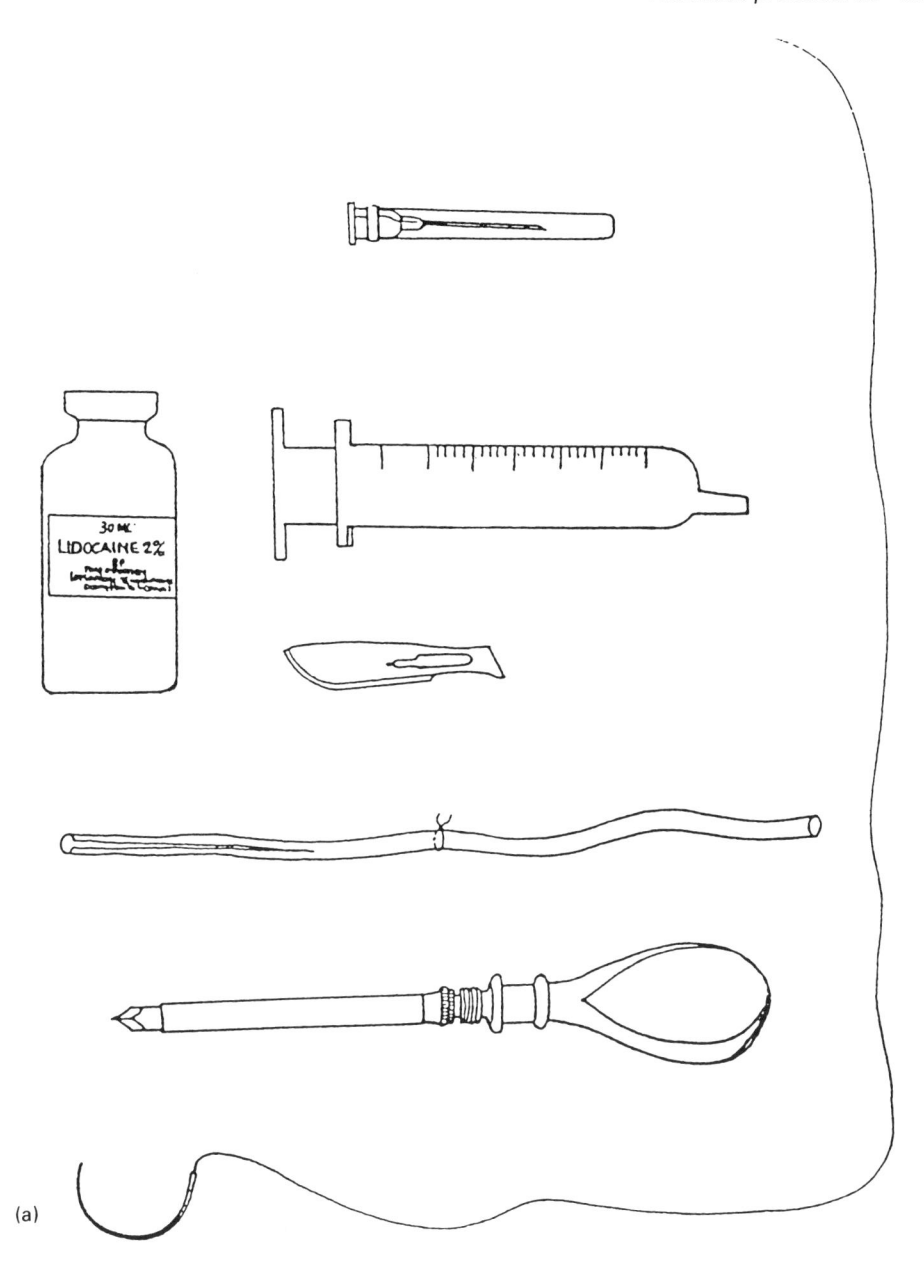

Figure P21 Suprapubic cystotomy.

3. Make a small incision, slightly larger than the diameter of the hydrocoele cannula, in the skin and linea alba.
4. Insert the trocar and cannula into the bladder with firm, steady pressure, perpendicular to the abdominal wall and strictly in the midline (Figure P21b). Entry into the bladder is associated with a characteristic sudden sensation of diminished resistance.
5. Remove the trocar. A large volume of urine inevitably escapes, which makes

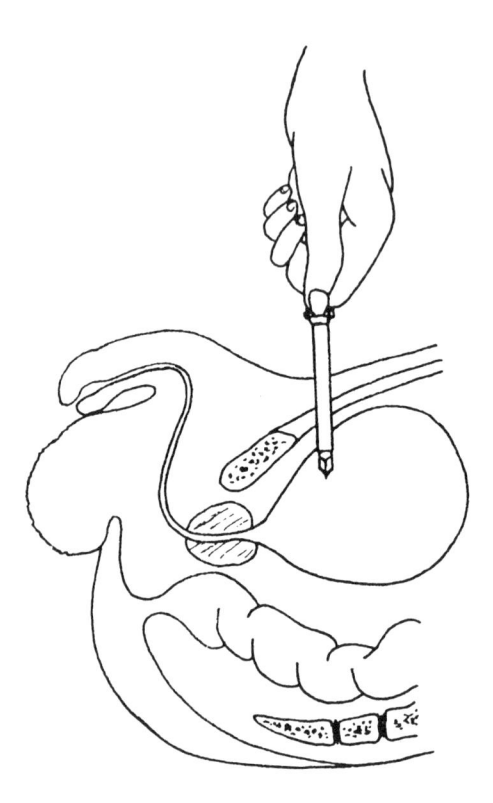

this stage of the procedure rather messy. The previously prepared tubing is inserted into the bladder through the cannula beyond the 15-cm mark.

6. Remove the cannula and gently withdraw the tubing until the silk marking tie at 15 cm is at the level of the skin.
7. Using the No. 1 silk suture through one edge of the incision, tie and secure the tubing. Tie several times around the tubing. Alternatively, make a butterfly type of collar with adhesive tape around the tube adjacent to the skin and secure it by taking the skin suture through one or both edges of the collar (Figure P21c). The drainage tube is further attached to the abdominal wall by a wide strip of adhesive.
8. The suprapubic tube is connected to urinary drainage bag by passing the tubing into the tubing of the drainage bag and securing the join with adhesive tape.
9. Systemic antibiotics and local dressings are unnecessary.

Complications and problems

1. The bladder is not distended: always perform puncture suprapubic cystotomy on a distended bladder, otherwise you may fail to enter the bladder or damage other structures. A lax bladder should be made palpably distended by filling the bladder with normal saline using a hypodermic needle placed directly into the bladder.
2. Injury to the preprostatic venous plexus may occur with alarming haemorrhage if the trocar is not inserted perpendicularly and in the midline. Do not insert the trocar in a downwards (inferior) or oblique direction.
3. There is a suprapubic scar: the puncture technique described above may cause damage to adherent bowel. In this situation a formal, operative suprapubic cystotomy is advised.

(b)

(c)

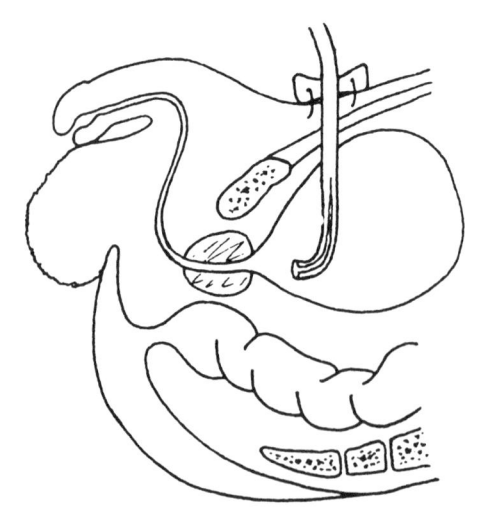

Figure P21 continued

Venous access and central venous pressure measurement (CVP)

The choice of a vein for venous access will depend on the urgency of the situation, and whether central venous access is required. Where seconds and minutes count and the peripheral veins are collapsed, cannulate a large central vein or perform a cutdown. Where there is more time use the methods below to improve your chance at cannulation of a peripheral vein. Use a central vein to measure the CVP and to administer certain infusions such as dopamine or for parenteral feeding.

Peripheral veins

Difficult peripheral vein cannulation

Cannulation can be made easier using the following methods, all of which take some time and are therefore suitable for difficult cases but not for urgent ones.
1. The best tourniquet is a blood pressure cuff inflated to about 30 mmHg below the systolic blood pressure. Keep it inflated for up to 5–10 min to give the veins time to fill with blood.
2. Immerse the limb in warm water for 10 min to cause venodilation.

If these methods fail, the technique of 'cutdown' cannulation can be used.

Cutdown cannulation

1. This takes about 20 min, but with practice it can be almost as fast as any other method. Suitable veins in adults and children are shown in Figure P22, where the necessary instruments are listed. The technique is shown in Figure P23.
2. Prepare the skin and inject 1 ml of local anaesthetic under the skin along the line of the incision, which should be about 2 cm long, across the line of the vein. Incise the skin with a scalpel, and separate the fat down to the vein using a pair of artery forceps (Figure P23a).
3. Clear a short length of the vein and put two slings of catgut under it, one at the top end and one at the lower end. One throw of a knot should be put in each of these but not tightened, and they can then be used for traction on the vein (Figure P23b).
4. Make a transverse cut in the wall of the vein (Figure P23c). This creates a very small hole in what is already a small constricted vein. Gently dilate the vein by inserting the tips of the fine-pointed scissors and opening them slightly (Figure P23d).
5. The cannula is then inserted through the skin below the wound (Figure P23e) (it is easier to cannulate the vein directly via the wound but this carries a higher risk of a subsequent wound infection). Insert the cannula with the needle still inside it but withdraw the needle as soon as the tip of the cannula is inside the vein, and then advance the cannula up the vein. At this point inject

Adult

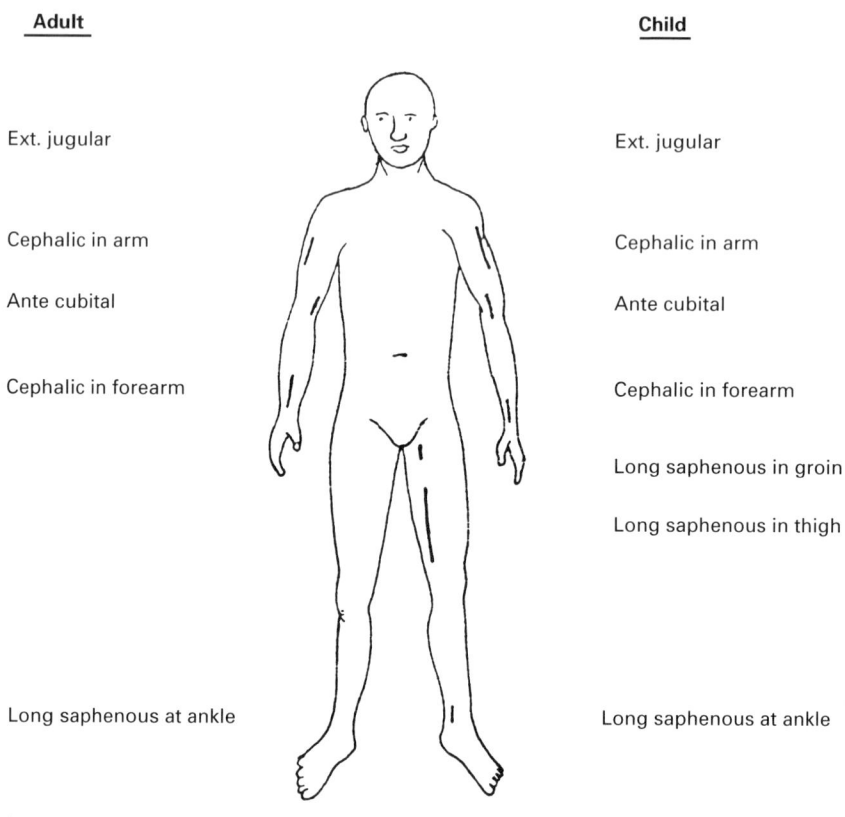

- Ext. jugular
- Cephalic in arm
- Ante cubital
- Cephalic in forearm
- Long saphenous at ankle

Child

- Ext. jugular
- Cephalic in arm
- Ante cubital
- Cephalic in forearm
- Long saphenous in groin
- Long saphenous in thigh
- Long saphenous at ankle

Instruments

1 Scalpel blade
3 Artery forceps
1 Fine pointed scissors
1 Catgut ligature 4/0 3/0 2/0
1 Skin suture on cutting needle
1 needle holders

Figure P22 Sites for cutdown.

some saline and repeat this every few minutes until the infusion is running. Tie the two catgut ligatures, one below the cannula and one (not tight) around the vein with the cannula in it. Suture the skin, leaving the suture ends long to tie around the cannula (Figure P23f).

6. Especially in the leg, the infusion will run very slowly at first. Use saline, preferably warmed, for at least the first hour, and do not start a blood transfusion until the drip is running well, except in hypovolaemic patients.

7. The main complication of cutdowns is infection, which can be minimised by using the method of cannula insertion described, and, more importantly, not leaving the cannula in place for too long. If possible change the drip site after a maximum of 48 h.

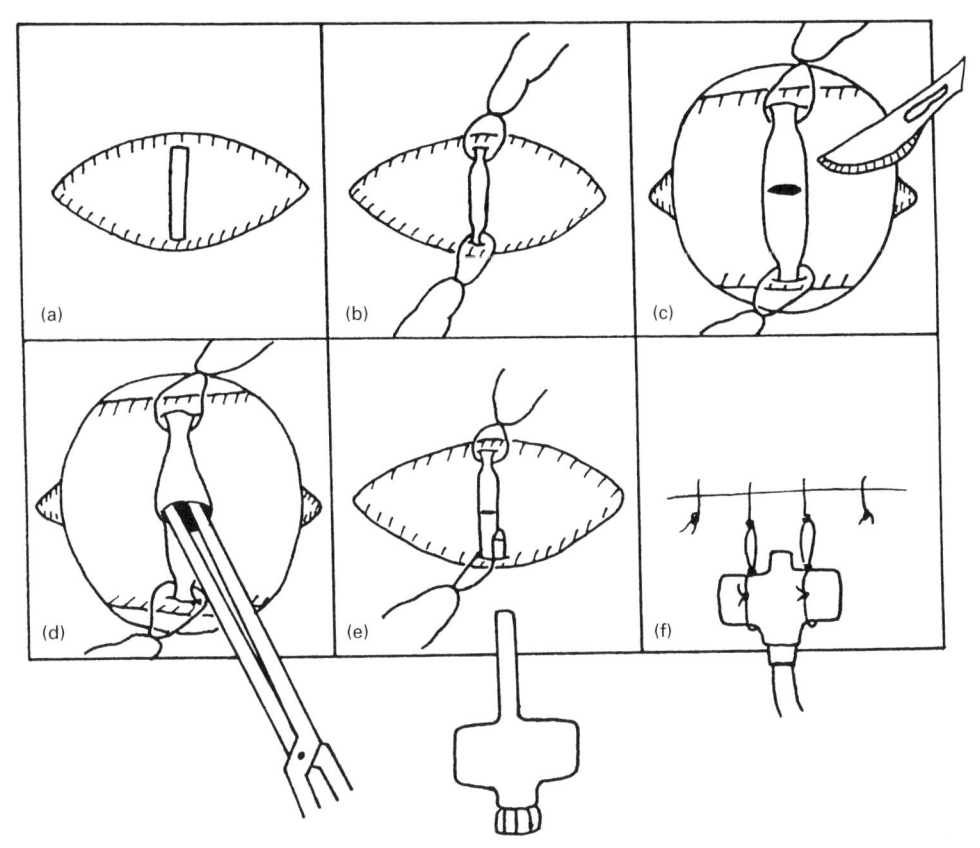

Figure P23 Performing a venous cutdown.

Children

All the methods and sites of venous cannulation can be used in children, but intraosseus infusion is often a better choice (p. 392).

Securing the drip

Many drips soon stop working. The usual reasons are that the cannula has dislodged or someone (never the person who had to start it) has turned off the drip.

Avoid this by making the drip very secure – if necessary put the limb in plaster of Paris – and instruct all staff not to let the drip stop at any time.

Central veins

These are the internal jugular, the subclavian, the external jugular and the femoral. The first two may be used to measure the CVP.

Equipment

1. Central venous catheter and introducing cannula.
2. Skin disinfectant and sterile drapes.
3. 1% lidocaine.
4. Syringe and needle.
5. Sterile swabs.
6. Intravenous giving set and fluids.

7. To measure CVP a three-way tap and manometer tubing are preferable, otherwise a butterfly cannula.
8. Skin suture and needle-holding forceps.

Indications

1. Hypovolaemia: To facilitate rapid infusion (femoral is easiest, particularly in children, but should not be used if there is intra-abdominal bleeding) and to guide fluid replacement.
2. Shocked patients from other causes such as septic shock or where cardiac failure may be a problem.
3. Inotropic drugs are to be used.
4. Oliguria or renal failure to guide fluid therapy.
5. Suspected cardiac tamponade following trauma.
6. Any patient in whom the correct fluid therapy is uncertain.
7. Pulmonary oedema. A CVP line may give useful information, but CVP readings may be normal in left-sided heart failure. A Swan–Ganz catheter is more helpful in this condition, but rarely available (p. 418).
8. Parenteral nutrition.

Special considerations

1. Is the operator trained in the procedure or supervised by someone who is?
2. What is the risk of pneumothorax, and are chest radiographs available to detect this complication? Undetected pneumothoraces are most dangerous in patients about to undergo anaesthesia or who require mechanical ventilation.
3. The chest X ray should confirm that the catheter tip is in the superior vena cava (SVC) or the right atrium.
4. Can the CVP line be safely supervised by the nurses?
5. Does the patient have a clotting defect? If so, clotting factors, platelets or fresh blood should be available in case of bleeding.

Preparation

Cannulation of any vein, particularly a central one, should be an aseptic procedure. Prepare the skin with antiseptic, use a towel to cover surrounding skin and hair and wear gloves if available. In an emergency this is not always feasible, so remove a potentially contaminated cannula as soon as possible afterwards.

Choose a suitable cannula and check that you are familiar with the method of insertion. (Most cannulae have instructions on the pack.) Use a 13–20 cm cannula for the internal jugular or subclavian vein; if these are not available then a cannula of normal length will do in an emergency. A few cannulae require trimming to make them the correct size.

Internal jugular vein cannulation
(Figure P24)

This vein runs along a line between the mastoid process and the sternoclavicular joint. It is contained in the carotid sheath along with the carotid artery and the vagus nerve. At first it is posterior to the carotid artery but becomes lateral and then anterolateral lower in the neck.

1. When attempting cannulation stand behind the patient, who should be positioned supine with head-down tilt. Use the right internal jugular vein (IJV) as it has a straight course to the superior vena cava (SVC).
2. Gently turn the patient's head to the left and ask him to relax his muscles. Palpate the lower border of the thyroid cartilage and then move your fingers laterally until the carotid pulsation is felt. Keep your fingers lightly on the carotid (which will help you to avoid cannulating it) and insert a 21 gauge (green) needle on a 5-ml syringe filled

with 1% lidocaine in the direction shown in Figure P24a. Aim lateral to the artery, pointing towards the nipple with the needle at an angle of 40° to the skin (Figure P24b). Inject small volumes of local anaesthetic into the tissues, aspirating frequently until you locate the vein. Do not insert the needle more than 4 cm in an adult. If the vein is not located on insertion, withdraw the needle slowly from the neck as the vein may be compressed on the way in, but open up on the way out (Figure P24c).

3. After locating the vein introduce the cannula in the same direction with a slight negative pressure on the syringe. When you aspirate blood, push the needle and cannula another 0.5 cm into the vein.
4. Now advance the cannula into the vein. When the cannula is finally positioned connect a drip set to prevent air embolus.
5. Run the drip to flush the line and then put the drip bag below the level of the bed with the drip switched on (Figure P25). If your cannula is correctly positioned blood will come back up the drip line, if it does replace drip and flush line again. Fix the cannula to the skin with adhesive tape or (preferably) sutures.

Problems

- Difficulty in finding the vein – try slightly more lateral with more head-down.
- If the carotid is punctured keep pressure on it for 10 min.
- If blood is aspirated from needle then the cannula will not pass, take out the needle, attach a syringe, slowly withdraw the cannula until blood is aspirated and then push the cannula gently into the vein. Occasionally it will not be possible to pass the cannula (1–2% of cases). If blood will not flow up the drip tubing then it is possible that the cannula is not in the vein. Check this

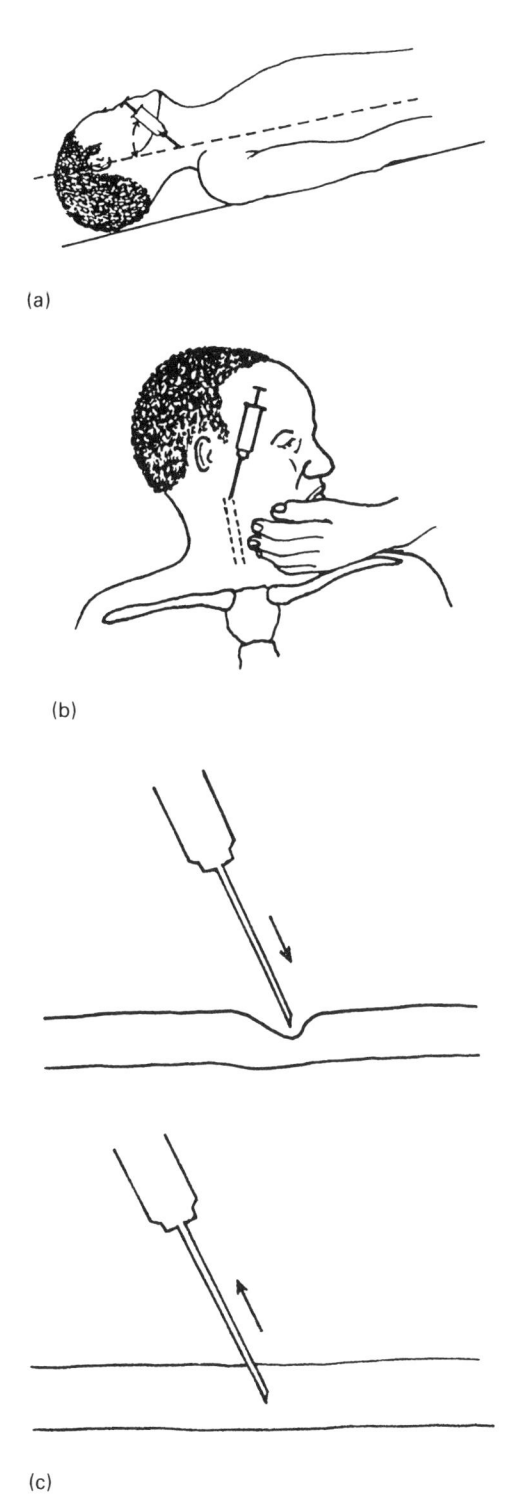

Figure P24 Internal jugular vein cannulation.

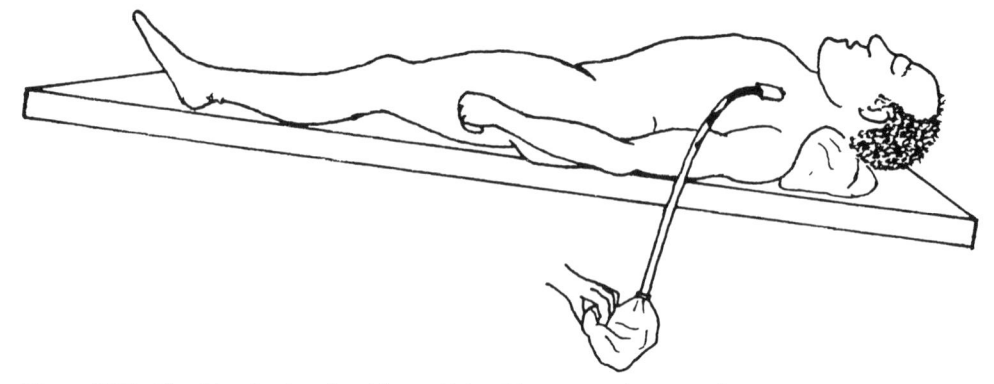

Figure P25 Checking for free backflow of blood in a central venous line.

by disconnecting the drip, flushing the line with 10 ml of saline and then aspirating. If blood still cannot be obtained withdraw the catheter 1 cm and try again.
- If you still have no success remove the cannula and recannulate.
- In children, a small pillow under the shoulders will help to position the child correctly.

Subclavian vein cannulation

1. Tilt the foot of the bed up 15–30.
2. The patient's head should be straight, looking towards the ceiling. His shoulders should be resting on the mattress, not hunched up. If they are get someone to pull on the arms.
3. The technique is the same for both sides, although the left subclavian is easier for right-handed people.
4. After putting on sterile gloves, clean the skin from across the midline to the acromion and from the neck to below the nipple. Drape the patient leaving the suprasternal notch, acromion and nipple visible.
5. Find the midpoint of the clavicle as measured between the suprasternal notch and the acromion. At the midpoint the clavicle is concave towards the foot of the bed.
6. Inject 1% lidnocaine without adrenaline, raising a skin bleb 2–3 cm inferior to the clavicle. Pass the needle towards the middle of the inferior surface of the clavicle and inject on the periosteum. Then inject under and behind the clavicle at its midpoint. Pass the needle medially towards the suprasternal notch, withdrawing and injecting as you go. You may or may not enter the vein, depending on the length of your needle.
7. Insert local anaesthetic at the point where you plan to suture the catheter to the anterior chest wall.
8. Local anaesthetic may not be necessary in comatose and moribund patients.
9. Make sure you are familiar with the type of central venous catheter you are using. Read the instructions. This description is based on the Cavafix catheter. The technique of insertion is similar for all catheters except that some connections are different with other catheters. There will be an introducing needle and cannula sheath to which you will connect a 5–10-ml syringe and there will be a central venous catheter with a stylet (Figure P26a).
10. Shorten (cut) the catheter at its distal end so that after insertion and securing to the skin the tip of the catheter will lie in the superior vena cava.

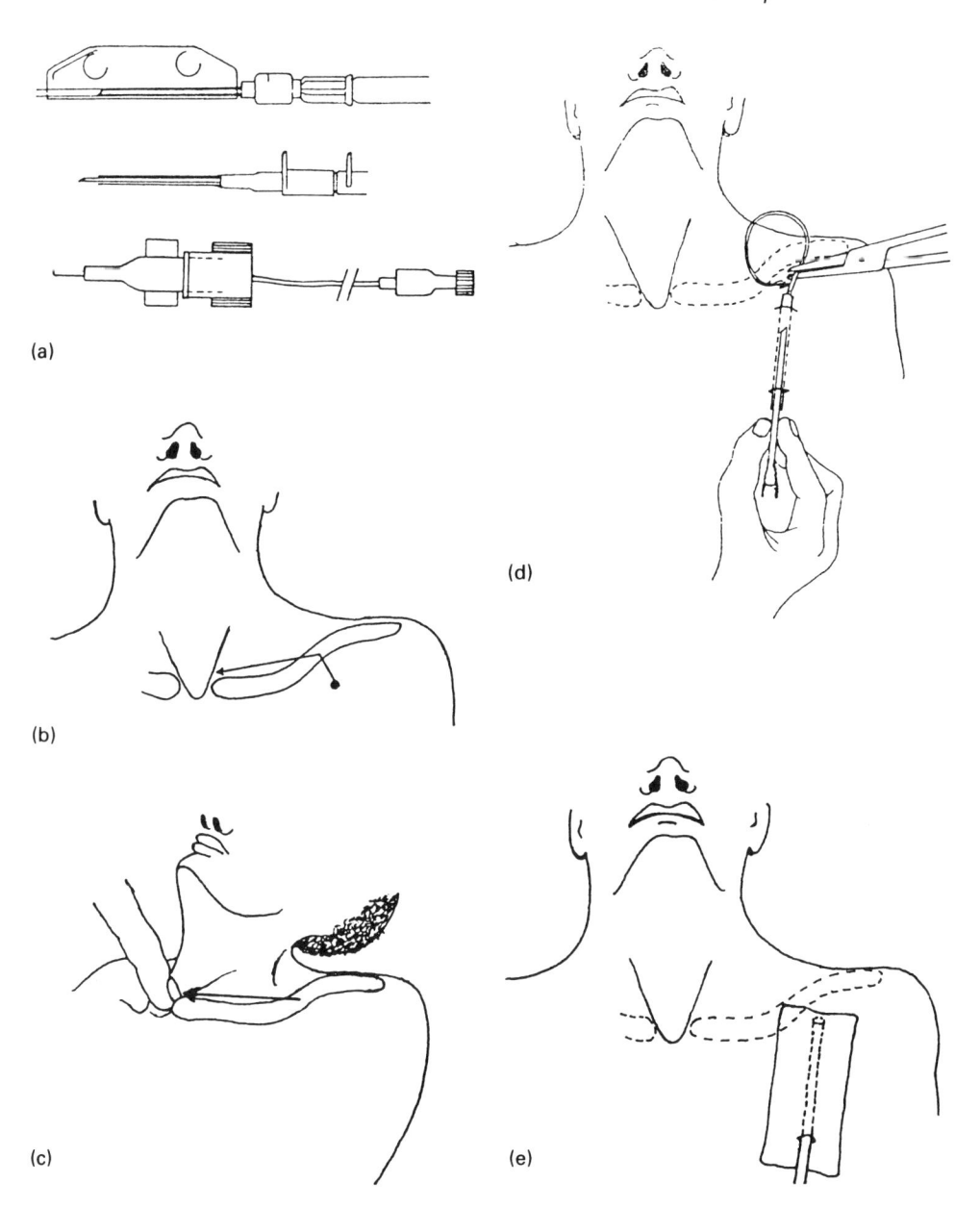

Figure P26 (a)–(e) Subclavian vein cannulation.

11. Attach a 10-ml syringe to the introducing cannula and needle and prick the skin at the point of local anaesthetic injection, 2–3 cm inferior to the midpoint of clavicle (Figure P26b).

12. Aim towards the midpoint of the clavicle, directing the needle towards the patient's chin. When you feel the tip of the needle against the middle of the clavicle walk the needle round under the

clavicle to its posterior surface, keeping right next to the clavicle at all times.
13. Once under the clavicle redirect the needle towards the top of your left index finger, which is placed in the suprasternal notch (Figure P26c). The point to aim for is 1–2 cm above the notch. Do not pass the needle more medially than the sternoclavicular joint. The needle and cannula should pass immediately beneath the clavicle as **horizontally** as possible. If the position of the patient's shoulders prevents this get an assistant to pull the shoulders down. You should not normally feel the first rib.
14. As you pass the introducing needle and cannula towards the top of your left index finger, withdraw on the syringe as you go. You will enter the vein about 1–2 cm before you reach the limit of the Cavafix introducer or just about at the limit of the Bardicath. The flow of blood into the syringe should be free and easy. Make sure the blood is venous and not arterial. There is a slight 'give' when you enter the vein. Sometimes you feel this but pass right through the vein. Pull back the needle by small amounts until you are able to withdraw blood freely.
15. *Problems*
(a) If you do not enter the vein first time, return to the spot behind the clavicle and aim for the middle of your index finger in the suprasternal notch. If this fails, aim for the suprasternal notch. If you are still unsuccessful, the next step is to remove the introducing needle and to go behind the clavicle 1 cm medially and then aim for the top of your left index finger again. If the more medial approach is not successful, try 1 cm more lateral to your original entry. **Ask for someone more experienced to help you** if you do not successfully enter the vein after one or two attempts. Do not keep trying, as you may have already caused a pneumothorax. Stop, get help and X-ray the chest, preferably in the erect position. Do not try on the other side without first being certain that there is no pneumothorax.
(b) You withdraw pulsating, aterial blood. In this case you have entered the subclavian artery. Withdraw; the artery is unlikely to suffer any permanent damage, but check the pulsation of the brachial pulse now and 4 h later.
(c) You withdraw air. You have probably punctured the lung. In which case withdraw the cannula. A large pneumothorax is unlikely to develop unless the patient is being ventilated or will have anaesthesia in the next 24 h. X-ray the chest and insert an intercostal drain if necessary. If you have a long introducing needle you may have punctured the oesophagus or trachea (this is much less likely than the pleura). You can decide if this is likely from the length of your cannula when laid across the front of the clavicle from the point of insertion. If it reaches the middle of the suprasternal notch you could have entered these structures. Usually there will be no sequelae but put the patient on antibiotics to prevent mediastinitis. If surgical emphysema in the absence of a pneumothorax develops, get surgical help as the neck may need to be drained.
16. Once you are in the vein remove the introducing needle with your right hand and hold the position of the cannula firmly with your left, keeping it horizontal (with the Bardicath the catheter is fed through the needle and there is no outer sheath cannula). Blood should flow out of the vein. Cover the entrance to the cannula with your left thumb to minimise bleeding. Providing the patient is head-down there will be no risk of air embolism.

17. Pick up the catheter (stylet still in place) from your tray, attach the yellow connector to the cannula and pass the catheter through the cannula into the vein as far as it will go, providing you have trimmed the catheter to the correct length. Make use of the plastic bag attached to the red connector. This is to allow you to feed in the catheter without touching it. The catheter should pass fairly easily, but sometimes the crumpling of the plastic bag gets in the way and then you need to pass the catheter using forceps, having removed the red connector and bag.
18. *Problems*
    (a) The cannula might be kinked under the clavicle. Make sure you are holding it securely and keep it horizontally. If the catheter still won't pass then remove the cannula and you will have to recannulate the vein.
    (b) The cannula may have moved. No blood will be coming out of the open cannula. If this is so then start again.
    (c) Very occasionally the tip of the cannula is right up against the inside wall of the vein. Pull the cannula back 1–2 mm and see if blood flows out. If it does and you can now pass the catheter you are likely to be all right.
19. If you are using a Cavafix remove the red connector and the plastic bag protecting the catheter. Pull out the yellow connector and prise it apart and secure the catheter and stylet in the hub of the cannula.
20. Pull the cannula out of the vein (to leave it in risks air embolism and haemorrhage if the catheter but not the cannula is accidentally removed). Remove the stylet and connect the intravenous line.
21. The drip should run freely. If it does take the infusion bag off the stand and hold it below the level of the bed. Blood should now run back into the tubing. This confirms that the catheter is in a large vein (Figure P25).
22. *Problems* If the drip does not run freely or there is no back flow, check that the drip control is open and that the three-way tap is in the correct position. If they are then stop the drip and disconnect the giving set. Inject 10 ml of saline down the catheter and then withdraw. Blood should be withdrawn if the catheter was blocked. Repeat this if necessary. If you cannot withdraw blood and blood will not flow back then the catheter may be kinked under the clavicle. Pull the catheter back 1 cm at a time flushing with saline until you produce a good back flow of blood. If all these measures are unsuccessful, the catheter is probably not in the vein and you should remove and start again.
23. Secure the catheter by strapping, suturing or an occlusive dressing to the chest wall. Instruct those nursing the patient in the care of the catheter and how to read central venous pressure.
24. If a subcutaneous tunnel is needed for parenteral nutrition then omit stage 23 and fashion the tunnel (Figure 26d) using an introducing cannula or scalpel and artery forceps. The skin at original insertion site 2–3 cm inferior to the clavicle should have 3–4 mm incision using a scalpel blade so that the catheter can be subcutaneous for 5–10 cm from this point. A Vygon or Hickman–Broviac catheter are best for long-term parenteral feeding. The technique of making the tunnel for each catheter is in the instructions.

After cannulating the IJV or the subclavian vein examine the chest regularly

---

KEY POINT

Check the position of the catheter tip on chest X-ray.

for evidence of a pneumothorax caused by puncturing the lung. A chest X-ray, preferably taken with the patient erect, will exclude this diagnosis and will confirm the position of the cannula.

Basilic approach

Another method of gaining access to the subclavian vein is via the basilic or median cubital vein at the antecubital fossa (Figure P27). The patient should lie with the arm abducted to 45° and a venous tourniquet applied. The head should be turned towards the site of the puncture. Use a 50–60-cm catheter.

External jugular vein

If the patient is positioned head-down, the external jugular vein is often seen passing across the side of the neck. It can be cannulated with a normal cannula as in a peripheral vein, which may be very useful in an emergency. It is not suitable for CVP measurement, as it has a valve at its junction with the subclavian vein. When cannulating ask someone to press gently on the lower end of the vein above the clavicle. This will disturb the vein and make cannulation easier.

Femoral vein cannulation
(Figure P28)

This is often the easiest vein to cannulate in a shocked child. Consider the intraosseus route (page 392) An ordinary cannula can be used. The vein lies medial to the femoral artery in the groin. Palpate the pulse and insert the cannula 1 cm medial and parallel to it, at or just below the groin crease, at about 45° to the skin. After entering the vein make the angle slightly shallower to help the cannula to pass up the vein more easily.

Never leave a cannula in the femoral vein for longer than necessary because thrombosis is a serious risk, and a disaster if it occurs.

Central venous pressure measurement

This can be measured by a catheter whose tip is in the internal jugular, subclavian, vena cava or right atrium. Connect a saline manometer between the cannula and drip

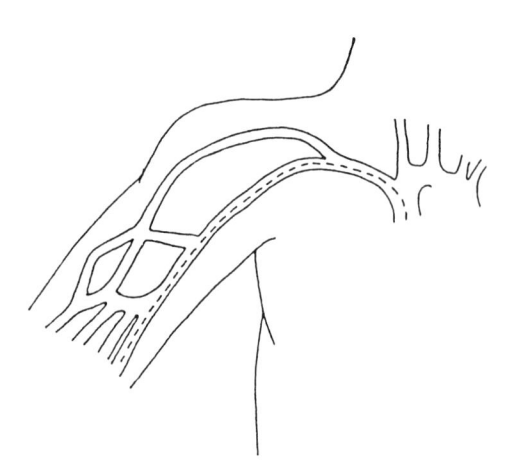

Figure P27 Basilic vein cannulation.

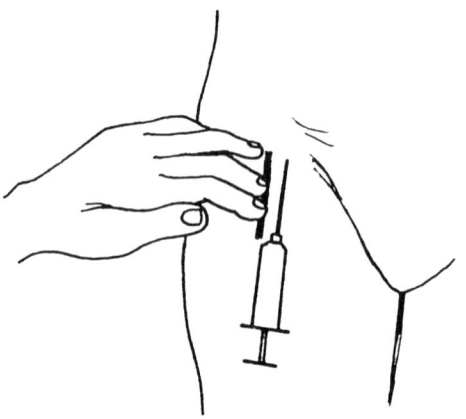

Figure P28 Femoral vein cannulation.

set as shown (Figure P29). Measure the CVP with the patient in the same position (preferably flat) each time, as posture may affect the reading.

Method

1. Check that the drip runs freely.
2. Position the zero point of the scale at the level of the right atrium (4th interspace, midway between the sternum and the back).
3. Fill the column with saline by turning the tap to connect the drip to the manometer and opening the drip.
4. Switch off the drip and turn the tap to connect the manometer to the patient. The level in the column falls until it stabilises. The CVP is the distance in centimetres above or below the zero point. If above, the CVP is 'plus', if below, the CVP is 'minus'. There should be a swing of at least around 0.5 cm of saline with the respiratory cycle.

Problems

The fluid in the column does not fall – check the position of the taps, check that the cotton wool at the top of the column isn't wet (if it is, take it out with a needle), aspirate or flush CVP aseptically in case of blockage.

Alternative method

When manometer tubing or three-way taps are not available use a butterfly cannula in

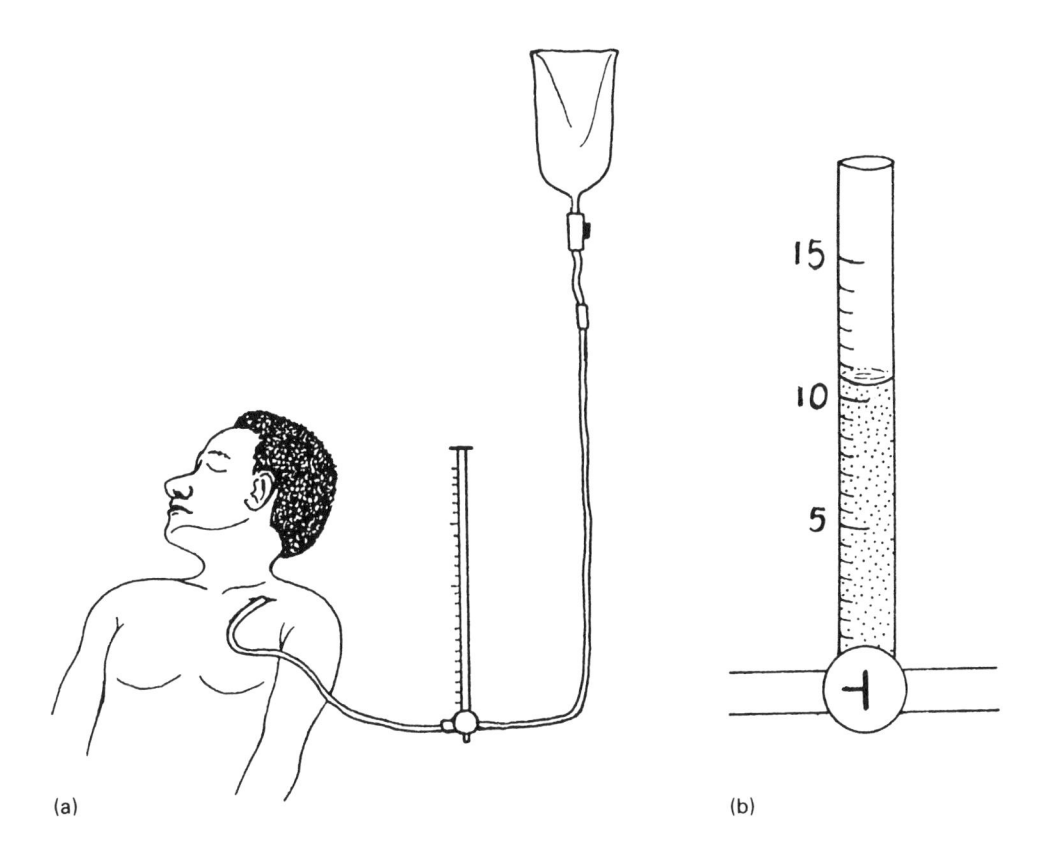

Figure P29 Central venous pressure measurement.

the rubber injection port of an ordinary i.v. giving set (Figure P30).

Interpretation

Central venous pressure is an accurate indicator of intravascular volume providing:
1. the tip of the catheter is in an intrathoracic vein – the fluid level should swing with respiration and not with the heart beat.
2. the catheter is not blocked or kinked (when recording CVP fluid should drop fairly quickly down the manometer tubing to the level of the CVP);
3. there is no right heart failure.

The normal CVP is 5–8 cmH$_2$O but this may be raised 3–5 cm in patients on ventilators.

The CVP may be normal despite hypovolaemia. This occurs because of the capacity of the venous side of the circulation to constrict in response to hypovolaemia. Examples are patients with pre-eclampsia and oliguric patients with a normal CVP who respond to a fluid challenge.

The rate of change in response to therapy is more important than a single reading. If the CVP fails to rise in response to fluid then venoconstriction compensating for

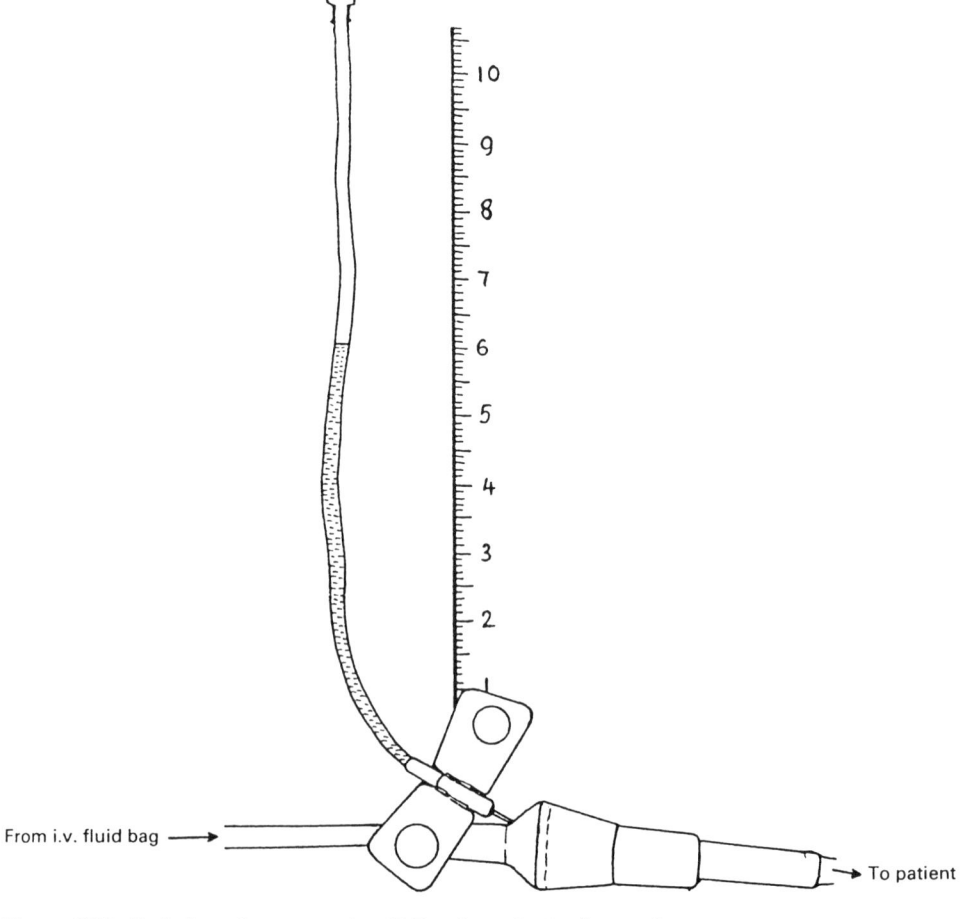

Figure P30 Technique for measuring CVP using a butterfly needle.

hypovolaemia can be assumed. On the other hand if the CVP rises by 4–5 cm in response to a few hundred ml of fluid or blood, fluid overload and cardiac failure are imminent if further fluids are not restricted.

A LOW CVP (<5 cmH$_2$O) implies hypovolaemia and the patient requires crystalloid, colloid or blood as appropriate.

A HIGH CVP (>10 cm) suggests fluid overload, cardiac failure, cardiac tamponade or increased intrathoracic pressure due to a tension pneumothorax. Note the patient on a ventilator may have a raised CVP as discussed above. In penetrating chest trauma a CVP above 30 cmH$_2$O is diagnostic of tamponade.

Unexpected result

Check the position of the catheter tip; check the fluid level in the manometer swings with respiration; ensure the catheter is not blocked or kinked by checking flow through the catheter and that (if the particular catheter allows) blood can be aspirated back through the catheter.

Unexpectedly high levels may be caused by the catheter being in the right ventricle (it will pulsate with each heart beat) or in an extrathoracic vein. Check by a chest X-ray when the tip of the line should be in an intrathoracic vein, preferably the SVC around the level of the sterno-manubrial junction.

Complications

These are minimised by good technique and vigilant nursing supervision once the line is in place. The complications associated with insertion and what is required to prevent, recognise or treat the condition are shown in Table P11.

Complications occuring during monitoring are shown in Table P12.

Kinking, blockage and inadvertent removal can be prevented only by good supervision of the line, taking care to avoid redundant tubing and always securing the line before moving the patient. A blocked catheter can be flushed with saline or sodium citrate providing the blockage is cleared within an hour or so of its occurrence. It is not advisable to unblock catheters after several hours since the clot may contain bacteria and dislodging the clot may cause septicaemia.

Contamination of the catheter tip with bacteria occurs in up to 20% of cases, 10%

Table P12 Problems and complications of central venous pressure monitoring

Kinking
Blockage
Inadvertent removal
Catheter sepsis and septicaemia
Catheter migration
Erosion of great vessels
Central vein thrombosis

Table P11 Complications of inserting central venous lines

Complication	Action
Arterial puncture	Stop bleeding by pressure. Rarely severe.
Pneumothorax	Chest X-ray to recognise. Intercostal drain to treat.
Hydrothorax	Chest X-ray to recognise. Intercostal drain to treat.
Oesophageal/tracheal injury	Treat conservatively.
Air embolism	Do not leave cannula in vein. Always have head-down tilt on insertion (prevention). Lie right-side-up, head-down.

of which have an associated bacteraemia. The risk of contamination and catheter-related sepsis is minimised by removing the line at 48 h, providing the patient is stable and venous access secure.

Erosion of the catheter tip through the wall of the superior vena cava or atrium is fortunately rare. Migration of the catheter into the superior vena cava, ventricle or pulmonary artery is also rare, and if it occurs then the catheter should be removed by the most simple means possible, which may involve cardiac catheterisation or surgical removal in a specialised centre.

Central vein thrombosis may complicate patients receiving cytotoxic drugs or hyperosmolar solutions on long-term parenteral nutrition (p. 288).

Removal

Remove the line as soon as it is no longer needed. The patient should be placed head down in 15° tilt and the catheter pulled briskly out after cutting any sutures. The catheter site can be covered with a swab or sticking plaster for 24 h. Send the tip of the catheter to your laboratory for a culture, if infection is suspected. Suspect a line infection in any patient with a fever and on central line.

Using a CVP transducer

The CVP can be continuously monitored using a disposable transducer on many modern monitors. This method allows a display of the waveform and the CVP is usually measured in mmHg (10 cmH$_2$O = 7.5 mm Hg).

Intraosseous infusions

(Figure P31)

The intraosseous route is suitable for children aged 6 years or younger. It is indicated where circulatory collapse is so severe that venous cannulation is impossible or difficult.

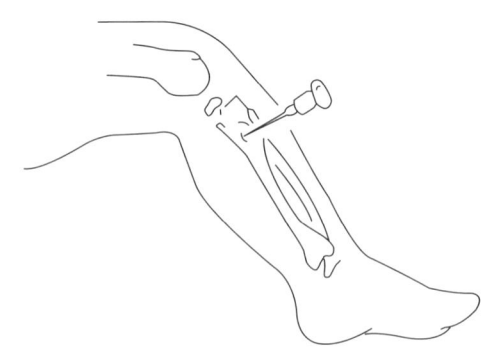

Figure P31 Tibial technique for intraosseous infusion.

The child should lie supine. Use local anaesthetic and an aseptic technique. A large calibre bone marrow aspiration needle (or a short 18G spinal needle with stylet) is inserted on the anteromedial surface of the tibia, 1–3 cm below the tibial tubercle. Penetrate the bone at 90°, then angle the bevel of the needle 45–60° towards the foot and away from the epiphyseal plate. Use a gentle twisting or boring action. Remove the stylet and attach a 10-ml syringe with 5 ml sterile saline. Aspiration of bone marrow into the syringe indicates successful cannulation of the medullary cavity. Inject the saline into the bone to flush away any clot. Failure to aspirate bone marrow does not always indicate a wrong position. If the needle remains upright and allows solution to flow freely it is probably correctly placed.

The intraosseous route should be used for up to 6 h by which time the patient should be well resuscitated and it will be possible to insert a peripheral venous cannula.

Potential complications include infections, penetration of the whole bone, subcutaneous infiltration, pressure necrosis of the skin, physical plate injury, haematoma.

Further reading

COLLIGNON P, SONI N, PEARSON I, SORRELL T, WOODS P. Sepsis associated with central vein catheters in critically ill patients. *Intensive Care Med* 1988;14:227–31.

DEEDAT AM, WILSON IH, WATTERS DAK. Central venous pressure monitoring for the critically ill in Zambia. *Trop Doct* 1990;20:74–6.

EGGLESTON FC. Simplified management of fluid and electrolyte problems. *Trop Doct* 1985;15:111–17.

HOCKING G. Central venous access and monitoring. *Update in Anaethesia* 2001;12:59–70. Also available on-line www.nda.ox.ac.uk/wfsa

McGEE DC, Gould MK. Preventing complications of central venous catheterisation. *N Engl J Med* 2003;348:1123–33.

Pericardial aspiration

Equipment

1. Long (8–10 cm) 16, 18 or 20 gauge needle; a safe alternative is a 20 gauge cannula and needle. 1% lidocaine local anaesthetic.
2. Iodine or hibitane solution.
3. Atropine 0.6 mg. (i.v. solution).
4. An ECG monitor or ECG machine.

Indications

1. Therapeutic aspiration for pericardial tamponade (see pp. 48 and 65).
2. Diagnostic aspiration for suspected pericardial effusion (see p. 49).

Contraindications

Restless or unco-operative patients, since there is a greater risk of trauma to cardiac vessels or myocardium. For life-threatening tamponade there are no contraindications.

Special considerations

1. If there is pericardial tamponade, aspiration is life-saving and can be attempted without the following precautions.
2. If echocardiography is available it should be used to confirm the presence of a pericardial effusion before aspiration. Urgent aspiration should not be delayed if the condition of the patient is unstable. It is preferable to use a cardiac monitor during the procedure if one is available.

Technique

The xiphisternal approach is described, as this is safer and easier in inexperienced hands.

1. Position the patient at 45° on pillows and explain the procedure to him.
2. Sedate the patient with 5–10 mg of diazepam i.v. if he is particularly anxious.
3. Premedicate with 0.5 mg atropine i.v. to prevent vagal slowing of the heart rate.
4. Connect the ECG electrodes to the back of the chest and ensure that you are getting a reliable trace on the monitor. Alternatively, connect the limb leads to the ECG machine and turn to standard lead II. Start the trace once you have entered the pericardium.
5. Shave, if necessary, and clean the skin in the xiphisternal area and infiltrate with 5–10 ml of lidocaine 1%.
6. With the needle/cannula connected to a 10-ml syringe puncture the skin just below the xiphisternum (Figure P32) and advance the needle at 45°, aiming for an imaginary point behind the left nipple or towards the left shoulder.
7. You will feel a definite 'give' as you puncture the central tendon of the diaphragm and at this point suck back on the syringe as you continue to slowly

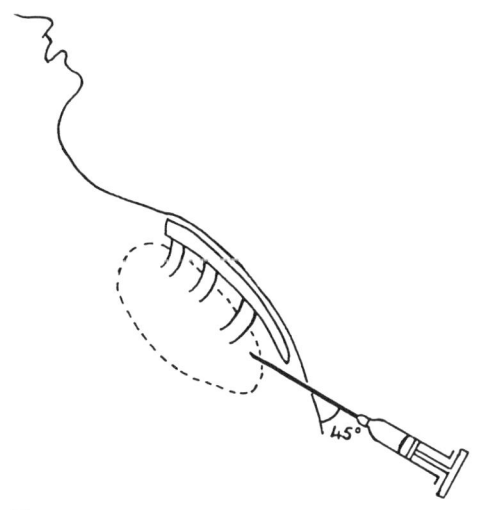

Figure P32 Pericardial aspiration using the xiphisternal approach. Note the angle of insertion of the needle below the xiphisternum.

advance the needle. Fluid, which may be bloodstained, purulent, clear or deep-brown in appearance will be aspirated as you enter the pericardial sac. If the fluid looks like blood, aspirate 10 ml and then leave it in a receiver to see if it clots; if it does not then it is safe to continue the procedure. If the blood clots you have penetrated either a vessel or the heart; in either case it is wiser to abandon the procedure unless you are dealing with tamponade, when a different angle may be successful.

8. Watch the monitor for ectopic activity or sudden S–T changes that indicate you are hitting the myocardial wall. This will also be appreciated by a 'scratchy' feel on the end of the needle and the needle may also be seen and felt to pulsate. Should any of these events occur withdraw the needle slightly and check again for fluid.
9. Withdraw the introducer needle if a cannula has been used.
10. Aspirate to dryness in the case of pericardial tamponade (there may be over 2 litres of fluid).
11. At the end of aspiration, if you are going to perform a check X-ray you may inject 20 ml of air into the pericardium to obtain a double contrast. This will demonstrate the true size of the heart post-aspiration and the air will be reabsorbed over the next few days with no effect on cardiac function. Do not inject more than this amount or you may provoke pneumopericardial tamponade. If air is injected into the heart itself then air embolism may result.

Monitoring

During the procedure an assistant should monitor the pulse rate, volume and rhythm and watch the cardiac monitor if available.

After the procedure, check the BP and pulse every 15 min on all patients for 2 h following the procedure.

The completeness of aspiration may be assessed by echocardiography.

Problems

1. Dramatic slowing of the heart rate caused by vagal stimulation. *Action*: stop the procedure and repeat the atropine injection (0.6 mg. i.v.).
2. Arrhythmias. *Action*: stop the procedure and check the blood pressure; if it fails and the arrhythmia persists then it will require specific treatment (p. 56). The majority of arrhythmias will cease on withdrawing the needle.
3. No fluid aspirated; this may occur if the pus is too viscid to be aspirated through a narrow-gauge needle. It may also occur if the original diagnosis was incorrect. *Action*: a wider-bore needle may be successful. In some instances surgical drainage using the xiphisternal approach is necessary to drain viscid effusions, pus or recurrent tamponade.

Management of cardiac arrest

Basic life support (BLS)

Cardiac arrest occurs when there is acute cessation of cardiac output. When this occurs for more than 3 min the brain becomes severely hypoxic and irreversibly damaged. If immediate resuscitation is carried out, up to 15% of patients may recover. The prognosis depends on the underlying cause, the efficiency of resuscitation and the general condition of the patient. The following guidelines are based on those of the Resuscitation Council (UK) – see further reading.

Adopt a SAFE approach

- Shout for help.
- Approach with care.
- Free the patient from immediate danger.
- Evaluate the patient's ABC.

Rescue breathing

- Each inflation should take about 1.5–2 sec.
- Resistance will be greater if inflation is too quick and less air will get into the lungs.
- Ideal V_t = 400–500 ml in an adult, about the amount required to produce visible lifting of the chest.
- Wait 2–4 seconds for full expiration before giving another breath. Ten breaths will therefore take about 40–60 sec.

Chest compressions

- **Finding the right place:** Using your index and middle fingers, identify the lower rib margins. Keeping your fingers together, slide them upwards to the point where the ribs join the sternum.

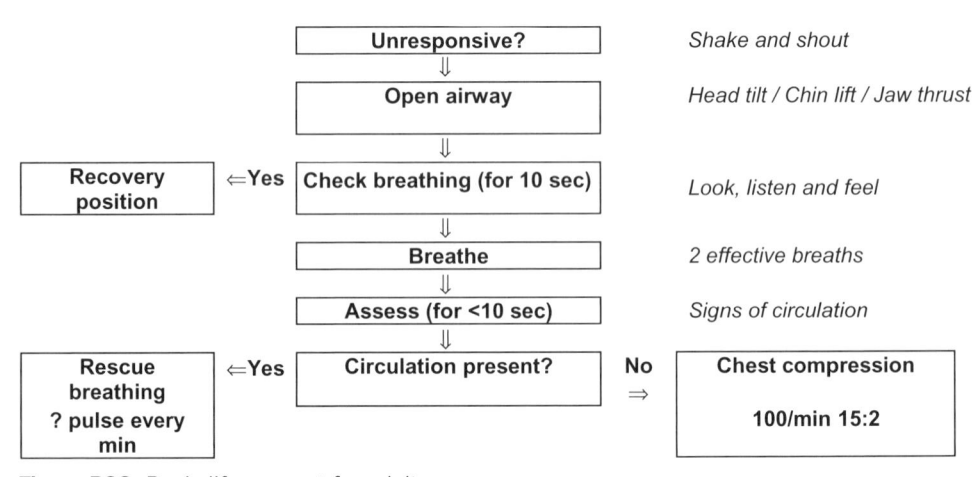

	Unresponsive?	Shake and shout
	⇓	
	Open airway	Head tilt / Chin lift / Jaw thrust
	⇓	
Recovery position ⇐Yes	Check breathing (for 10 sec)	Look, listen and feel
	⇓	
	Breathe	2 effective breaths
	⇓	
	Assess (for <10 sec)	Signs of circulation
	⇓	
Rescue breathing ? pulse every min ⇐Yes	Circulation present? No ⇒	Chest compression 100/min 15:2

Figure P33 Basic life support for adults.

With your middle finger on this point, place your index finger on the sternum. Slide the heel of your other hand down the sternum until it reaches your index finger; this should be the middle of the lower half of the sternum. Place the heel of one hand there, with the other hand on top of the first. Interlock the fingers of both hands and lift them to ensure that pressure is not applied over the victim's ribs. Do not apply any pressure over the upper abdomen or bottom tip of the sternum.
- **Aim to depress the sternum approximately 4–5 cm** and apply only enough pressure to achieve this.
- At all times the pressure should be firm, controlled and applied vertically. Erratic or violent action is dangerous.
- The recommended rate of compression is a rate and not the number of compressions which are to be given in a minute; this will depend upon interruptions for rescue breathing.
- About the same time should be spent in the compression phase as in the released phase.

Advanced life support (ALS)

Defibrillation

- First cycle = 200 J 200 J 360 J. All subsequent shocks should be 360 J.
- Electrode polarity is unimportant. Use defibrillation pads to improve electrical contact. One paddle is placed below the right clavicle in the midclavicular line, the other over the lower left ribs in the mid/anterior axillary line (outside the position of the normal cardiac apex), avoiding placement over the breast tissue in female. Transdermal patches should be removed to prevent arcing, and defibrillator pads/paddles should be placed 12–15 cm away from implanted pacemakers.
- For safety reasons, charge the defibrillator only when the paddles are in contact with the patient. Hold the oxygen mask away from the patient during actual defibrillation.
- VT and pulseless VT are the commonest causes of reversible cardiac arrest in adults. These are the most 'recoverable' rhythms and it is therefore always worthwhile persisting with cardio-pulmonary resuscitation (CPR) whilst they are present. However, successful resuscitation does depend on *early defibrillation*. BLS, i.v. access and airway control should not delay delivery of shocks. There is no point in palpating for a pulse between shocks if the ECG rhythm still shows VF since it will only delay delivery of the next shock.

Ventilations

- Once the trachea is intubated, chest compressions should continue uninterrupted (except for pulse checks and defibrillation) at a rate of 100 per minute whilst ventilations are administered simultaneously at a rate of 12 per minute.
- A pause in chest compressions allows coronary perfusion pressure to fall substantially and is followed with a delay before the original perfusion pressure is restored after compressions are recommenced.
- Over one minute you should have completed about five cycles of 15:2 compressions:breaths.

Bicarbonate

- Is best administered on the basis of arterial blood gasses (ABGs). Currently it is recommended in the presence of severe acidosis (arterial pH <7.1, base excess ≤10) as a dose of 50 mmol (50 ml of 8.4% sodium bicarbonate).

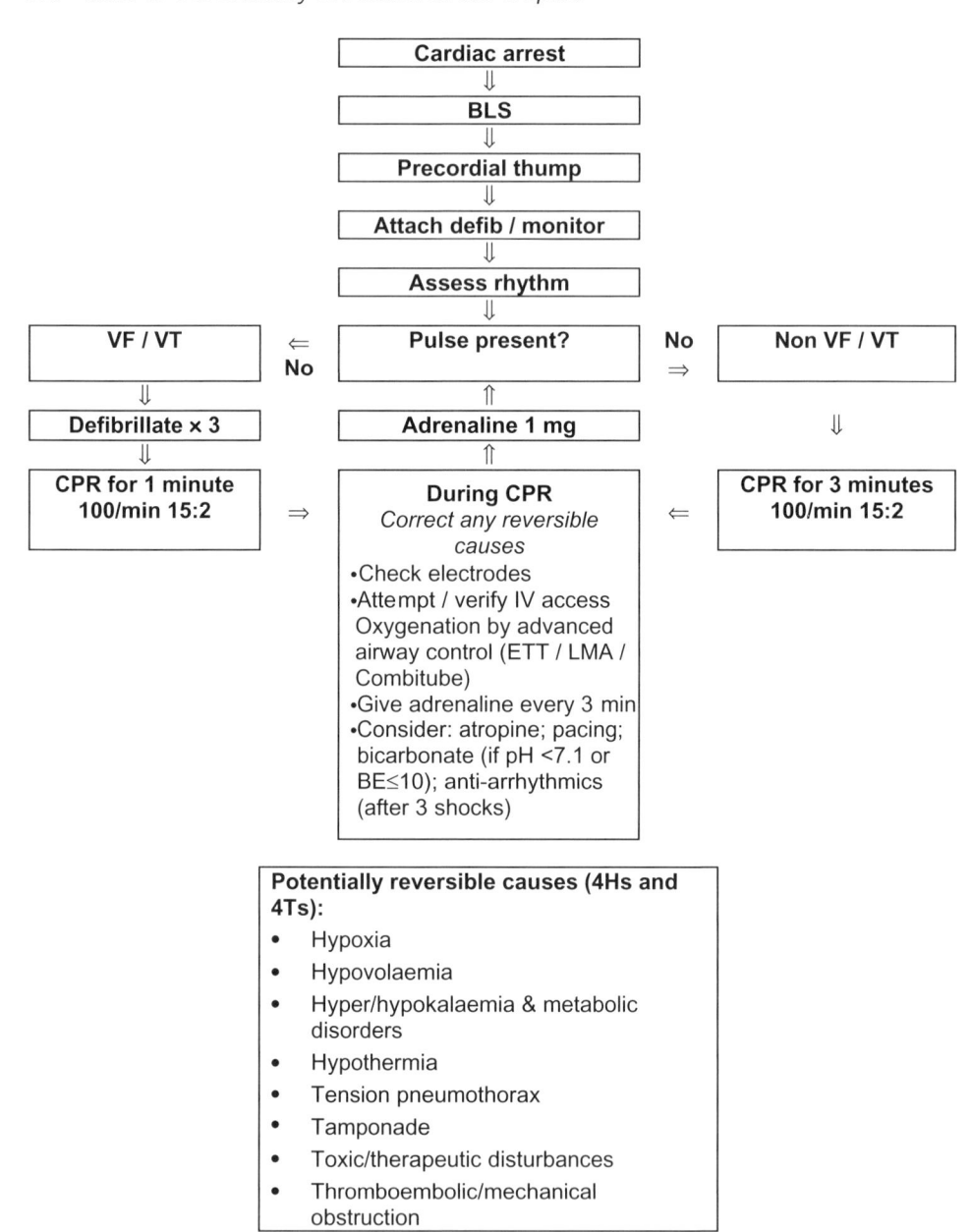

```
                    ┌─────────────────┐
                    │ Cardiac arrest  │
                    └────────┬────────┘
                             ⇓
                    ┌─────────────────┐
                    │      BLS        │
                    └────────┬────────┘
                             ⇓
                    ┌─────────────────┐
                    │ Precordial thump│
                    └────────┬────────┘
                             ⇓
                    ┌─────────────────────┐
                    │ Attach defib/monitor│
                    └──────────┬──────────┘
                               ⇓
                    ┌─────────────────┐
                    │  Assess rhythm  │
                    └────────┬────────┘
                             ⇓
```

```
   VF / VT      ⇐ No    Pulse present?     No ⇒     Non VF / VT
     ⇓                         ⇑                         ⇓
Defibrillate × 3         Adrenaline 1 mg
     ⇓                         ⇑
CPR for 1 minute    ⇒     During CPR       ⇐      CPR for 3 minutes
 100/min 15:2        Correct any reversible         100/min 15:2
                            causes
                      •Check electrodes
                      •Attempt / verify IV access
                      Oxygenation by advanced
                      airway control (ETT / LMA /
                      Combitube)
                      •Give adrenaline every 3 min
                      •Consider: atropine; pacing;
                      bicarbonate (if pH <7.1 or
                      BE≤10); anti-arrhythmics
                      (after 3 shocks)
```

Potentially reversible causes (4Hs and 4Ts):
- Hypoxia
- Hypovolaemia
- Hyper/hypokalaemia & metabolic disorders
- Hypothermia
- Tension pneumothorax
- Tamponade
- Toxic/therapeutic disturbances
- Thromboembolic/mechanical obstruction

Figure P34 Advanced life support for adults.
VF, ventricular fibrillation; VT, ventricular tachycardia; ETT, endotracheal tube; LMA, laryngeal mask airway; BE, base excess.

- If ABG analysis is impossible it may be reasonable to give bicarbonate after about 20 min of CPR.

Anti-arrhythmics

- Amiodarone should be considered (150 mg i.v. over 10 min then 300 mg

Practical procedures

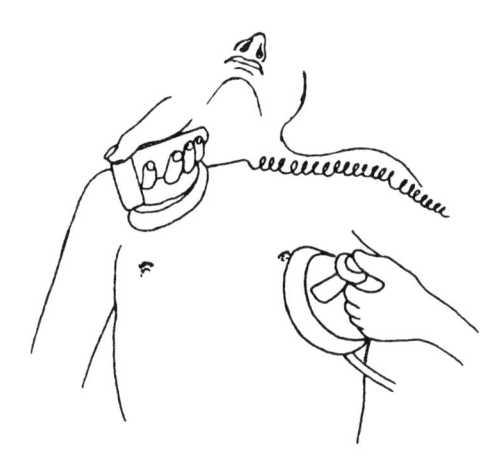

Figure P35 Defibrillator paddles in place.

i.v. over 1 h) in cardiac arrest due to VF or pulseless VF after the third shock.
- Consider lidocaine as second-line treatment for VF/VT after 12 unsuccessful shocks (4 loops). A starting dose of 50–200 mg (5–20 ml of 1% lidocaine) is reasonable, followed by a maintenance dose of 2 mg/min.
- Bretylium is no longer recommended.

After resuscitation

General

Try to determine the cause of the cardiac arrest to assess whether specific management of an underlying disorder is required. Some causes are shown in Table P13.

Specific

A cardiac arrest may be followed by serious complications, and patients need close observation for several hours.

Cerebral hypoxia results in cerebral oedema and is likely to have occurred if a patient does not regain full consciousness following successful resuscitation. Mannitol 1 g/kg may be given and if there is any respiratory problem the patient should be ventilated for at least 6–8 h. The head should be in a neutral position and the head of the bed should be raised a little.

Cardiac output may be low and require inotropic support. Renal failure may also occur and should be managed as described on p. 91. Occasionally damage to the chest or abdomen may occur and a chest X-ray should be taken to exclude pneumothorax, fractured ribs, haemothorax, or tamponade. Intra-abdominal bleeding may occasionally be caused and may present with the signs of unexpected hypovolaemia.

When to stop resuscitation

If after 15–20 min of resuscitation there is no spontaneous cardiac or respiratory activity

Table P13 Causes of cardiac arrest

Hypoxia	Respiratory failure
Cardiac	Ischaemia
	Failure
	Arrhythmias
Drugs	Many drugs in overdose
Metabolic	Hyper/hypokalaemia
	Acidosis
Temperature	Ventricular fibrillation at 28–30°C
Trauma	Head injury
	Tension pneumothorax
	Tamponade
	Myocardial injury
	Hypovolaemia

and the pupils are fixed and dilated then resuscitation should be abandoned except in the case of hypothermic patients, who are sometimes resuscitated successfully after long periods of arrest when rewarmed.

Whom to resuscitate?

It is inappropriate to attempt resuscitation of a patient who has developed a cardiac arrest as a result of a long-term uncurable illness such as advanced cancer. Equally, it is unacceptable to resuscitate anyone who cannot expect a reasonable quality of life because of illness if successfully resuscitated. These are often difficult decisions to make at the time of arrest and if you are in doubt it is safer to attempt resuscitation. In some hospitals clinicians in charge of patients with long-term illnesses make recommendations on whether resuscitation is appropriate should cardiac arrest occur. When these decisions are made they should be communicated to the nursing and medical staff caring for the patient.

Further reading

UK Resuscitation Council Guidelines 1998. http://www.resus.org.uk

ZIDEMAN D. Paediatric Life Support. *Update in Anaesthesia* No 10. http:www.nda.ox.ac.uk/wfsa

Autotransfusion

An autologous blood transfusion, or autotransfusion, is a procedure in which blood is collected from a patient and is then subsequently reinfused. This means that the blood donor and recipient are the same person.

There are three main methods of autotransfusion:
1. Pre-deposit of blood.
2. Haemodilution at induction of anaesthesia.
3. Salvaging of blood at operation.

Pre-deposit of blood

This method involves the collection by venesection of the patient's own blood in the period leading up to elective surgery. The blood is then stored (deposited) under appropriate conditions until it is required for transfusion at the time of operation. Pre-depositing of blood in this manner relies on the fact that in most reasonably fit and healthy patients the deficit of blood volume and haemoglobin caused by venesection is physiologically corrected within a relatively short space of time. If 500 ml of blood are venesected from the patient the deficit is normally corrected within 3 to 5 days.

In practice it is advisable to ensure that the haemoglobin concentration of the patient lies within the normal range before venesection takes place. Collect only 500 ml of blood every 5 days and re-check the haemoglobin concentration immediately prior to operation to ensure that the patient has been able to compensate for the deficit. A preoperative haemoglobin above 10 g/dl is generally acceptable. If necessary, it is possible to collect up to 2 litres of blood from a patient within the space of 3 weeks. It is important to prescribe oral iron supplements to venesected patients to prevent depletion of this important blood component and to ensure maximum bone marrow activity.

Pre-depositing of blood for operations and other procedures is useful:
1. where there is a reluctance or refusal of patients who may require transfusion to accept blood which has been donated by others;
2. where patients requiring transfusion possess a rare blood group and donors of compatible blood cannot be found or there are cross-matching difficulties;
3. where there are no or only limited blood bank facilities available or its services are unreliable.

Haemodilution at induction of anaesthesia

This method of autotransfusion involves the venesection and collection of the patient's own blood at the time of induction of anaesthesia. The blood volume deficit is immediately corrected by the infusion into the patient of crystalloid or colloid fluid in a volume equivalent to that of the blood collected. This results in haemodilution, which in healthy patients with a normal preoperative haemoglobin level will cause no adverse effect. The collected blood is then available for transfusion back into the patient during the course of the operation.

Although not as satisfactory as the pre-deposit method, venesection and haemodilution does provide a means of ensuring blood is available for transfusion and can be useful in situations where only a limited amount of blood loss is expected at operation but where blood for transfusion may be needed.

The patients selected for this method of autotransfusion should be healthy and have a normal haemoglobin level. It is recommended that no more than 500 ml of blood be venesected at induction, unless continuous monitoring of the haematocrit is available, when venesection and dilution to a haematocrit of 30% is possible.

Salvaging of blood at operation

The salvaging of blood lost into body cavities and its subsequent re-infusion back into the patient can be a life-saving procedure. It is particularly useful in situations where there is severe blood loss at operation and where there are delays in obtaining sufficient compatible blood from other donors. Two common examples of this situation are a ruptured spleen and a ruptured ectopic pregnancy.

The salvaging procedure requires the co-operation of the surgeon and scrub nurse. One method is as follows:
1. In theatre have a number of pre-prepared stoppered sterile glass bottles with an approximate volume of 500 ml and which contain a suitable anticoagulant. In practice the anticoagulant can be 2 g of sodium citrate and 3 g of dextrose made up to 120 ml with sterile water for each 500 ml bottle. Alternatively, the anticoagulant content from purpose-designed venesection bags can be decanted into the glass bottles.
2. Ask the surgeon to collect the blood from the body cavity into a kidney dish (approximately 400–500 ml of blood per dish).
3. The scrub nurse should then pour the anticoagulant from the pre-prepared bottles into the kidney dish and mix the salvaged blood and anticoagulant well.
4. The mixture of blood and anticoagulant should then be filtered through 4 or 5 layers of gauze, to remove any clots, into the glass bottles. The bottles are then stoppered and handed to the anaesthetist.
5. The anaesthetist should then connect a filtered blood-giving set through the stopper of the bottle, fit an air inlet, and commence the transfusion. If a fine gauge (40 μm) blood filter is available it should be used.

There should be no contamination of the transfused blood. This means that the procedure should be conducted under aseptic conditions and that the blood being salvaged should be sterile and not have come into contact with the contents of the bowel or any other source of infection.

It has been suggested that, due to accumulation of microaggregates and an increased tendency to haemolysis, the amount of blood transfused by this method should be limited to one-fifth of the patient's total blood volume.

However, it must be appreciated that the salvaging of blood at operation and its subsequent re-infusion is often a life-saving procedure and experience has shown that even when much larger volumes than this are re-infused these disadvantages do not constitute a major problem.

Carotid angiography at the bedside

Aim

To demonstrate the position of the intracranial vessels and show if there is a space-occupying lesion within the skull in the absence of CT scanning.

Indications

1. A head-injured patient who is deteriorating.
2. An unconscious patient in whom the diagnosis is unclear.

Equipment

1. Any X-ray machine that can take an X-ray of the skull is satisfactory.
2. A stationary grid.
3. An oxygen supply and some means of ventilating the patient is required.
4. Angiogram tray: towels, sharp 18G lumbar puncture needles, 10-ml syringes, 30-cm plastic connection tubes with ends, kidney bowls.
5. Facilities for general anaesthesia.

X-ray technique

With the patient supine, extend the neck slightly by raising the shoulder, but not too much or there will be difficulty in getting a good X-ray projection. The X-ray should be taken along the plane of the superior orbital ridge, sphenoid ridge and petrous ridge for the best view of the vault of the skull and its enclosed vessels. To achieve this, the X-ray tube should be angled at about 11° above the baseline of the skull (lateral orbital margin and external auditory meatus). A film and stationary grid are placed beneath the skull for AP views (the most important) or at the side for lateral views. X-rays will be taken as the operator finishes the injection of dye to enable the maximum filling of the arterial system to take place – if the circulation is slow for any reason (usually increased intracranial pressure) then the moment of exposure must be correspondingly delayed.

Anaesthesia

If general anaesthesia is to be used, an endotracheal tube is mandatory – general anaesthesia will be necessary when there is impairment of ventilation and an anaesthetist must be present.

Careful sedation and local anaesthesia are extremely satisfactory. Local anaesthesia should be applied to the cervical plexus where it emerges 3 cm below the mastoid process along the posterior border of the sternomastoid muscle. Infiltrate into that area (not into the carotid artery or the jugular vein) and also raise a small bleb on the skin on the neck where the injection needle will enter. This method can be used without sedation where the patient is very drowsy.

Injection technique

1. Conray 280 is the contrast of choice. Do not use stronger solutions or spasm of the cerebral vessels will result.
2. If you are right-handed, stand on the right side of the patient and vice versa.
3. Right carotid:
    (a) Put the first two fingers of the left hand just medial to the junction of the lower and middle third of the sternomastoid – feel the artery and push it slightly towards the trachea – not so much that it is compressed but enough to put it slightly on the stretch so that it does not slide about.
    (b) Push the needle through the anaesthetised skin and attempt to transfix the artery; do not try to enter the vessel as one would in a venepuncture – go right through it (Figure P36).
    (c) Remove the trochar (it need only be used when the skin is being perforated) and slowly withdraw the needle; as the point leaves the distal wall and reenters the vessel you will feel a 'click' and blood will spurt out of the needle.
    (d) If you do not enter the vessel, do not remove the needle from the skin but, when the point is obviously clear of the vessel, steady the artery as before, and try again. Eventually you will enter the vessel.
4. Left carotid:
    (a) A similar technique is used except that the artery is pushed slightly away from the trachea for the operator on the right side.
    (b) Once the needle is in the vessel do **not** try to advance it up the lumen; there is a great danger of stripping off the intima or making a subintimal injection.
5. Connect the plastic tube to the needle and gently irrigate the needle with normal saline or some similar electrolyte solution.
6. Check the position of the head (true AP or true lateral), the tube, and the film.

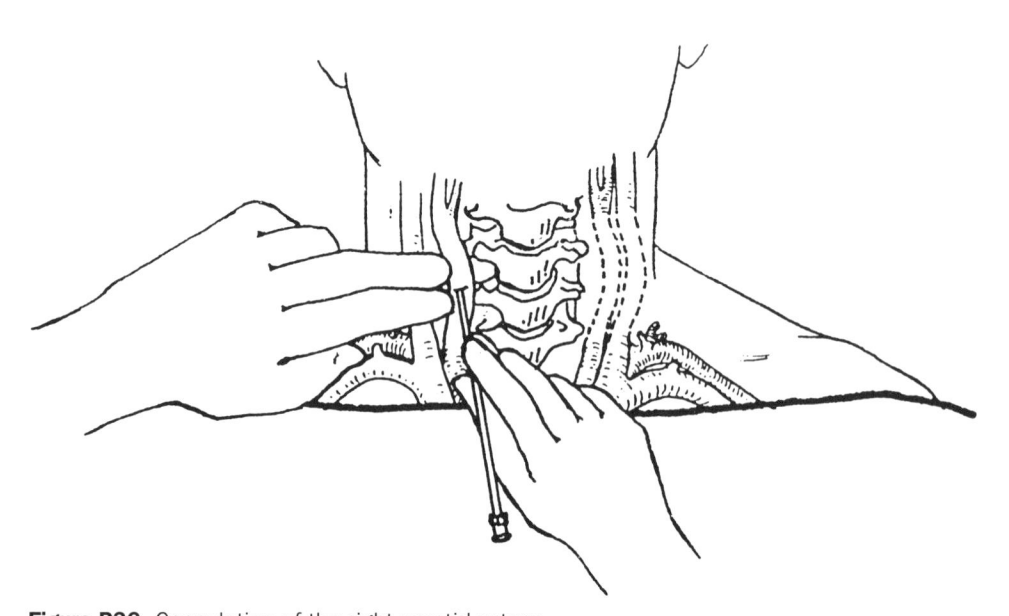

Figure P36 Cannulation of the right carotid artery.

7. Fill a 10-ml syringe with Conray, connect it to the plastic tube, make certain there is a good flow of blood into the tube and that it flows in and out easily, rotate the anode of the X-ray tube and inject as fast as possible (all in 1–2 sec).
8. Shout 'shoot' as the last millilitre enters the tube.
9. After the procedure, remove the needle and apply gentle manual pressure.

This technique should provide satisfactory pictures of the AP and lateral arterial phases. Should circulation be slow or it be wished to show arteriolar, capillary or venous phases, the injection is done as before but instead of shouting 'shoot' as the syringe empties the operator counts 'one, two, three' slowly or 'one ... six' before giving the exposure call.

Problems

These arise when the needle is not properly in the vessel and blood escapes into the tissues and causes swelling. This is rarely serious but if it occurs bilaterally it might compress the trachea, so that if it occurs the procedure should be terminated. Injections into the tissues are not serious. Sometimes the needle, having been in the vessel, seems to have come out; always push it in before removing it and starting again. Sometimes it is lying in the wall and just needs a slight push; if you pull it out first, you will lose it.

Be absolutely certain that you do not inject any air bubbles into the artery as an air embolus and a stroke will result.

Interpretation

Four angiograms taken with a portable X-ray plant and a stationary grid are shown in Figures P37–P40. Interpretations are given in the accompanying captions.

Removal

Pull the cannula out and press for 5 min.

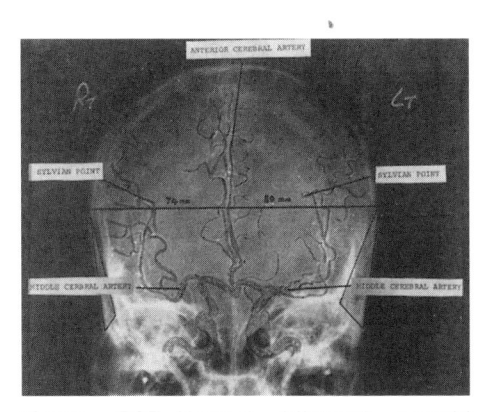

Figure P37 Normal bilateral carotid angiogram. The anterior cerebral artery should be seen in the midline equidistant from the outside of the skull (acceptable range of variation: up to 2.5 mm from the midpoint). In this picture the head is turned slightly to the right (the right orbit is less visible than the left, the right zygomatic arch is easily seen, the left is hidden, the sagittal suture is angled slightly to the left and the triangle consisting of the lateral border of the orbit, the lateral end of the sphenoid ridge and the outside of the skull (as marked) are more obvious on the side from which the head is rotated). Thus the anterior cerebral arteries are carried slightly to the right side. Hence on the right side the distance from the outer wall of the skull to the anterior cerebral artery is 74 mm, while on the left it is 80 mm; that is, a 'shift' of 3 mm – this degree of shift is easily accounted for by the rotation of the head noted above.

At the posterior end of the Sylvian fissure the middle cerebral artery turns laterally and runs outwards towards the surface. The point at which it makes the turn is known as the Sylvian point. This should lie between 35 and 45 mm from the outside of the skull.

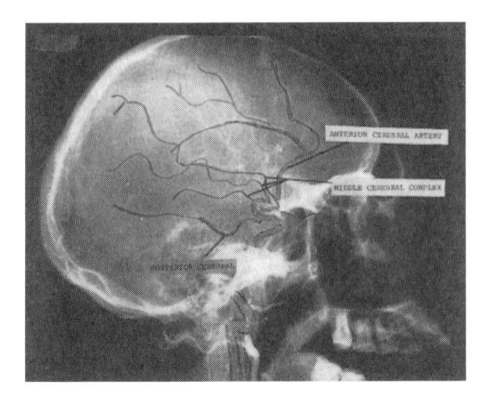

Figure P38 Lateral cartoid angiogram. The anterior cerebral artery runs in a curved fashion over the corpus callosum. If the rising portion of the artery (A_2 segment) has a slightly posterior convexity then the liklihood is that it is normally placed. The middle cerebral artery runs obliquely upwards and backwards. The posterior cerebral artery runs horizontally – if it dips downwards in its course close to the point of origin from the internal carotid artery this suggests temporal lobe herniation. Apart from this, the lateral view is not of great importance in the diagnosis of head injuries.

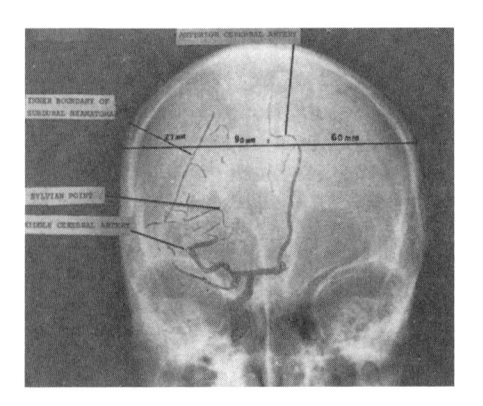

Figure P39 The subdural haematoma. The anterior cerebral artery is pushed across to the left by 15 mm. The Sylvian point is pushed downwards and medially. The surface of the brain is pushed 27 mm from the inner wall of the skull by a totally avascular area, the subdural haematoma. Always remember that subdural haematomas may be bilateral. If there is a large haematoma and a small shift of the anterior cerebral artery, suspect a second lesion on the other side. Always inject the opposite vessel or make a burr hole to establish the presence or absence of such a lesion.

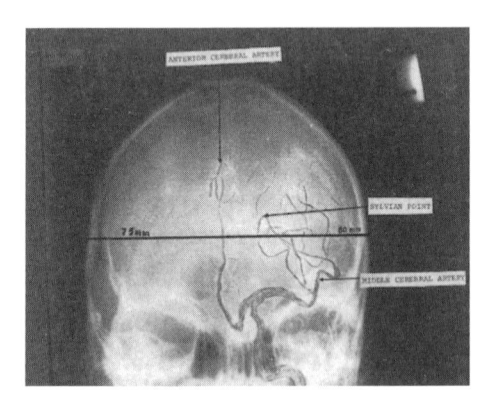

Figure P40 The extradural haematoma. These lesions are not as easily demonstrated as the classical subdural haematoma. This figure shows a posteriorly placed extradural haematoma (though the diagnosis of EDH vs. SDH cannot be made on the basis of the angiogram – it can only be said that there is a large mass, probably placed posteriorly). Anteriorly placed lesions cause a smooth, round sideways curve of the anterior cerebral artery. Posterior lesions produce a straighter shifting of the anterior cerebral artery, with more medial displacement of the Sylvian point than is found in anteriorly placed masses. If a mass is placed anterior or posterior to the maximum diameter of the skull it will not be seen as a surface lesion on the X-ray because it will be hidden by the blood vessels coming to the surface at that point.

Burr holes

Intracranial exploration of a deteriorating head-injured or unconscious patient

Protocol

The patient has been admitted suffering from a head injury or with a deteriorating level of consciousness for which no cause can be found. He has been assessed and subsequently you are worried because he has started to deteriorate further – that is, there is a reduction in his conscious level, or he is developing focal signs (weakness on one side of the body), or one pupil which formerly was small and reactive has now become large and fixed. If you have the facilities you have done a CT scan or a cerebral angiogram and know there is something pressing on the brain with increasing severity and you are making a burr hole to relieve it. If you do not have angiographic or some other similar facility you are making diagnostic burr holes to establish whether there is a surface clot and to relieve it if present.

Preparation

1. It is inadvisable for the untrained person to start such a procedure without the following:
   (a) some form of diathermy;
   (b) a supply of cotton wool pledgets for the easy control of bleeding;
   (c) suction.
2. Endotracheal anaesthsia is preferable, but if the patient is deeply unconscious, with a clear airway and adequate respiration, local anaesthesia may be used. However, airway control is paramount and an ET tube is strongly advised. It is essential that someone is present who will monitor the patient's cardiorespiratory function. This is best done by the anaesthetist.
3. Shave the whole head.
4. Drape the whole head so that both sides are easily accessible unless a previous test has shown that only one side is involved.
5. You may like to give i.v. mannitol at the time you start, to reduce the intracranial pressure and by making more space for you to work make it easier to drain the haematoma. You can give 1 g/kg over about 20 min. Ensure that a urinary catheter is in place.

Method

1. For a complete exploration, six burr holes will need to be made if no previous diagnosis has been established and this can be the tedious part. Make the first burr holes on the same side as the dilated pupil or on the side opposite the paralysis if present. In unilateral lesions you will be correct 80% of the time. Frontal and parietal burr holes should be made first. These should be between 3 and 4 cm from the midline, the frontal one being in the region of the coronal suture (which is relatively easily

palpated in most people) and the parietal just behind the easily visible parietal eminence, in order to straddle the motor area. The incisions should be made in the sagittal plane. If these explorations prove negative, or if for adequate drainage it should be necessary to make a third burr hole, this should be made in the temporal region just in front of the ear and about 2 cm above the zygomatic arch through a vertical incision. This is a convenient location because if it becomes necessary for a small bone flap to be turned or a craniectomy performed, these three skin incisions and their underlying burr holes can easily be joined (Figure P41).

2. If the operation is being done under local anaesthesia infiltrate the skin adequately, in particular the level just superficial to the galea aponeurotica, which contains the nerves and vessels.

3. Make an incision 3–4 cm long down to the bone, hold the wound open and control the bleeding with a self-retaining (mastoid type) retractor. If bleeders have to be cauterised be careful not to burn the skin edge, or necrosis and infection may result later. It is best to do all steps of the frontal and parietal burr holes together so that the dura mater is exposed at the same time in each burr hole.

4. Push the periosteum off the bone.

5. Take the perforator and drill the bone. The perforator is wedge-shaped, so that the shoulders protect it and prevent it plunging through. None the less, care must be exercised because sometimes the skull bone is soft and disasters can happen. When the point of the perforator has just penetrated the inner table change to a burr. Burrs are shaped to cut on the side and will drill out the conical cavity produced by the perforator into a 'well-shaped' hole. When the burr has gone as far as it needs you will feel a resistance, as it tends to 'lock'. It can be forced on but is in danger of 'plunging' if that happens so do not push it (Figure P42).

6. If there is bleeding from the walls of the burr hole, plug this with bone wax. Remove the small fragments of bone at the base. You are now ready to open the dura mater in both burr holes.

7. Cauterise the dura mater in a cruciate fashion. If you have been unfortunate enough to make one of your burr holes over an obvious branch of the middle meningeal artery you can cut across it, but do not cut along it or you may have difficulty in controlling the haemorrhage. Carefully incise the dura mater with an 11 or 15 blade. One of several things may be seen (Figure P43):

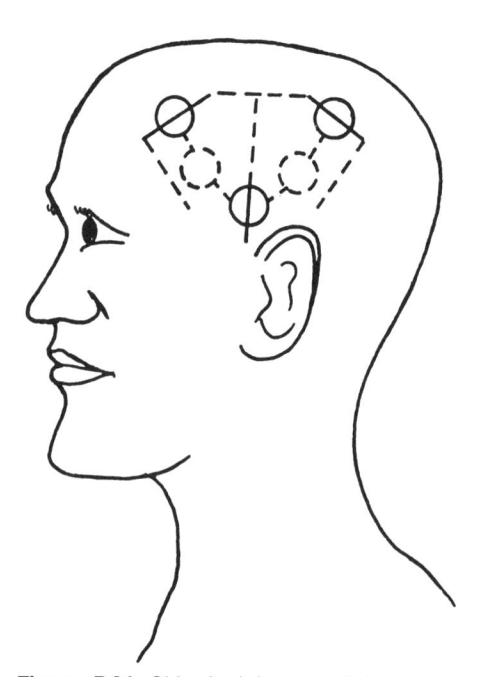

Figure P41 Skin incisions and burr hole sites. Dotted lines show how to convert the skin incisions into a horseshoe or 'T' flap and the burr holes into a flap which will be turned down onto a temporis muscle.

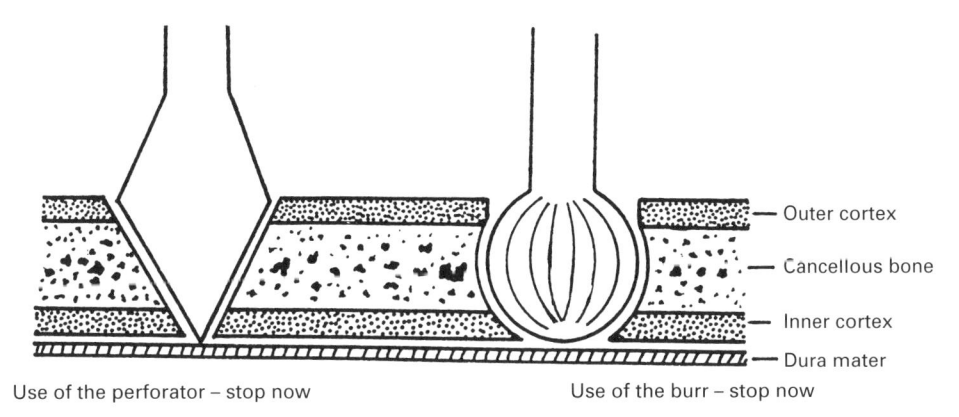

Figure P42 Use of the perforator and burr.

(a) The arachnoid may be seen, possibly with the brain tightly pushed against the inner surface of the burr hole. The latter means there is no surface clot but there is increased pressure.
(b) There may be a flow of dark-brown fluid – this suggests a subdural haematoma and you should wash the fluid out by passing in a small rubber catheter and running warm saline from one burr hole to another. Make sure you did not cut a surface vein – it is unlikely but can happen and may cause confusion.
(c) You may see a grey-green membrane below the dura mater. This is likely to be a chronic subdural membrane and it will have to be incised. If you are uncertain what to do the best thing is to take a syringe and a 21-gauge (green) needle and pass it into the 'membrane'. If it is a subdural membrane, you should encounter old, brown blood within 1 cm in which case you can confidently incise it, open it up with a blunt instrument, and then wash out the fluid. Using a needle and syringe can be a wise precaution if you are in doubt, because sometimes the arachnoid beneath the dura mater can be opaque in colour and misleading. There are virtually no large vessels in the subdural membrane, but there are vessels in the arachnoid, so you must be sure what you are cutting, though arachnoidal bleeding can easily be controlled by Sterispon, collagen or Surgicell and light pressure using a small cotton wool pledget and the diathermy.

8. Whether there is or is not a subdural membrane, wash the blood out by gently depressing the brain if it is close to the dura mater and irrigating the space with warm saline. Never inject saline into the subdural space without being sure that there is a way out for it, or it will become trapped and the intracranial pressure will be forced up.
9. The frontal and parietal burr holes should be adequate to drain most subdural haematomas, but sometimes a low-lying one may need a temporal burr hole to complete the drainage.
10. Whether burr holes are negative or positive on the suspected side, at least one hole must be made on the other side because a sizeable percentage of subdurals are bilateral.
11. When you are satisfied you have got all blood out, or that the exploration is negative, you will close the wound. Do not try to close the dura mater,

(a) When you open the dura mater

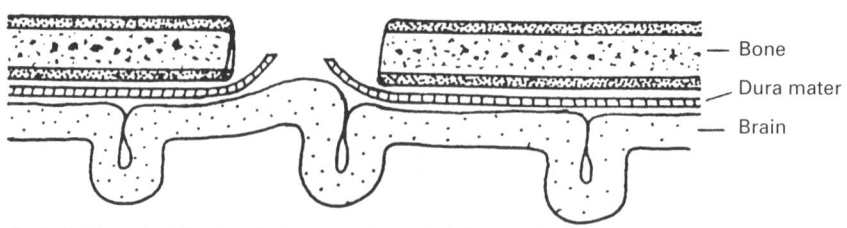

Bone
Dura mater
Brain

Brain tight against the burr hole – no subdural clot here – but if the brain is bulging into the hole there is either diffuse swelling or pressure somewhere else.

(b) This is a subdural haematoma – wash it out with warm saline

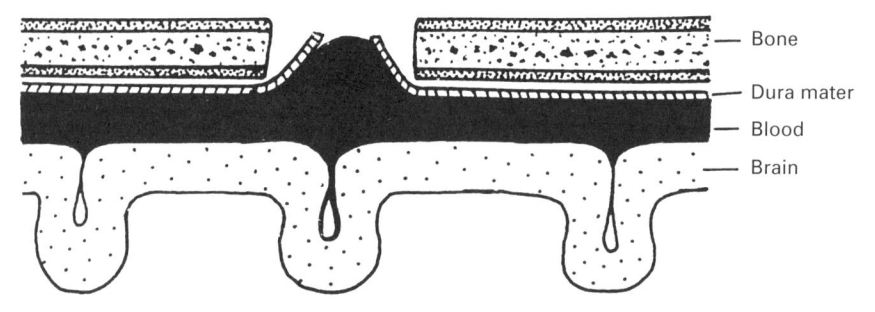

Bone
Dura mater
Blood
Brain

(c) This is a thick subdural membrane – put a needle in and then incise the membrane to let the blood out

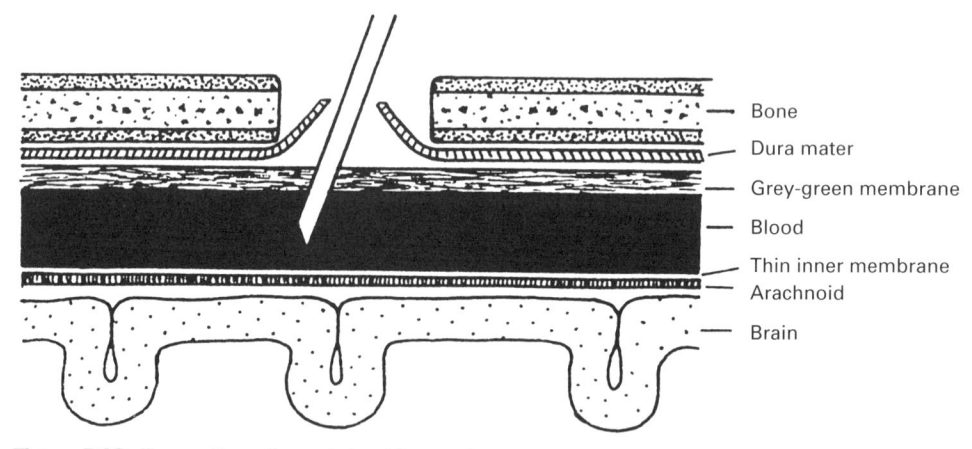

Bone
Dura mater
Grey-green membrane
Blood
Thin inner membrane
Arachnoid
Brain

Figure P43 Evacuation of a subdural haematoma.

(a) because you will not be able to do so; and
(b) because you want to leave it open, so that any subdural fluid remaining may escape into the subcutaneous tissues and be absorbed or aspirated.

12. Ensure there is no bleeding between the dura mater and the bone by cauterising the junction of the bone and dura mater to make them adhere to one another or by laying a strip of Sterispon round the edge while leaving the centre open.

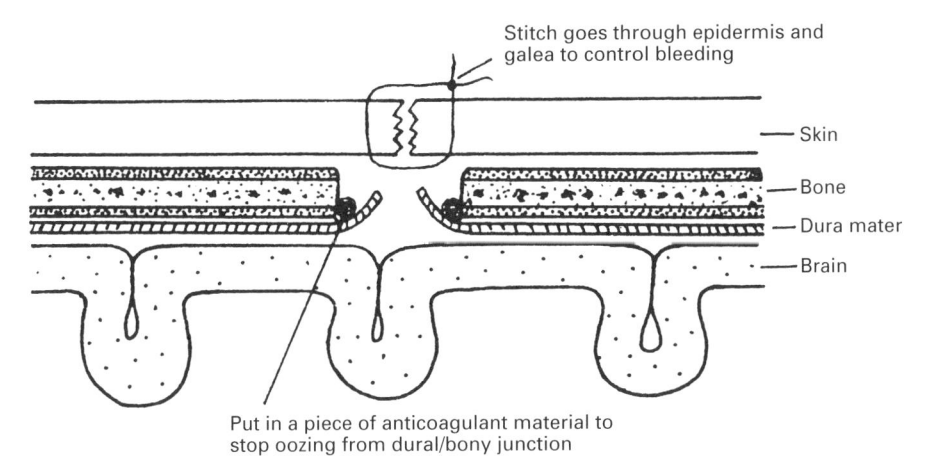

Stitch goes through epidermis and galea to control bleeding
— Skin
— Bone
— Dura mater
— Brain

Put in a piece of anticoagulant material to stop oozing from dural/bony junction

Figure P44 Closing the burr hole.

13. Close the skin in one layer ensuring the stitch passes through both the epidermis and the galea and to control haemorrhage (Figure P44).
14. If you make a burr hole and find blood *before* you open the dura mater (Figure P45), you are dealing with an *extradural haematoma* and the chances are that it must be dealt with by you or the patient will die. There are two courses open to you:

    (a) You make a formal craniotomy, drain the blood and stop the bleeding. This is not as difficult as it sounds.
    (b) You enlarge the burr holes, drain the blood and stop the bleeding.

Let us assume you find an epidural clot under both burr holes; you should immediately make a temporal burr hole and confirm the presence of the clot in that region.

The extradural haematoma

You make the burr hole and there is the blood!

— Bone
— Blood
— Dura mater
— Brain

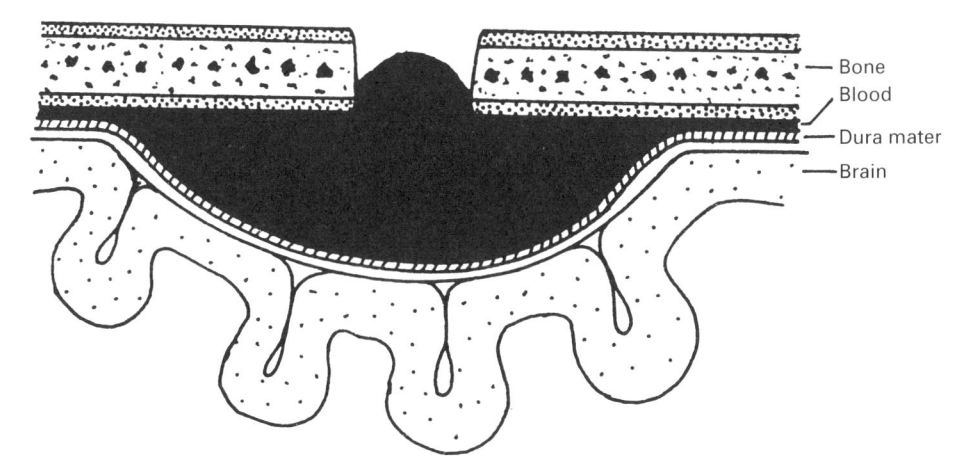

Figure P45 Extradural haematoma.

15. Join the two frontal and parietal skin incisions and convert them either into an inverted horseshoe or a 'T' skin incision based on the temporal burr hole (Figure P41). It is very important to get sufficient bone away to give yourself room to deal with the clot and the bleeder. If you have a Gigli saw and a saw guide you can join the three burr holes or make two others and give yourself a loose bone flap which you can replace (Figure P41). If you do not have such a device then any bone-nibbling instrument you possess should be used to remove bone. Discard the bone; it does not matter how much you remove – it can always be replaced later; the prime objective is to get the clot out and stop the bleeding. If there is a fracture line follow that. The bleeder is likely to be somewhere along the line or nearby. Remove an area of bone about 7 cm in diameter (you should be able to manage through that) and stop the bone bleeding with wax.
16. Start to remove the clot and see if you can get it all out. It will extend under the bone for quite a long distance but you can scoop it out. The bleeding vessel is likely to be somewhere near the centre of the clot and if you find it there are two ways of dealing with it:
    (a) try to catch it in a stitch which passes right through the dura mater (mind the brain underneath); or
    (b) incise the dura mater and catch the whole vessel in an artery forceps (Figure P46).
    It can then be cauterised or stitched. Do not try to cauterise the bleeding vessel on the surface of the dura mater, as it will burn back along the vessel and continue bleeding. If this were all you could do the chances are that you would save the patient's life.
17. There is always some secondary bleeding from the lateral edge of the clot – control this by removing all the clot, pushing in some Sterispon and suturing the dura mater up against the bone around the opening (Figure P47). In order to do this you will certainly have to incise the dura mater itself to let some air under it, or you will not be able to

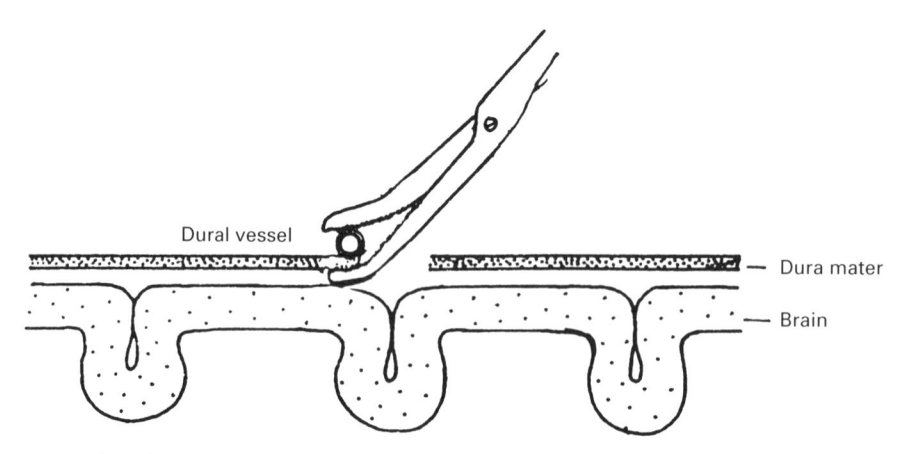

Stopping a large dural bleeder can be difficult – don't try to coagulate on the surface – make a cut in the dura mater next to the vessel, catch it with an artery forceps and cauterise it or put a stitch round it.

Figure P46

Tenting up the dura mater to the bone to stop bleeding

Skin

Bone

Stitch holding up the dura mater

– Dura mater

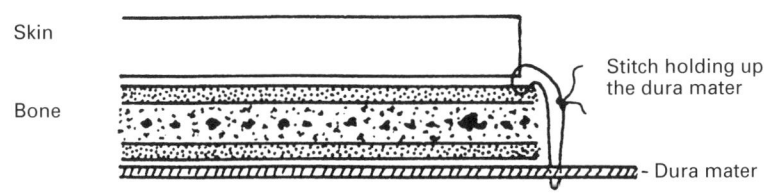

Figure P47

lift it up. The brain is very compressed and will not immediately expand.

When you have tented up the dura mater all round the bone edge, the likelihood is that all bleeding will stop. You probably will not be able to close your dural incision. This does not matter; graft it or cover the defect with Sterispon. Do not worry about the collapsed brain under the dura mater; just leave the space there filled with air – it will re-expand.

You can then close the skin and if you wish to use a suction bottle drain; there is no contraindication, but remember not to raise the suction pressure too high – if the dura mater has been opened you will be applying suction pressure directly onto the brain.

If the patient had a lucid interval before becoming unconscious prior to your operation, the chances are that he will do very well – if he had no lucid interval this means that he has associated brain damage and the outlook is not so good.

The depressed fracture

Protocol

The patient has suffered a depressed fracture which is either
1. compound – or suspected of being so; or
2. is associated with underlying focal signs and therefore presumably brain damage.

Preparation

1. Endotracheal anaesthesia.
2. Shave the head and prepare and drape the area.
3. Expose the fracture by making a longitudinal incision across the site using one of the limbs of the skin tear. Hold the wound open by a self-retaining retractor. Scrape the periosteum off the undamaged bone and demonstrate the limits of the fracture.
4. Elevate the bone. When bone is pushed in it tends to fracture in two planes – vertically to the surface and along the plane of the cancellous bone giving two layers. All pieces of bone tend to impact on each other, jamming the fracture in very tightly (Figure P48).
5. You may be able to insert an instrument somewhere along the fracture line and start levering it up. However, it may be so tightly jammed that this is not possible, in which case you must make a burr hole adjacent to the depression and then use a punch to move towards the depressed bone and lift it up. When you grab hold of pieces of bone make sure you do not push them inwards.
6. Remove all the fragments of bone and make sure none remains underneath the free edges of the fracture area as they will push the dura mater away from the bone and cause haemorrhage. Remember that when the dura mater lies close to bone there is no bleeding.

Figure P48 Treatment of a depressed fracture.

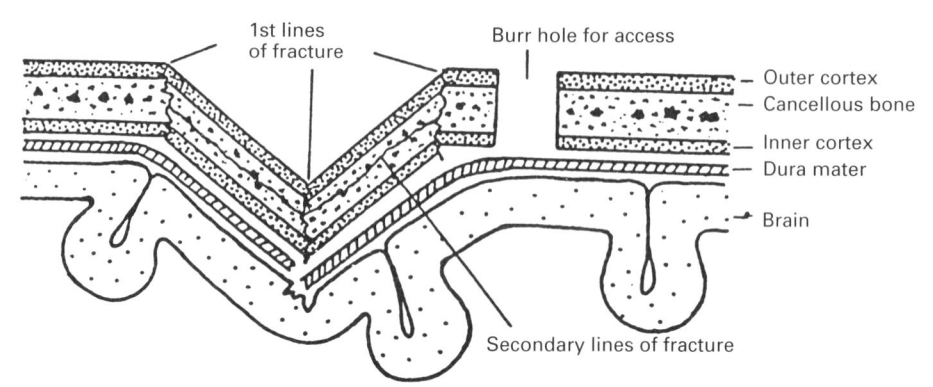

The depressed fracture – if you cannot get under the fragments make a burr hole at the side and come in from there. Do not forget the bone usually fractures in two planes.

Control bleeding from the bone edge with bone wax and remove excess from between bone and dura mater.

7. Examine the dura mater for tears; if there are none proceed to Point 9. If there is a tear then examine the underlying brain for damage. It is very easy to see this: the pia and arachnoid maters are torn and bruised brain is seen below. It may be that portions of bone are embedded in the brain; if so, *they, and areas of dead brain, must be removed*. Damaged brain sucks very easily (normal brain is not easy to aspirate with the sucker); damaged brain rarely bleeds and then only on the surface. Open the dura mater further and gently stroke the damaged area with a small sucker and dead brain will come away easily. Follow this down until you have removed all fragments of bone and removed the dead brain as well. Any oozing in the base of the cavity will soon stop with the application of Sterispon held in place by sloppy cotton.

8. When you have haemostasis you can shake 0.5 g streptomycin powder into the cavity and then close the dura mater. It may be necessary to take a small graft of fascia to close a tear in the dura mater (though small defects can be covered by Surgicell or similar); I usually use 4/0–5/0 black silk for suturing, but anything will do.

9. Ensure haemostasis outside the dura mater as follows:
   (a) Remove any pieces of depressed bone.
   (b) Remove any pieces of bone wax which have got into the space between the bone and the dura mater.
   (c) Wax the bone.
   (d) Lay on Sterispon.
   (e) Tent up the dura mater to compess it to against the bone by stitching the dura mater to the outside periosteum (Figure P47).

10. Put the rest of the streptomycin into the bony defect and close the skin, making sure your suture passes through the galea aponeurotica (Figure P44). Give the drug systemically as well.

11. If the defect is large, cranioplasty may have to be done later, but not until the wound has settled down and healed completely.

12. It is not this author's practice to give prophylactic anticonvulsants.

Managing the serious head injury with a GCS <9 and intracranial pressure monitoring

The general approach presented here represents aggressive therapy which is now standard practice in the developed world. It can easily be adapted for use in the developing world, even in the absence of CT scanning.

Intubate the patient in the emergency room using an anaesthetic induction technique. Preferably not with muscle relaxant or sedative alone. Then, ventilate, paralyse and sedate. Continued coughing and straining will cause severe and prolonged rises in ICP. Do not use excessive or prolonged hyperventilation. Aim for a $PaCO_2$ level around 35.

Treat the other injuries as is appropriate. It is very important to correct shock and hypotension by replacing blood loss urgently. Aim for a systolic blood pressure >90 mmHg, and preferably >100 mmHg.

Perform exploratory burr holes (see operative surgery section), to exclude an extracerebral collection. Insert intracranial pressure monitor if measurement is feasible. Elevate head end of the bed 20° if the blood pressure is adequate. Preferably manage the patient in the intensive care unit.

Anticonvulsants: status epilepticus cannot be diagnosed clinically if the patient is paralysed and sedated. Administer a loading dose of phenytoin, then a maintenance dose.

Control of ICP

A. With an ICP monitor in situ

- Maintain cerebral perfusion pressure (CPP) >70 mmHg. CPP is calculated by subtracting intracranial pressure from mean arterial pressure.
- Check blood gases – ensure that PaO_2 is >100 mmHg, and $PaCO_2$ is 30–40, preferably 35.
- Check neck posture – ensure the neck isn't twisted which would obstruct venous return.
- Mannitol 0.5 g/kg 4–6 hourly p.r.n. Monitor serum osmolality. Keep <310. Watch urine output.
- Acute hyperventilation for 30 sec – this is usually done by hand-bagging the patient, i.e. connecting the ventilatin circuit to a rubber bag, and manually breathing the patient.
- Venting CSF – 1–2 ml by opening the vent tap. If you drain too much the ventricle may collapse. The ICP trace may then be lost, and venting will fail particularly if the brain is very swollen with small slit-like ventricles, which is often the case after a diffuse brain injury.
- Barbiturate – thiopentone infusion.
- Hypothermia using ice bags, or preferably a cooling blanket with intramuscular chlorpromazine to stop shivering, to a level of 35°C. There is some controlled

scientific evidence that hypothermia improves the early outcome of severe head injury, but not definitely the long term outcome.
- Treat if ICP >20 mmHg for >2 min, preferably with venting +/−, and mannitol rather than prolonged hyperventilation. The policy now is to maintain the CO_2 level at about 35 mmHg (i.e. low range of normal). Do not allow the $PaCO_2$ to stay persistently below 25 mmHg.
- Unilateral or bilateral temporal craniectomy has a small role in allowing the brain to expand out of the cranial cavity in an attempt to lower an otherwise uncontrollable ICP. This is still unproven and may save a patient's life only to leave a neurologically damaged individual.

If the ICP stays above 30 mmHg. The patient is likely to die.

B. Without ICP monitor in situ

Paralysis and sedation are helpful for control of ICP, but you will lose any ability to neurologically assess the patient, except for the pupil size and reaction. As a compromise use sedation without paralysis, so you can assess the patient's responses when the drugs wear off.

Regular mannitol – 0.25 to 0.5 g/kg 4–6 hourly i.v.

Maintain $PaCO_2$ level at about 35.

It is difficult to manage a very restless, agitated head injury patient who cannot be controlled without sedation. Sedation will render the patient very difficult to assess clinically for deterioration. The dilemma is either you will have to observe the patient closely, and operate if there is further neurological deterioration; or preferably sedate and operate early with exploratory burr holes to detect and evacuate any extra-cerebral collection.

Intracranial pressure monitoring

Indication

1. This will usually be done for severe head injury patients who cannot be monitored clinically or who will be ventilated, paralysed/sedated, especially if multiple injuries are present and a prolonged period of ventilation is to be anticipated.
2. Post-craniotomy for evacuation of acute extra axial collection.

Strategy

Intracranial pressure cannot be monitored without breaching the skull. The simplest method of measuring the pressure is to place an infant feeding tube in the ventricle, bring it out through the burr hole and connect it to a pressure transducer, similar to that used to measure blood pressure, by filling the infant feeding tube with fluid. The advantage of this technique is that CSF can be vented to help reduce the raised intracranial pressure. The disadvantage is the increased infection rate if the tube is left in for more than 48 h. There is no clear evidence that prophylactic antibiotics would reduce the risk of this infection. The CSF should be cultured regularly to make sure no infection is developing when this technique is used.

Alternative methods of measuring ICP are: to place a catheter in the subdural space, but the disadvantage of this is that when the brain is very swollen and tight the catheter may be occluded. Epidural transducers are prone to inaccuracy due to damping. Similarly the old bolt method where a hollow metal bolt (Richmond bolt) is screwed into a burr hole to allow fluid communication between the subdural space and a pressure transducer is also prone to inaccuracy due to damping. Neither of the last two methods is recommended. There are fibre-optic transducers that can be placed directly in the brain tissue (e.g. Camino™) catheter or small electrical transducers which can be placed in the brain tissue or attached to a ventricular catheter (e.g. Codman™). These newer devices are significantly more expensive and are usually not available in the developing world. The simpler fluid-filled systems described are quite satisfactory.

Interpreting the result

The normal intracranial pressure is 10–15 mmHg. Once the brain becomes tense and turgid brain compliance is reduced and pressure waves may appear. Plateau waves are the most dangerous (ICP elevations of >50 mmHg for 5–20 min) and urgent treatment is required. β-waves have amplitudes of 20–30 mm and occur rhythmically every 30 sec to 2 min. A sustained pressure above 20 mmHg for more than 2 min warrants urgent treatment.

Technique

1. **Subdural catheter.** The infant feeding tube can be placed in the subdural space for evacuation of a collection and this is then brought out through a separate stab incision in the scalp. If there has been no craniotomy, a burr hole is placed usually in the right frontal region above the hairline and away from the midline. The dura is opened with a cruciate incision. The catheter is passed gently over the cortical surface, filled with Ringer's or saline solution and brought out through a separate stab incision.

2. **Ventricular catheter.** A burr hole is placed in the line of the pupil just behind the hair line usually on the right side. The dura is opened with a cruciate incision. Initially a brain needle is passed directly into the frontal horn of the lateral ventricle and if the brain needle is passed directly perpendicular to the burr hole it should enter the ventricle. Aiming for the inner canthus of the eye on the same side is an alternative trajectory. You will feel a release in resistance when the catheter passes through the ependyma into the CSF. The stylet is then removed and CSF will escape. The stylet is replaced and the brain needle removed. Immediately on doing this, the infant feeding tube is passed down the track to reach the ventricle. Confirm that CSF is escaping adequately and then tunnel the catheter and bring it out through a separate stab incision. Anchor it to the scalp and close the scalp in two layers.

Troubleshooting

If the catheter becomes blocked with a small amount of debris or clot, it can be syringed with a millilitre of saline trying to extract what is put in.

If ventriculitis develops the ICP monitor should normally be removed. Give 5 mg gentamicin into the CSF and remove the catheter. Continue systemic antibiotics for 7 days, including cover for both Gram positive and negative organisms, e.g. gentamicin and flucoxacillin or vancomycin, if staphlococcal resistance is a problem. If the IC catheter needs to remain, treat the CSF with daily gentamicin and systemic antibiotics. If the ventriculitis starts to clear in 48 h remove the catheter and re-site on the opposite side.

Advanced investigative and monitoring techniques in shock

Core–peripheral temperature

This measures the difference between core temperature using a rectal thermometer and peripheral skin temperature of the big toe. The greater the difference the worse the peripheral circulation and so the shock. Core–peripheral temperature difference is a selective guide to the state of the circulation. A large difference indicates a constricted systemic circulation with poor peripheral perfusion. Good response to therapy in shock will be accompanied by a decrease in the core and peripheral temperature difference.

Swan–Ganz catheterisation

This uses a catheter with a small balloon and pressure transducer at its tip, which is inserted into the subclavian or jugular vein and passed through the heart into the pulmonary artery, guided by the balloon in the flow of blood (Figure P49). Changing pressure waves are recorded as the catheter is passed through the right atrium, right ventricle, into the pulmonary artery. When in the pulmonary artery the balloon is inflated, the small pulmonary artery in which the catheter tip sits is occluded and the distal 'pulmonary capillary wedge pressure' is recorded. The wedge pressure reflects the pressure of blood in the left

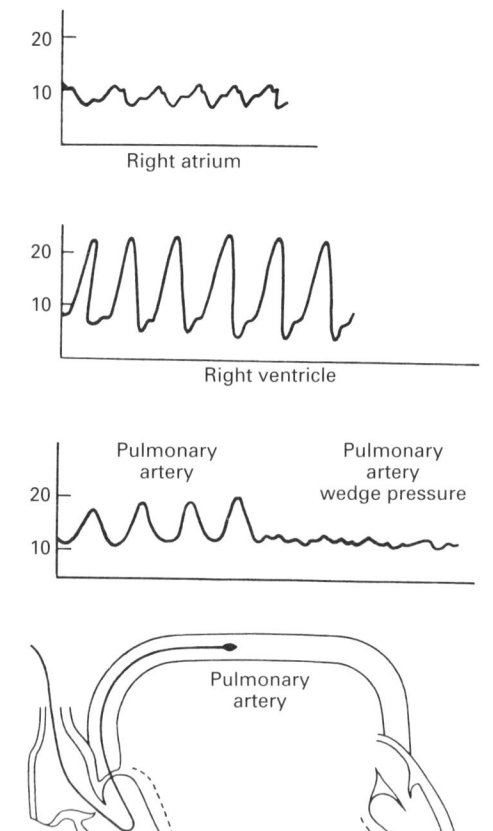

Figure P49 The Swan–Ganz catheter and pressure measurements.

atrium. The main indication for use in shocked patients is where one is not sure how effectively the left side of the heart is pumping. Some benefit has been demonstrated with their use in severe septic shock, and they provide excellent teaching facilities, but are expensive, costing about $US80, and need electronic pressure transducers, monitors and computers. Their role in the developing world is likely to be fairly limited at present.

Cardiac output

Cardiac output can be calculated with a Swan–Ganz catheter by a thermodilution technique. The dose of inotropes (dopamine and dobutamine) and vasodilators (nitroprusside and glyceryl trinitrate) can be titrated to optimise cardiac output.

Knowing the cardiac output allows measurement of tissue oxygen delivery and consumption which can be of benefit in critical illness, particularly when using vasoactive drugs such as inotropes.

Intra-aortic balloon pump

This complex apparatus consists of a computerised unit attached to a catheter which is passed up the aorta from the femoral artery. The tip of the catheter sits in the descending aorta and the computer controls the inflation of a balloon, at its tip. Inflation in diastole improves coronary perfusion and deflation reduces afterload during systole. They are of benefit following cardiac surgery. There is no evidence of any benefit in other types of heart failure and the catheters cost US$600 each.

Transoesophgeal echocardiography

This technique allows echocardiography with particularly good information about the left ventricle function. It is unavailable in many centres and requires training to use the technique. The probes cost $US50,000.

Arterial cannulation and direct pressure measurement

Indications

In patients who have very unstable blood pressures in whom immediate knowledge of the pressure is important, e.g. during major arterial surgery. Also used where regular blood gas analysis is required.

Method

Normally a disposable electronic transducer is connected using specially designed, rigid, high-pressure tubing to a 20 gauge Teflon cannula in the radial, brachial or femoral artery. The system is flushed continuously with heparinised saline (1 unit heparin/ml saline) at a rate of about 3 ml/h. Specialised continuous flushing devices are available for this purpose.

Where direct arterial pressure monitoring is required but a transducer is not available a simple system can be made up to measure mean arterial pressure (MAP). Mean arterial pressure is the average pressure in the arterial side of the circulation and is approximately the diastolic blood pressure plus one-third of the difference between diastolic and systolic pressures. Thus, e.g., a patient with a pressure of 110/80 would be expected to have a mean pressure of around

$$80 + \frac{110 - 80}{3} = 80 + \frac{30}{3} = 90 \text{ mmHg MAP}$$

Figure P50 shows the layout of the system. All components must be sterile. Proceed as follows:

1. Make up a 20-ml syringe with heparinised saline (1 unit heparin/ml saline) and connect this to a three-way tap.
2. Connect the female limb of the three-way tap to an aneroid blood pressure gauge or mercury column with a piece of tubing about $\frac{1}{2}$ to 1 metre long. Inject saline up this tube until the gauge reads 200 mmHg and then close the tap to the gauge.
3. Connect the male end of the three-way tap to a piece of connecting tubing and flush the air out with the heparinised saline in the syringe.
4. Carefully sterilise the skin over the artery and if the patient is conscious infiltrate round the selected artery with a little 1% lidocaine.
5. Gently cannulate the artery with a 20 gauge (preferably Teflon) and connect it to the three-way tap via the prepared tubing.
6. Flush the cannula with the syringe at the three-way tap and then turn the tap to connect the artery with the aneroid gauge. The gauge will fluctuate around the mean arterial pressure. The gauge and tubing should be at heart level to give an accurate reading.

Problems

Remember that the reading in the gauge is mean pressure and **not** systolic. If you fail to cannulate the artery put pressure on it

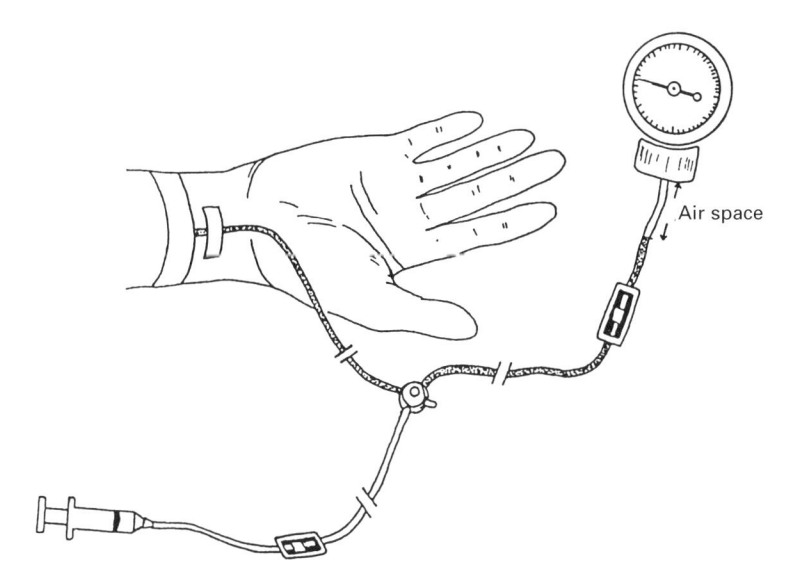

Figure P50 Simplified method of measuring arterial pressure using a 3-way tap and an aneroid sphygmomanometer.

for 5 min to stop bleeding. Do not allow blood to come up the tubing (it will clot in the cannula) – flush the tubing every few minutes with 1 ml of saline then turn the tap off to the syringe. A syringe pump set to deliver 3–5 ml/h of heparinised saline into the line is a good way of doing this. Do not allow heparinised saline to come into the gauge; this will ruin it. Do not allow air to enter the artery. Ensure sterility at all times. Check the accuracy of the aneroid gauge regularly. Continuous observation of the system is essential and its use is mostly suited to the operating theatre. Be careful that you do not flush clots into the artery or give an injection into the line by accident. Many i.v. drugs cause distal gangrene if injected into an artery.

Checking the accuracy of an aneroid gauge

This should be done regularly as part of your equipment maintenance and immediately if the aneroid gauge has been dropped or is possibly damaged in some way.

Connect the aneroid gauge to a mercury sphygmomanometer as shown in Figure P51. Slowly pump the bulb and check that the readings on the mercury column and the aneroid gauge are the same at 50, 100, 150, 200 and 250 mmHg. If there are differences the aneroid gauge is likely to be faulty.

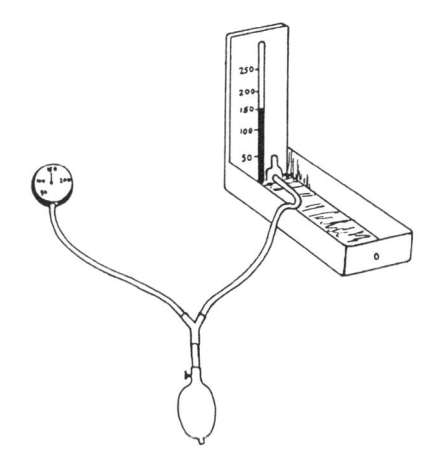

Figure P51 Checking the accuracy of an aneroid gauge.

A to Z of ventilation

This section explains some of the terms used when ventilating patients. A guide to the functional classification of ventilators is included and some advice on basic control settings.

alarm A safety device which indicates a fault in the ventilator or circuit. Assess the patient and ventilator immediately you hear an alarm, as it usually indicates a serious problem.

Ambu bag A self-filling lung inflation bag which can be used with a mask or endotracheal tube to provide intermittent positive pressure ventilation. Oxygen may be added via a connection at the back of the bag. Before use check the bag and valve by putting your thumb over the patient connection and attempt to expel the air from the bag (Figure V1). If the valve and bag are working you will be unable to do this; if either is faulty the bag will empty easily. In this book the term *Ambu bag* is used throughout to indicate a self-inflating bag.

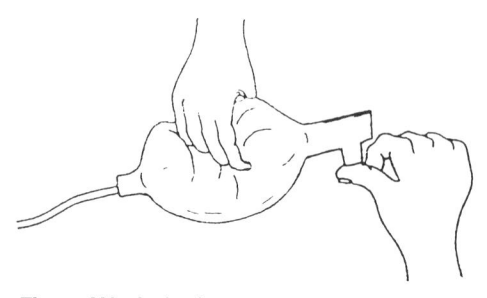

Figure V1 Ambu bag.

analogue See **display**.

assisted breathing. A ventilator function which makes the machine assist the patient's inspiration whenever the patient starts to breathe in. Usually used with a trigger or sensitivity control which determines the amount of effort the patient needs to make to activate the ventilator. This function is also called pressure support or assist control.

bag and suck Coughing is inefficient in patients who have an endotracheal tube or a tracheostomy, and bagging and sucking is a method of chest physiotherapy used in these patients to help clear sputum from their airways. One nurse gives the patient oxygen from an Ambu bag for several breaths and then a second nurse suctions the trachea in an aseptic fashion (see p. 352). The technique is often done with the physiotherapist and may be combined with percussion, tapping and other forms of physiotherapy.

The diameter of the catheter which you use for sucking down an endotracheal tube should always be less than half the diameter of the endotracheal tube (Figure V2). If you use too large a catheter you will suck oxygen out of the lung and cause immediate and serious hypoxia.

bellows The part in certain ventilators, e.g. East Radcliffe or Oxford, which contains the air and oxygen which is then used to inflate the patient's lungs.

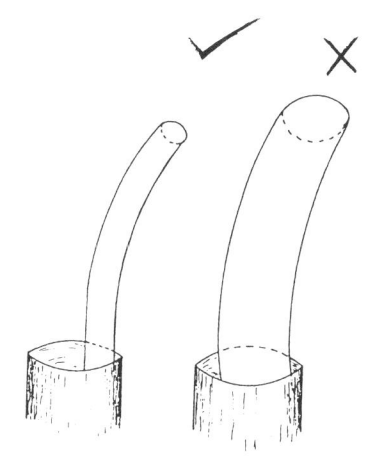

Figure V2 Bag and suck; the suction tubing should be less than half the diameter of the endotracheal tube.

Bennett A manufacturer of powerful electrical ventilators which can ventilate either adults or children.

Bird A compact gas-driven ventilator which may be used for short-term ventilation in adults (see **ventilator**) and is often used in intubated patients for positive pressure breaths with physiotherapy.

carina The part of the trachea where it divides into the two main bronchi.

catheter mount The connection (Figure V3) between an endotracheal tube and the ventilator tubing (see **connectors**).

compliance An expression of the effort required to inflate the lungs measured as ml of lung inflation per cmH_2O pressure. Normally the ventilator uses around 15–30 cmH_2O during inflation, but a patient with low compliance may require considerably higher inflation pressures, as there is difficulty in expanding the lungs.

compressor A machine which pressurises ambient air to drive certain apparatus such as ventilators. Most compressors depend on electricity to power them. In humid climates it may be necessary to dry the air after compression to prevent damage to the equipment being supplied by the compressor. An alternative supply of dry compressed air is from medical air cylinders.

connectors These should be a firm fit between ventilator tubes and not require sticky tape to hold them together. This is best achieved by using International Standards Organisation (ISO) sized fittings as much as possible. These are 22 mm and 15 mm. Unfortunately there are a variety of other sized connectors available which may make the situation difficult. Always check connections before putting a patient on a ventilator.

control mode A term used on some ventilators to describe standard intermittent positive pressure ventilation (IPPV). Also called controlled ventilation.

CPAP Continuous positive airway pressure, which may be used in intubated patients breathing spontaneously. A small pressure, usually around 4–10 cmH_2O, is applied to the

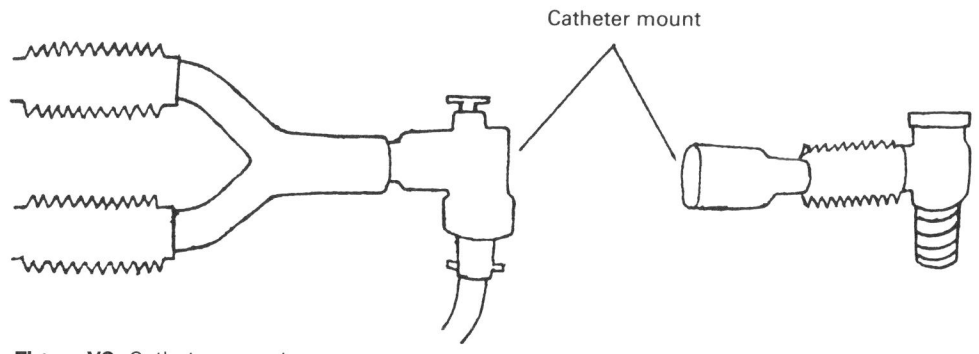

Figure V3 Catheter mount.

breathing circuit and is present throughout all the cycles of respiration. It has the effect of adding a small amount of inspiratory assist and expiratory resistance. It is useful during weaning and may improve oxygenation. It is sometimes used in neonatal practice employing a sealed headbox or nasal CPAP cannula. It can also be administered, using special masks, to adults who are not intubated.

cricoid pressure During induction of anaesthesia, firm backward pressure on the cricoid cartilage occludes the oesophagus, preventing regurgitation. It should be applied at the moment consciousness is lost until the trachea is intubated and the cuff inflated.

cuff See **endotracheal tube**.

cuirass ventilator A ventilator which is worn like a jacket and assists ventilation using the principle of negative pressure ventilation like an iron lung.

cycling The term used to describe the ventilator changing from inspiration to expiration and back.

dead space 1. Anatomical: the conducting passages of the respiratory tract which take no part in gas exchange, i.e. from the nose to the smallest bronchioles.

2. Apparatus: the part of the ventilator tubing that remains filled with alveolar gas at the end of expiration, which is rebreathed during the next inspiration. This usually comprises the endotracheal tube and the catheter mount. If this dead space is too high then ventilation will be less effective and will cause CO_2 retention. This can be an important problem in paediatric ventilation.

3. Physiological: in the lungs some alveoli may have no blood flow in the capillaries around them and so do not exchange any gases. This creates extra dead space which is termed physiological dead space.

display On most ventilators there are dials or gauges monitoring certain parameters. They may be in analogue or digital form. (See Figure V4.)

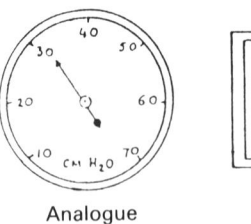

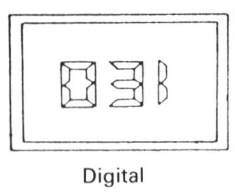

Analogue   Digital

Figure V4 Display.

East Radcliffe A simple, robust, electrically driven ventilator which can also be powered by turning a handle on the side in the event of an electricity failure. A 12 volt battery may also be used as a power supply.

endotracheal tube (ETT, ET tube) The tube that is placed in the patient's trachea to provide a route for ventilation. Such tubes should always be of the plastic type (i.e. PVC) if ventilation is expected to last for more than 24 h.

The position of the tube should always be checked by auscultation to ensure that ventilation is reaching both lungs, and this can usefully be confirmed by taking a chest X-ray where the tip of the tube should be in the mid-trachea.

The cuff on the tube is designed to seal the trachea so that air cannot leak past it, causing loss of ventilation, or pharyngeal fluids bypass it leading to inhalation pneumonia. It should be inflated with just enough air to prevent leakage of air on inspiration during positive pressure ventilation. Inflate the cuff while listening carefully for the leak to stop while the ventilator is inflating the lungs. Some people measure cuff pressure and try to keep the pressure below 30 cmH_2O. Desirable pressure is 15–25 cmH_2O.

There are two types of cuff on endotracheal or tracheostomy tubes (see Figure V5). A standard cuff, which requires a relatively high pressure to inflate a small-volume cuff as in standard red rubber tubes used in anaesthesia, and a high-volume, low-pressure cuff found on some PVC

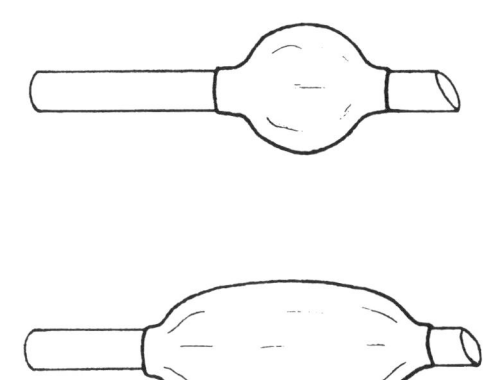

Figure V5 Endotracheal tube cuffs.

tubes designed for use on ICU. Overinflation of the cuff produces excess pressure on the tracheal mucosa, causing ischaemia, inflammation and oedema of the trachea, which may eventually result in severe tracheal damage. To avoid this, tubes with low-pressure, high-volume cuffs are better for prolonged intubation. Overinflation of the cuff may also cause the cuff to protrude over the end of the endotracheal tube and obstruct air flow.

When a patient with an endotracheal tube develops a leak around the tube it is usually fixed by a small amount of extra air in the cuff. When this does not work, check that the cuff is not damaged or coming out of the larynx.

Children below the age of 10 years should not have a cuffed endotracheal tube, as this is more likely to cause damage to the trachea at the cricoid ring and the resistance to breathing will increase because of the smaller internal diameter of a cuffed tube. A guide to the sizes and lengths of endotracheal tubes is given in Table P1, p. 330.

expiratory time this is the period of time given to a ventilated patient for expiration.

extubation Removal of the endotracheal tube (see p. 334).

fighting Patients on ventilators may become restless for various reasons, including hypoxia, hypercarbia, pain, full bladder, hypotension, following general anaesthesia, endotracheal tube positioned against the carina, uncomfortable positioning or emotional distress. When this occurs it is vital not to automatically give sedation but to assess whether there is anything serious happening to the patient which requires treatment.

filter A disposable filter is commonly used in the patient circuit to protect the patient and ventilator from bacterial/viral contamination. Many of these filters also act as condenser humidifiers.

FiO_2 Fractional inspired oxygen; a patient receiving 100% oxygen is said to have an $FiO_2 = 1$, while someone breathing air, which has 21% oxygen, has an FiO_2 of 0.21. If you multiply the FiO_2 by 100 this will give you the percentage of oxygen being delivered to the patient.

frequency Respiratory rate, i.e. number of breaths taken in a minute.

humidifier Normally, the nose and upper respiratory tract are responsible for humidifying or moisturising the dry air which we breathe, to make it suitable for the lungs. When a patient has an endotracheal tube or a tracheostomy, this must be done artificially to prevent drying of secretions and subsequent dangerous blockage of the tube. There are several methods:

1. Condenser humidifiers (Figure V6a) trap moisture in the expired air and then humidify the next inspiration using this moisture. These are cheap and usually disposable after 24 h of use. Different sizes are available for children and adults and many also act as filters.

2. Kettle or hot-water humidifiers (Figure V6b) add water vapour from heated water to the inspired gases. These usually run at a temperature of 55–60°C, which compensates for the cooling effect

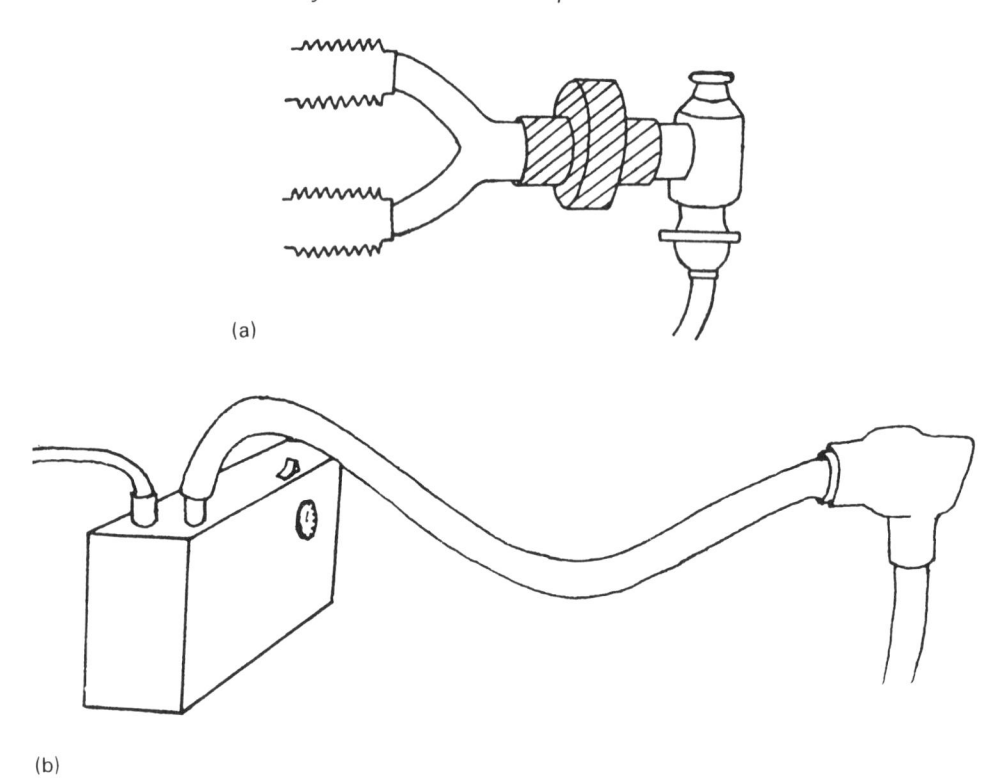

Figure V6 Types of humidifier: (a) condenser (shaded); (b) kettle.

due to the length of the inspiratory tubing after the humidifier. The best heated humidifiers monitor the temperature of the inspired gases at the patient end. If the temperature exceeds 37°C then the humidifier temperature is reduced. Where this facility is not available, feel the temperature of the gases at the patient end and check that they are not too hot. As the air cools on its way to the patient some water condenses in the ventilator tubing, which should be drained regularly into the water traps provided. The ventilator tubes from the humidifier should always be arranged, so that the excess water formed by condensation tends to run back into the humidifier and not into the patient. Always mount the humidifier below the level of the patient so as to minimise the risk of water entering the lungs.

See also **nebuliser**.

hypercarbia An increased amount of CO_2 in the blood leading to respiratory acidosis usually caused by ventilatory failure.

hypocarbia A decreased amount of CO_2 in the blood, which is usually secondary to hyperventilation.

hypoxia A low level of oxygen in the blood and tissues.

IMV Intermittent mandatory ventilation is a mode of intermittent positive-pressure ventilation (q.v.) used during the weaning process. A reduced small number of ventilator breaths are delivered to the patient (3–8 each minute) and the patient is allowed to take as many extra spontaneous breaths as he wishes through the ventilator. This technique may be of help when someone is not ready to breathe completely on their own, but does not need to be fully ventilated. Note that the ventilator does not assist the patient during inspiration, unlike the assist mode. Some patients do not adapt easily to this mode of ventilation, and certain ventilators have a high resistance when used in this mode which patients may not tolerate. Synchronised IMV (SIMV) is a newer version of this technique in which the ventilator avoids giving an inspiration when the patient is breathing out.

intermittent negative pressure ventilation (INPV) See **iron lung**.

inspiratory time The period of time taken for the ventilator to deliver a breath to the patient.

inspiratory : expiratory ratio The ratio of the time taken for inspiration in relation to expiration, sometimes shortened to I : E ratio. It is usually around 1 : 2.

IPPV Intermittent positive-pressure ventilation is the technique employed in modern ventilators to deliver gas to the patient. Air usually mixed with oxygen is delivered to the patient under a small positive pressure (usually 15–30 cmH$_2$O) which inflates the lungs. At the end of inspiration the lungs recoil naturally causing the air to leave the lungs (expiration).

iron lung An early ventilator developed in the polio epidemics in the 1950s. The patient is placed in a large, rigid container which is sealed around the neck. At regular intervals some air inside the container is withdrawn, causing a fall in the pressure surrounding the patient resulting in expansion of the lungs. When the negative pressure in the container is returned to normal the lungs recoil and the patient breathes out. This is termed intermittent negative-pressure ventilation (INPV).

jacket ventilators See **cuirass ventilator**.

larynx – local anaesthesia This is a useful technique for intubating poor-risk patients or those with airway problems. If there is time, give a drying premedication (atropine) to prevent excessive salivation. Spray the inside of the mouth with 2–4% lidocaine and ask the patient to move the solution around the mouth for 30 sec before swallowing it. Gently introduce a laryngoscope as far as is comfortable, spray the back of the tongue and the epiglottis (if visible), and remove the laryngoscope. When the patient has settled re-introduce the laryngoscope and spray below the epiglottis, including the cords if visible (it may take several sprays until the patient will tolerate deep laryngoscopy). Proceed gently and slowly until the cords are anaesthetised and then intubate. Take care not to exceed the maximum recommended dose of lidocaine (see A to Z of Drugs, p. 449).

leak A leak occurs when air passing from the ventilator to the patient escapes. This is one of the most dangerous situations during ventilation as it may cause underventilation leading to hypoxia and hypercarbia. Common sites for leaks to develop are shown in Figure V7.

limits During IPPV it is customary to set some parameters that you wish the ventilator to deliver to the patient, e.g. tidal volume 700 ml. The machine is designed to work within these settings (sometimes called limits) and if the required parameter is not achieved an alarm is triggered. Limits that may be set are different for individual ventilators, common ones being tidal volume, minute volume and inspiratory pressure.

Manley Multivent A new gas driven ventilator designed for use in theatre and ICU in developing countries. Made by Penlon UK. (See **ventilator**.)

Mapleson C circuit An anaesthetic circuit which can be used for manually ventilating the patient or to allow him to breathe a high concentration of oxygen (Figure V8). When the circuit is used for IPPV the valve must be partly closed so that you can inflate his lungs but should be

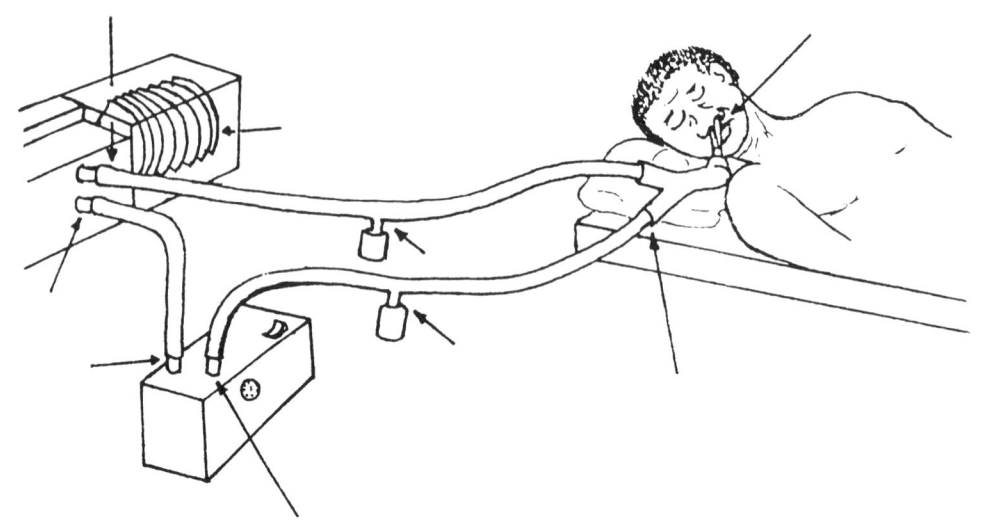

Figure V7 Common sites for leaks.

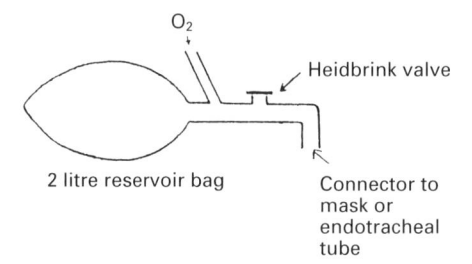

Figure V8 Mapleson C circuit.

left open during spontaneous ventilation. It is essential that the circuit has enough gas flow going through it to prevent rebreathing, and in an adult you should use around 150 ml/kg/min. In unskilled hands an Ambu bag is a safer way of ventilating a patient than a Mapleson C circuit.

minitracheostomy A technique of placing a small endotracheal tube (size 4.0 mm) through the cricothyroid membrane to allow suction of secretions in patients who are unable to cough adequately but who do not require a formal tracheostomy. The patient still breathes spontaneously through his nose and mouth because the tube is small. It can also be used for emergency oxygenation.

minute volume The amount of air breathed by the patient in one minute. This can be calculated by measuring the tidal volume and multiplying it by the number of breaths taken in a minute (respiratory rate). Thus, e.g., a patient with a tidal volume of 500 ml who is breathing 12 times a minute has a minute volume of $500 \times 12 = 6000$ ml.

minute volume divider A type of ventilator which is powered by gas flow via air and oxygen flow meters. The volume of gases supplied to the ventilator should be equal to the minute volume of the patient. After the tidal volume is set the ventilator divides the fresh gas flow up into breaths and delivers it to the patient.

nasal intubation An endotracheal tube may be inserted either via the mouth or through the nose. Although they are more difficult to fix than oral tubes, tying them in is usually satisfactory. Suturing them to the nose is another method, but is uncomfortable for the patient and should never be done to the nasal septum. Contraindications include severe facial injuries, base-of-skull fractures and coagulation failure. Although nasal tubes are more comfortable than oral tubes and do not cause mouth ulceration, some believe that they may cause bacteraemia and sinusitis.

nebuliser Certain drugs, such as salbutamol and terbutaline, can be absorbed directly via the bronchial tree. When the drug comes into contact with the bronchi they cause local bronchodilation, without the systemic effects of giving the drugs i.v. or i.m. The drug must be delivered to the bronchi as very small particles which are produced as a fine mist by a nebuliser. Some specialised nebulisers have been used to humidify inspired gases.

negative pressure Some ventilators (e.g. the East Radcliffe) are capable of producing a slight negative pressure in the patient circuit during expiration to assist with exhalation. In theory this also helps to return blood to the heart during the expiratory phase. However, negative pressure is not used nowadays, as it is thought that it can cause atelectasis. Note that negative end expiratory pressure (NEEP) is the opposite of positive end expiratory pressure (PEEP).

Oxford A gas-driven ventilator manufactured by Penlon that is fairly simple to maintain and can be driven by a source of compressed gas. It is easily adapted for small children.

oximeter A device which measures the percentage of haemoglobin saturated with oxygen. The sensing probe is placed on the ear lobe or finger and the monitor continuously displays the percentage of Hb carrying oxygen. Normally this should be above 95%. These devices are very useful in detecting hypoxia, and in the critically ill patient may be used to guide oxygen therapy, ventilation and weaning.

oxygen Oxygen is required for life and is in the atmosphere in a concentration of around 21%. Patients who are being ventilated usually require extra oxygen because of lung abnormalities. You can work out how much

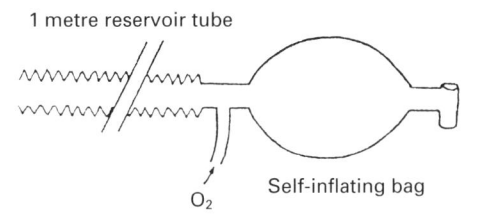

Figure V9 Oxygen.

oxygen a patient is receiving if you know the minute volume and the flow of oxygen (See Table P3 p. 346). Oxygen may be added to the ventilator or Ambu bag either by attaching it to a special port (Figure V9) or by making a T-piece in the air inlet. See **T-piece**.

oxygen concentrator This is a device which separates oxygen from room air by means of a special filter called a molecular sieve. It is powered by electricity and produces oxygen without requiring oxygen cylinders. They are produced in many different sizes, ranging from a domestic model which produces up to 4 litres per minute of 80% oxygen to large models which can supply an entire hospital. The output of oxygen from these machines should be monitored in case of internal failure. It is practical to keep some oxygen cylinders in reserve in case of power cuts.

PEEP Positive end expiratory pressure is when a small amount of positive pressure is used during the expiratory phase (usually 2–10 cmH$_2$O). This helps to keep the alveoli open and may also improve the efficiency of blood flow through the lungs. PEEP is normally given to most patients on IPPV at around 5 cmH$_2$O. Levels are increased as required. Avoid PEEP in asthma/COAD. PEEP elevates the CVP because it raises intrathoracic pressure, and tends to reduce the venous return for the same reason. This may reduce cardiac output so close cardiovascular monitoring must be carried out. It is also useful in patients with pulmonary oedema, near drowning and ARDS. See **CPAP** and Figure V10.

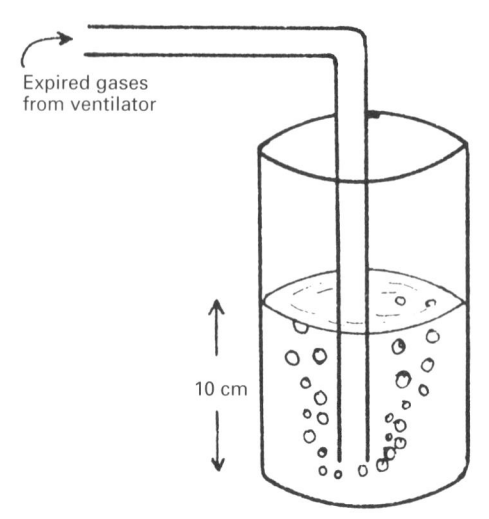

Figure V10 10 cm PEEP produced by leading expired gases from ventilator under water; cm depth under water = cm PEEP.

Portex A manufacturer of polyvinylchloride (PVC) endotracheal tubes suitable for long-term ventilation. See **endotracheal tube**.

positive pressure The force used by a ventilator to drive air into the patient's lungs.

pre-oxygenation The process of giving a patient 100% oxygen via an anaesthetic circuit for 5 min before he is intubated or suctioned. This has the effect of replacing the nitrogen in the lung with oxygen so that the patient is less liable to develop hypoxia during the procedure because of the extra oxygen stored in the lungs.

pressure control See **ventillator**.

PVC Polyvinyl chloride – a non-irritant type of plastic used for making endotracheal or tracheostomy tubes.

rate The number of breaths given to the patient each minute.

red rubber This is the material used in the red-coloured endotracheal tubes which is rather irritant to the tracheal tissues. It is recommended that where possible this type of tube should be replaced by a PVC tube if intubation is required for more than 24 h. If no PVC tubes are available then early tracheostomy is advised.

resistance Undersized endotracheal tubes, dirty or sticky valves and multiple connections in the ventilator circuit all increase the resistance to breathing. Ensure that resistance in the circuit is as low as possible so that the work of breathing is kept to minimum. This is of particular importance in children.

respiration 1. The process in which oxygen is transported from the air to the blood and into the cell.
2. The process with which cells utilise oxygen.

respiratory failure When there is failure of respiration (see Chapter 1). Definition usually refers to the type of respiration defined under 'respiration 1' (see above).

sedation When a patient is being ventilated drugs may be used to enable him to tolerate the endotracheal tube (see p. 338) and **ventilator**.

sensitivity See **assisted breathing**.

settings See **ventilator**.

shunt This occurs when the alveolus is not filled with air and the blood flows past it without becoming oxygenated (e.g. pulmonary oedema, lung consolidation). This leads to severe hypoxia.

Another type of shunt occurs in patients with congenital heart disease when the blood passes through a congenital abnormality such as a ventricular septal defect or a patent ductus arteriosus. If systemic venous blood flows through a shunt into the left side of the heart it will bypass the lungs and result in cyanosis (right-to-left shunt). In a left-to-right shunt there is increased pulmonary blood flow from a proportion of the blood in the left side of the heart passing into the pulmonary circulation.

SIMV See **IMV**.

suction This is important to keep the airway clear and helps to prevent atelectasis of the lung due to retained secretions. A sucker must always be available for a ventilated patient, especially during intubation or endotracheal tube changes. See **bag and suck**.

T-piece A simple arrangement to allow high concentrations of oxygen to be delivered from an Ambu bag, drawover anaesthetic circuit or ventilator. The oxygen is connected via a T-shaped connector to the equipment end and the other limb of the T is connected to a metre of ventilator tubing which is open at the end. This tubing acts as a reservoir and prevents the oxygen spilling out to the room air during expiration.

tidal volume The amount of gas in a breath, usually expressed in ml. The normal is around 10 ml/kg. Patients on ventilators need larger tidal volumes (up to 15 ml/kg.)

time cycled See **ventilator**.

tracheostomy Access to the airway via the trachea (see p. 359).

units of pressure measurement Pressure may be described in several units. The following conversion factors may be used:
1 mmHg = 0.13 kPa
1 kPa = 7.5 mmHg
1 kPa = 10 cmH$_2$O
1 torr = 1 mmHg
1 atmosphere = 14.7 lbf/in^2 = 760 mmHg

valves Devices which direct the flow of gases. Usually they prevent the patient rebreathing his expired air and are of three main types (Figure V11). Some, like type A, are only useful for IPPV; others, like type B, can be used for IPPV or spontaneous ventilation, e.g. in a weaning circuit or drawover anaesthesia. Type B valves always have two cusps. A type C value is a Heidbrink value and is used in the Mapleson C circuit. During IPPV it must be partly closed, and open for spontaneous ventilation.

ventilation The process of inspiration and expiration whether spontaneous or IPPV.

ventilation/perfusion (V/Q) ratio Normally the supply of air to an alveolus and the blood flow around it are well balanced. If interruption to either of these is upset there is said to be V/Q mismatch, which results in deterioration of respiratory function. A high V/Q ratio develops with good ventilation but low blood flow.

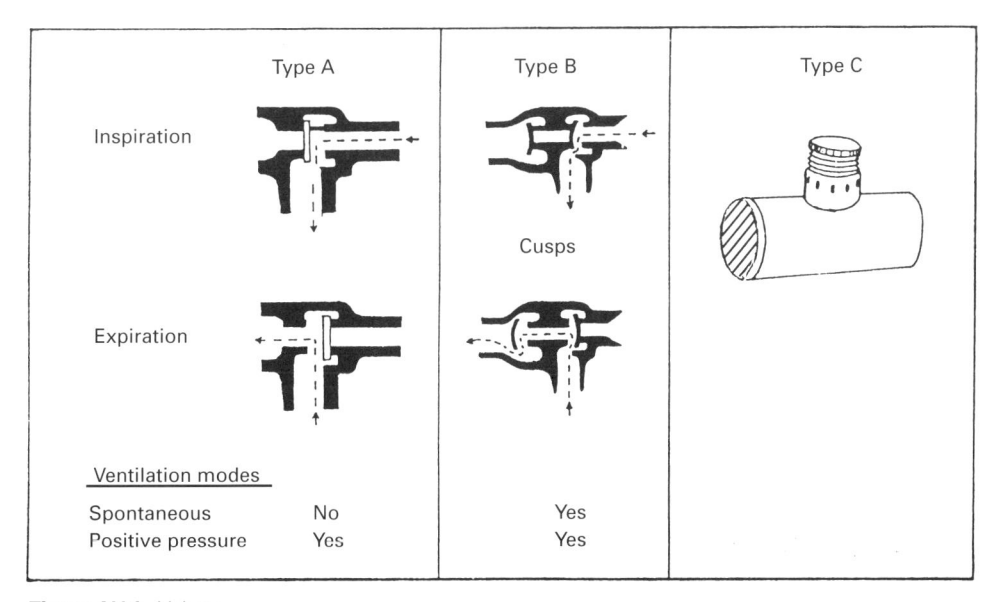

	Type A	Type B	Type C
Inspiration			
		Cusps	
Expiration			
Ventilation modes			
Spontaneous	No	Yes	
Positive pressure	Yes	Yes	

Figure V11 Valves.

A low V/Q happens when the reverse happens. *See also* **shunt**.

ventilator Understanding how different ventilators work will help you understand the limitations of particular models.

If you ventilate a patient with a resuscitation bag such as an Ambu bag, you generate a flow of gases into the patient's lungs, called IPPV. If you had to do this for any length of time you would wish to know how often to ventilate (respiratory rate), how hard to squeeze the bag (the pressure you should generate), how much air to give to the patient for each breath from the bag (tidal volume), and how much oxygen to add to the circuit (FiO_2). After determining the answers to these questions you would be able to ventilate the patient accurately to his requirements.

All ventilators work in principle like an Ambu or self-inflating bag, some using an electric motor to 'squeeze' the bag, others compressed air. When you put a patient on a ventilator you need to give the ventilator instructions for the parameters discussed above. There are a number of controls on a ventilator which you set to give this sort of information, and the values you enter will be determined by the age, size and condition of the patient (Table V1).

Although all ventilators are used for inflating the patient's lungs, there are some important differences between models, making some more suitable for certain patients. For example, not all ventilators can produce a small enough tidal volume to ventilate babies, and some specialised paediatric ventilators cannot be used for ventilating adults.

Table V1 Initial settings for ventilator controls

Function	Normal setting		Action
Tidal volume	8–10 ml/kg		Sets size of breath
Minute volume	Tidal volume × rate		Sets volume breathed/minute
Frequency or rate	Adult	12–20/minute	
	Child 9–15 years	15–20/minute	
	2–8 years	15–25/minute	
	0–1 years	20–30/minute	
Oxygen	See nomogram, p. 337		Add oxygen to the circuit as clinically indicated
Sensitivity or trigger	Normally set at minimum; −20 cmH$_2$O stops triggering; −1 to −3 allows triggering		Allows or stops patient triggering ventilator
Pressure limit	Set at 30 cmH$_2$O child Set at 40 cmH$_2$O adult		Prevents ventilator producing too much pressure in circuit
I:E ratio	Usually adjust to 1:2		
Driving gas flow rate: Minute volume dividers	Set at minute volume		Sets the minute volume, which is then divided into breaths by the ventilator
Pressure setting (pressure generators)	Adequate to allow acceptable tidal volume		Sets ventilator inspiratory pressure

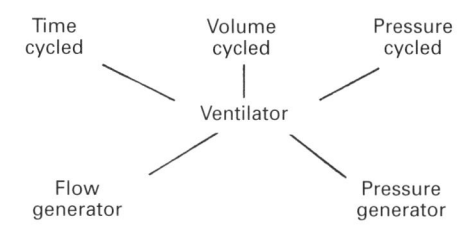

Figure V12 Ventilator types.

Ventilators are classified by:
1. the method of cycling from inspiration to expiration and back again;
2. the pattern of gas flow used to inflate the lungs (See Figure V12).

These differ as follows:
1. *Cycling* is most commonly based on a time set by the operator, either directly by specifying, for example, 1 sec for inspiration and 2 sec for expiration, or indirectly, for example, by setting 20 breaths per minute at a normal I:E ratio (1:2) which will give an inspiratory time of 1 sec. Although the controls differ from one ventilator to another the end result is the same – after a 1 sec inspiratory time the ventilator will change to expiration for 2 sec.

    Other ventilators only cycle from inspiration to expiration when they have delivered a certain tidal volume (volume cycled) or reached a certain airway pressure (pressure cycled). Sometimes ventilators have the cycling dependent on a combination of these factors.
2. *Gas flow*: ventilators differ in the way that they deliver air to the patient's lungs. Some ventilators always deliver the set tidal volume over a certain period of time and are called volume preset or flow generators. If the patient develops stiff lungs (low compliance) or a kinked endotracheal tube this type of ventilator is useful, as it will automatically increase the inspiratory pressure to drive the same tidal volume into the patient.
3. Pressure present ventilators (or pressure generators) are set to deliver gases at a certain pressure. On some ventilators such as the Manley Multivent the inspiratory pressure is set by adding weights to the arm pressing down on the bellows. On other ventilators a control is set to a pressure which provides adequate respiratory pressure to expand the lung. This mode of ventilation is becoming the standard on ICU to avoid excess airway pressures.
4. Paediatric ventilators are often pressure generators, so that the dangers of high airway pressures can be avoided. The limitation with this type of ventilator is if the tube starts to block or the patient's lung compliance changes that he will be underventilated. Some pressure generators can supply high flows of gases and are able to compensate to some extent for leaks in the patient circuit (e.g. due to a deflated endotracheal tube cuff). Always know the limitations of your ventilator and use it accordingly. For patients with normal lungs (e.g. Guillain–Barré syndrome), most types of ventilator can be used.

ventilatory failure Insufficient minute volume, causing retention of CO_2 and usually hypoxia. In a spontaneously breathing patient this can be caused by various problems such as opiate respiratory depression, muscle weakness as in Guillain–Barré, or any condition reducing the minute volume (see Chapter 1). In a ventilated patient it may be due to an incorrectly set ventilator, or a fault such as a leak developing in the patient circuit.

volume cycled See **ventilator**.

weaning The term used to describe the process by which a ventilated patient comes off the ventilator and breathes spontaneously. While intubated the patient must be attached to a circuit

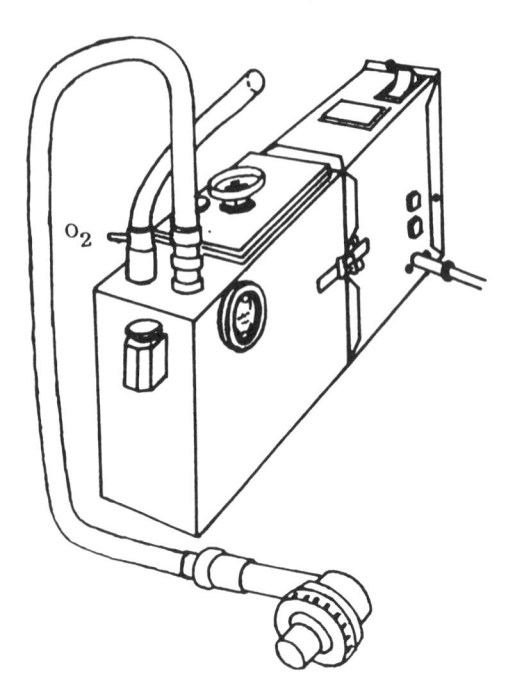

Figure V13 The patient breathes warm, humidified, oxygen-enriched air via a hot-water humidifier. A non-rebreathing valve (type B, p. 431) connects the circuit to the endotracheal tube and oxygen is added via a T-piece.

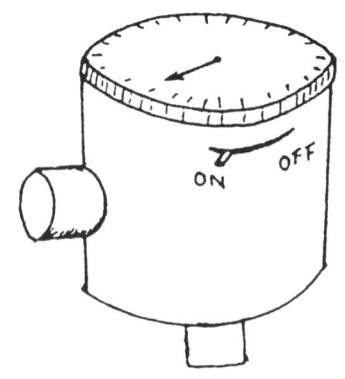

Figure V14 Wright's respirometer.

during this period which can keep him humidified and administer oxygen. A suitable circuit for adults and children over 10 years is shown in Figure V13. If available, condenser or blower humidifiers are better alternatives.

Wright's respirometer A device (Figure V14) which can be connected to a ventilator or to a spontaneously breathing patient which measures the tidal and minute volumes. It should not be left in the expiratory limb of the ventilator for more than 15 min at a time as it will become wet inside and less accurate. This is especially important when using the East Radcliffe ventilator which has a respirometer permanently on the machine activated by a lever.

Yankaur A type of rigid sucker end which is useful for sucking out the pharynx.

Drugs for critical care

Drugs in critical care

Staff who prescribe and administer drugs to critically ill patients must be aware of their actions, side effects, indications and contraindications. This section describes the way drug doses are expressed and lists the common drugs used in critical care.

Doses

These are measured in the following ways:
1. Drug mass units:
    gram (g); milligram (mg); microgram (μg);
        1 g = 1000 mg = 1 000 000 μg.
2. Solutions units:
    litre (l); millilitre (ml);
        1 l = 1000 ml.
    1 ml = 15 drops of saline in a normal i.v. infusion;
    1 ml = 60 microdrops in a paediatric microdrop i.v. giving set.
3. Percentages:

> To find the number of mg in each ml of a solution multiply the % strength by 10; e.g. 1% × 10 = 10 mg/ml.

4. Ratios:
    1 : 1 000 is the same as a 0.1% solution;
    1 : 1 000 solution contains 1 mg in 1 ml;
    1 : 10 000 solution contains 0.1 mg in 1 ml.
5. Other units:
    milli-equivalents (mEq), e.g. sodium bicarbonate;
    millimoles (mmol), e.g. sodium in saline. Take care when converting mEq to mmol and vice-versa – the values are the same with monovalent ions but not with bivalent ions, e.g. Ca or Mg, in which 1 mmol = 2 mEq, (see p. 85) or trivalent ions in which 1 mmol = 3 mEq.

Percentage strength of drug	Number of grams or milligrams				
	1 ml	10 ml	100 ml	500 ml	1000 ml
0.5%	5 mg	50 mg	500 mg	2.5 g	5 g
1%	10 mg	100 mg	1 g	5 g	10 g
2%	20 mg	200 mg	2 g	10 g	20 g
5%	50 mg	500 mg	5 g	25 g	50 g
10%	100 mg	1 g	10 g	50 g	100 g
20%	200 mg	2 g	20 g	100 g	200 g
50%	500 mg	5 g	50 g	250 g	500 g

Recommended drug doses

These are given in two forms, usually related to body weight in kilograms (kg):
1. The therapeutic dose is the amount of drug required to produce a clinical action; e.g. 5–20 mg diazepam i.v. for control of convulsions.
2. The maximum safe dose is the amount of drug which if exceeded could produce side effects; e.g. 3 mg/kg of lidocaine is the maximum dose of plain lidocaine that should be used in a 4-h period to avoid toxicity from the drug.

Key points in drug administration

Check the drug, dose and route carefully. Check for any history of drug reactions or contraindications to proposed therapy, e.g. propranolol (a beta-blocker) should never be given to asthmatics.

When giving drugs by injection use only sterile equipment and carefully disinfect the site of injection with a suitable antiseptic. This is especially important if you are injecting into a drip.
1. *Intravenous drugs.* Inject slowly, watching the patient for any side effects or signs of allergic reactions. When using sedatives or analgesics, inject until the desired effect is obtained and then stop. Regular i.v. drugs are best given via an intravenous infusion.
2. *Intramuscular drugs.* Try to make the patient relax during injection. Use only sites shown in Figure 16.5; i.m. injections are not absorbed in patients who are shocked. Check that the needle is not in a vein by aspirating before injection.
3. *Infusion drugs.* Check that the dilution is correct and the drip reliable. Many of the drugs used by infusion have serious side effects if given too quickly. Be certain that there is an adequate method of controlling the rate of infusion such as a syringe driver or gate clamp, dial-a-flow, electronic drip counter or pump. Ensure that the patient has adequate supervision and monitoring for the drug being used. *Infusion doses* may be calculated as μg/kg/minute, μg/minute, mg/hour or drops per minute (d.p.m.). Often a range of doses is suggested and you should start the drug at the lowest dose first and then increase it until the required effect is achieved.

How much to use

When using regimens of μg/kg/min there is an easy way of working out how much solution to use:
1. Estimate the patient's body weight in kg.
2. Take this number and multiply it by 3.
3. Add this number of mg to 5% dextrose (or other solution) to make a total volume of 50 ml.
4. Administer this through a syringe pump.
5. 1 μg/kg/min = 1 ml/h.

Example – to give a 60 kg patient 5 μg/kg/min of dopamine
1. Body weight = 60 kg.
2. Number of mg = 60 × 3 = 180 mg.
3. Add to 180 mg of dopamine dextrose 5% to make 50 ml volume.
4. Administer through a syringe pump.
5. 5 ml/h = 5 μg/kg/min.

Principles of antibiotic therapy[1]

Antibiotic therapy should be used when:
- the micro-organism is likely to be sensitive;
- it will improve the patient's disease;
- it will reach the tissues which are infected;
- the benefits of therapy outweight the risk of side effects;
- the patient is not allergic to the drug; and
- potential drug interactions have been considered.

1 Antibiotic doses are dealt with in Chapter 8.

Antibiotics are abused if the above conditions are not met.

1. **Use the correct antibiotic** Do not prescribe penicillin for staphyloccocal infections, since over 90% of hospital and 80% of rural staph aureus isolates are resistant to penicillin. Flucloxacillin, which is resistant to breakdown by penicillinase-producing staphylococci, is effective in up to 90% of cases.
2. **Give antibiotics only when there is likely to be benefit** To give flucloxacillin for the treatment of a subcutaneous abscess after surgical drainage is unwise since antibiotics do not normally improve the outcome of abscesses which have been incised and drained. The treatment of an abscess is not antibiotics but rather drainage. An antibiotic is indicated if there is coexistent septicaemia or the infection is situated in complex tissue spaces such as in the hand or foot.

   Also to give an antibiotic 'just in case it might do some good' is not only a waste of money but also dangerous since it needlessly risks side effects of therapy.
3. **Ensure the drug will reach the site of infection**. It is best not to prescribe gentamicin for meningitis because gentamicin does not enter CSF very well. A knowledge of tissue penetration by antibiotics is important. Chloramphenicol penetrates CSF well, as does penicillin when the meninges are inflamed.

> **KEYPOINT**
>
> Will the antibiotic prescribed reach the site of infection?

4. **Consider allergy, side effects and drug interactions** Always ask about a history of allergy. If cloxacillin is given to a patient with allergy to penicillin any reaction could be fatal. In staphylococcal infection such as septic arthritis a non-penicillin group drug should be given (e.g. gentamicin) if the patient is allergic to penicillins.

> **KEYPOINT**
>
> Always enquire about a history of allergy before prescribing an antibiotic.

   Gentamicin is potentially nephrotoxic and ototoxic. If cephalosporins are being given to the same patient the risk of hearing loss is increased. Urine output and urea must be carefully monitored if patients are receiving these drugs together. Gentamicin should not normally be given for more than 5 days unless it is possible to measure gentamicin levels (a rare facility in the tropics). Metronidazole may potentiate the action of warfarin, leading to a severe haemorrhage if the prothrombin time is not monitored. Common interactions between antibiotics and other drugs are shown in Table D1.
5. **Whenever possible follow an antibiotic policy** There should be an antibiotic policy which is based on the likely pathogens and known resistance patterns. Records of resistance patterns of bacteria should be kept to enable infected patients to be treated immediately with the antibiotics most likely to be successful. Keep records in a notebook or on a wall chart. An antibiotic policy will allow rational prescribing of antibiotics, by guiding health workers and doctors as to costs, sensitivity patterns of micro-organisms and the likely causes of infection. Large sums of money could be saved by hospitals and governments if antibiotic policies based on local data were established. Limited and expensive antibiotics should be saved for those most likely to benefit.

Local anaesthetics in critical care

Local anaesthetics are commonly used drugs in critically ill patients. The most

Table D1 Effects of potential drug interactions with antibiotics[1]

Antibiotic	Interacting drug	Effects
Aminoglycosides	Cephalosporins	Nephrotoxicity
Aminoglycosides	Furosemide	Ototoxicity and nephrotoxicity
Aminoglycosides	Curare	Prolongs neuromuscular blockade
Ampicillin	Oral contraceptive	Contraceptive failure
Cephalosporins	Furosemide	Nephrotoxicity
Metronidazole	Warfarin	Potentiates warfarin
Sulphonamides	Warfarin	Potentiates warfarin
Sulphonamides	Phenytoin	Phenytoin toxicity
Sulphonamides	Tolbutamide	Hypoglycaemia
Rifampicin	Tolbutamide	Hypoglycaemia
Chloramphenicol	Phenytoin	Penytoin toxicity
Chloramphenicol	Tolbutamide	Hypoglycaemia
Isoniazid	Warfarin	Potentiates warfarin
Isoniazid	Phenytoin	Phenytoin toxicity
Tetracycline	Antacids	Tetracycline failure

1 These are examples of drug interactions with antibiotics. For a full listing of drug interactions, refer to a textbook of pharmacology.

common drugs in use are bupivacaine and lidocaine, details of which are to be found on pp. 442 and 449. When used correctly they are safe drugs but they may result in serious reactions if given incorrectly.

Precautions in the use of local anaesthetics

Toxicity results from an overdose of milligrams rather than of volume:
1. Check the concentration of the drug carefully.
2. Check whether adrenaline has been added and whether it is required. It is contraindicated for blocks on the fingers, penis and toes.
3. Always aspirate before injecting.
4. During infiltration, keep the needle tip moving.
5. Always be prepared for reactions to local anaesthetic drugs with the correct equipment and drugs immediately available. When using large doses it is safest to have an indwelling needle for immediate venous access.

Toxic reactions to local anaesthetics

Signs and symptoms

Dizziness, restlessness, drowsiness, blurred vision, circumoral paraesthesia, tremors, convulsions, fall in blood pressure, cardiac arrest.

Treatment

Immediately stop the injection. If there are mild symptoms only, observe the patient and insert the i.v. line if you have not already done so. Treat serious side effects by controlling the airway, administering oxygen and giving i.v. fluids to counteract hypotension, and follow this with ephedrine 10 mg i.v. if this is not rapidly effective. Treat convulsions with i.v. diazepam, or a small dose of thiopental if you are in theatre. If convulsions are not controlled immediately, give suxamethonium and intubate and ventilate the patient.

Adding adrenaline to local anaesthetics

Adrenaline should be added to make a concentration of 1:200 000. To do this, add 1 ml of 1:10 000 adrenaline to 19 ml of plain local anaesthetic.

A to Z of drugs

This section gives specific details on the administration of drugs in critically ill patients. When using this guide check for any special recommendations regarding drug dosage under specific disease entries. The descriptions are not comprehensive and extra information may be obtained from standard books.

Adenosine

Effects	Slows conduction through AV node.
Indications	Treatment of acute paroxysmal SVT (including WPW) or differentiation of SVT from VT.
Dose	3 mg fast i.v. bolus, increasing to 6 mg then 12 mg at 2 min intervals as necessary.
Length of action	10 sec.
Side effects	Flushing, dyspnoea, headache – all transient.
Caution	Second or third degree heart block, asthma.

Adrenaline epinephrine

Effects		Increases heart rate and BP, vasoconstriction, bronchodilation via sympathetic nervous system alpha and beta receptors.
Preparation		1 : 1000 and 1 : 10 000 ampoules for injection. Also with local anaesthetics in concentrations of 1 : 80 000 to 1 : 400 000.
Indications		Asystole, anaphylaxis, status asthmaticus in children (s/cut), croup, additive to local anaesthesia, heart failure, vasoconstrictor.
Adult dose	i.v.	Cardiac arrest 1 mg, other uses 0.1 ml/kg of 1 : 10 000 titrated slowly against response.
	Infusion	5 mg in 50 ml dextrose 5%. Start at 5 ml/h via syringe pump and increase until effective.
	s.c., i.m.	0.1–0.5 ml of 1 : 1000 (may repeat after 10 min).
	ET	Twice i.v. dose.
	Nebulised	3–5 ml of 1 : 1000 made up to 5 ml with 0.9% saline.
Paediatric dose	i.v.	0.1 ml/kg of 1 : 10 000.
	s.c., i.m.	0.01 ml/kg of 1 : 1000 (may repeat after 15 min).
Length of action		Short, few minutes only if i.v.

440 Care of the Critically Ill Patient in the Tropics

Side effects	Hypertension, arrhythmias, cardiac ischaemia, ventricular fibrillation.
Caution	Care in patients with pre-existing cardiac disease or arrhythmias. Patients on infusion must be monitored closely (preferably with an arterial line), and the drug given via a central line. The infusion must be controlled as described on p. 436.

Alfentanil Rapifen

Effects	Short acting opiate.
Indications	Anaesthesia or ICU sedation.
Dose	Anaesthesia 5–10 µg/kg with induction; ICU sedation usually 1–3 mg/h.
Length of action	5–10 min from bolus dose. Even after infusion wears off rapidly. Does not accumulate in renal failure therefore useful for ICU sedation in this group of patients.
Side effects	Profound respiratory depressant, bradycardia occasionally.

Aminophylline

Effects		Bronchodilation, mild inotropic and chronotropic action, produces mild diuresis.
Preparation		Ampoule 250 mg in 10 ml.
Indications		Bronchospasm from any cause including congestive cardiac failure.
Dose	i.v.	5 mg/kg i.v. over 20 min.
	Infusion	Give loading dose if patient not already taking theophylline preparation and then infuse at 0.5 mg/kg/h. Reduce dose in the elderly, patients with cirrhosis or heart failure and those receiving erythromycin or cimetidine.
	Oral	100–300 mg three to four times daily.
	Rectal	360 mg suppository once or twice daily.
Length of action		6–12 h.
Side effects		Cardiac arrhythmias, vomiting, diuresis, CNS excitation.
Caution		Patients who are taking a theophylline drug by mouth should not be given a bolus dose of aminophylline i.v., but may be given infusion without the loading dose. Theophylline levels may be measured in some laboratories and should be 10–20 mg/l.

Amiodarone Cordarone X

Effects	Antiarrhythmic drug.
Preparation	50 mg/ml.
Indications	Treatment of supraventricular and ventricular arrhythmias.

Dose		5 mg/kg over 1 h dilute in 5% dextrose only. Do not dilute to less than 600 μg/ml. Maximum 1.2 g in 24 h. Cardiac arrest 150 mg in 10 min.
Length of action		Long acting.
Side effects		Thyroid dysfunction, photosensitivity, pulmonary fibrosis.
Caution		Except in emergency give via CVP line as irritant if drip tissues. Thyroid dysfunction and pregnancy.

Atracurium Tracrium

Effects		Non-depolarising muscle relaxant.
Preparation		10 mg/ml
Indications		Muscle relaxation.
Dose	i.v.	0.3–0.6 mg/kg.
	Infusion	0.4 mg/kg/h.
Length of action		20–40 min.
Side effects		Higher doses cause histamine release.
Caution		Length of action is not increased by renal failure. Avoid in status asthmaticus.

Atropine

Effects	Increases heart rate, dries mouth and reduces gastrointestinal motility through its effect on the paraysmpathetic nervous system (especially the vagus nerve).
Preparation	0.5–1 mg/ml
Indications	Bradycardia treatment and prevention, drying of secretions, organophosphate poisoning.
Adult dose	0.6–1.2 mg (give twice dose if via ET).
Paediatric dose	20 μg/kg.
Length of action	1–4 h.
Side effects	Pyrexia in small children, arrhythmias, urinary retention, CNS side effects (e.g. confusion) in elderly if used in very high doses.
Caution	Avoid if possible in pyrexial children in hot climates.

Bicarbonate (sodium bicarbonate)

Effects	Neutralises acidosis, alkalinises urine, reduces plasma K^+.
Preparation	4.2% or 8.4% (1 ml of 8.4% contains 1 mEq or 1 mmol).
Indications	Following cardiac arrest or other causes of severe acidosis, hyperkalaemia.
Dose	1 mEq/kg following cardiac arrest. Metabolic acidosis 0.5 mEq/kg, repeat as indicated.
Length of action	Variable depending on situation; at cardiac arrest give after 20 min.

Side effects	Alkalosis, fluid overload (due to high concentration of Na which is present).

Bupivacaine Marcain

Effects	Local anaesthetic drug.
Preparation	0.25%, 0.5%, 0.75% plain or + adrenaline.
Indications	Infiltration, plexus, epidural, spinal anaesthesia.
Dose	Do not exceed 2 mg/kg in any 4-h period with any preparation.
Length of action	2–8 h.
Side effects	Local anaesthesia toxicity.
Caution	Never give i.v. even for Bier's blocks.

Calcium

Effects	Mild inotrope, decreases depressant effect of citrate on the heart during massive blood transfusion, counteracts tetany due to low Ca levels.
Preparation	Ca gluconate and chloride (both 10%).
Indications	During massive blood transfusion (faster than 1 unit/5 min in an adult), hyperkalaemia, tetany.
Dose	2–4 mg/kg of chloride preparation, 4–8 mg/kg of gluconate (which contains less ionised Ca).
Side effects	Bradycardia, irritating to veins and tissues.
Caution	Do not give in the same giving set as blood.

Chlorpromazine Largactil

Effects		Major tranquilliser with sedative effect, also antiemetic action and useful in treating persistent hiccups. A mild vasodilator and alters temperature homeostasis.
Preparation		Ampoules 25 mg/ml.
Indications		Emergency control behavioural disturbance, persistent vomiting, tetanus, persistent hiccup.
Dose	i.m.	25–50 mg 4–8 hourly.
	i.v.	5 mg sometimes used to produce mild vasodilating effect.
Side effects		Extrapyramidal symptoms, hypotension, tachycardia, drowsiness.
Caution		Elderly and debilitated patients – reduce dose.

Cimetidine Tagamet

Effects	Histamine-2 receptor antagonist thereby reducing gastric acid output.
Preparations	Injection 100 mg/ml in 2 ml ampoules. Tablets 200, 400, 800 mg.

Indications		Benign gastric and duodenal ulceration, reflux oesophagitis, prevention of stress ulceration.
Dose	i.v.	200 mg over 2 min diluted in saline 6 hourly
	Oral	400 mg b.d. or as a single 800 mg evening dose for 4–6 weeks.
Length of action		3–6 h.
Side effects		Never inject rapidly intravenously as it may cause arrhythmias. Also confusional states, drug interactions (potentiates warfarin, phenytoin, aminophylline), rarely gynaecomastia.

Dexamethasone

Effects	Steroid.
Preparation	4 mg/ml.
Indications	Raised intracranial pressure.
Dose	4 mg i.v. / oral 6 hourly.
Side effects	See hydrocortisone.

Diazepam Valium

Effects		Centrally acting sedative, potent anticonvulsant.
Preparation		0.5% solution either in plain solution or as Diazemuls, which is less damaging to the veins.
Indications		Premedication, sedation, anticonvulsant, e.g. in eclampsia, antispasmodic for tetanus, after ketamine to prevent hallucinations.
Adult dose	i.v.	5–20 mg. Effect variable on different patients, elderly may be very sensitive. When giving i.v. inject slowly, watching the patient's response.
	Infusion	Assess the dose of diazepam required and add this to an acceptable volume of fluid. A common starting regimen is 80 mg of diazepam in each litre of i.v. fluid given over 8 hours.
Paediatric dose	i.v.	0.1–0.25 mg/kg
	p.r.	0.1 mg/kg
Length of action		Depends on dose, 15 min to several hours.
Side effects		Undue sleepiness, lack of co-operation, respiratory depression or obstruction especially in the elderly, occasional hypotension. Metabolites of diazepam may accumulate if used by infusion in high doses over several days. Gradual reduction of the dose judged by clinical response is advised. Midazolam more widely used in ICU.
Caution		i.v. use may produce damage to veins and if prolonged use is expected central venous administration is advised or a change to the Diazemuls preparation.

i.m. injection should never be done as it is poorly absorbed and painful.

Digoxin

Effects		Decreases the rate of conduction of impulses through the atrioventricular node. Also increases the force of contraction of the heart (positive inotropic effect).
Preparation	Injection	250 µg/ml.
	Tablets	62.5, 125 and 250 µg.
Indications		Supraventricular arrhythmias, especially atrial fibrillation, heart failure.
Dose	i.v.	0.5 mg over 15 min and repeated after 6 h. Thereafter maintenance by oral route.
	Orally	For fast digitalisation give 0.75–1.5 mg stat followed by 0.25 mg at 6-hourly intervals until fibrillation is controlled. Thereafter maintain on 0.125–0.25 mg daily. For slow digitalisation give 0.25–0.75 mg daily until benefits are seen, when the dose may be reduced. Some laboratories can measure digoxin levels to guide dosage. Therapeutic range 1–2 µg/l.
Length of action		Half-life: 34–51 h but increased in renal failure.
Side effects		Patients with decreased renal function or hypokalaemia (often secondary to diuretics) are particularly prone to toxic side effects. These include nausea and vomiting, arrhythmias (supraventricular, bradycardias and heart block), headaches and visual disturbances. Gynaecomastia rarely.
Caution		i.v. digoxin should be given slowly or by infusion and only in emergency situations. The dose should be reduced if the patient has received any cardiac glycoside within 72 h. Avoid i.m. digoxin – poorly absorbed.

Dobutamine Dobutrex

Effects		Powerful inotropic agent that increases heart rate and strength of contraction via sympathetic beta receptors in heart. Increases cardiac output.
Preparation		250 mg ampoules for dilution.
Indications		Cardiac failure.
Dose	Infusion	Dilute 3 mg/kg to 50 ml with 5% dextrose and start at 2.5 ml/h (= 2.5 µg/kg/min). Best administered via a central vein, though a large peripheral vein may be used in an emergency.
Length of action		A few minutes.
Side effects		Tachycardia, hypertension, arrhythmias, cardiac ischaemia.

A to Z of drugs   445

Caution		Patients on infusion must be monitored closely (preferably with an arterial line), and the drug is best given via a central line. The infusion must be controlled as described on p. 436.

Dopamine

Effects		Powerful inotropic drug with variable effects depending on dose level. At low doses (1.5–5 µg/kg/min) increases splanchnic (especially renal) blood flow via stimulation of the dopaminergic receptors. At medium doses (5–10 µg/kg/min) increases strength and rate of contraction of the heart via sympathetic nervous system beta receptors; at high doses (>15 µg/kg/min) stimulation of alpha receptors causing vasoconstriction and reduction in renal blood flow.
Preparation		200 mg ampoules.
Indications		Hypotension in certain situations.
Dose	Infusion	Dilute 3 mg/kg to 50 ml with 5% dextrose. Infuse at 2–15 µg/kg/min titrated against response.
Length of action		A few minutes.
Side effects		Hypertension, tachycardia, arrhythmias, myocardial ischaemia, tissue necrosis may occur if extravasates through a peripheral vein. Administer via a central vein.
Caution		Patients on infusion must be monitored closely (preferably with an arterial line), and the drug given via a central line. The infusion must be controlled. Renal dopamine not now used in ICU!

Ephedrine

Effects		Vasopressor causing vasoconstriction of blood vessels, increase in heart rate and contractility via sympathetic alpha and beta receptors causing a rise in BP and cardiac output. Also mild bronchodilator.
Preparation		3 or 5% solution, 1 ml ampoules.
Indications		Hypotension caused by vasodilation, e.g. following spinal or epidural anaesthesia or drug overdoses. Fluid depletion should always be treated before using a vasopressor. Safe for emergency use in pregnancy as it does not reduce placental blood flow.
Adult dose	i.v.	5–10 mg; repeat until effective.
Length of action		5–10 min, repeated doses less effective.
Side effects		Hypertension, arrhythmias, myocardial ischaemia, CNS stimulation.
Caution		Care in ischaemic heart disease.

Esmolol Brevibloc

Effects	Short acting, cardioselective beta-blocker.
Preparation	10 mg/ml (and 250 mg/ml for dilution).
Indications	Supraventricular tachycardia or intraoperative hypertension.
Dose	SVT: 0.5 mg/kg over 1 min, then 50–200 µg/kg/min. Hypertension: 25–100 mg, then 50–300 µg/kg/min.
Length of action	Very short.
Side effects	Hypotension, bradycardia.
Caution	Asthma, heart failure, AV block, verapamil treatment.

Flumazenil Anexate

Effects		Benzodiazepine receptor antagonist.
Preparation		100 µg/ml.
Indications		Benzodiazepine overdose.
Dose	i.v.	200 µg then 100 µg at 60-sec intervals (up to maximum 1 mg).
	Infusion	100–400 µg/h.
Length of action		45–90 min.
Side effects		Arrhythmia, seizures.
Caution		Benzodiazepine dependence (acute withdrawal).

Furosemide Lasix

Effect	Potent diuretic acting on the loop of Henle.
Preparation	1% solution, other strengths available.
Indications	Pulmonary oedema, cardiac failure, fluid overload. Oliguria is not an indication until is has been established that the patient is not fluid depleted.
Dose	Normally 0.3–1 mg/kg i.v. In certain renal disorders higher doses are required.
Length of action	2–4 h.
Side effects	In people with reduced circulatory volume, e.g. eclampsia, indiscriminate use may worsen the hypovolaemia by causing a brisk diuresis and a degree of vasodilation. Also dehydration and electrolyte imbalance (particularly hypokalaemia).

Glyceryl trinitrate GTN

Effects		Smooth muscle relaxation causing vasodilation of venous capacitance vessels, and, in higher doses, arterioles. Coronary vasodilation.
Preparation		Tablets 0.3 mg, i.v. infusion.
Indications		Myocardial ischaemia, cardiac failure.
Dose	Sublingual	0.3–0.6 mg sublingual as required.
	Infusion	1 mg/ml in dextrose. Start at 2 ml/h and titrate against response.

Length of action		Short, although sustained release tablets may be available.
Side effects		Tachycardia, hypotension, headache.
Caution		Active drug may be absorbed onto plastic i.v. tubing. Patients on infusion must be monitored closely (preferably with an arterial line), and the drug is best given via a central line. The infusion must be controlled as described on p. 436.

Heparin

Effects		Potent parenteral anticoagulant that works by potentiating the inhibition of several coagulation factors, including thrombin and factor X. Effectiveness is measured by the laboratory activated partial thromboplastin time (APTT).
Preparations		5 ml vials containing 1000 units/ml, 5000 units/ml, 10 000 units/ml, and 25 000 units/ml. (100 units = 1 mg.) Low molecular weight heparins are also available.
Indications		Prevention and treatment of deep vein thrombosis, for the prevention of thrombus formation on prosthetic valves, for the treatment of pulmonary embolus. For therapeutic effect, aim for a prothrombin time of 2–3 times normal. (This does not apply to low-dose prophylaxis for deep-vein thrombosis.)
Dose	i.v.	5000 units i.v. stat. followed by an infusion of 40 000 units over 24 h or 10 000 units i.v. 6 hourly.
	s.c.	5000 units prior to surgery then 5000 units 8–12 hourly until ambulant for prevention of DVT.
Length of action		4–6 h.
Side effects		Haemorrhage is the major side effect. Because of the short half-life of heparin, stopping the drug will often be effective. For serious haemorrhage protamine sulphate will reverse the effects of heparin (1 mg neutralises 100 units of heparin when given within 15 min; for a longer interval a smaller dose is sufficient).
Caution		Do not give to patients with an active bleeding source including peptic ulcer. Use with caution in those with hepatic or renal dysfunction.

Hydralazine Apresoline

Effects	Direct arteriolar vasodilator causing a reduction in blood pressure.
Preparation	Powder 20 mg in ampoule.
Indications	Hypertension; drug of choice for eclampsia.

Adult dose	i.v.	5–10 mg as a bolus and repeat after 15 min if not effective. Hydralazine reaches its peak effect after 20 minutes; therefore patience is required.
	i.m.	20 mg repeated every 2–4 h.
	Infusion	40 mg in 1000 ml of 5% dextrose. Initially 200 µg/min, maintenance 50–150 µg/min.
Length of action		2–4 h.
Side effects		Tachycardia, occasional severe hypotension.

Hydrocortisone

Effects		The suppression of inflammatory reactions; raises the blood sugar and also has a weak mineralocorticoid action.
Preparations	i.v.	As powder in 100 mg vials for reconstitution with 2 ml of water.
	Tablets	10 mg, 20 mg.
Indications		Acute asthma, anaphylactic shock, allergic reactions including severe drug reactions, transfusion reactions, replacement therapy for adrenal insufficiency, suppression of inflammation in many disease processes including connective tissue disorders, pericardial TB, Crohn's disease and ulcerative colitis.
Adult dose	i.v.	By infusion or slow injection 100–500 mg 6–8 hourly as required.
	Oral	For replacement therapy, 20–30 mg/day in divided doses.
Paediatric dose	i.v.	up to 1 year 25 mg; 1–5 years 50 mg; 6–12 years 100 mg.
Length of action	i.v.	Onset of action, 2 h; duration of action, 12 h.
Side effects		Long-term treatment may result in: hypertension, muscle weakness, osteoporosis, diabetes, peptic ulceration. Mental state changes including euphoria and dysphoria. Growth suppression in children. Tuberculosis and other infections may be masked by steroids in their presentation. Adrenal suppression occurs in patients taking >10 mg prednisolone/day, for longer than one month. Caution on withdrawing therapy is required in such patients with gradually reduced dosages being given over weeks or months.

Isoprenaline

Effects	Increase in heart rate and contractility via sympathetic nervous system beta receptors resulting in a rise in BP and cardiac output. Also potent bronchodilator.
Preparation	2 mg ampoules.

A to Z of drugs

Indications		Complete heart block, cardiac failure, bronchospasm, overdose beta-blocker.
Adult dose	Infusion	Add 2 mg to 500 ml dextrose 5% and start at 2–4 µg, titrate against response.
Paediatric dose		0.1 µg/kg/min
Length of action		Rapidly metabolised.
Side effects		Tachycardia, arrhythmias, hypertension, cardiac ischaemia.
Caution		Patients on infusion must be monitored closely (preferably with an arterial line), and the drug is best given via a central line. The infusion must be controlled as described on p. 436.

Labetalol Trandate

Effects		Sympathetic nervous system antagonist at the beta receptors causing a slowing of the heart and reduction in the force of contraction. It also has some blocking action at the alpha receptors, which results in vasodilation of blood vessels. Both these effects cause a fall in BP.
Preparation		20 ml ampoule 0.5%.
Indications		Hypertension: may be used in eclampsia, pre-eclampsia, and supraventricular arrhythmias.
Adult dose	i.v.	10 mg increments i.v. to a maximum of 200 mg.
	Infusion	Commence at 20 mg/h and increase to maximum of 150 mg/h.
	Oral	100–200 mg twice daily.
Length of action		1–6 h.
Side effects		Bradycardia (treat excessive bradycardia with atropine), bronchospasm, hypotension.
Caution		**Do not use in asthmatics** or patients with heart block.

Lidocaine Xylocaine

Effects		Local anaesthetic; also stabilises cell membranes of excitable tissue such as myocardium which gives it an anti-arrhythmic action.
Preparation		0.5%, 1%, 2%, 4%, 5%, 10%.
Dose	LA	Maximum safe dose in a 4-h period: 3 mg/kg plain. 7 mg/kg with adrenaline 1 : 200 000.
	i.v.	For ventricular arrhythmias give 1–1.5 mg/kg i.v. plain solution as a bolus and follow with an infusion if necessary.
	Infusion	4 mg/min for 30 min than 2 mg/min for 2 h then 1 mg/min until not required. Start with i.v. loading dose.
Side effects		Local anaesthetic toxicity.

Mannitol

Effects		Osmotic diuretic.
Preparation		10–20% for infusion.
Indications		Cerebral oedema, prevention of acute renal failure, forced diuresis.
Dose	Infusion	Depends on indication 0.25–1 g/kg sufficient for most indications except acute renal failure. Should be administered over 15–20 min to gain a rapid rise in plasma osmolality which will produce most effective diuresis.
Side effects		Fluid overload, cardiac failure, loss of effect if excessive amounts are used, fever.
Caution		In heart failure, established renal failure. Shake container well before use to ensure all drug is dissolved.

Metaraminol Aramine

Effects	Alpha agonist.
Preparation	10 mg/ml for dilution in saline 0.9% 10–20 ml.
Indications	Hypotension particularly during anaesthesia.
Dose	0.5–1 mg.
Length of action	5–15 min.
Side effects	Hypertension, reflex bradycardia, arrhythmias.
Caution	MAOIs.

Methyldopa Aldomet

Effects		Centrally acting hypotensive.
Preparations	Tablets	125, 250, 500 mg.
	Infusion	Solution 50 mg/ml in 5 ml ampoule.
Indications		Moderate to severe hypertension.
Adult dose	Oral	250 mg: b.d. increasing to a maximum of 3 g daily.
	i.v.	Infusion 250–500 mg 6 hourly in 5% glucose, repeated if necessary.
Paediatric dose		3 mg/kg increasing to maximum of 15 mg/kg/8 h.
Length of action	Oral	8–48 h.
	i.v.	Onset from 4–6 hours maintained up to 16 h.
Side effects		Haemolytic anaemia, sedation, hypotension, impotence.

Midazolam

Effects		Short acting benzodiazepine sedative.
Preparation		2 mg/ml or 5 mg/ml.
Indications		Sedation.
Dose	i.v.	0.5–5 mg, titrate to effect.
	Infusion	2–10 mg/h.
Length of action		20–60 min.

Side effects	Hypotension, respiratory depression, apnoea.
Caution	Reduce dose in elderly (very sensitive). May accumulate with ICU infusions.

Morphine

Effects	Opiate analgesic brain and spinal cord.
Preparation	1% solution, 1 ml ampoules.
Indications	Severe pain. May be given i.v., i.m. or s.c.
Adult dose	10–15 mg. If giving i.v. dilute to 10 ml and titrate against effect.
Paediatric dose	0.1–0.2 mg/kg.
Length of action	2–6 h depending on route of administration.
Side effects	Vomiting, respiratory depression, smooth muscle contraction, occasionally causing biliary colic; may worsen pain of renal colic; sedation.
Caution	<5 kg, head injury, respiratory disease, elderly sensitive.

Naloxone Narcan

Effects		Reverses effects of opiate drugs.
Preparation		Adult 400 μg/ml; neonate 20 μg/ml.
Indications		Opiate overdose, neonatal depression from maternal opiate.
Adult dose	i.v.	100–400 μg titrated to effect required.
Paediatric dose	i.v./i.m.	10 μg/kg
Length of action		30–60 min.
Side effects		If naloxone has been used to reverse an overdose of analgesia then pain from the original problem will become a problem if too much naloxone is given. If this is a problem with your patient do not give more opiate as it will not work, except in very high doses, which may depress breathing seriously once the effect of naloxone has worn off.

Nifedipine Adalat

Effects		Peripheral and coronary vasodilatation.
Preparations	Oral	5, 10 mg tablets
	Oral	20 mg tablets sustained release
Indications		Hypertension, angina.
Dose		For hypertension 20–40 mg b.d. sustained-release tablets.
		For angina 10–20 mg t.d.s. tablets.
		In emergency management of hypertension 10 mg sublingual – may result in sudden hypotension.
Side effects		Minor: flushing, headaches and ankle oedema.

Noradrenaline Levophed

Effects	Blood vessel vasoconstriction via alpha receptors, increase in BP.
Preparation	1 mg/ml; 4 ml ampoules.
Indications	Hypotension due to widespread vasodilation.
Dose Infusion	Mix 4 mg to 40 ml with 5% dextrose. Start at 3–5 ml/h.
Length of action	Short, must be given by infusion.
Side effects	Hypertension, excesive vasoconstriction, myocardial ischaemia, arrhythmias.
Caution	Patients on infusion must be monitored closely (preferably with an arterial line), and the drug given via a central line. The infusion must be controlled as described on p. 436.

Omeprazole Losec

Effects	Proton pump inhibitor. Reduction in gastric acid secretion.
Preparation	10 mg, 20 mg, 40 mg tablets and 40 mg ampoule.
Indications	Increase gastric pH.
Dose	20–40 mg o.d.
Side effects	Headache, diarrhoea.

Pancuronium

Preparation	4 mg in 2 ml ampoules.
Effects	Muscle relaxant (non-depolarising) producing paralysis of all muscles including those of respiration.
Dose i.v.	0.1 mg/kg; supplementary doses a quarter of the original dose.
Length of action	40–60 min.
Side effects	Tends to cause a tachycardia and rise in BP. This quality makes it a useful relaxant in shock. It does not release histamine, which is useful for asthmatics.
Caution	Do not use in renal failure as pancuronium will accumulate.

Pethidine

Effects	Opiate analgesic, brain and spinal cord.
Preparation	50 mg/ml; 1 or 2 ml ampoules for injection.
Indications	Severe pain. Give i.v. or i.m.
Adult dose	1–1.5 mg/kg. If giving i.v., dilute to 10 ml and titrate against effect.
Paediatric dose	1–1.5 mg/kg.
Length of action	2–4 h depending on route of administration.
Side effects	Vomiting, respiratory depression.

A to Z of drugs

Caution		<5 kg body weight, head injury, respiratory disease, elderly sensitive.

Phenytoin Epanutin

Effects		Anticonvulsant that reduces seizure frequency by stabilising seizure threshold and preventing spread of seizure activity.
Preparations	Capsules	25, 50 and 100 mg.
	Suspension	30 mg/5 ml.
	Injection (i.v., i.m.)	250 mg in 5 ml ampoules.
Indications		The prevention and control of grand mal and temporal lobe seizures; also effective in the control of fits in eclampsia.
Paediatric dose	Oral	5–9 mg/kg/day.
Adult dose	Oral	150–300 mg/day
	i.v.	13–15 mg/kg loading dose (not faster than 50 mg/min) then 100 mg 6 hourly.
Length of action		Orally, 12–24 hours; i.v. onset of action is rapid.
Side effects		Acute toxic side effects include ataxia, nystagmus, and slurring of speech. Hirsutism, generalised lymphadenopathy, and gingival hyperplasia may occur with chronic therapy. Avoid if possible in pregnancy, especially the first trimester.

Propofol Diprivan

Effects		Intravenous induction agent.
Preparation		10 mg/ml or 20 mg/ml.
Indications		Anaesthesia / ICU sedation.
Dose	i.v.	Anaesthesia induction 1–3 mg/kg (3–5 mg/kg children)
	Infusion	Sedation 0.3–4 mg/kg/h. Not recommended for children <16 years for sedation in ICU.
Length of action		Short.
Side effects		Pain on injection, tachyphylaxis on infusion. Best given with an opiate. Hypotension, myoclonic spasms occasionally.

Propranolol Inderal

Effects	Sympathetic nervous system antagonist at the beta receptors, causing a slowing of the heart and reduction in the force of contraction.
Preparation	0.1% solution, 1 ml ampoules.
Indications	Hypertension, tachyarrhythmia.
Adult dose	0.5–3 mg slowly i.v. titrating against effect.
Length of action	1–2 hours i.v.
Side effects	Bradycardia, hypotension, bronchospasm.
Caution	**Do not use in asthmatics** or heart block.

Ranitidine Zantac

Effects		Similar action to cimetidine.
Preparation		Tablets 150 mg, 300 mg; injection 50 mg.
Indications		As cimetidine.
Dose	Oral	150 mg b.d.
	Injection	50 mg t.d.s. i.v./i.m.
Length of action		6–8 h.
Side effects		Few reactions, should be injected slowly i.v.

Salbutamol Ventolin

Effects		Potent bronchodilator via sympathetic nervous system beta 2 receptors. Also relaxes uterus.
Preparation		Aerosol inhaler, nebuliser (asthma), injection, tablets.
Indications		Bronchospasm, premature labour.
Adult dose	Aerosol	1–2 puffs 4 hourly.
	Nebuliser	2.5–5 mg 2–6 hourly.
	i.m./s.c.	500 µg 4 hourly; i.v. 250 µg slowly
	Infusion	3–20 µg/minute titrated against effect.
	Tablets	2–4 mg three or four times daily.
Paediatric dose	Aerosol	As above.
	Nebuliser	As above.
	Tablets	Age 2–5 years 1–2 mg 3–4 times daily.
		Age 6–12 years 2 mg 3–4 times daily.
Length of action		Oral/inhaled 3–6 hours.
Side effects		Tachycardia, tremor, headache, hypokalaemia on infusion.

Suxamethonium Scoline, Anectine

Effects		Muscle relaxant (depolarising) producing paralysis of all muscles including those of respiration.
Preparation		100 mg in 2 ml ampoule.
Indications		When short duration of paralysis is required e.g. for endotracheal intubation before going on a ventilator.
Dose	i.v.	1–1.5 mg/kg.
Length of action		3–5 min, may prolong block by giving increments (quarter of first dose) or infusion. Always atropinise patient before a second dose of suxamethonium as severe bradycardia may be caused by repeat doses.
Side effects		Bradycardia if atropinisation inadequate, muscle pains day after use and poor return of muscle power if the total dose of suxamethonium used in an intermittent technique exceeds 8 mg/kg.
Caution		Hyperkalaemia in spinal cord injury, massive burns and should not be used from 5 days after the injury until 6 months after the injury. Avoid in renal failure if the

Vecuronium Norcuron

Effects	Non-depolarising muscle relaxant.
Preparation	10 mg ampoule.
Indications	Muscle relaxation.
Dose	Intubation: 80–100 µg/kg.
	Maintenance: 20–30 µg/kg.
Length of action	20–40 min.
Caution	May accumulate with infusion and action prolonged with renal failure.

Prior text (top of page): K^+ is raised. In these conditions a dangerous elevation of K^+ may occur leading to a possible cardiac arrest.

Verapamil Cordilox

Effects		Increases the refractory period of heart muscle: decreases conduction velocity in the conducting tissue.
Preparations	Injection	2.5 mg/ml in 2 ml ampoules
	Tablets	40, 80, 120, 160 mg.
Indications		Supraventricular arrhythmias, angina.
Dose	i.v.	5 mg slowly repeated after 5 min until the arrhythmia is controlled. Maximum 10–15 mg.
	Oral	For arrhythmias 40–120 mg t.d.s., for angina 80–120 mg t.d.s.
Length of action		4–8 h.
Side effects		Hypotension, bradycardia, heart block and asystole after i.v. injection. nausea, vomiting and constipation with tablets.
Caution		Do not give verapamil and beta-blockers concurrently as fatal heart block may occur.

Warfarin

Site/mode of action	Anticoagulant, antagonising the effects of vitamin K.
Effects	Prolongs coagulation of blood as measured by the laboratory prothrombin time or INR.
Preparation	Oral tablets 1 mg, 3 mg, 5 mg.
Dose	A typical loading dose of 10 mg daily for three days should be followed by a daily dosage of between 2 and 8 mg, depending on the APTR. This should be maintained between two to three times normal.
Indications	Deep vein thrombosis, pulmonary embolism, atrial fibrillation (when there is risk of embolisation), and patients with prosthetic heart valves.
Length of action	36 h for the initial anticoagulant effect to be noted and 3 days to be fully anticoagulated (given adequate doses).

Side effects	The major risk of overdosage is haemorrhage. This may be seen as haemorrhage in the gums, mouth and gastrointestinal tract, haematuria, skin haemorrhages and in severe cases haemoptysis and cerebrovascular accident. Haemorrhage is treated by withdrawing warfarin, giving vitamin K, 10 mg, orally or i.v., and in severe cases giving fresh frozen plasma. Warfarin is teratogenic and should be avoided in the first trimester of pregnancy.
Caution	Alcohol and many drugs (e.g. aspirin, phenobarbital, phenylbutazone, some antibiotics, and phenytoin) potentiate the effects of warfarin increasing the bleeding tendency. Patients on warfarin should be reviewed regularly with monitoring of the prothrombin time. Should monitoring not be available the benefits of anticoagulation must be weighed against the risks of haemorrhage.

Table of normal values

Laboratory normal values vary. This table is a guide to assist with the understanding of this book.

Haematology
Haemoglobin	13–16 g/dl
Red cell count	$3.8–6.5 \times 10^{12}/l$
White cell count	$4.0–11.0 \times 10^9/l$
Mean corpuscular volume	75–95 fl
Reticulocytes	0.2–2.0%
Platelets	$150–400 \times 10^9/l$
Packed cell volume	Male 0.4–0.54
	Female 0.35–0.47

Blood Chemistry
Sodium	132–144 mmol/l
Potassium	3.5–5.0 mmol/l
Urea	2.5–6.6 mmol/l
Chloride	95–105 mmol/l
Glucose	2.5–6.0 mmol/l
Creatinine	62–124 µmol/l
Iron	14–29 µmol/l
Total iron binding capacity	45–72 µmol/l
Urate	0.12–0.42 mmol/l
Bicarbonate	24–32 mmol/l
Calcium	2.12–2.55 mmol/l
Calcium (ionised)	1.05–1.30 mmol/l
Magnesium	0.7–1.0 mmol/l
Phosphate	0.8–1.4 mmol/l
Bilirubin	5–17 µmol/l
AST (asparate amino-transferase)	5–40 U/l
ALT (alanine amino-transferase)	5–40 U/l
LDH (lactase dehydrogenase)	55–200 U/l
Alkaline phosphatase	40–100 U/l
Albumin	35–45 g/l
Total protein	60–80 g/l
Amylase	10–100 U/l
Creatin kinase	< 200 U/l
(CK-MB	< 10 µg/l)
INR	0.9–1.2
Troponin I	<0.4 µg/l

Blood Gases
pH	7.36–7.44
PaO_2	11–13 kPa (83–98 mmHg)
$PaCO_2$	4.8–6.0 kPa (36–45 mmHg)
Bicarbonate	22–26 mmol/l

Urine
Specific gravity	1.008–1.030
pH	4.8–7.5
Sodium	50–100 mmol/l
Urea	250–500 mmol/l
Osmolality	70–1200 mmol/kg H_2O

Cerebrospinal Fluid
Pressure CSF	50–150 mm
Protein	up to 0.4 g/l
Glucose	2.5–3.9 mmol/l
Chloride	120–128 mmol/l
Lymphocytes	up to $4/mm^3$

To convert blood glucose mmol/l to mg/100 ml multiply by 18.

To convert blood gases kPa to mmHg multiply by 7.5

Further reading

ALLMAN KG, WILSON IH. *Oxford Handbook of Anaesthesia*. Oxford University Press, 2002.

ANDERSON ID. *Care of the Critically Ill Surgical Patient*. London: Arnold, 1999.

BERSTEN A, SONI N (eds) *Oh's Intensive Care Manual*. 5th edn. Oxford: Butterworth Heinemann, 2003.

ELLIS BW, PATERSON-BROWN S (eds) *Hamilton Bailey's Emergency Surgery*. 13th edn. London: Arnold, 2001.

MACKWAY-JONES K, MOLYNEUX E, PHILLIPS B, WIETESKA S (eds). Advanced Life Support Group. *Advanced Paediatric Life Support. The practical approach*. 3rd edn. London: BMJ Books, 2001. ISBN 0-7279-1554-1.

PARRY E, GILLIANO G, GODFREY R, MABEY D. *Principles of Medicine in Africa*. 3rd edn. Cambridge University Press, 2003.

ROSENFELD JV, WATTERS DAK. *Neurosurgery in the Tropics and Subtropics*. Basingstoke: Macmillan, 2000.

SHANN F, BIDDULPH J, VINCE J. *Paediatrics for Doctors in Papua New Guinea*. DWU Press, Department of Health, Papua New Guinea, 2003.

SOUTHALL D, COULTER B, RONALD C, NICHOLSON S, PARKE S (eds). Child Advocacy International. *International Child Health Care. A practical manual for hospitals worldwide*. London: BMJ Books, 2002. ISBN 0-7279-1476-6.

WARRELL DA. *The Oxford Textbook of Medicine*. 4th edn. Oxford University Press, 2003.

WATTERS DAK (ed.) Surgery in the tropics. *Bailliere's Clin Trop Med Commun Dis* 1988;3(2):173–389.

WATTERS DAK, KIIRE CF. *Gastroenterology in the Tropics and Subtropics*. Basingstoke: Macmillan, 1995.

WHO. *Management of severe malnutrition: a manual for physicians and other senior health workers*. Geneva: World Health Organization, 1999. ISBN 92-4-154511-9.

Some useful web addresses

http://www.nda.ox.ac.uk/wfsa
World Anaesthesia/WFSA/Update in Anaesthesia

http://www.aagbi.org/
Association of Anaesthetists of Great Britain and Ireland

http://www.anzca.edu.au/
Australian and New Zealand College of Anaesthetists

http://www.asahq.org/homepageie.html
American Society of Anesthesiologists

http://www.rcoa.ac.uk/
Royal College of Anaesthetists of UK

http://www.oaa-anaes.ac.uk/
Obstetric Anaesthetists Association

http://www.aaic.net.au/
Anaesthesia & Intensive Care

http://www.anesthesiology.org/
Anesthesiology

http://www.anesthesia-analgesia.org/
Anesthesia and Analgesia

http://www.bja.oupjournals.org/
British Journal of Anaesthesia

http://www.cja-jca.org
Canadian Journal of Anaesthesia

http://www.bmj.com/
British Medical Journal

http://www.thelancet.com/
The Lancet

http://www.nejm.org
New England Journal of Medicine

http://www.cochrane.org/
Cochrane Collaboration

http://www.virtual-anaesthesia-textbook.com/
Virtual Anaesthesia Textbook

http://www.frca.co.uk
Self assessment for anaesthesia exams

http://www.eguidelines.co.uk/
eGuidelines

http://www.ncbi.nlm.nih.gov/PubMed/
PubMed

http://www.ohsu.edu/cliniweb/
Cliniweb

http://www.medexplorer.com/
MedExplorer

http://www.medimatch.com
MediMatch

Index

abdomen
  multiple injuries 199–200
  postoperative care 261
  trauma 210–14
  wounds 218
  X-ray 212
  see also peritonitis
abortion 271, 272, 276, 278
abscess 135
  adnexal 278
  brain 181
  intra-abdominal 160
  intracranial 181–2
  pancreatic 45
  retropharyngeal 154
  subphrenic 162
acidosis 1, 20, 34, 94, 125, 281
acute respiratory distress syndrome: see ARDS
adenosine 439
adrenaline 31, 438, 439
advanced life support 397–399
Advanced Trauma Life Support 196
aerocoele 192
Agpar score 279–80
airway
  cervical spine 197, 253
  CPAP 342, 343, 423–4
  cricoid 17
  neonates 280–1, 282
  obstructed 1, 3, 5, 194, 196
  reflexes 254
  suction 352–4
alcohol poisoning 119, 121
alfentanil 440
alkalosis 358
Ambu bag 337, 422
aminophylline 440
amiodarone 65, 440–1
amniotic fluid embolism 275–6
amoxycillin 153
ampicillin 153
amputation, traumatic 218
anaemia 51
  anaesthetics 271
  haemolysis 35, 37, 144
  malnutrition 290
  microangiopathic haemolytic 36
  preoperative care 251
  renal failure 91, 94–5
anaesthesia 437–8
  anaemia 271
  carotid angiography 403
  diabetes 107
  haemodilution 401–2
  intubation 268
  larynx-local 427
  postoperative care 253–6
  problems 248, 256
  tracheostomy 360–1
analgesia 229, 232, 242, 257–8
anaphylaxis 26, 27
aneroid gauge 421
angina 65–6, 68
angioplasty 67
animal bites 219
antacids 30
antibacterial agents 235, 236 7, 245
antibiotics 436–7
  brain abscess 181
  drugs 438
  infection 135, 278–9
  prophylactic 192, 202, 217
anticoagulants 34, 69, 74, 250
anticonvulsants 179
antidiuretic hormone 192
antidotes to poisoning 119, 120
antimalarial therapy 145–8
antiretrovirals 165
anti-tetanus toxoid 240
antivenom 128, 129
anuria 89
aorta dissection 51–2, 75
aortic aneurysm 71
aortic valve regurgitation 70
APACHE II 324
apnoea test 184
arachnoid 409
ARDS 5, 9, 10, 14–15, 27, 218, 343
arrhythmia 48, 52–4, 56–7
  drugs 67, 119, 398–399
  ECG 57–61, 300
  pericardial aspiration 395
  preoperative care 249
  pulmonary oedema 59–60
  tachycardia 57–8
artemisins 145–6
arteries 355, 356, 420–2
arteriography 215
artery cannulation 420–2
asphyxia 279–80, 282–3
aspirin 74, 75, 126
asthma 11–12, 18–19, 251–2, 338
atelectasis 258, 261, 262
atracurium tracrium 441
atropine 123–4, 427
auscultation 136
autograft 237
autoimmune disease 36
autonomic neuropathy 107
autotransfusion 25, 31–2, 402–3
AVPU scale 198

bacteraemia 29–30, 262, 392
bag and mask 281, 282
bag and suck 337, 422, 423
balloon pump 419
balloon tamponade 42–3
barrier nursing 140, 305
basic life support (BLS) 396
basilic vein 388
bedside equipment 314–15, 326, 327
bellows 422
benzyl penicillin 157
beta-blockers 67, 73, 74, 250
bicarbonate 356, 397, 441–2
blackwater fever 143, 144–5
bladder, ruptured 213
blast lung 218
bleeding 34–5, 40–1
  arachnoid 410
  liver failure 101
  oesophageal varices 42–3
  renal failure 95
  umbilical cord 281
blood
  arterial 356
  chemistry of 457–8
  coagulation 34–5, 192
  glucose 78, 103, 244

459

460 *Index*

storage 34
volume 76
blood gases 6, 10–11, 34, 338, 343, 352, 355–8, 458
blood loss 201, 268
blood pressure: *see* hypertension; hypotension
blood substitutes 33
blood transfusion
 autotransfusion 25, 31–2, 401–2
 burns 239, 245
 cardiac failure 33–4
 checks 296
 haemolysis 35, 37–8
 infection 33
 renal failure 94–5
blood urea 93–4, 244
body fluid 76, 78–9
 burns 227–8, 232–3
 drains 257
 overload 270
 postoperative care 257
bolus injections 287, 302
bomb explosions 218
bone marrow suppression 144
bowels 295
box jellyfish stings 131
brachial artery 355
bradycardia 1–2, 281, 338, 340
brain damage 192–3
brain stem 183–4, 186
breast feeding 240, 270
breathing
 assisted 422
 inadequate 3, 4, 9–10
 multiple injuries 196, 197–8
 rescue 396
 resistance 430
 sedation 342
breathing exercises 349
British Burn Association 227
bronchiolitis 19
bronchodilator drugs 348
bronchopleural fistula 209
bronchopneumonia 262
bronchospasm 31, 252
bruising 205
bullet wounds 210–11, 214–16
bupivacaine 442
burns 229–32
 analgesia 229, 232, 242
 blood transfusion 239, 245
 body fluid 227–8, 232–3
 cervical spine 226
 chest physiotherapy 240–1
 depth of damage 227, 228, 230–2
 explosions 226–7
 exposure 235–6
 fluid therapy 226, 233–4
 gastrointestinal tract 239–40
 hands 238–9
 history of patient 229, 230

hypermetabolic state 227, 228–9, 237–8
hypovolaemic shock 228
infection 229, 244–5, 304
malaria 245
metabolic changes 228–9
nutrition 239–40, 246, 286
poisoning 238
renal failure 243
respiratory complications 229, 232
resuscitation 226–7, 242–3
sepsis 227
shock 226–7, 228
surgery 237
weight loss 229, 243
wounds 235
burr holes 188–9, 217, 407–13

calcium 85, 86, 442
cannula 209, 234
cannulation
 arteries 420–2
 children 381, 388
 complications 391–2
 cutdown 379–81
 veins 382–8
carbon dioxide 356
carbon monoxide 121–2, 226
cardiac arrest 58, 59–60, 396–400
cardiac enzymes 49–50
cardiac failure 30, 31, 46–8
 blood transfusion 33–4
 drugs 55 (fig)
 hypertension 48, 51, 73–4
 left side 46, 47, 48, 52–5
 preoperative care 249
 renal failure 89
 right-sided 46, 48, 55–6
cardiac tamponade 208, 210
cardio-pulmonary resuscitation 59–60, 308, 397
cardiodiomyopathies 48
cardiogenic shock 52
cardiorespiratory arrest 308
cardiotoxic drugs 119
carina 423
carotid angiography 181, 182, 188, 403–6
carotid endarterectomy 75
catabolism 228, 284
catheters
 Cavafix 384, 386, 387
 fluid therapy 234
 infection 134, 244
 mount 423
 nasopharyngeal 369–70
 peritoneal lavage 372
 removal 373
 subdural 418
 urethral 297
 ventricular 418
central venous lines 134, 252–3, 324, 384

central venous pressure (CVP) 15, 26, 243, 297, 301, 388–92
 see also cannulation
cephalosporins 153
cerebrospinal fluid 460
 brain abscess 181
 cloudy 156–7
 intracranial pressure 417
 leaking 191, 199
 poliomyelitis 138
 reduction of volume 188
 subarachnoid haemorrhage 182–3
cerebrovascular accident 9, 74
cervical collar 202, 203, 292, 293
cervical spine 186–7, 194, 197, 204, 205, 226, 253
charts and protocols, ICU 317–22
chest
 flail segment 9, 207–8
 infection 150
 penetrating wounds 218
 postoperative care 258, 261
 trauma 16, 199, 205, 207–8
chest compressions 396–7
chest physiotherapy 8, 240–1, 261, 299, 349–51
chest vibration 350
chest X-ray 6, 333, 375
children
 cannulation 381, 388
 convulsions 180
 dehydration 83
 electrolyte disorders 86
 endotracheal intubation 330
 hypovolaemic shock 22, 23–6
 inhaled foreign body 7, 16–17
 intraosseous infusions 392
 intravenous fluid therapy 80–2
 malnutrition 286, 290
 nutrition 240, 241
 peritoneal dialysis 374
 poisoning 122
 respiratory problems 16–19
 rheumatic fever 70, 71
 tracheostomy 17
Chlamydia pneumoniae 136
Chlamydia trachematis 279
chloramphenicol 153, 157, 278
chloroquine 124, 146–7
chlorpromazine 112, 442
cholera 27
choriocarcinoma 271–2
Christmas disease 34
chronic obstructive airways disease (COAD) 343, 347, 429
cimetidine 442–3
ciprofloxacin 153
circulation 196, 198

Index 461

clinical sickness score 324, 325
clopidogrel 75
Clostridium tetani 148
Clostridium welchi 303
co-trimoxazole 153
coagulation 34–5, 192, 266
colectomy 41
colloid solutions 23, 25, 33
coma 165–70
  causes 102, 103, 170–4
  convulsions 177–81
  diagnostic approach 174
  errors in diagnosis 170
  fluid balance 176
  heat stroke 111
  hypercarbia 177
  hyperglycaemia 102, 107
  intracranial pressure 176–7
  non-ketotic 102, 107, 110
  nutrition 176
  physiotherapy 176
  positioning patient 175–6
  pre-eclampsia 270
  respiration 3, 5
  stroke 74
  see also Glasgow Coma Scale
communication 308–10
compartment syndrome 219
compressor 423
congenital heart disease 50, 69–70
coning 168, 194
conjunctivitis 293
constipation 295
continuous positive airways pressure 342, 343, 423–4
convulsions 177–81, 266–7
coronary artery bypass 67, 69
corticosteroids 38, 157
Corynebacterium diphtheriae 138
coughing, assisted 350–1
cranioplasty 414
creatinine 89, 93–4
cricoid airway 17
cricoid pressure 424
cricothyroid stab 197
cricothyrotomy 7, 359, 362–3
cross-infection 305
croup 18
crush injuries 219
cryoprecipitate 33
crystalloid solutions 23, 25
CT scan 45, 75, 160, 174, 188–9
culdocentesis 271, 272, 276
cyanide 122, 226
cyanosis 50, 51
cystogram 213
cystoscopy 91
cystotomy, suprapubic 376–8
cystourethroscopy 91
cytotoxic venom 128

dantrolene 114
death 317, 323
debridement 216
deep vein thrombosis 262–3
defibrillation 64, 65, 397, 399
degloving injuries 218–19
dehydration 38–40, 77–8, 82, 83, 113
delirium tremens 116–17
depressed fractures 199, 413–14
desferrioxamine 126, 127
dexamethasone 181, 443
dextran 251
diabetes 101–4, 107–10
diabetes insipidus 192
diabetes mellitus 111
diabetic ketoacidosis 78, 102, 104–6
dialysis 95, 96
diaphragm, ruptured 212
diarrhoea 243–4, 261, 295
diazepam 443–4
  chloroquine 124
  convulsions 266–7
  fits 179, 191
  phenobarbital 282
  tetanus 149–50
  thrombophlebitis 151
  ventilation 258
diazoxide 73, 268
dieticians 321
digoxin 65, 444
diphtheria 138
diplopia 138
disaster treatment 222–4
disinfection 140, 307
disseminated intravascular coagulation 34, 266
diuresis, forced alkaline 127
diuretics 30, 52, 101, 188
dobutamine 444–5
dopamine 445
drains 257, 395
  see also intercostal drain
dressings 217, 235–6, 237, 262
drips 80, 287, 382
drug errors 296
drugs
  administration 301–2, 438
  antibiotics 438
  cardiac fusion 55
  doses 435–6
  ICU 315, 321, 328
  intramuscular 301, 436
  intravenous 302, 436
dyspnoea 2, 5, 50, 59, 143, 292

Early Management of Severe Burns 227
ears 238
ECG 51, 58, 59, 300
echocardiography 51, 52, 70, 418
echoencephalography 188
eclampsia 264–5, 267–8
ectopic pregnancy 271
electrical sockets 314–15

electrolyte balance 257, 373
electrolyte disorders 84–6
electrolytes 76–8, 79–80, 94, 244, 290
emergency rehearsals 223–4
emergency surgery 109, 252–3
emphysema 208
empyema 10, 367–8
encephalitis 154–8
encephalopathy 9, 72, 97–9, 100–1
endocarditis 70, 250
endoscopy 41, 42
endotoxaemia 30
endotracheal intubation 329–35
endotracheal tubes 297–8, 329, 330, 424–6, 430
ephedrine 445
epidural analgesia 257–8, 267, 268
epiglottis 17–18
epilepsy 117, 178, 248
ergometrine 268, 275
escharotomy 232, 233, 245
Escherichia coli 303
esmolol 446
essential fatty acids 289
ethanol 121
ethical problems 344
excision 216, 245
explosions 226–7
extubation 254, 334–5, 341, 425
eye care 186, 293, 307
eye injuries 205, 206, 238

facial injuries 202
fainting 113
Fansidar 147
fasciotomy incisions 220
femoral artery 355
femoral vein 387
femur fractures 221–2
fetal heart rate monitoring 282
fibrillation 57, 65, 75
fits 143, 177–9, 181, 191, 194, 282
  see also convulsions
fluid balance 76, 89, 93, 176, 295
  see also body fluid
fluid overload 77–8, 82–3
fluid therapy 188, 226, 233–4
flumazenil 446
folic acid deficiency 144
Fournier's gangrene 163
fractures 199, 205, 207, 221–2, 253, 412–13
fumigation 307
fundoscopy 179
furosemide 52, 54, 446

gangrene 163, 219–20, 276, 278
Gardiner–Wells tongs 203

gas exchange, inadequate 1, 4, 5, 10–11
gas gangrene 219–20, 276
gastric lavage 119, 124
gastric ulcers 41
gastroenteritis 81, 290
gastrointestinal tract 40–3, 79, 153, 239–40, 261, 287
gentamicin 278, 437
Glasgow Assessment Schedule 194
Glasgow Coma Scale 166–7, 170, 192–3, 300, 320
  conscious level 248
  deteriorating 189–90
  head injuries 186, 324
  ICU 317
  multiple injuries 198, 199
glomerular filtration rate 87
glomerulonephritis 89, 91
glucose 77, 78, 103, 244
glucose-6-phosphate dehydrogenase deficiency 35–6, 37, 144
gluteraldehyde 307
glyceryl trinitrate 66, 68, 446
glycosuria 102
gonoccal infection 278–9
grand mal convulsions 117, 178
Guillain–Barré Syndrome 139, 359

haematology 457
haematoma 189, 194, 274–5, 406, 409, 410, 411
haematuria 266
haemo-pneumothorax 207
haemodilution 401–2
haemofiltration 95
haemoglobinuria 37, 234
haemolysis 35–8, 144, 251
haemophilia 33, 34
Haemophilus influenzae 17, 154
haemorrhage
  ante-partum 35, 272–4
  cerebral 74
  gastrointestinal 40–3
  liver failure 99
  obstetrical 270–1
  post-partum 274–5
  subarachnoid 182–3
  uterus 272
haemorrhoids 41
haemothorax 10, 209–10
haemotoxic venom 128
hand-washing 303, 305, 307–8
hands, burns 238–9
head injuries 185–7
  airway 194, 354
  cervical spine 194
  CT scan 188–9
  fits 194
  fluid therapy 188
  Glasgow Coma Scale 186, 324

Glasgow Outcome Scale 193
hypotension 185–6, 194
hypoxia 185, 248
intracranial pressure 248, 414–16
mortalities 193
positioning patient 187
sedation 194
ventilation 190
see also burr holes
health workers 305–6
heart
  afterload 30, 55
  conduction pathways 56
  contractility 30
  dying 63
  hypovolaemic shock 30
  irregular 64–5
  output 418
  preload 30
heart disease 50, 65–8, 69–70, 71
  see also cardiac failure
heat exhaustion 112–13
heat stroke 110–12
heat syncope 113
hemiplegia 74–5, 192
heparin 38, 69, 250, 355, 447
hepatic cirrhosis 42
hepatitis, viral 97
hepatitis B 33, 305–6
hernia 211
hips, fractures 221
HIV infection 33, 164–5, 306
human chorionic gonadatrophin 271
human immune globulin 150
humerus 222
humidification 347, 425–6, 434
hydralazine 73, 268, 447–8
hydration 8, 78
hydrocortisone 114, 115, 448
hydrogen peroxide 307
hydronephrosis 91, 93
hyperbaric oxygen 122
hyperbilirubinaemia 38
hypercalcaemia 85
hypercapnia, permissive 343
hypercarbia 1, 2, 3, 5, 6, 177, 248, 426
hyperglycaemia 101, 102, 107, 287–8
hyperkalaemia 34, 85, 86, 94, 111
hypermetabolic state, burns 227, 228–9, 237–8
hypernatraemia 84, 86, 94
hyperpyrexia 113–14, 145, 150
hypertension
  anaesthesia 367
  cardiac failure 48, 51, 74
  cerebrovascular accident 74
  eclampsia 267–8
  encephalopathy 9, 72

  epidural analgesia 268
  malignant 72
  pre-eclampsia 265, 267–9
  pregnancy 264
  preoperative care 250
  pulmonary oedema 51
  renal failure 73–4, 91, 95
  tachycardia 150
hyperthyroidism 116
hyperventilation 110, 111
hypoadrenalism 115–16
hypocalcaemia 34, 85, 86
hypocarbia 428
hypoglycaemia 98–9, 143, 144, 281
hyponatraemia 84, 86
hypophosphattaemia 111
hypotension 72–3
  asthma 12
  head injuries 185–6, 194
  hypovolaemic shock 28
  malaria 144
  poisoning 119
  positioning patient 291–2
  postoperative care 258, 259–60
  ventilation 340
hypothermia 26, 34, 114–15, 258
hypothyroidism 116
hypovolaemic shock 20–3, 250
  burns 228
  children 22, 23–6
  heart 30
  hypotension 28
  intestine 29–30
  kidneys 29
  lungs 29
  oliguria 26, 28, 29, 92, 143
  pancreatitis 44
  renal failure 89
  resuscitation 23–6
  tachycardia 20
hypoxaemia 177
hypoxia 1, 2, 3, 5, 6, 426
  bradycardia 338
  cellular 121, 142, 143
  cerebral 400
  head injuries 185, 248
  liver failure 99
  oxygen therapy 345
  pneumonia 39
  pulmonary infarction 39
  renal 87
  sickle cell disease 40
  tissue 20–1
hysterectomy 272, 275

Inappropriate ADH Secretion (SIADH) 86
incentive spirometry 351
infection 133, 303, 304–5
  antibiotics 135, 278–9
  blood transfusion 33
  burns 229, 244–5, 304

Index 463

catheters 134, 244
central venous lines 134
chest 150
eradication 150
exogenous/endogenous 303
gonoccal 278–9
health workers 305–6
intravenous fluid therapy 295–6
nutrition 151
paralysis 137–9
peritoneum 373
prevention 240, 303, 305
renal failure 94
secondary 145
skin trauma 304
tachycardia 134, 150, 159
wounds 261–2
insulin deficiency 101
insulin treatment 103–5, 106
intensive care unit
 bedside equipment 326, 327
 benefits 312–13
 care levels 313–14, 315
 charts and protocols 317–22
 clinical responsibilities 317
 design and location 314–16
 drugs 315, 321, 328
 effectiveness 323–4
 equipment care 321, 326
 investigations 328
 nurses 312–13
 organisation 316–17, 322
 paraclinical departments 320–1
 patient selection 323
 planning/costs 313–14
 specific requirements 325–6
 standard software 328
 teaching/training 324–5
 treatment/monitoring 316
 unit equipment 326
 wastage of resources 324
intercostal drain 9, 205, 207, 365–8
intestine 29–30
intracranial pressure (ICP) 176–7, 415–17
Intralipid 288
intraosseous infusions 392
intravenous fluid therapy 80–2, 295–6
intravenous lines 80
intravenous urography 91, 212
intubation 7, 14, 268, 281, 331–2
intubation trolley 327–8
iron lung 429
iron poisoning 126–7
Irukandji syndrome 131
ischaemia 39, 49–50, 293–4, 304
isoprenaline 448–9

jaundice 34, 35, 37, 99, 252

jellyfish stings 131
jugular venous pressure 25–6, 56, 82–3

ketoacidosis 27, 109
 diabetic 78, 102, 104–6
ketones 285
kidneys 29, 87
 see also renal failure

labetalol 73, 449
laparoscopy 276
laparotomy 134, 160, 210, 211, 253, 278
laryngeal oedema 31, 334–5
laryngectomy 359
laryngoscopy 331, 334–5
laryngospasm 14, 254
laryngotracheobronchitis 18
larynx 359
Lassa fever 140
Legionnaires' disease 136
lidocaine 64, 449
liver 42–3, 97, 205
liver failure 97–99, 100
 bleeding 101
 cerebral function 98
 chronic 34
 hypoxia 99
 nutrition 101
 pregnancy 97
 respiratory function 99
 urine output 101
localising signs, false 168–9
lumbar puncture 170
lumbar vertebrae 293
lungs 6, 29, 343

mafenide 245
magnesium 85–6
magnesium sulphate 266, 267
magnesium trisilicate 239–40
malaria 140, 141, 145–8
 burns 245
 cerebral 141, 142–3
 haemolysis 37
 hypoglycaemia 144
 hypotension 144
 life-threatening 140–8
 parasites 244
 pyrexia 262
 renal failure 143
malnutrition 86, 284–5, 286, 290
maloprim 148
mannitol 188, 282, 450
Mapleson C circuit 427–8
masks 345, 347
mastoiditis 181
matron's report 319
meconium aspiration 282
medical venesection 54
mefloquine 148
meningism 143

meningitis 154, 156–7
metabolic acidosis 111, 358
metabolic alkalosis 358
metaraminol aramine 450
methanol 125
methyldopa 73, 269, 450
midazolam 258, 450–1
minitracheostomy 362–3, 428
mitral regurgitation 70
mole 76
monoplegia 192
morphine 338
mouth 199
mouth cleaning 293
mouth to face resuscitation 281
multiple injuries
 abdomen 199–200
 Alert/Verbal/Pain/Unresponsive scale 198
 blood loss 201
 breathing 196, 197–8
 chest 199
 circulation 196
 Glasgow Coma Scale 198, 199
 limbs 201
 management 196–201
 pelvis 201
 resuscitation 196
 secondary survey 198–9
murmurs 250
muscle cramps 112
muscle relaxants 338–9
Mycoplasma 136
myocardial infarction 66, 68, 249–50
myocardial ischaemia 49, 68
myocarditis 51
myoglobinuria 112, 234

naloxone 9–10, 451
nasal intubation 430–1
nasal spectacles 345
naso-pharyngeal cannula 345–6
nasogastric tubes 261, 287, 288, 295, 297, 374–5
nasopharyngeal catheter 369–70
nasotracheal intubation 330
near-drowning 15–16
nebulisers 348, 429
neck spasms 154
necrosectomy 45
necrosis 293–4
necrotising fasciitis 163–4
needle-stick injuries 306
Neisseria meningitidis 154
neonates
 asphyxia 282–3
 blood volume 76
 convulsions 267
 haemolysis 35
 hyperbilirubinaemia 38
 intubation 281
 resuscitation 279–82
 tetanus 151–2

464 Index

nephrectomy 213
nephrostomy 93
nephrotoxic drugs 93, 96
neurogenic pulmonary oedema 192
neurotoxic venom 128
newborn babies: *see* neonates
nifedipine 73, 451
nimodipine 182
noradrenaline 452
normal values table 457–8
nurse-to-patient ratio 316
nurses 312–13, 332–3
nursing critical illness 291, 299–301, 302–3, 310–11
nursing report 310, 311, 318
nutrition 93–4, 286
  adults 240, 241
  assessment 285
  burns 239–40, 246, 286
  catabolism 284
  children 240, 241
  coma 176
  critically ill 294–5
  enternal 287–8
  infection 151
  parenteral 244, 288–9, 294–5
  support discontinued 289–90

obstetrics 268–9, 270–1, 276–9
  see also pregnancy
octreotide 42
oesophageal transection 42–3
oliguria 92
  hypovolaemic shock 26, 28, 29, 92, 143
  pre-eclampsia 269
  renal failure 89
omental protrusion 210, 211
omeprazole 454
opiates 338
oral hypoglycaemics 104
oral rehydration solution (ORS) 81
oral therapy 234
orbital cellulitis 181
organophosphate compounds 123–4
oropharyngeal airway 253
osmolality 77
osmolarity 77
osteomyelitis 324
oximetry 336, 338, 418, 429
oxygen 337, 356, 370–1, 429
oxygen concentrator 429
oxygen cylinders 315, 326
oxygen therapy 8, 12–13, 345, 346–7
oxytocics 275
oxytocin 279

palsy 168–9, 359
pancreas 45
pancreatitis 44–5

pancurionium 339, 452
papilloedema 169–70
paracentesis 65, 160, 210, 211
paraffin oil 122
paralysis 137–9
paralytic ileus 239–40, 261
paraplegia 39
parasites 142, 244
parasympathetic dysautonomia 131
patient deterioration 340–1
patient history, burns 229, 230
patient's family 308–10
PEEP (positive end expiratory pressure) 10, 15, 29, 218, 343, 347, 429
pelvis 201, 213, 277
peptic ulcer 41
percutaneous tracheostomy 364
perfluorocarbons 33
perfusion 431–2
pericardial aspiration 394–5
pericardial paracentesis 65, 210
pericardial tamponade 48–9, 52, 65
perineum 238
peripartum cardiomyopathy 51, 71
peritoneal aspiration 211
peritoneal dialysis 371–3
peritoneal lavage 211, 371–3
peritoneum 373
peritonitis 158–61, 276
pesticides 122–3
pethidine 452
pH 94, 356
pharmacotherapy 237–8
pharyngitis 138
phenobarbital 179, 181, 191, 282
phenytoin 179, 191, 267, 282, 453
physiotherapist 321
physiotherapy for coma 176
placenta praevia 272–4
placental abruption 272–4
plasma 32, 77
plasmaphoresis 139
Plasmodium falciparum 141
plaster casts 220
platelets 32–3, 34
pneumonia 2–3
  aspiration 13–14, 287–8
  bacterial 135
  chest physiotherapy 261
  Chlamydia pneumoniae 136
  hypoxia 39
  Mycoplasma 136
  oxygen therapy 12–13
  viral 135–6
  white blood cell count 136
pneumonitis 122
pneumothorax 3, 9, 11, 205, 207–9, 341, 368

poisoning 118–19
  antidotes 119, 120
  burns 238
  carbon monoxide 121–2
  children 122
  chloroquine 124
  cyanide 122
  ethanol 121
  hypotension 119
  iron 126–7
  methanol 125
  organophosphate compounds 123–4
  paraffin oil 122
  resuscitation 119
  salicylates 126
  through skin 119, 124
  vomiting 119
poliomyelitis 137–8
polycystic disease 91
polyneuropathy, acute ascending 139
polyuria 91
positioning patient 187, 291–2, 343
post-mortems 323–4
postoperative care 255, 258
  abdomen 261
  anaesthesia 253–6
  analgesia 257–8
  body fluid 257
  chest 258, 261
  gastrointestinal motility 261
  hypotension 258, 259–60
  monitoring 256–7
  surgery 256–63
  unconscious patient 293–4
  wounds 261–2
post-partum collapse 275–6
postural drainage 349–50
potassium 84, 85, 86, 94, 106
pre-eclampsia 72, 264–6
  coma 270
  delivery 267–8
  hypertension 265, 267–9
  oliguria 269
  placental abruption 272–4
  post-delivery 270
  pulmonary oedema 269
  renal failure 269–70
pregnancy
  complication 145
  ectopic 271
  fits 181
  heart disease 71
  hypertension 264
  liver failure 97
  urine glucose 103
  see also eclampsia; pre-eclampsia
preoperative care 248–9, 250–2
pre-oxygenation 432
pressure sores 176, 293–4
prickly heat 111

procaine 114
propofol 453
propranolol 453
prostate, enlarged 91
protective clothing 306
protein 93–4, 286
proteinuria 265, 266
pseudocyst 45
puffer fish 131
pulmonary embolism 50, 69, 263
pulmonary infarction 39
pulmonary oedema 143–4
  acute 54, 72
  arrhythmia 59–60
  dyspnoea 89
  hypertension 51
  left heart failure 47
  pre-eclampsia 269
  ventilation 15
pulse, absent 58
pupils 168, 186, 199
PVC 432
pyelography, retrograde 91
pyelonephritis 91
pyloroplasty 41
pyosalpinx 278
pyrexia 5, 117, 134, 262

quinine 145–6, 147

radial artery 355
ranitidine 454
rehydration 81
relaparotomy 162
renal failure 87–90
  acidosis 94
  acute 88–9, 90–2, 94–5
  anaemia 91, 94–5
  bleeding 95
  blood transfusion 94–5
  burns 243
  cardiac failure 89
  causes 88, 90
  chronic 88, 91, 95–6
  crush injuries 219
  haemoglobinuria 37, 234
  haemolytic crisis 35
  hypertension 73, 91, 95
  hypovolaemic shock 89
  infection 94
  malaria 143
  myoglobinuria 234
  oliguria 89
  post-renal 88, 89–90, 91, 93
  pre-eclampsia 269–70
  preoperative care 252
  pre-renal 87, 89, 91, 92–3
  renal 88, 89, 91, 93
renal injury 212–13
respiration 2–3, 5, 430
respiratory acidosis 357–8
respiratory alkalosis 111, 358
respiratory failure 1–7, 8, 430
  blood gases 6, 10–11, 352

burns 229, 232
chest physiotherapy 8
children 16–19
hydration 8
neuromuscular causes 14–17
observation chart 321
paralysis 137–8
preoperative care 251
tetanus 14
tracheostomy 7
see also ventilation
respiratory injuries 234–5
resuscitation
  aftercare 399–400
  bag and mask 281, 282
  burns 226–7, 242–3
  cardio-pulmonary 59–60, 308, 397
  choosing patients 400
  fluids 23, 24, 25, 81
  hypovolaemic shock 23–6
  multiple injuries 196
  neonates 279–82
  poisoning 119
  prognosis 308
  stopping 399–400
Resuscitation Council (UK) 396
resuscitation trolley 308
rheumatic fever 70, 71
rhonchi 47
rib fractures 205, 207

salbutamol 454
salicylates 126
Salmonella typhi 152–4, 154
salpingitis 278
sanitation 137
SARS (Severe Acute Respiratory Syndrome) 136
scalp wounds 189–91, 199
scorpion stings 130–1
sedation 194, 338–9, 342
self-extubation 341
Sengstaken–Blakemore tube 42, 43
sepsis
  burns 227
  obstetrical 276–9
  pelvic 277
  peritonitis 158
  puerperal 278
  recurrent 109–10
  source 135
  tubo-ovarian 278–9
  wounds 262
septic abortion 276, 278
septic shock 20, 21, 27, 133–5
septicaemia 35, 37, 133–5, 134, 144, 262
septicaemic shock 162–3
shellfish poison 131
shock
  anaphylactic 27, 30–1
  burns 226–7

cardiogenic 21, 52
  investigations 418–9
  irreversible 21, 28
  septic 20, 21, 27, 133–5
  septicaemic 162–3
  see also hypovolaemic shock
shunt 430
sickle cell disease 36, 37, 38–40, 136, 251
silver sulphadiazine 236
SIMV 343
sinusitis 181
skin grafts 163, 164, 237
skin trauma 304
skull 187, 190–1, 193, 217–18
  see also burr holes
smoke inhalation 226
snake bites 93, 127–30, 139
sodium 84, 86, 94, 233
sodium nitroprusside 73
space-occupying lesion (SOL) 181, 402
specific gravity 77
spectrophotometric examination 145
sphygmomanometer 420
spider bites 130–1
spinal injuries 202–5
spiritual care 310
spleen 205
splenectomy 35
splints 238–9
sputum removal 352–4
stab wounds 210, 211
Staphylococcus aureus 303
sterilising equipment 301, 307–8
steroids 26, 27, 148, 181, 282
Stevens–Johnson syndrome 148
streptococcal infection 163–4
Streptococcus pneumoniae 154
Streptococcus viridans 303
stress ulceration 29–30, 43
stridor 335
strokes 74–5, 404
subarachnoid haemorrhage 182–3
subphrenic abscess 162
suckling 279
suction 315, 337, 430–1
suction tray 326
suicide 119
suppository 295
suprapubic cystotomy 376–8
surgery
  brain abscess 181
  burns 237
  diabetes 107–10
  emergency 109, 252–3
  postoperative care 256–63
sutures 217, 261
suxamethonium 339, 454
Swan–Ganz catheter 30, 71, 417–19
sweating 110

syntometrine 268, 275

tachycardia
  arrhythmia 57–8
  artrial 61
  hypovolaemic shock 20
  infection 134, 150, 159
  obstetrics 268–9
  sinus 61
  supraventricular 64
  ventilation 340
  ventricular 60, 64
tachypnoea 134
TB meningitis 157
teeth 199
temperature, core–peripheral 418
tetanus 14, 85, 148–50, 151–2, 190–1, 217, 276
tetanus toxin 149
tetracycline 148
thirst 82
thoracic aorta 210
thoracic vertebrae 293
thoractomy 208, 210
thrombocytopaenia 34, 134
thromboembolism 250–1
thrombolysis 75
thrombophlebitis 150–1, 296
thrombosis 50, 291
thyroid crisis 116
thyroid stimulating hormone (TSH) 116
thyrotoxicosis 51, 116
tibia 222
tissue ischaemia 39
tongue 199
tonsilitis 138
tourniquet damage 219
toxin neutralisation 150
trace elements 287
tracheal stenosis 334–5
tracheal tug 1
tracheostomy 197, 359–63, 431
  anaesthesia 360–1
  children 17
  percutaneous 364
  procedure 360, 361–2
  respiratory failure 7
traction 205, 222, 292
transducers, fibre-optic 416
triage 223–4
trocar introducer 365–6
tropical anhydrosis 111
tubo-ovarian sepsis 278–9
tubocurarine 339
tubular necrosis 29, 87, 90, 91, 93
typhoid 152–4

ulcers 29–30, 41, 43, 153, 239–40

ultrasound 45, 49, 87, 160
umbilical cord 281, 282
unconscious patient 293–4
  see also coma
units of pressure measurement 431
uraemia 89, 95
urea 78, 89
ureters 90
urethra, ruptured 213
urethral catheters 297
urethrogram 213–14
urinary problems 150, 262
urine 458
  glucose 77, 103
  ketones 285
  osmolality 77
  output 101, 243
  urethral catheters 297
  see also oliguria
uterus 272, 275, 278

vaccination 137, 151
vagotomy 41
valves 433
valvular disease 48, 50, 69
vasa praevia 274
vaso-occlusive crisis 39–40
vasoconstriction, peripheral 28
vasodilation 30, 110, 144
vasopressin 42
vecuronium norcuron 455
vegetative patients 193–4
veins 379–81, 382–8
venous thrombosis 291
ventilation 8–9, 336–44, 397
  alarm 422
  asthma 12
  compliance 423
  connectors 423
  control mode 423
  cycling 424, 433
  dead space 424
  diazepam 258
  display 424
  duration 342–3
  equipment 337
  ethics 344
  expiratory time 425
  fighting patients 425
  filter 425
  fractional inspired oxygen 425
  frequency 425
  head injuries 190
  hypotension 340
  inspiratory time 427
  intermittent 426–7
  inverse ratio 343
  investigations 338
  leaking 427
  lung protection 343

management 336–9
minute volume 428
monitoring 337–8
negative pressure 429
non-invasive 343
patient deterioration 340–1
positive pressure 430
pulmonary oedema 15
rate 430
sedation 338–9
SIMV 343
suction 337
T-piece 431
tachycardia 340
tidal volume 431
weaning off 433–4
ventilators
  control settings 432
  pressures 341
  setting up 336
  types 423, 424, 427, 429, 431, 433
ventilatory failure 433
ventricular failure 53
ventricular infarction 49–50
ventriculitis 417
verapamil 455
viral haemorrhagic fevers 139–40
viral hepatitis 97
visiting times 310
vitamins 287
vomiting 119, 243–4

warfarin 34, 75, 250, 455–6
weight loss 229, 243
white blood cell count 111, 134, 136, 139, 181
wounds
  abdomen 218
  bullets 210–11, 214–15, 216
  burns 235
  cleaning 215–16
  closure 216–17
  dressings 217, 262
  excision 216, 245
  infection 261–2
  sepsis 262
  vascular injury 215
Wright's respirometer 6, 434

X-ray
  abdomen 212
  carotid angiography 181, 182, 188, 403–6
  cervical spine 186–7, 204
  chest 6, 333, 375
  skull 187
xiphisternal drainage 395

Yankaur sucker end 434